Toward Brain-Computer Interfacing

Neural Information Processing Series
Michael I. Jordan and Thomas Dietterich, editors

Advances in Large Margin Classifiers, Alexander J. Smola, Peter L. Bartlett, Bernhard Schölkopf, and Dale Schuurmans, eds., 2000

Advanced Mean Field Methods: Theory and Practice, Manfred Opper and David Saad, eds., 2001

Probabilistic Models of the Brain: Perception and Neural Function, Rajesh P. N. Rao, Bruno A. Olshausen, and Michael S. Lewicki, eds., 2002

Exploratory Analysis and Data Modeling in Functional Neuroimaging, Friedrich T. Sommer and Andrzej Wichert, eds., 2003

Advances in Minimum Description Length: Theory and Applications, Peter D. Grunwald, In Jae Myung, and Mark A. Pitt, eds., 2005

Nearest-Neighbor Methods in Learning and Vision: Theory and Practice, Gregory Shakhnarovich, Piotr Indyk, and Trevor Darrell, eds., 2006

New Directions in Statistical Signal Processing: From Systems to Brains, Simon Haykin, José C. Príncipe, Terrence J. Sejnowski, and John McWhirter, eds., 2007

Predicting Structured Data, Gökhan Bakir, Thomas Hofmann, Bernard Schölkopf, Alexander J. Smola, Ben Taskar, S. V. N. Vishwanathan, eds., 2007

Toward Brain-Computer Interfacing, Guido Dornhege, José del R. Millán, Thilo Hinterberger, Dennis J. McFarland, Klaus-Robert Müller, eds., 2007

Large Scale Kernel Machines, Léon Bottou, Olivier Chapelle, Denis DeCoste, Jason Westman, eds., 2007

Toward Brain-Computer Interfacing

edited by
Guido Dornhege
José del R. Millán
Thilo Hinterberger
Dennis J. McFarland
Klaus-Robert Müller

foreword by
Terrence J. Sejnowski

A Bradford Book

The MIT Press
Cambridge, Massachusetts
London, England

For information about special quantity discounts, please email special_sales@mitpress.mit.edu.

This book was set in LaTex by the authors.

Printed and bound in the United States of America.

Library of Congress Cataloging-in-Publication Data
Toward brain-computer interfacing / edited by Guido Dornhege ... [et al.] ; foreword by Terrence J. Sejnowski.
  p.;   cm.   – (Neural information processing series)
"A Bradford book."
Includes bibliographical references and index.
ISBN 978-0-262-04244-4 (hardcover : alk. paper)
1. Brain-computer interfaces. I. Dornhege, Guido. II. Series.
[DNLM: 1. Brain Mapping. 2. User-Computer Interface. 3. Brain–physiology. 4. Psychomotor Performance. 5. Rehabilitation–instrumentation. WL 335 T737 2007]
QP360.7.T69 2007
612.8'2–dc22

                                                                            2007000517

10 9 8 7 6 5 4 3 2 1

Contents

Foreword

The advances in brain-computer interfaces in this book could have far-reaching consequences for how we interact with the world around us. A communications channel that bypasses the normal motor outflow from the brain will have an immediate benefit for paraplegic patients. Someday the same technology will allow humans to remotely control agents in exotic environments, which will open new frontiers that we can only dimly imagine today.

The earliest systems to be developed were based on noninvasive electroencephalographic (EEG) recordings. Because these systems do not require invasive surgical implants, they can be used for a wide range of applications. The disadvantage is the relatively low rate of signaling that can be achieved. Nonetheless, advances in signal processing techniques and the development of dry electrodes make this an attractive approach.

Three separate research areas have contributed to major advances in invasive brain-computer interfaces. First, the neural code for motor control was uncovered based on recordings from single neurons in different cortical areas of alert primates. The second was the development of mathematical algorithms for converting the train of spikes recorded from populations of these neurons to an intended action, called the decoding problem. Third, it was necessary to achieve stable, long-term recordings from small, cortical neurons in a harsh aqueous environment.

For both invasive and noninvasive BCIs interdisciplinary teams of scientists and engineers needed to work closely together to create successful systems.

Success in brain-computer interfaces has also depended on the remarkable ability of the brain to adapt to unusual tasks, none more challenging than "mind control" of extracorporeal space. We are still at an early stage of development, but the field is moving forward rapidly and we can confidently expect further advances in the near future.

Terrence J. Sejnowski
La Jolla, CA

Preface

The past decade has seen a fast growing interest to develop an effective communication interface connecting the human brain to a computer, the "brain-computer interface" (BCI). BCI research follows three major goals: (1) it aims to provide a new communication channel for patients with severe neuromuscular disabilities bypassing the normal output pathways, (2) it provides a powerful working tool in computational neuroscience to contribute to a better understanding of the brain, and finally (3)—often overseen—it provides a generic novel independent communication channel for man-machine interaction, a direction that is at only the very begining of scientific and practical exploration. During a workshop at the annual Neural Information Processing Systems (NIPS) conference, held in Whistler, Canada, in December 2004, a snapshot of the state of the art in BCI research was recorded. A variety of people helped in this, especially all the workshop speakers and attendees who contributed to lively discussions. After the workshop, we decided that it would be worthwhile to invest some time to have an overview about current BCI research printed.

We invited all the speakers as well as other researchers to submit papers, which were integrated into the present collection. Since BCI research has previously not been covered in an entire book, this call has been widely followed. Thus, the present collection gathers contributions and expertise from many important research groups in this field, whom we wholeheartedly thank for all the work they have put into our joint effort. Note, of course, that since this book is the outcome of a workshop, it cannot cover all groups and it may—clearly unintentionally—contain some bias.

However, we are confident that this book covers a broad range of present BCI research: In the first part we are able to present overviews about many important noninvasive (that is, without implanting electrodes) BCI groups in the world. We have been also able to win contributions from a few of the most important invasive BCI groups giving an overview of the current state of the invasive BCI research. These contributions are presented in the second part. The book is completed by three further parts, namely an overview of state-of-the-art techniques from machine learning and signal processing to process brain signals, an overview about existing software packages in BCI research, and some ideas about applications of BCI research for the real world.

It is our hope that this outweighs the shortcomings of the book, most notably the fact that a collection of chapters can never be as homogeneous as a book conceived by a single author. We have tried to compensate for this by writing an introductory chapter (see chapter 1) and prefaces for all five parts of the book. In addition, the contributions were carefully refereed.

Guido Dornhege, José del R. Millán, Thilo Hinterberger, Dennis J. McFarland, and Klaus-Robert Müller

Berlin, Martigny, Tübingen, Albany, August 2006

Acknowledgments

Guido Dornhege and Klaus-Robert Müller were funded by BMBF (FKZ 01IBE01A, 16SV2231, and 01GQ0415), EU PASCAL. Guido Dornhege furthermore acknowledges the support by the Fraunhofer Society for the BCI project. José del R. Millán acknowledges support from the European IST Programme FET Project FP6-003758, the European Network of Excellence "PASCAL," and the Swiss National Science Foundation NCCR "IM2." Thilo Hinterberger was supported by the German Research Society (DFG, SFB 550, and HI 1254/2-1) and the Samueli Institute, California. Dennis McFarland was supported by NIH (NICHD (HD30146) and NIBIB/NINDS (EB00856)) and by the James S. McDonnell Foundation. Klaus-Robert Müller also wishes to thank, for warm hospitality during his stay in Tübingen at the Max-Planck Institute for Biological Cybernetics, the Friedrich Miescher Laboratory and the Department of Psychology at University of Tbingen, where part of this book was written. Klaus-Robert Müller furthermore acknowledges generous support by the Fraunhofer Society for the BCI endeavor and in particular his sabbatical project.

Finally, we would like to thank everybody who contributed toward the success of this book project, in particular to Mel Goldsipe, Suzanne Stradley, Robert Prior, to all chapter authors, and to the chapter reviewers.

1 An Introduction to Brain-Computer Interfacing

Andrea Kübler
Institute of Medical Psychology and Behavioural Neurobiology
Eberhard-Karls-University Tübingen, Gartenstr. 29
72074 Tübingen, Germany

Klaus-Robert Müller
Fraunhofer–Institute FIRST   *Technical University Berlin*
Intelligent Data Analysis Group (IDA)   *Str. des 17. Juni 135*
Kekuléstr. 7, 12489 Berlin, Germany   *10 623 Berlin, Germany*

1.1 Abstract

We provide a compact overview of invasive and noninvasive brain-computer interfaces (BCI). This serves as a high-level introduction to an exciting and active field and sets the scene for the following sections of this book. In particular, the chapter briefly assembles information on recording methods and introduces the physiological signals that are being used in BCI paradigms. Furthermore, we review the spectrum from subject training to machine learning approaches. We expand on clinical and human-machine interface (HMI) applications for BCI and discuss future directions and open challenges in the BCI field.

1.2 Overview

Translating thoughts into actions without acting physically has always been material of which dreams and fairytales were made. Recent developments in brain-computer interface (BCI) technology, however, open the door to making these dreams come true. Brain-machine interfaces (BMI[1]) are devices that allow interaction between humans and artificial devices (for reviews see e.g. Kübler et al. (2001a); Kübler and Neumann (2005); Lebedev and Nicolelis (2006); Wolpaw et al. (2002)). They rely on continuous, real-time interaction between living neuronal tissue and artificial effectors.

Computer-brain interfaces[2] are designed to restore sensory function, transmit sensory information to the brain, or stimulate the brain through artificially generated electrical signals. Examples of sensory neuroprostheses are the retina implant (e.g. Eckmiller (1997); Zrenner (2002)) and the cochlear implant, which circumvents the nonfunctioning auditory hair cells of the inner ear by transmitting electrically processed acoustic signals via implanted stimulation electrodes directly to the acoustic nerve (e.g., Zenner et al. (2000); Merzenich et al. (1974); Pfingst (2000)). Further, with an implanted stimulating neuroprosthesis, hyperactivity of the subthalamic nuclei can be inhibited to improve Parkinsonian symptoms (e.g., Mazzone et al. (2005); Benabid et al. (1991)).

Brain-computer interfaces provide an additional output channel and thus can use the neuronal activity of the brain to control artificial devices, for example, for restoring motor function. Neuronal activity of few neurons or large cell assemblies is sampled and processed in real-time and converted into commands to control an application, such as a robot arm or a communication program (e.g., Birbaumer et al. (1999); Müller-Putz et al. (2005b); Taylor et al. (2002); Hochberg et al. (2006); Santhanam et al. (2006); Lebedev and Nicolelis (2006); Haynes and Rees (2006); Blankertz et al. (2006a); Müller and Blankertz (2006)).

Brain activity is either recorded intracortically with multielectrode arrays or single electrodes, epi- or subdurally from the cortex or from the scalp. From the broad band of neuronal electrical activity, signal detection algorithms filter and denoise the signal of interest and decoded information is commuted into device commands.

Over the past twenty years, increased BCI research for communication and control has been driven by a better understanding of brain function, powerful computer equipment, and by a growing awareness of the needs, problems, and potentials of people with disabilities (Wolpaw et al. (2002); Kübler et al. (2001a)). In addition to addressing clinical and quality of life issues, such interfaces constitute powerful tools for basic research on how the brain coordinates and instantiates human behavior and how new behavior is acquired and maintained. This is because a BCI offers the unique opportunity to investigate brain activity as an independent variable. In traditional psychophysiological experiments subjects are presented with a task or stimuli (independent variables), and the related brain activity is measured (dependent variable). Conversely, with neurofeedback by means of a BCI, subjects can learn to deliberately increase or decrease brain activity (independent variable) and changes in behavior can be measured accordingly (dependent variable). Studies on regulation of slow cortical potentials, sensorimotor rhythms, and the BOLD response (see below) yield various specific effects on behavior, such as decreased reaction time in a motor task after activation of contralateral motor cortex (Rockstroh et al. (1982)), faster lexical decisions (Pulvermüller et al. (2000)), or improved memory performance as a function of deactivation of the parahippocampal place area (Weiskopf et al. (2004b)). In these examples, the link between activation and deactivation of a specific cortical area and changes in behavior is quite evident. More general effects on learning such as better musical performance in music students (techniques and subjective interpretation) and better dancing performance in dance students (technicality, flair, overall execution) were observed after regularization of alpha and theta activity (Gruzelier and Egner (2005); Raymond et al. (2005))

An often overlooked direction of BCI applications beyond clinical and basic research aspects is the yet unexplored use of BCI as an additional independent channel of man-machine interaction (see chapters 23, 24 and 25 for first examples in this direction of research). In particular, brain signals can provide direct access to aspects of human brain state such as cognitive workload, alertness, task involvement, emotion, or concentration. The monitoring of these will allow for a novel technology that directly adapts a man-machine interface design to the inferred brain state in real-time.

Furthermore, BCI technology can in the near future serve as an add-on when developing new computer games, for example, fantasy games that require the brain-controlled mastering of a task for advancing to the next game level.

A variety of technologies for monitoring brain activity may serve as a BCI. In addition to electroencephalography (EEG) and invasive electrophysiological methods, these include magnetoencephalography (MEG), positron emission tomography (PET), functional magnetic resonance imaging (fMRI), and optical imaging (functional near infrared spectroscopy, fNIRS). As MEG, PET, and fMRI are demanding, tied to the laboratory, and expensive, these technologies are more suitable to address basic research questions and short-term intervention for location of sources of brain activity and alteration of brain activity in diseases with known neurobiological dysfunction. In contrast, EEG, NIRS, and invasive devices are portable, and thus may offer practical BCIs for communication and control in daily life.

Current BCIs for human users have been mainly used for cursor control and communication by means of selection of letters or items on a computer screen (e.g., Birbaumer et al. (1999); Blankertz et al. (2006a); Hochberg et al. (2006); Obermaier et al. (2003); Wolpaw and McFarland (2004)). An overview of BCI applications in clinical populations is given in chapter 22.

Interfaces between machine and the animal brain have been used to control robotic arms (e.g., Taylor et al. (2002); Wessberg et al. (2000), and for a review, see Lebedev and Nicolelis (2006)). However, before BCIs can be utilized across a wide range of clinical or daily life settings, many open technological issues must be resolved. Sensors are the bottleneck of todays invasive and noninvasive BCIs: invasive sensors can last only a limited time before they lose signal (Hochberg et al. (2006); Nicolelis et al. (2003)), and noninvasive sensors need long preparation time due to the use of conductive gel. More neurobiological and psychological research is necessary to understand the interaction between neurons and behavior related to the use of BCIs. Already machine learning and advanced signal processing methods play a key role in BCI research as they allow the decoding of different brain states within the noise of the spontaneous neural activity in real-time (see chapters 9, 11, 12, 13, 14, 15, 16, and 18). There is, however, a need for continuous improvement; in particular, higher robustness, online adaptation to compensate for nonstationarities, sensor fusion strategies, and techniques for transferring classifier or filter parameters from session to session are among the most burning topics.

1.3 Approaches to BCI Control

Two separate approaches to BCI control exist, while almost all BCIs realize a mixture of both approaches: (1) Learning to voluntarily regulate brain activity by means of neurofeedback and operant learning principles. Following subject training, in which the subject learns to regulate a specific brain activity by means of feedback, different brain states can be produced on command and, thus, become suitable as control commands. (2) Machine learning procedures that enable the interference of the statistical signature of specific brain states or intentions within a calibration session (see chapter 5).

1.3.1   The Biofeedback Approach—Voluntary Control of the Brain Response

Biofeedback is a procedure that, by means of feedback of a (seemingly) autonomous parameter, aims at acquiring voluntary control over this parameter. Participants receive visual, auditory, or tactile information about their cardiovascular activity (heartrate, blood pressure), temperature, skin conductance, muscular activity, electrical brain activity (EEG, MEG), or the blood oxygen level dependent (BOLD) response (with fMRI). In discrete or continuous trials, the participants are presented with the task to either increase or decrease the activity of interest. By means of the feedback signal, participants receive continuous information about the alteration of the activity. At the end of the trial, participants are informed about their performance (e.g., by highlighting a correctly hit target) and correct trials may be positively reinforced by a smiling face (Kübler et al. (1999); see also chapter 3) or by earning tokens that can be exchanged later for toys (e.g., training of children with ADHD in first author's affiliation). If participants are repeatedly trained, they learn to manipulate the activity of interest, which is then—at least to a certain extent—under voluntary or conscious (cortical) control.

1.3.2   The Machine Learning Approach—Detection of the Relevant Brain Signal

A somewhat opposite approach[3] is the machine learning approach to BCI, where the training is relocated from the subject to the learning algorithm. Thus, decoding algorithms are individually adapted to the users that perform the task. For obtaining a qualitative impression about the variability that is to be compensated, see chapter 13, figures 13.1 and 13.2, where different individuals perform finger tapping or motor imagery. Note that even the intraindividual variance between sessions is high. Learning algorithms require examples from which they can infer the underlying statistical structure of the respective brain state. Therefore, subjects are first required to repeatedly produce a certain brain state during a calibration session (e.g., for the BBCI, this calibration session takes approximately twenty minutes, see chapter 5). Even from such a small amount of data, current learning machines can extract spatiotemporal blueprints of these brain states, which are readily usable in the subsequent feedback session. The tackling of the enormous trial-to-trial variability is a major challenge in BCI research. We believe that advanced techniques for machine learning are an essential tool in this endeavor. The use of state-of-the-art learning machines enables not only the achievement of high decision accuracies for BCI (e.g., chapters 5, 6, 9, 12, 13, and 14), but also, as a by-product of the classification, the few most salient features for classification are found, which can then be matched with neurophysiological knowledge. In this sense, machine learning approaches are useful beyond the pure classification or adaptive spatiotemporal filtering step, as they can contribute to a better interpretation and understanding of a novel paradigm per se (see Blankertz et al. (2006b)). Thus, machine learning can be usefully employed in an exploratory scenario, where (1) a new paradigm is tested that also could generate unexpected neurophysiological signals, (2) a hypothesis about underlying task relevant brain processes is generated automatically by the learning machine through feature extraction, and (3) the paradigm can be refined, and thus a better understanding of the brain processes could be achieved (see figure 13.8). In this sense, a machine learning method offering explanation can be of great use in the semiautomatic exploration loop for testing new paradigms. Note that this holds also for data analysis beyond decoding of brain signals.

1.3.3   Integration of the Two Approaches

The two last paragraphs reflect opposite positions. In practice, BCIs will neither rely solely on feedback learning of the users nor only on machine learning. For example, in the BBCI (see chapter 5) that has no *explicit* user biofeedback training, a user's brain activity will adapt to the settings of the decoding algorithm when using the BCI in feedback mode, such that the most successful EEG activity pattern will be repeatedly produced. Thus, a coadaptation of the learning user and algorithm occurs inevitably. However, it remains unclear how to optimally bring these two interacting learning systems into synchrony; a thorough study is still missing. Experimentally, the two learning systems can be coupled using online learning (see chapter 18 for discussion).

It is furthermore important to note that in a proportion of the subject population, typically in 20 percent of the users, one is unable to successfully classify the brain activation patterns. We refer to this group as the BCI illiterates. This finding holds no matter whether machine learning or biofeedback is used to train the subjects. Further research is needed to fully understand and overcome the BCI illiteracy phenomenon.

1.4   Clinical Target Groups—Individuals in Need of a BCI for Motor Control and Communication

A variety of neurological diseases such as motor neuron diseases, spinal cord injury, stroke, encephalitis, or traumatic brain injury may lead to severe motor paralysis, which may also include speech. Patients may have only a few muscles to control artificial devices for communicating their needs and wishes and interacting with their environment. We refer to the locked-in state if some residual voluntary muscular movement, such as eye or lip movement, is still possible. People who lost all voluntary muscular movement are referred to as being in the complete locked-in state (see also chapter 22 and Birbaumer (2006a)). In the realm of BCI use, it is of particular importance how and how much the brain is affected by disease. To provide a detailed discussion of all diseases that may lead to the locked-in syndrome would go beyond the scope of this introduction. Thus, we will refer to only those diseases that have been repeatedly reported in the BCI literature, that is amyotrophic lateral sclerosis, high spinal cord injury, and stroke; all three diseases have quite different effects on the brain.

1.4.1   Amyotrophic Lateral Sclerosis

Amyotrophic lateral sclerosis (ALS) is a progressive neurodegenerative disease involving the first and second motoneurons and the central nervous system (see also chapter 22). Patients with ALS show global brain atrophy with regional decreases of grey matter density being highest in right-hemispheric primary motor cortex and left-hemispheric medial frontal gyrus (Kassubek et al. (2005)). White matter reduction is found along the corticospinal tracts, in the corpus callosum, and in frontal and parietal cortices. Clinical symptoms are atrophic paresis with fasciculations mostly starting in hands and lower arms. With progressive neuronal degeneration, patients become severely physically impaired. In later stages of the disease, speech, swallowing, and breathing are also affected. Patients succumb to respiratory failure unless they choose artificial ventilation via tracheotomy. Patients with tracheotomy may render the locked-in state with only residual muscular movement or even the completely locked-in state. Cognitive impairment has been reported repeatedly (Hanagasi et al. (2002); Ringholz et al. (2005)), but improved learning has also been shown (Lakerfeld et al. (submitted); Rottig et al. (2006)). Emotional processing seems to be altered such that positive and negative extremes are attenuated (Lulé et al. (2005)). Quality of life in ALS patients is surprisingly high and within the range of patients with nonfatal diseases such as diabetes or irritable bowl syndrome (Kübler et al. (in preparation)). One important component of individual quality of life repeatedly mentioned by patients, specifically as the disease progresses, is the ability to communicate.

1.4.2   Cervical Spinal Cord Injury

Most often spinal cord injury follows trauma. It may also occur due to acute ischaemia in the arteria spinalis-anterior or acute compression. Acute symptoms are spinal shock with atonic paresis below the lesion, atonic bladder, paralysis of the rectum, disturbed sensitivity in all qualities (pain, pressure, temperature) and vegetative dysfunction. These symptoms continue into the post-traumatic phase and are endorsed by painful, involuntary stretching and bending of extremities (so-called spinal automatisms). Cervical spinal cord injury has been shown to be accompanied by local cortical grey matter reduction in somatosensory areas (S1) bilaterally located posterior to the hand region in M1. Atrophy also occurred in the right leg area and extended to parietal BA5 in the left hemisphere (Jurkiewicz et al. (2006)). Several years post trauma, patients may be well adapted to a life with impairment, experience a balanced emotional life, and lead an intact social life. Pain contributes to poorer quality of life, and gainful employment is related to high quality of life (Lundqvist et al. (1991)). Clinically relevant symptoms of depression occur specifically in the first year post injury (Hancock et al. (1993)).

1.4.3   Brain Stem Stroke

The classic locked-in syndrome as defined by Bauer and colleagues is characterized by total immobility except for vertical eye movement and blinking (Bauer et al. (1979); Smith and Delargy (2005)). Most often the locked-in syndrome is of cerebrovascular origin such that thrombotic occlusion of the arteria basilaris leads to infarction in the ventral pons (Katz et al. (1992); Patterson and Grabois (1986)). As a result, corticobulbar and cortical spinal tracts are interrupted as are both the supranuclear and postnuclear oculomotor fibers. If movements other than vertical eye movement is preserved, the locked-in syndrome is referred to as incomplete, and if no movement, and thus no communication, is possible as total (Bauer et al. (1979)). Higher cortical areas or subcortical areas besides the brain stem are not affected. Consequently, consciousness and cognition are usually unimpaired in such patients. A survey on quality of life in chronic locked-in patients (more than one year after diagnosis) with no major motor recovery, revealed no differences to healthy controls in the perception of mental and general health (Laureys et al. (2005)). In a survey ($N = 44$) by Leon-Carrion et al., less than 20 percent of the patients described their mood as bad (5 percent) or reported to be depressed (12.5 percent) and 81 percent met with friends more than twice a month (Leon-Carrion et al. (2002)). Many locked-in patients return home from hospital and start a different but meaningful life (Laureys et al. (2005)).

1.5   Brain-Computer Interfaces for Healthy Subjects

Applications of BCI technology go beyond rehabilitation. Although BCI for healthy subjects is pursued much less, it is of high industrial relevance. It is less the desire to communicate for the healthy: this is much more easily done via keyboard, computer mouse, speech, or gesture recognition devices. It is this additional independent channel "BCI" for man-machine interaction (see chapters 23, 24 and 25 for first examples in this direction of research) that has remained unexplored. Brain signals read in real-time on a single trial basis could provide direct access to human brain states, which can then be used to adapt the man-machine interface on the fly. One application field could be *monitoring* tasks such as alertness monitoring, where the brain holds the key to access information that can otherwise not be easily acquired. Signals of interest to be inferred from brain activity are cognitive workload, alertness, task involvement, emotion, or concentration. For instance, workload could be assessed in behavioral experiments by measuring reaction times. However, this would give very indirect and therefore imprecise measures with respect to temporal resolution, quality, and context. The online monitoring of cognitive workload could contribute to construct better systems in safety critical applications (see chapter 24). A further direction is the *direct use* of brain states in computer applications or as novel features for computer gaming (see figure 1.1). The latter is an interesting challenge since the game interfaces should be able to compensate for the imperfect signal of a BCI. In other words, if the classification rate of a BCI is 95 percent, then the respective computer game interface will have to be robust with respect to the 5 percent errors that will inevitably occur. Tetris, although already successfully played with the BBCI system, is a good example of a game where small errors can seriously spoil the course of the game.

The current state of EEG sensor technology and the price of EEGs are major obstacles for a broad use of BCI technology for healthy users. However, once fashionable, cheap, contactless EEG caps are available—for example, in the shape of baseball caps—a wide market and application perspective will immediately open.

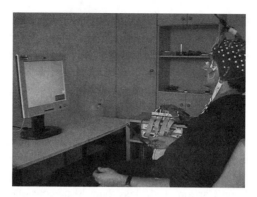

Figure 1.1   The simple game of Pong is revived in a new technological context: imagination of the right hand moves the cursor to the right, imagination of the left hand pushes the cursor to the left. In this manner, the ball that is reflected from the sides of the game field can be hit by the brain-racket. Thus, the user can use his intentions to play "Brain Pong." Dornhege (2006); Krepki (2004); Krepki et al. (2007).

1.6   Recording Methods, Paradigms, and Systems for Brain-Computer Interfacing

Current BCIs differ in how the neural activity of the brain is recorded, how subjects (humans and animals) are trained, how the signals are translated into device commands, and which application is provided to the user. An overview of current noninvasive BCIs is provided in chapters 2–7, while invasive BCIs are discussed in chapters 8–12. An overview of existing software packages is found in chapters 20 and 21.

1.6.1   Noninvasive Recording Methods for BCI

The electrical activity of the brain can be recorded noninvasively with electroencephalography (EEG) (e.g., Birbaumer et al. (1999); Pfurtscheller et al. (2000b); Wolpaw et al. (2003); Blankertz et al. (2006a)). The current produced by neural activity induces a magnetic field that can be recorded with magnetoencephalography (MEG) (Birbaumer and Cohen (2005)). Increased neural activity is accompanied by locally increased glucose metabolism, resulting in increased glucose and oxygene consumption. As a consequence of glucose consumption, cranial arteries dilate, allowing for increased blood flow, that results in hyperoxygenation of the active tissue. Imaging techniques make use of the different magnetic and optical properties of oxygenated and deoxygenated hemoglobin. The different magnetic properties of the ferrous on the heme of oxy- and deoxyhemoglobin are the basis of the blood oxygen level dependent (BOLD) response measured with functional magnetic resonance imaging (fMRI) (Chen and Ogawa (2000)). Oxy- and deoxyhemoglobin have different optical properties in the visible and near infrared range. The changes in the ratio of oxygenated hemoglobin to blood volume due to neural activity is measured with near infrared spectroscopy (NIRS) (Bunce et al. (2006)). In the following sections, we briefly review noninvasive BCIs categorized according to the recording techniques.

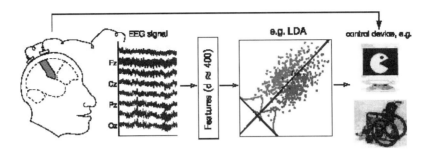

Figure 1.2   Generic noninvasive BCI setup: signals are recorded, e.g., with EEG, meaningful features are extracted and subsequently classified. Finally, a signal is extracted from the classifier that provides the control signal for some device or machine.

1.6.1.1   Brain Signals Recorded from the Scalp (EEG-BCIs)

In a typical BCI setting, participants are presented with stimuli or are required to perform specific mental tasks while the electrical activity of their brains is being recorded by EEG (see figure 1.2 for a general setup of a noninvasive BCI). Extracted and relevant EEG features can then be fed back to the user by so-called closed-loop BCIs. Specific features of the EEG are either regulated by the BCI user (slow cortical potentials (SCP), sensorimotor rhythms (SMR)) or are elicited by visual, tactile, or auditory stimulation (event-related potentials, namely the P300 or steady-state [visually-]evoked potentials (SS[V]EP)). In the following paragraphs we provide a short description of the physiology of these features and their use for brain-computer interfacing.

Slow Cortical Potentials (SCP)

Research over the past thirty years on SCPs and their regulation led to the excitation-threshold-regulation theory (Birbaumer et al. (1990, 2003); Strehl et al. (2006)). The vertical arrangement of pyramidal cells in the cortex is essential for the generation of SCP (see figure 1.3). Most apical dendrites of pyramidal cells are located in cortical layers I and II. Depolarization of the apical dendrites giving rise to SCP is dependent on sustained afferent intracortical or thalamocortical input to layers I and II, and on simultaneous depolarization of large pools of pyramidal neurons. The SCP amplitude recorded from the scalp depends upon the synchronicity and intensity of the afferent input to layers I and II (Speckmann et al. (1984)). The depolarization of cortical cell assemblies reduces their excitation threshold such that firing of neurons in regions responsible for specified motor or cognitive tasks is facilitated. Negative amplitude shifts grow with increasing attentional or cognitive resource allocation. Cortical positivity may result from active inhibition of apical dendritic neural activity or simply from a reduction of afferent inflow and subsequent reduced postsynaptic activity. In any case, positive SCPs are considered to increase the excitation threshold of upper cortical layers via a negative feedback loop involving the basal ganglia and the reticular nucleus of the thalamus. Increasing cortical negativity is accompanied by increased activation of inhibitory striatal nuclei that leads to an increase

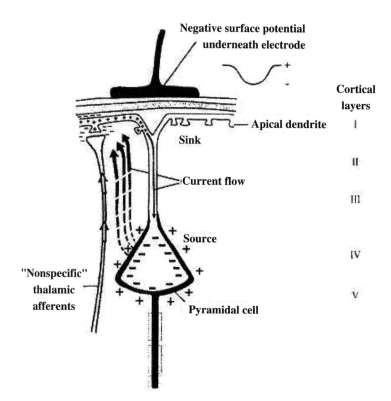

Figure 1.3 Negative slow cortical potentials at the surface of the cortex originate from afferent thalamic or cortical input to the apical dendrites in layers I and II. The extracellular surrounding of the dendrites is electrically negative, leading to current flow into the cell mediated by positive sodium ions (sink). Intracellularly, the current flows toward the soma (source). This fluctuation of ions generates field potentials that can be recorded by electrodes on the scalp (from Kübler et al. (2001a), figure 4, with permission).

of the excitation threshold of upper cortical layers, thereby preventing overexcitation (Birbaumer et al. (2003); Hinterberger et al. (2003c); Strehl et al. (2006)).

A strong relationship among self-induced cortical negativity, reaction time, signal detection, and short-term memory performance has been reported in several studies in humans and monkeys (Lutzenberger et al. (1979, 1982); Rockstroh et al. (1982)). Tasks requiring attention are performed significantly better when presented after spontaneous or self-induced cortical negativity.

Slow Cortical Potentials as Input for a BCI (SCP-BCI)

The SCP-BCI requires users to achieve voluntary regulation of brain activity. Typically, the SCP-BCI presents users with the traditional S1-S2 paradigm, which in the sixties led Walter and colleagues to the detection of the contingent negative variation (CNV) (Walter et al. (1964)): a negative SCP shift seen after a warning stimulus (S1) two to ten seconds before an imperative stimulus (S2) that requires participants to perform a task (e.g., a

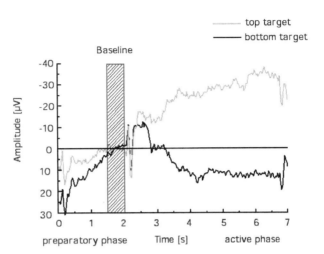

Figure 1.4   Course of slow cortical potentials (SCP) averaged across 600 trials (amplitude as a function of time). The grey line shows the course of SCP when cortical negativity has to be produced to move the cursor toward the target at the top of the screen, the black line when cortical positivity is required to move the cursor toward the bottom target. Negative and positive SCP amplitudes clearly differ between the two tasks providing a binary response. At the beginning of a trial the task is presented, accompanied by a high-pitched tone (S1—warning stimulus) indicating that two seconds later the active phase will start providing SCP feedback to the user. The active phase is introduced by a low-pitched tone (S2—imperative stimulus). Between S1 and S2 a contingent negative variation (CNV) develops, which indicates that the user is preparing to perform the task.

button press or cursor movement). The CNV (see figure 1.4) indicates depolarization and, thus, resource allocation for task performance as described above. Similarly, the SCP-BCI presents users with a high-pitched tone (S1) that indicates to the user that two seconds later, simultaneously with a low-pitched tone (S2), feedback of SCPs will start either visually as cursor movement on a monitor or by auditory means with instrumental sounds (Hinterberger et al. (2004a); Kotchoubey et al. (1997); Kübler et al. (1999)). Users are presented with two tasks, for example, cursor movement into targets either at the top or bottom of the screen, or an increase or decrease in the pitch of tones. To perform the task, BCI users have to produce positive and negative SCP amplitude shifts as compared to a baseline (see figure 1.4). SCP amplitude shifts must be above or below a predefined threshold to be classified as negative or positive. Severely paralyzed patients communicated extended messages with the SCP-BCI (Birbaumer et al. (1999); Neumann et al. (2003)) (see chapter 3).

Sensorimotor Rhythms (SMR)

Sensorimotor rhythms include an arch-shaped μ-rhythm (see figure 1.5), usually with a frequency of 10 Hz (range 8–11 Hz), often mixed with a β (around 20 Hz) and a γ component (around 40 Hz) recorded over somatosensory cortices, most preferably over C3 and C4. Spreading to parietal leads is frequent and also is seen in patients with

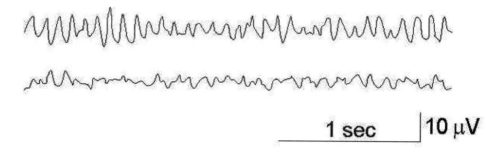

1 sec   10 μV

Figure 1.5 Upper trace: μ-rhythm over sensory motor areas. Lower trace: desynchronization of μ-rhythm through movement imagery.

amyotrophic lateral sclerosis (Kübler et al. (2005a)). Recently, an ALS patient showed left-hand movement-imagery-related SMR modulation at P4, which is in accordance with increased parietal activation during hand movement imagery in ALS patients as measured with functional magnetic resonance imaging (Kew et al. (1993); Lulé et al. (in press)). The SMR is related to the motor cortex with contributions of somatosensory areas such that the beta component arises from the motor and the alphoid μ-component from sensory cortex. SMR is blocked by movements, movement imagery, and movement preparation; thus, it is seen as an "idling" rhythm of the cortical sensory region. In cats, μ-rhythm-like activity has been shown to originate from the nucleus ventralis posterior of the thalamus. Usually μ-rhythm activity is not readily seen in scalp-recorded spontaneous EEG activity and it thus historically has been believed to occur in only a small number of adult persons. However, with better signal processing it has been shown to be ubiquitous in adults. Immediately, scalp-detectable μ-rhythm may, however, be an indicator of pathology. It was reported to accompany autonomic and emotional dysfunction such as migrane, bronchial asthma, tinnitus, anxiety, aggressiveness, and emotional instability. It is also often seen in patients with epilepsy. Three theories for the neurophysiological basis of the μ-rhythm exist: (1) it could be the correlate of neuronal hyperexcitability as specifically expressed in pathology, (2) it could be a sign of cortical inhibition, which would explain the blocking of μ-rhythm by movement or movement imagery, or (3) it may be interpreted as somatosensory "cortical idling," adding the component of afferent input (summarized according to Niedermeyer (2005b)).

Sensorimotor Rhythms as Input for a BCI (SMR-BCI)

Sensorimotor rhythms (SMR) decrease or desynchronize with movement or preparation for movement and increase or synchronize in the postmovement period or during relaxation (Pfurtscheller et al. (1999)). Furthermore, and most relevant for BCI use by locked-in patients, they also desynchronize with motor imagery. Thus, to modulate the SMR amplitude no actual movement is required. Many BCI groups choose SMR as input signal because—at least in healthy participants—they are easy to regulate by means of motor imagery (see figure 1.6 and chapters 2–5). Modulation of SMR can be achieved within the first training session where the subjects are instructed to imagine left and right hand and foot movement (e.g., Blankertz et al. (2006a), see also chapter 5). After

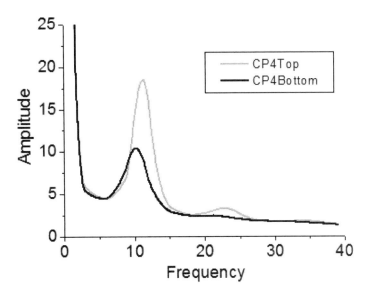

Figure 1.6   EEG frequency spectrum of an ALS patient at electrode position Cp4 as a function of amplitude averaged over about 160 trials. The grey line shows the averaged EEG when the cursor has to be moved into the top target at the right-hand-side margin of the screen, the black line when the cursor has to be moved into the bottom target. Downward cursor movement is achieved by motor imagery (in this case left-hand movement leading to SMR modulation at Cp4), upward cursor movement by "thinking of nothing." During downward cursor movement, the SMR amplitudes decrease (desynchronize) in the α and β band leading to a binary signal.

subsequent machine learning (about two minutes on a standard PC) and visual inspection, individualized spatiotemporal filters and classifiers are ready to be used for feedback. Good subjects are then able to achieve information transfer rates of fifty bits per minute in asynchronous BCI mode (for a comparison of different evaluation criteria, see chapter 19). Even under the extremely challenging conditions of life demonstrations at CeBit 2006 in Hanover, Germany, subjects were able to achieve on average a selection rate of five to eight letters per minute in a spelling task (see chapter 5 and Müller and Blankertz (2006)).

To achieve similar EEG patterns of imagined movements as compared to actual movements, it is important to instruct participants to imagine movement kinesthetically, meaning to "feel and experience" the movement instead of simply visualizing a movement (Neuper et al. (2005)). As with the SCP-BCI, to operate the SMR-BCI subjects are required to regulate the SMR amplitude and are thus provided with visual (Pfurtscheller et al. (2006c); Wolpaw et al. (2003)) or auditory feedback (Hinterberger et al. (2004a); Nijboer et al. (in press)) (see also chapter 3). Typically, subjects are shown two or more targets on a monitor in which the cursor has to be moved by means of SMR amplitude modulation (see also chapters 2, 4, and 5). In a recent study with four ALS patients, it was shown that SMR regulation is possible despite considerable degeneration of cortical and spinal motor neurons (Kübler et al. (2005a)). However, the SMR amplitude is much lower in patients as compared to healthy individuals.

Event-Related Potentials

Event-related potentials (ERPs) are electrocortical potentials that can be measured in the EEG before, during, or after a sensory, motor, or psychological event. They have a fixed time delay to the stimulus and their amplitude is usually much smaller than the ongoing spontaneous EEG activity. The amplitudes are smaller because ERPs are more localized in the corresponding cortical areas. They are less frequent than the spontaneous EEG waves with similar shape and amplitude (Birbaumer and Schmid (2006)). To detect ERPs, averaging techniques are used. An averaged ERP is composed of a series of large, biphasic waves, lasting a total of five hundred to thousand milliseconds. Error monitoring of the brain is also accompanied by evoked potentials referred to as error related potentials. These deflections in the EEG may be used for error detection in a BCI (see chapter 17). In the following two paragraphs, a short overview is provided of the P300 component of the event-related potential and the visually (and sensorily) evoked potential for BCI use. BCIs on the basis of visually evoked potentials and visual P300 require intact gaze.

P300

The P300 is a positive deflection in the electroencephalogram (EEG) time-locked to auditory or visual stimuli (see figure 1.7). It is typically seen when participants are required to attend to rare target stimuli presented within a stream of frequent standard stimuli (Squires et al. (1977)), an experimental design referred to as the oddball paradigm (Fabiani et al. (1987)). The P300 amplitude varies as a function of task characteristics such as discriminability of standard and target stimuli (Johnson and Donchin (1978)), loudness of tones (Squires et al. (1977)), overall probability of the target stimuli, the preceding stimulus sequence (Squires et al. (1976)), and the electrode position (Squires et al. (1977)). Mostly observed in central and parietal regions, it is seen as a correlate of an extinction process in short-term memory when new stimuli require an update of representations.

P300 as Input Signal for a BCI (P300-BCI)

As early as the late eighties, Farwell and Donchin had shown that the P300 component of the event-related potential can be used to select items displayed on a computer monitor (Farwell and Donchin (1988)). The authors presented their participants with a 6 x 6 matrix where each of the 36 cells contained a character or a symbol. This design becomes an oddball paradigm by first intensifying resp. flashing each row and column for 100 ms in random order and second by instructing participants to focus attention to only one of the 36 cells. Thus, in one sequence of 12 flashes (6 rows and 6 columns are highlighted), the target cell will flash only twice, constituting a rare event compared to the 10 flashes of all other rows and columns and therefore eliciting a P300 (see figure 1.7). Selection occurs by detecting the row and column that elicit the largest P300 (see also chapter 2). The P300-BCI does not require self-regulation of the EEG. All that is required from users is that they are able to focus attention and gaze on the target letter albeit for a considerable amount of time.

Over the past five years, the P300 has received increasing amounts of attention as a BCI control signal. For example, a number of offline studies have been conducted to improve

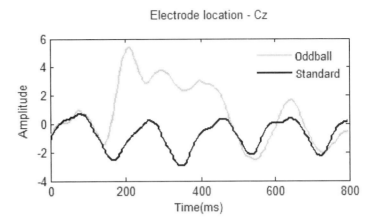

Figure 1.7   Averaged EEG at the vertex electrode (Cz) of an ALS patient using a 7 x 7 P300 spelling matrix. The black line indicates the EEG response to 2448 standard stimuli and the grey line to 51 target letters (oddball) that have to be selected from the spelling matrix. A positive deflection as a response to targets can be seen in the time window between 200 and 500 ms.

the classification rate of the P300 Speller (Kaper et al. (2004); Serby et al. (2005); Xu et al. (2004); He et al. (2001); Thulasidas et al. (2006)). Using a support vector machine classifier, Thulasidas et al. report online selection of three characters per minute with 95 percent accuracy (Thulasidas et al. (2006)). Bayliss showed that the P300 also can be used to select items in a virtual apartment, provided presentation of targets constitute an oddball paradigm (Bayliss et al. (2004)). In 2003, Sellers, Schalk, and Donchin published the first results of an ALS patient using the P300 Speller (Sellers et al. (2003)). In recent studies, Sellers et al. and Nijboer et al. presented results of the P300 speller used by ALS patients indicating that ALS patients are able to use the P300-BCI with accuracies up to 100 percent (Nijboer et al. (submitted); Sellers et al. (2006b)). It was also shown that the P300 response remains stable over periods of twelve to more than fifty daily sessions in healthy volunteers as well as in ALS-patients (Nijboer et al. (submitted); Sellers and Donchin (2006)). Piccione et al. tested the P300 as a control signal for a BCI in seven healthy and five paralyzed patients (Piccione et al. (2006)). As in the other studies, task completion and good performance was achieved after little time, thus there was no need for time-consuming training. However, the patients' performance (68.6 percent) was worse than that of healthy participants (76.2 percent). In particular, those patients who were more impaired performed worse than did healthy participants, whereas there was no difference between less impaired patients and healthy participants (Piccione et al. (2006)). Recently, Vaughan et al. introduced a P300-BCI for daily use in a patient's home environment (Vaughan et al. (2006)). Auditorily presented oddball paradigms may be used for patients with restricted or lost eye movement and are currently being investigated (Sellers and Donchin (2006); Hill et al. (2005)).

SSVEP

After visual stimulation (e.g., an alternating checkerboard), evoked potentials can be recorded from the visual cortex in the occipital lobe (O1, O2, Oz—according to the international 10-20 system). A visually evoked potential becomes steady if the presentation rate of stimuli is above 6 Hz (Gao et al. (2003b)). When participants focus their gaze on a flickering target, the amplitude of the steady-state visually evoked potential (SSVEP) increases at the fundamental frequency of the target and second and third harmonics (Wang et al. (2006); Müller-Putz et al. (2005b)). Amplitude and phase of the SSVEP depend on stimulus parameters such as repetition rate and contrast. The frequency resolution of the SSVEP is about 0.2 Hz and the bandwidth in which the SSVEP can be detected reliably is between 6 and 24 Hz (Gao et al. (2003b)).

SSVEPs as Input Signal for a BCI (SSVEP-BCI)

Like the P300-BCI, the SSVEP-BCI requires attention and intact gaze but no user training as the cortical response is elicited via external stimulation (see chapter 4). To elicit SSVEPs, targets with different flickering frequencies are presented on a monitor (Wang et al. (2006)) or on a board with light emitting diodes (LED) (Müller-Putz et al. (2005b); Gao et al. (2003b)). The number of targets realized in a BCI varies from 4 (Müller-Putz et al. (2005b)) up to 48 (Gao et al. (2003b)). Classification accuracies of more than 90 percent correct are often reported (Kelly et al. (2005); Nielsen et al. (2006); Trejo et al. (2006)). In a 9-target SSVEP-BCI, healthy participants spelled out their phone number and birth date with a spelling rate of 7.2–11.5 selections per minute (information transfer rate of 18.37–27.29 bits/min) (Nielsen et al. (2006)), and in an 11-target SSVEP-BCI with an average accuracy of 83.3 percent (23.06 bits/min) (Lee et al. (2006)).

A caveat of all SSVEP approaches to BCI control is their dependence on intact gaze, which renders them unsuitable for patients with restricted eye movement. Two studies address this issue. Kelly et al. investigated classification accuracies when users were not required to focus gaze on the flickering targets but on a fixation cross between two targets— a condition the authors refer to as covert attention (Kelly et al. (2005)). A decrease in accuracy was observed from about 95 percent when targets were fixated directly to about 70 percent in the covert attention condition. Thus, at least a rather simple two-target SSVEP paradigm might be used by locked-in patients albeit with reduced accuracy. A BCI based on steady-state evoked potentials completely independent of vision was introduced by Müller-Putz and colleagues (Müller-Putz et al. (2006)). The authors used vibratory stimulation of left- and right-hand fingertips to elicit somatosensory steady-state evoked potentials (SSSEP, see figure 1.8). The EEG was recorded from central electrodes (C3, Cz, and C4—according to the international 10-20 system). In each trial, both index fingers were stimulated simultaneously at different frequencies and participants were instructed via arrows on a computer screen to which finger they should pay attention. Online accuracies of four participants varied between 53 (chance level) and 83 percent correct, but offline classification was between 65 and 88 percent correct. Albeit not yet as reliable as the SSVEP-BCI the SSSEP-BCI may become an option for patients with impaired vision.

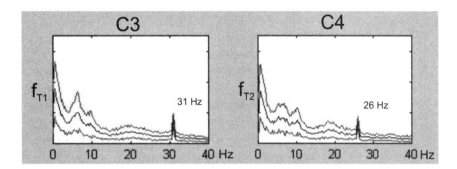

Figure 1.8   Peak at 31 Hz recorded at C3 when focusing attention on stimulation of right index finger (left panel) and 26 Hz at C4 when focusing on stimulation of left index finger. Both peaks reflect the stimulation frequency correctly (We thank Dr. Gernot Müller-Putz from the Laboratory of Brain-Computer Interfaces Institute for Knowledge Discovery at the Technical University of Graz, Austria, for this picture and the permission of reproduction).

1.6.1.2   Combinations of Signals

It is a well-known fact that different physiological phenomena, for example, slow cortical potential shifts such as the premovement Bereitschaftspotenzial or differences in spatiospectral distributions of brain activity (i.e., focal event-related desynchronizations), code for different aspects of a subject's intention to move. While papers noted the potential of combining these multiple modalities, it was first explored systematically by Dornhege et al. (2004a). Their work showed that BCI information transfer rates can be boosted significantly when combining different EEG features. From a theoretical point of view, feature combination is most beneficial if the features of the single modalities have maximal statistical independence. High mutual independence can be measured in EEG features and thus subject dependent improvements of up to 50 percent relative classification performance gain are observed when using combined features in an offline evaluation (Dornhege et al. (2004a); Dornhege (2006)). The use of robust well-regularized classifiers is mandatory in this "sensor-fusion" process because otherwise the model complexity is hard to control in such high dimensional feature spaces (see chapter 13). We conjecture that not only combinations between different EEG modalities but also between different recording technologies will be useful in the future, for example, between fMRI and EEG, or between local field potentials and spike data. Machine learning will be challenged by fusing different time-scales and their underlying statistical processes.

1.6.1.3   The Magnetic Activity of the Brain

The magnetic field generated by electrical brain activity can be measured by means of magnetoencephalography (MEG). To date, this method is used only in laboratory settings and is consequently not suitable for a BCI for communication and control in the patient's home environment. However, the advantages of MEG as compared to EEG, namely better spatial resolution leading to a precise localization of cortical activation related to a specific task or sensory stimulation and higher signal-to-noise ratio, especially for higher frequency activity like gamma band activity, render it a viable tool for short-term intervention and rehabilitation (see chapter 14). In a study with three tetraplegic patients after cervical spinal cord injury, Kauhanen et al. achieved the same classification accuracies in MEG data as compared to EEG data (Kauhanen et al. (2006)). The patient's task was to attempt finger movement, and data were analyzed offline. Lal et al. showed that regulation of the magnetic activity of the brain by means of motor imagery can be used to select letters on a computer screen, but participants were not yet provided with online feedback of MEG activity; instead they were provided with feedback of results, that is, a smiling face after correct classification or selection of the correct letter (Lal et al. (2005b)). Mellinger et al. even provide online MEG feedback for healthy participants during motor imagery (Mellinger et al. (under revision)). Three of five participants achieved cursor control of 90 percent accuracy or more within the first training session. Thus, learning to regulate brain activity by means of MEG feedback and achieved accuracies were comparable to EEG (Blankertz et al. (2006a)). MEG may be used to localize the focus of activity during motor imagery if EEG provides no clear results (see chapter 22). Currently, MEG feedback during motor imagery is used to train chronic stroke patients to reactivate the paralyzed limb provided that not the entire motor cortex or pyramidal tracts are lesioned. Chronic stroke patients undergo an MEG feedback training such that their paralyzed limb is provided with an orthosis that opens and closes the paralyzed hand (Birbaumer and Cohen (2005)). Motor imagery opens the orthosis whereas relaxation (thinking of nothing) closes it. This training provides the patients with self-induced sensory feedback of the paralyzed limb. The idea behind this being that activation of a sensorimotor network enables patients to relearn motor functions (Braun et al. (submitted)) (see also chapter 22).

1.6.1.4   The Blood Oxygen Level Dependent Response (BOLD)

For the past approximately five years it has been possible to use the blood oxygen level dependent (BOLD) response as input signal for a BCI. Local concentration of deoxygenated hemoglobin in brain tissue depends on neuronal activity and metabolism and changes can be measured with functional magnetic resonance imaging (fMRI). Compared to EEG, fMRI allows spatial resolution in the range of millimeters and a more precise allocation of neuronal activity. Additionally, activation in subcortical areas can be recorded. Due to recent advances in acquisition techniques, computational power, and algorithms, the functional sensitivity and speed of fMRI was increased considerably (Weiskopf et al. (2004b)) and the delay of feedback could be reduced to below two seconds (Weiskopf et al. (2003)), which allows the use of this technique as real-time fMRI. Target areas for feedback were sensory (S1, e.g., Yoo et al. (2004)) and motor areas (M1, e.g., DeCharms et al. (2004); SMA Weiskopf et al. (2004b)), the parahippocampal place area (Weiskopf et al. (2004b)), the affective and cognitive subdivision of the anterior cingulate cortex (ACC) (Weiskopf et al. (2003)), and rostral ACC (DeCharms et al. (2005)). Learning of self-regulating the BOLD response was reported in all studies that included subject training to regulate the BOLD response, and some reported behavioral effects in relation to activation or deactivation of target areas: Increase of activation in the affective subdivision of the ACC led to higher valence and arousal ratings of the subjective affective state (Weiskopf et al. (2003)). Better encoding of words after down regulation of the parahippocampal place area (as compared to the supplementary motor area) and decreased reaction time in a motor task after upregulation of the supplementary motor area (as compared to the parahippocampal place area) was demonstrated (Weiskopf et al. (2004b)). Regulation of the insula, an area involved in emotional processing, also proved possible and was shown to increase the negative valence of participants when confronted with negative stimuli such as pictures of violence or mutilated bodies (Sitaram et al. (2006)). Recently, specific effects on pain perception as a function of self-regulation of the rostral part of the ACC was reported in the first clinical study including patients with chronic pain. In healthy subjects, the authors controlled for effects of repeated practice, brain region, feedback, and intervention. In chronic pain patients, only feedback was controlled such that one group received feedback of the BOLD response in the rostral ACC and another of skin conductance, heart rate, and respiration. Healthy participants were presented with nociceptive heat stimuli. Only in those healthy participants and pain patients who received real-time feedback of the BOLD response in the rostral ACC, an area known to be involved in pain perception, were changes in pain ratings found (DeCharms et al. (2005)). This study already demonstates the possible power of the fMRI-BCI for treating clinical groups if the neurobiological basis of the disorder is known. For example, hypoactivation in orbitofrontal and limbic areas involved in emotional processing were found in psychopaths (Birbaumer et al. (2005)), and hypofunction in dorsolateral and dorsomedial prefrontal cortex and the pregenual part of the ACC is consistently found in depressed patients (Davidson et al. (2002)). Even more complex cognitive functions as needed for the game of paper, rock, and scissors could be decoded successfully with fMRI by Kamitani and Tong (2005). Most recently, Owen et al. successfully distinguished activation patterns to motor imagery (playing tennis) and spatial navigation (through one's own house starting at the front door) in a patient diagnosed with persistent vegetative state, and could thus show that she was consciously aware (Owen et al. (2006)). For further reference, see also the review by Haynes and Rees (2006).

1.6.1.5   *Near Infrared Spectroscopy (NIRS) as a Recording Method for BCI*

The advantage of functional MRI as compared to EEG is its 3D spatial resolution. However, fMRI is expensive and bound to the laboratory. Near infrared spectroscopy offers a comparable spatial resolution albeit restricted to cortical areas (depth 1–3 cm) with much less technical effort and costs. Moreover the NIRS-BCI is portable and could thus be used in a patient's home environment.

The NIRS-BCI system presented by Sitaram and colleagues incorporates the so-called continuous wave technique. Regional brain activation is accompanied by increases in regional cerebral blood flow (rCBF) and the regional cerebral oxygen metabolic rate (rCMRO$_2$). The increase of rCBF exceeds that of rCMRO$_2$ resulting in a decrease of deoxygenated hemoglobin in venous blood. Thus, the ratio of oxygenated to deoxygenated hemoglobin is expected to increase in active brain areas and is measured with NIRS. The continuous wave approach uses multiple pairs or channels of light sources and light detectors operating at two or more discrete wavelengths. The light source may be a

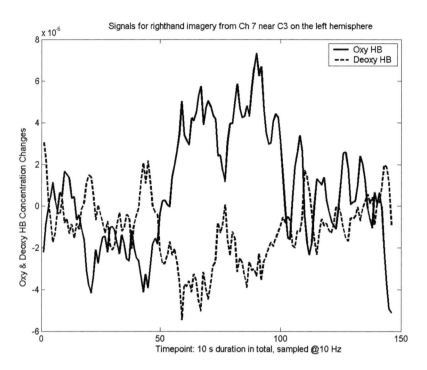

Figure 1.9 Exemplary data from a healthy participant performing motor imagery (right hand movement). The solid line indicates course of oxygenated (Oxy HB; HB = hemoglobin) and the dashed line of deoxygenated hemoglobin (Deoxy HB) averaged across a full session (80 trials) from channel 7 on the contralateral (left) hemisphere (close to the C3 electrode position as per the 10-20 system) for the duration 0–140 time points after stimulus presentation. 140 time points are equal to 10 s of execution of the motor imagery task at a sampling rate of 14 Hz. (We thank Ranganatha Sitaram from the Institute of Medical Psychology and Behavioural Neurobiology, University of Tübingen, for this picture and the permission of reproduction).

laser or a light emitting diode (LED). The optical parameter measured is attenuation of light intensity due to absorption by the intermediate tissue. The concentration changes of oxygenated and deoxygenated hemoglobin are computed from the changes in the light intensity at different wavelengths (Sitaram et al. (2007)). It has been shown already that brain activation in response to motor movement and imagery can be readily detected with NIRS (see figure 1.9, Coyle et al. (2004); Sitaram et al. (2005, 2007)).

1.6.2 Invasive Recording Methods for BCI

Invasive recording methods either measure the neural activity of the brain on the cortical surface (electrocorticography, ECoG) or intracortically from within the (motor) cortex (see figure 1.10 for general setup). These methods have strong advantages in terms of signal quality and dimensionality. However, they require surgery and the issues of long-term stability of implants and protection from infection arise (Hochberg et al. (2006)). The decision of a BCI user for the one method over the other will strongly depend on

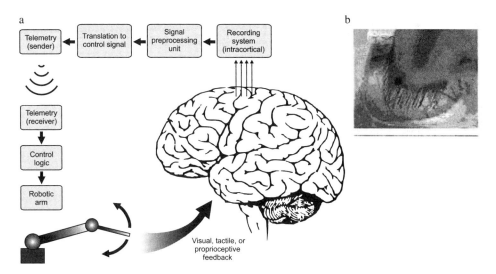

Figure 1.10   Generic setup of an invasive BCI (left) and picture of an array electrode placed into the monkey cortex (right). Figure (b) from Nicolelis (2001) by permission.

the purpose of BCI use; for example, multidirectional neuroprosthesis control may only be possible with intracortical recordings, whereas communication at a speed of approximately ten selections per minute can be achieved with noninvasive methods. We might speculate that invasive methods have to proof substantially better than noninvasive methods to become attractive for possible users.

1.6.2.1   *Brain Signals Recorded from the Surface of the Cortex (ECoG)*

The electrocorticogram (ECoG) uses epidural or subdural electrode grids or strips to record the electrical activity of the cortex. It is an invasive procedure that requires craniotomy for implantation of electrodes (see Leuthardt et al. (2006b)). However, the procedure becomes less invasive when less electrodes are required (strips instead of grids) because strips may be inserted via a small hole in the scalp. The main advantages of ECoG are a higher spatial resolution than the EEG (tenths of millimeters versus centimeters), broader bandwidth (0–200 Hz versus 0–40 Hz) that allows also recording of γ band activity, and higher amplitude (50–100 μV versus 5–20 μV) and less vulnerability to artifacts such as electromyogram (Leuthardt et al. (2004)). Commonly, ECoG is used to localize seizure activity in patients with epilepsy before they undergo surgery. Studies on the feasibility of ECoG for BCI were thus largely conducted with epilepsy patients and are reviewed in detail in chapter 8. To our knowledge, only one ALS patient consented to grid implantation for the purpose of controlling a BCI for communication, but communication was not achieved (Birbaumer (2006a,b), see chapter 22). Most of these studies performed offline open-loop analysis of ECoG data (Huggins et al. (1999); Levine et al. (1999)). Using Distinction Sensitive Learning Vector Quantization (DSLVQ) for offline classification of data recorded during self-paced middle finger extension, Scherer et al. reported accuracies between 85 and 91 percent (Scherer et al. (2003)). Hill et al. applied autoregressive models and support vector machine classification to data obtained during motor imagery and achieved accuracies around 75 percent (Hill et al. (2006)). Few studies closed the loop and provided feedback of ECoG to the participants (Felton et al. (2005); Leuthardt et al. (2004, 2006a); Wilson et al. (2006)). In each study by Leuthardt et al., the ECoG of four patients was recorded with electrode grids or strips over prefrontal, temporal, sensorimotor, and speech areas. Patients were required to perform and imagine motor and speech tasks such as opening and closing the right or left hand, protruding the tongue, shrugging shoulders, or saying the word *move*. Each task was associated with a decrease in μ- and β-rhythm and an increase of gamma-rhythm amplitudes over prefrontal, premotor, sensorimotor, or speech areas. The spatial and spectral foci of task-related ECoG activity were similar for action and imagery. Frequency bands in the gamma range were most often chosen for online control, and during movement imagery accuracies achieved within a brief training of 3–24 minutes were between 73 and 98 percent. Wilson et al. proposed to use multimodal imagery for cursor control and showed that cursor control can be achieved with nonmotor imagery such as auditory imagery (a favorite song, voices, phone) (Wilson et al. (2006)). In a completely paralyzed ALS patient implanted with a 32-electrode grid, classification of signals related to motor imagery was at the chance level (Birbaumer (2006a); Hill et al. (2006); see also chapter 22). More than one year after implantation approximately 50 percent of the electrodes provide stable and clear signal recording (unpublished data from first author's affiliation).

1.6.2.2   Brain Signals Recorded from Within the Cortex

Intracortical signal acquisition can be realized with single, few, or multiple electrodes (arrays) that capture the action potentials of individual neurons. Electrode tips have to be in close proximity to the signal source and the arrays have to be stable over a long period of time. With two exemplary ALS patients, Kennedy and Bakay showed that humans are able to modulate the action potential firing rate when provided with feedback (Kennedy and Bakay (1998)). The authors implanted into the motor cortex a single electrode with a glass tip containing neurotrophic factors. Adjacent neurons grew into the tip and after a few weeks, action potentials were recorded. One patient was able to move a cursor on a computer screen to select presented items by modulating his action-potential firing rate (Kennedy et al. (2000, 2004)). In Mehring et al. (2003), it was demonstrated that hand movements could be estimated from local field potentials.

Multielectrode arrays for intracortical recording are still to be improved for clinical application (Nicolelis (2003); Nicolelis et al. (2003), see figure 1.10). They have been used in animals with stable recordings for up to two years (Nicolelis et al. (2003); Donoghue (2002)). Recent results by Hochberg et al. (2006) for human patients show that stable long-term recordings are possible but at the expense of losing signal at a large number of electrodes. Several groups use multielectrode recording to detect activation patterns related to movement execution in animals (Carmena et al. (2003); Paninski et al. (2004); Taylor et al. (2003); Chapin et al. (1999)). The action-potential firing rate in motor areas contains sensory, motor, perceptual, and cognitive information that allows the estimation of a subject's intention for movement execution, and it was shown that 3D hand trajectories can be derived from the activity pattern of neuronal cell assemblies in the motor cortex by appropriate decoding (Serruya et al. (2002)). For example, Taylor et al. realized brain-controlled cursor and robot arm movement using recordings from a few neurons (18 cells) in the motor cortex only (Taylor et al. (2002)). Rhesus macaques learned first to move a cursor into eight targets located at the corners of an imaginary cube with real hand movements. Accompanying neural activity patterns were recorded and used to train an adaptive movement prediction algorithm. After sufficient training of subjects and algorithm, subjects' arms were restricted and cursor movement was performed by brain control. Similarly, rhesus monkeys were trained to move a brain-controlled robot arm in virtual reality (Taylor et al. (2003)) and then to feed themselves with a real robot arm (Schwartz (2004b)).

Recently, Musallam et al. presented data from three monkeys that were implanted with electrode arrays in the parietal reach area, area 5, and the dorsal premotor cortex (Musallam et al. (2004)). Subjects were first trained to reach for targets at different positions on a screen after a delay of 1.2 to 1.8 seconds following cue presentation. Neural activity during the memory period was correctly decoded with an accuracy of about 64 percent. The authors then trained subjects to associate visual cues with the amount, probability, or type of reward (orange juice versus water). Neural activity was then found to alter as a function of expected reward and thus represented additional information for classification. Accordingly, classification results could be improved by 12 percent.

Santhanam et al. (2006) used a 96-electrode array implanted in the monkey dorsal premotor cortex and report selection rates of 6.5 bits per second. This astonishing high information transfer rate was achieved in an instructed delay reach task with ultra-short trial lengths around 250 ms. Integration over spike activity in very short time windows was enough for these excellent decoding results.

Hochberg et al. (2006) report on a study where an array of 96 electrodes was implanted in a *human* subject diagnosed with tetraplegia three years after high spinal cord injury. With the array position being the primary motor cortex, it could be demonstrated that spike patterns were modulated by hand movement intention. A decoding algorithm based on a linear filter provided a "neural cursor" to the subject, who was then able to operate the TV, to open or close a prosthetic hand even while in a conversation, or to accomplish other tasks. The authors furthermore report a considerable loss of recorded units after 6.5 months, which again underlines the necessity to advance sensor technology. It is important to note that this was the first pilot clinical trial with an intracortical array implantation in humans.

These and other experimental works reveal that it is possible to derive limb or cursor movement directly from the neural activity patterns of the cortex with appropriate decoding algorithms (see also Lebedev and Nicolelis (2006)).

Finally, a simultaneous stimulation of the reward area and the sensory area in the rat allowed the control over movement patterns of the rat (Talwar et al. (2002)). A more recent work by Chapin studies how to perform a stimulation of the sensory areas to ultimately supply artificial sensory feedback for neuroprosthetics (Chapin (2006)).

1.7   Concluding Discussion

Brain-Machine Interfacing—be it invasive or noninvasive—has witnessed a recent explosion of research. The reason for this increased activity is the wide application potential that the field is bearing. (1) Clinical applications of BCI (such as those outlined in chapter 22) become evident, and work in the invasive BMI community shows the potential for future use in neuroprosthetics (Leuthardt et al. (2006a)). This is in particular underlined by the first successful human clinical trial reported by Hochberg et al. or a recent monkey study by Santhanam et al. that explores the "speed-limit" of invasive brain-computer interfacing (Hochberg et al. (2006); Santhanam et al. (2006)). Similar success can be seen in noninvasive BCIs, where two-dimensional cursor control allows a richer repertoire of communication and higher information transfer rates (ITR) (Wolpaw and McFarland (2004)). The Berlin BCI system is now able to almost completely dispense with subject training, an important progress that nevertheless has yet to be verified for disabled users. Event-related potentials such as the P300 and the steady-state visually evoked potential provide to date the highest ITR for noninvasive BCIs (Nijboer et al. (submitted); Nielsen et al. (2006); Lee et al. (2006)). The Tübingen, Albany, and Graz BCIs are used for rehabilitation in exemplary patients. Overall, there is about a factor of ten in information transfer rate between invasive and noninvasive BCIs and it will depend on each individual patient whether the risk of surgery and potential inflammation incurred in the invasive methods will justify this gain. (2) Although clinical application in rehabilitation will always serve as a main motivation and driving force for BCI research, it is the fascination for the brain itself and the urge to better understand its function that also drives BCI researchers. In fact, BCIs are a unique new tool that have emerged over the past years to analyze seminal questions in brain research such as plasticity, dynamics, representation, neural coding, intention, planing, and learning in a very direct manner. Invasive BMIs can now record from several hundreds of electrodes and can thus directly study, for example, the change of neural code during learning. Noninvasive BCIs allow researchers to watch how the brain alters and instantiates behavior and cognition in real-time. (3) Finally, there is a variety of applications that incorporate advanced signal processing, such that single trial data can be classified robustly. This step forward allows BCI researchers to contribute to general topics in the domain of human-machine interaction. The exploration of the novel independent communication and control channel BCI to assess the users state in a direct manner opens a broad field and it remains to be seen how far the BCI channel will prove to be useful when considering typical HMI applications like assessment of cognitive workload (see chapter 24), alertness, task involvement, emotion, or concentration. Clearly new systems that can use BCI for navigating or gaming in virtual worlds (see chapter 23) and for enhancing and improving man-machine interaction are on the way (see chapter 24). It is important to note that the above applications will be limited to the noninvasive EEG based systems due to their comparatively low risk and cost.

Many open problems remain on the path toward better brain-computer interfacing and broader applicability of the BCI technology. As very extensively outlined by, for example, Lebedev and Nicolelis (2006); Nicolelis (2001) and Nicolelis et al. (2003), it will be important to advance recording and transmission technology such that chronical implants become possible that can persist for a long time with very low risk and telemetrically transmit signals to BCI. A better understanding of basic neuroscience issues like representation, plasticity, and learning will allow the construction of better BMIs. Similar reasoning also holds for noninvasive BCIs where contactless wearable sensors are a necessary condition for a wide applicability of BCIs even outside medical domains, for example, for computer gaming and general man-machine interfacing applications such as usability studies. Overall, it will be essential to advance signal processing and machine learning technology to build faster, better, more adaptive, and most important more robust systems. What we defined as the phenomenon of BCI-illiteracy has to be investigated in more depth to understand whether there will always be a part of the population that is unable to operate a BCI and for what reasons. Knowing the amazing possibility of humans to learn a task and observing the considerable inter- and intraindividual signal variances, it seems reasonable to make BCIs fully adaptive. Unsolved, however, is how we can get these two complex learning systems—the machines and the human brains—in synchronicity such that stable BCI control becomes the rule and not the exception. To investigate long-term stability of BCI systems clearly, more long-term clinical trials are necessary. Gradual improvement in all these directions will be indispensible for the future success of this lively and vigorous field.

Acknowledgments

We thank Boris Kotchoubey, Michael Schröder, and Guido Dornhege for valuable comments on the manuscript. This work is funded by the Deutsche Forschungsgemeinschaft (DFG), the National Institutes of Health (NIH), the *Bundesministerium für Bildung und Forschung* (BMBF), and the IST Programme of the European Community. This publication reflects only the authors' views.

Notes

(1) BCI and BMI are used as synonyms.
(2) We distinguish here between brain-computer interfaces that listen to the neural code and computer-brain interfaces that are also able to transmit information from the computer toward the brain.
(3) Popularized under the slogan "let the machines learn" by the Berlin Brain-Computer Interface group (BBCI).

I   BCI Systems and Approaches

Introduction

This part provides an insight into a representative variety of BCI systems that are currently being pursued in research labs.

A distinctive feature in BCI studies is the paradigm used for the interaction between user and computer. On one hand there are systems that require an active and voluntary strategy for generating a specific regulation of an EEG parameter such as the motor-related μ-rhythm or the self-regulation of slow cortical potentials (SCP). On the other hand there are passive paradigms, where participants only have to passively view an item for selection. Those systems detect the evoked responses such as P300 as presented in chapter 2 or make use of steady-state evoked potentials (SSVEP) as presented in chapter 4.

Finally, one distinction between BCI labs is based on the realization of the system. Most groups, as introduced in chapters 2, 3, and 7, use extensive subject training. So, users have to adapt their brain signals to a fixed decoding algorithm, that is, the learning is on the subject side. Over the past five years, the Berlin group has established a paradigm change, where learning is now done by the computer, following the motto "let the machines learn." Now several groups have adopted this principle. Examples for this approach are discussed in chapters 4, 5, and 6. Note that even if a pure machine learning approach was intended, the subject will inevitably learn once feedback has started, so in principle BCI systems will always have both aspects: subject and machine training.

In this section six major BCI labs introduce their systems. For further ideas we refer to Babiloni et al. (2004), Gao et al. (2003b), Sykacek et al. (2003), Thulasidas et al. (2006), Kauhanen et al. (2006), and Kaper et al. (2005). Note that this list can never be complete.

Chapter 2 outlines the Albany BCI, where a user is trained to manipulate his μ and β rhythms to control a cursor in 1- or 2D. Furthermore, BCI control based on the P300 paradigm is shown.

Similar to Albany, the Tübingen BCI, outlined in chapter 3, train their subjects to adapt to the system using slow cortical potentials. The group uses BCI as a means for communication of ALS patients with the outside world and as the design of this interaction. Further BCI systems discussed in the chapter are P300 and μ-rhythm-based BCIs, an interesting new BCI paradigm based on auditory stimulation and the use of invasive techniques like ECoG for BCI.

In chapter 4 the main research directions of the Graz BCI are depicted. The group is broadly exploring the whole BCI field from sensors, feedback strategies, and cognitive aspects to novel signal processing methods, with excellent results. The Graz BCI is shown to be not only of use for patients but also it contributes to general man-machine interaction as demonstrated for a moving in a VR environment. Typically, only a few electrodes and machine learning techniques combined with user adaptation are employed to achieve BCI control.

Chapter 5 introduces the Berlin BCI. Compared to training times of weeks or even months in other BCIs, the BBCI allows for subject control after 30 minutes. This drastic decrease in training time became possible by virtue of advanced machine learning and signal processing technology. The chapter presents online feedback studies based on the physiological signals' preparatory potential and μ-rhythm modulation. The study shows that after less than one hour, five of six untrained subjects were able to achieve high performances when operating a variety of different feedbacks.

Similar to the Berlin approach, the Martigny BCI introduced in chapter 6 tries to relocate the effort from the subject training to the machine by using machine learning techniques and online adaptation to realize a BCI. In particular, online adaptation is an important direction to compensate for the intrinsic nonstationarities found in EEG signals.

Finally, the ideas of the Vancouver BCI are introduced in chapter 7. The main focus here is to establish an asynchronous BCI for patients, that is, a system that detects whether a user is intending something or not. To achieve this goal, the authors also use machine learning techniques that adapt the machine to the user.

The cheapest, most popular, and thus most commonly used measuring device for non-invasive BCI is certainly EEG, but recently also BCI experiments using fMRI (cf., e.g., Weiskopf et al. (2004a); Kamitani and Tong (2005)) and MEG were conducted successfully (cf. Mellinger et al. (2005); Kauhanen et al. (2006)). So far fMRI and MEG are too expensive for a broad use in BCI, but they have been very important for a better understanding of the physiological phenomena in the context of BCI control (cf. Haynes and Rees (2006)).

Thilo Hinterberger, Guido Dornhege, and Klaus-Robert Müller

2 Noninvasive Brain-Computer Interface Research at the Wadsworth Center

Eric W. Sellers, Dean J. Krusienski, Dennis J. McFarland, and Jonathan R. Wolpaw
Laboratory of Nervous System Disorders
Wadsworth Center
New York State Department of Health
Albany, NY 12201-0509

2.1 Abstract

The primary goal of the Wadsworth Center brain-computer interface (BCI) program is to develop electroencephalographic (EEG) BCI systems that can provide severely disabled individuals with an alternative means of communication and/or control. We have shown that people with or without motor disabilities can learn to control sensorimotor rhythms recorded from the scalp to move a computer cursor in one or two dimensions and we have also used the P300 event-related potential as a control signal to make discrete selections. Overall, our research indicates there are several approaches that may provide alternatives for individuals with severe motor disabilities. We are now evaluating the practicality and effectiveness of a BCI communication system for daily use by such individuals in their homes.

2.2 Introduction

Many people with severe motor disabilities require alternative methods for communication and control because they are unable to use conventional means that require voluntary muscular control. Numerous studies over the past two decades indicate that scalp-recorded EEG activity can be the basis for nonmuscular communication and control systems, commonly called brain-computer interfaces (BCIs) (Wolpaw et al. (2002)). EEG-based BCI systems measure specific features of EEG activity and translate these features into device commands. The most commonly used features have been sensorimotor rhythms (Wolpaw et al. (1991, 2002); Wolpaw and McFarland (2004); Pfurtscheller et al. (1993)), slow cortical potentials (Birbaumer et al. (1999, 2000); Kübler et al. (1998)), and the P300 event-related potential (Farwell and Donchin (1988); Donchin et al. (2000); Sellers and

Donchin (2006)). Systems based on sensorimotor rhythms or slow cortical potentials use components in the frequency or time domain that are spontaneous in the sense that they are not dependent on specific sensory events. Systems based on the P300 response use time-domain EEG components that are elicited by specific stimuli.

At the Wadsworth Center, our goal is to develop a BCI that is suitable for everyday use by severely disabled people at home or elsewhere. Over the past 15 years, we have developed a BCI that allows people, including those who are severely disabled, to move a computer cursor in one or two dimensions using μ and/or β rhythms recorded over sensorimotor cortex. More recently, we have expanded our BCI to include use of the P300 response that was originally described by Farwell and Donchin (1988). Fundamental to the efficacy of our system has been BCI2000 (Schalk et al. (2004)), the general-purpose software system that we developed and that is now used by more than one hundred BCI laboratories around the world (see chapter 21 for a complete description of the BCI2000 system).

2.3   Sensorimotor Rhythm-Based Cursor Control

Users learn during a series of training sessions to use sensorimotor rhythm (SMR) amplitudes in the μ (8–12 Hz) and/or β (18–26 Hz) frequency bands over left and/or right sensorimotor cortex to move a cursor on a video screen in one or two dimensions (Wolpaw and McFarland (1994, 2004); McFarland et al. (2003)). This is not a normal function of this brain signal, but rather the result of training. The SMR-based system uses spectral features extracted from the EEG that are spontaneous in the sense that the stimuli presented to the subject provide only the possible choices and the contingencies are arbitrary.

The SMR-based system relies on improvement of user performance as a result of practice (McFarland et al. (2003)). This approach views the user and system as the interaction of two dynamic processes (Taylor et al. (2002); Wolpaw et al. (2000a)), and can be best conceptualized as coadaptive. By this view, the goal of the BCI system is to vest control in those signal features that the user can most accurately modulate and optimize the translation of these signals into device control. This optimization is presumed to facilitate further learning by the user.

Our first reports of SMR use to control a BCI used a single feature to control cursor movement in one dimension to hit a target located at the top or bottom edge of a video monitor (Wolpaw et al. (1991)). In 1993 we demonstrated that users could learn to control the same type of cursor movement to intercept targets starting at a variable height and moving from left to right across the screen (McFarland et al. (1993)). Subsequently, we used two channels of EEG to control cursor movement independently in two dimensions so users could hit targets located at one of the four corners of the monitor (Wolpaw and McFarland (1994)). We also evaluated using one-dimensional cursor control with two to five targets arranged along the right edge of the monitor (McFarland et al. (2003)). This task is illustrated in figure 2.1a. Cursor control in these examples was based on a weighted sum of one or two spectral features for each control dimension. For example, an increase in the amplitude of the 10Hz μ rhythm, located over the sensorimotor cortex (electrode C3), could move the target up and a decrease in the amplitude of this μ-rhythm could serve to

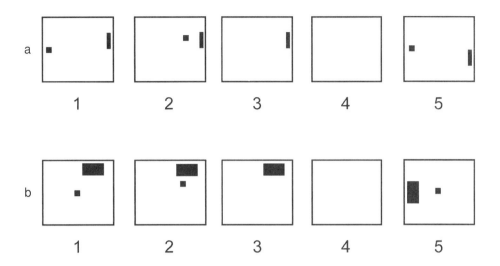

Figure 2.1 (a) One-dimensional four-target SMR control task (McFarland et al. (2003)). (b) Two-dimensional eight target SMR control task (Wolpaw and McFarland (2004)). (1) The target and cursor are present on the screen for 1 s. (2a) The cursor moves steadily across the screen for 2 s with its vertical movement controlled by the user. (2b) The cursor moves in two dimensions with direction and velocity controlled by the user until the user hits the target or 10 s have elapsed. (3) The target flashes for 1.5 s when it is hit by the cursor. If the cursor misses the target, the screen is blank for 1.5 s. (4) The screen is blank for a 1-s interval. (5) The next trial begins.

move the target down. In this case, feature selection was based on inspection of univariate statistics.

We found that a regression approach is well suited to SMR cursor movement since it provides continuous control in one or more dimensions and generalizes well to novel target configurations. The utility of a regression model is illustrated in the recent study of SMR control of cursor movement in two dimensions described in Wolpaw and McFarland (2004). An example trial is shown in figure 2.1b. A trial began when a target appeared at one of eight locations on the periphery of the screen. Target location was block-randomized (i.e., each occurred once every eight trials). One second later, the cursor appeared in the middle of the screen and began to move in two dimensions with its movement controlled by the user's EEG activity. If the cursor reached the target within 10 s, the target flashed as a reward. If it failed to reach the target within 10 s, the cursor and the target simply disappeared. In either case, the screen was blank for one second, and then the next trial began. Users initially learned cursor control in one dimension (i.e., horizontal) based on a regression function. Next they were trained on a second dimension (i.e., vertical) using a different regression function. Finally the two functions were used simultaneously for full two-dimensional control. Topographies of Pearson's r correlation values for one user are shown in figure 2.2, where it can be seen that two distinct patterns of activity controlled cursor movement. Horizontal movement was controlled by a weighted difference of 12-Hz μ-rhythm activity between the left and right sensorimotor cortex (see figure 2.2, left topography). Vertical movement was controlled by a weighted sum of activity located

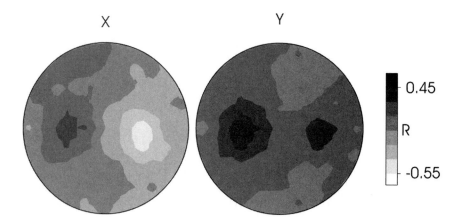

Figure 2.2   Scalp topographies (nose at top) of Pearson's r values for horizontal (x) and vertical (y) target positions. In this user, horizontal movement was controlled by a 12-Hz μ-rhythm and vertical movement by a 24-Hz β-rhythm. Horizontal correlation is greater on the right side of the scalp, whereas vertical correlation is greater on the left side of the scalp. The topographies are for R rather than R2 to show the opposite (i.e., positive and negative, respectively) correlations of right and left sides with horizontal target level (Wolpaw and McFarland (2004)).

over left and right sensorimotor cortex in the 24-Hz β-rhythm (see figure 2.2, right topography). This study illustrated the generalizability of regression functions to varying target configurations.

This 2004 study also determined how well users could move the cursor to novel locations. Targets were presented at sixteen possible locations consisting of the original eight targets and eight additional targets that were on the periphery in the spaces between the original eight and not overlapping with them. Target location was block-randomized (i.e., each occurred once in sixteen trials). The average movement times to the original locations was compared with the average movement times to the novel locations. In the first of these sessions, movement time was slightly but not significantly longer for the novel targets, and this small difference decreased with practice. These results illustrated that ordinary least-squares regression procedures provide efficient models that generalize to novel target configurations. Regression provides an efficient means to parameterize the translation algorithm in an adaptive manner that smoothly transfers to different target configurations during the course of multistep training protocols. This study clearly demonstrated strong simultaneous independent control of horizontal and vertical movement. This control was comparable in accuracy and speed to that reported in studies using implanted intracortical electrodes in monkeys (Wolpaw and McFarland (2004)).

We have also evaluated various regression models for controlling cursor movement acquired from a four-choice, one-dimensional cursor movement task (McFarland and Wolpaw (2005)). We found that using more than one EEG feature improved performance (e.g., C4 at 12Hz and C3 at 24Hz). In addition, we evaluated nonlinear models with linear regression by including cross-product (i.e., interaction) terms in the regression function. While the translation algorithm could be based on either a classifier or a regression function, we concluded that a regression approach was more appropriate for the cursor

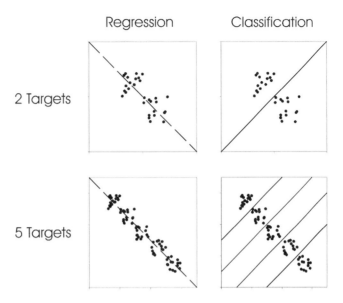

Figure 2.3 Comparison of regression and classification for feature translation. For the two-target case, both methods require only one function. For the five-target case, the regression approach still requires only a single function, while the classification approach requires four functions (see text for full discussion).

movement task. Figure 2.3 compares the classification and regression approaches. For the two-target case, both the regression approach and the classification approach require that the parameters of a single function be determined. For the five-target case, the regression approach still requires only a single function when the targets are distributed along a single dimension (e.g., vertical position on the screen). In contrast, for the five-target case the classification approach requires that four functions be parameterized. With even more and variable targets, the advantage of the regression approach becomes increasingly apparent. For example, the positioning of icons in a typical mouse-based graphical user interface would require a bewildering array of classifying functions, while with the regression approach, two dimensions of cursor movement and a button selection serve all cases.

We have conducted preliminary studies that suggest users are also able to accurately control a robotic arm in two dimensions by applying the same techniques used for cursor control. A more recent study shows that after encountering a target with the cursor, users are able to select or reject the target by performing or withholding hand-grasp imagery (McFarland et al. (2005)). This imagery evokes a transient response that can be detected and used to improve the overall accuracy by reducing unintended target selections. As these results illustrate, training of SMRs has the potential to be extended to a variety of applications, and the control obtained for one task can transfer directly to another task.

Our current efforts toward improving the SMR paradigm are refining the one- and two-dimensional control procedures with the intention of progressing to more choices and to higher dimensional control. This includes the identification or transformation of EEG features so that the resulting control signals are as independent, trainable, stable, and

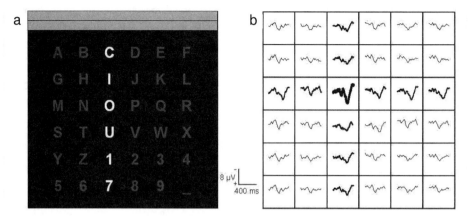

Figure 2.4   (a) A 6 × 6 P300 matrix display. The rows and columns are randomly highlighted as indicated by column 3. (b) Average waveforms for each of the 36 cells contained in the matrix from electrode Pz. The target letter "O" (thick waveform) elicited the largest P300 response, and a smaller P300 response is evident for the other characters in column 3 or row 3 (medium waveforms) because these stimuli are highlighted simultaneously with the target. All other cells indicate nontarget stimuli (thin waveforms). Each response is the average of 30 stimulus presentations.

predictable as possible. With control signals possessing these traits, the user and system adaptations should be superior, and thus the required training time should be reduced and overall performance improved.

2.4   P300-Based Communication

We have also begun to use and further develop the potential of the P300 class of BCI systems. In the original P300 matrix paradigm introduced by Farwell and Donchin (1988), the user is presented with a 6 × 6 matrix containing 36 symbols. The user focuses attention on the desired symbol in the matrix while the rows and columns of the matrix are highlighted in a random sequence of flashes. A P300 response occurs when the desired symbol is highlighted. To identify the desired symbol, the classifier determines the row and the column that the user is attending to (i.e., the symbol that elicited a P300) by weighting specific spatiotemporal features that are time-locked to the stimulus. The intersection of this row and column defines the selected symbol. Figure 2.4 shows a typical P300 matrix display and the averaged event-related potential responses to the intensification of each cell. The cell containing the letter "O" was the target cell and elicited the largest P300 response when highlighted. To a lesser extent the other characters in the row or the column containing the O also elicited a P300 because these cells are simultaneously highlighted with the target cell.

Our focus has been on improving matrix speller classification. These studies examined variables related to stimulus properties, presentation rate, classification parameters, and classification methods. Sellers et al. (2006a) examined the effects of matrix size and interstimulus interval (ISI) on classification accuracy using two matrix sizes (3 × 3 and

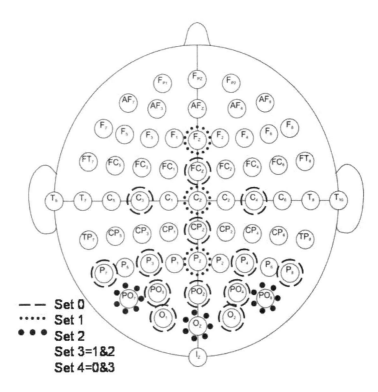

Figure 2.5 Montages used to derive SWDA classification coefficients. Data were collected from all 64 electrodes; only the indicated electrodes were used to derive coefficients (see text).

6×6), and two ISIs (175 and 350 ms). The results showed that the amplitude of the P300 response for the target items was larger in the 6×6 matrix condition than in the 3×3 matrix condition. These results are consistent with a large number of studies that show increased P300 amplitude with reduced target probability (e.g., Duncan-Johnson and Donchin (1977)).

Our lab has tested several variables related to classification accuracy using the stepwise discriminant analysis (SWDA) method (Krusienski et al. (2005)). We examined the effects of channel set, channel reference, decimation factor, and the number of model features on classification accuracy (Krusienski et al. (2005)). The factor of channel set was the only factor to have a statistically significant effect on classification accuracy. Figure 2.5 shows examples of each electrode set. Set 1 (Fz, Cz, and Pz) and set 2 (PO7, PO8, and Oz) performed equally, and significantly worse than set 3 (set 1 and set 2 combined). In addition, set 4 (which contained 19 electrodes) was no better than set 3 (which contained 6 electrodes).

These results demonstrate at least two important points: First, 19 electrode locations appear to provide no more useful information beyond that provided by the 6 electrodes contained in set 3. Second, electrode locations other than those traditionally associated with the P300 response provide unique information for classification of matrix data. Occipital

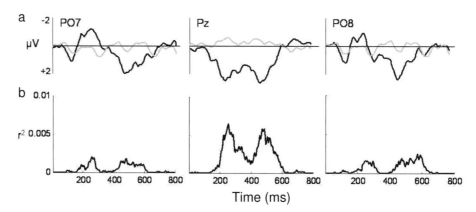

Figure 2.6 (a) Example waveforms for target (black) and nontarget (grey) stimuli for electrodes PO7, Pz, and PO8. The target waveform represents the average of 480 stimuli and the nontarget waveform represents the average of 2400 stimuli. The P300 response is evident at Pz and a negative deflection preceding the P300 is evident at PO7 and PO8. (b) r^2 values that correspond to the waveforms shown in panel a.

electrodes (e.g., Oz, PO7, and PO8) have previously been included in matrix speller data classification (Kaper et al. (2004); Meinicke et al. (2002)). In addition, Vaughan et al. (2003a) showed that these electrode locations discriminate target from nontarget stimuli, as measured by r^2, but the nature of the information provided by the occipital electrodes has not been rigorously investigated. Examination of the waveforms suggests that a negative deflection preceding the P300 response provides this additional unique information (see figure 2.6a).

While a relationship to gaze cannot be ruled out at this time, it is likely that the essential classification-specific information recorded from the occipital electrodes is not produced because the user fixates the target item. An exogenous response to a stimulus occurs within the first 100 ms of stimulus presentation and appears as a positive deflection in the waveform (Skrandies (2005)). In contrast, the response observed at PO7 and PO8 is a negative deflection that occurs after 200 ms. The r^2 values remain near zero until approximately 200 ms, also suggesting a negligible exogenous contribution. Moreover, whether or not this negativity is specific to the matrix style display or also present in standard P300 tasks is yet to be determined.

While it is reasonable to assume that the user must be able to fixate for the response to be elicited, Posner (1980) has shown that nonfixated locations can be attended to. To our knowledge, P300-BCI studies that examine the consequences of attending to a location other than the fixated location have not been conducted. Furthermore, one may also assume that fixating a nontarget location may have a deleterious effect on performance because it is harder to ignore distractor items located at fixation than it is to ignore distractor items located in the periphery (Beck and Lavie (2005)). At the same time, fixation alone is not sufficient to elicit a P300 response. Evidence for this is provided by studies that present target and nontarget items at fixation in a Bernoulli series (e.g., Fabiani et al. (1987)). If fixation alone were responsible for the P300, both the target and nontarget items would produce equivalent responses because all stimuli are presented at fixation. Hence, we argue that a visual P300-BCI is not classifying gaze in a fashion analogous to the Sutter (1992) steady-state visually evoked potential system.

To be useful a BCI must be accurate. Accurate classification depends on feature extraction and the translation algorithm being used for classification (Krusienski et al. (2005)). Currently, we are testing several alternative classification methods in addition to SWDA. To date, we have tested classifiers derived from linear support vector machines, Gaussian support vector machines, Pearson's correlation method, Fisher's linear discriminant, and SWDA. The preliminary results reveal minimal differences among several different classification algorithms. The SWDA method we have been using for our online studies perform as well as, or better than, any of the other solutions we have tested offline (Krusienski et al. (2006)).

2.5 A Portable BCI System

In addition to refining and improving SMR- and P300-BCI performance we are also focused on developing clinically practical BCI systems. We are beginning to provide severely disabled individuals with BCI systems to use in their daily lives. Our goals are to demonstrate that the BCI systems can be used for everyday communication and that using a BCI has a positive impact on the user's quality of life (Vaughan et al. (2006)). In collaboration with researchers at the University of Tübingen and the University of South Florida, we have conducted many experimental sessions at the homes of disabled individuals (e.g., Kübler et al. (2005a); Sellers and Donchin (2006); Sellers et al. (2006c)). This pilot work has identified critical factors essential for moving out of the lab and into a home setting where people can use a BCI in an autonomous fashion. The most pressing needs for a successful home BCI system are developing a more compact system, making the system easy to operate for a caregiver, and providing the user with effective and reliable communication applications.

The current home system includes a laptop computer, a flat panel display, an eight-channel electrode cap, and an amplifier with a built in A/D board. The amplifier has been reduced to $15 \times 4 \times 9$ cm, and we anticipate a smaller amplifier in the future. We have addressed making the system more user-friendly by automating some of the processes in the BCI2000 software and employing a novice user level that allows the caregiver to start the program with a short series of mouse clicks. Thus, the caregiver's major task is placing and injecting gel into the electrode cap, which takes about five minutes. We have also modified the BCI2000 software to include a menu-driven item selection structure that allows the user to navigate various hierarchical menus to perform specific tasks (e.g., basic communication, basic needs, word processing, and environmental controls) in a more expedient manner than earlier versions of the SMR (Vaughan et al. (2001)) and P300 (Sellers et al. (2006c)) software. In addition, we incorporated a speech output option for users who desire this ability. A more complete description of the system is provided in Vaughan et al. (2006).

Finally, we have provided one severely disabled user with an in-home P300 system that he uses for daily work and communication tasks. He is a 48-year-old man with amyotrophic lateral sclerosis (ALS) who is totally paralyzed except for some eye movement. Since installation, the BCI has been used at least five times per week for up to eight hours per day. The format is a 9×8 matrix of letters, numbers, and function calls that operates as a keyboard and makes the computer and Windows-based programs (e.g., Eudora, Word, Excel, PowerPoint, Acrobat) completely accessible via EEG control. The system uses an ISI of 125 ms with a stimulus duration of 62.5 ms, and each series of intensifications lasts for 12.75 s. On a weekly basis the data is uploaded to an ftp site and analyzed in the lab, and classification coefficients are updated via our previously described SWDA procedure (Krusienski et al. (2005); Sellers and Donchin (2006); Sellers et al. (2006a)). The user's average classification accuracy for all experimental sessions has been 88 percent. These results have demonstrated that a P300-BCI can be of practical value for individuals with severe motor disabilities, and that caregivers who are unfamiliar with BCI devices and EEG signals can be trained to operate and maintain a BCI (Sellers et al. (2006c)). We plan to enroll additional users in the coming months.

2.6   Discussion

The primary goal of the Wadsworth BCI is to provide a new communication channel for severely disabled people. As demonstrated here, the SMR and P300 systems employ very different approaches to achieve this goal. The SMR system relies on EEG features that are spontaneous in the sense that the stimuli presented to the user provide information regarding SMR modulation. In contrast, the P300 response is elicited by a stimulus contained within a predefined set of stimuli and depends on the oddball paradigm (Fabiani et al. (1987)). The SMR system uses features extracted by spectral analysis while the P300 system uses time-domain features. While the P300 can be characterized in the frequency domain (e.g., Cacace and McFarland (2003)), to our knowledge, this has not been done for P300-BCI use.

We use regression analysis with the SMR system and classification for the P300 system. The regression approach is well suited to the SMR cursor movement application since it provides continuous control in one or more dimensions and generalizes well to novel target configurations (McFarland and Wolpaw (2005)). In contrast, the classification approach is well suited to the P300 system where the target is treated as one class and all other alternatives are treated as the other class. Done in this way, a single discriminant function generalizes well to matrices of differing sizes.

Finally, these two BCI systems differ in terms of the importance of user training. BCI users can learn to control SMRs to move a computer cursor to hit targets located on a computer screen. This is not a normal function of this brain signal, but, rather, is the result of training. In contrast, the P300 can be used for communication purposes without extensive training. The SMR system relies on improvement of user performance as a result of practice (McFarland et al. (2003)), while the P300 system uses a response that appears to remain relatively constant across trials in terms of waveform morphology (Cohen

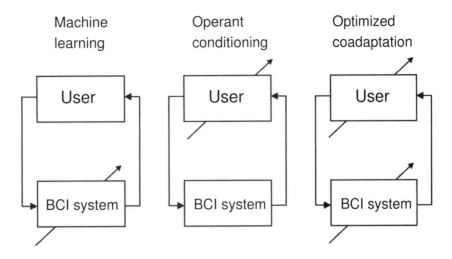

Figure 2.7   Three concepts of BCI operation. The arrows through the user and/or the BCI system indicate which elements adapt in each concept.

and Polich (1997); Fabiani et al. (1987); Polich (1989)) and classification coefficient performance (Sellers and Donchin (2006); Sellers et al. (2006a)). An SMR-BCI system is more suitable for continuous control tasks such as moving a cursor on a screen; although Piccione et al. (2006) have shown that a P300 system can be used to move a cursor in discrete steps, albeit more slowly than with an SMR system.

While most BCI researchers agree that coadaptation between user and system is a central concept, BCI systems have been conceptualized in at least three ways. Blankertz et al. (e.g., Blankertz et al. (2003)) view BCI to be mainly a problem of machine learning; this view implicitly sees the user as producing a predictable signal that needs to be discovered. Birbaumer et al. (e.g., Birbaumer et al. (2003)) view BCI to be mainly an operant conditioning paradigm, in which the experimenter, or trainer, guides or leads the user to encourage the desired output by means of reinforcement. Wolpaw et al. (2000a) and Taylor et al. (2002) view the user and BCI system as the coadaptive interaction of two dynamic processes. Figure 2.7 illustrates these three views of BCI. The Wadsworth Center SMR system falls most readily into the coadaptive class, while the Wadsworth Center P300 system is most analogous to the machine learning model. Ultimately, determining which of these views (or other conceptualizations of BCI systems) is most appropriate must be empirically evaluated for each BCI paradigm.

We feel that one should allow the characteristics of the EEG feature(s) to dictate the BCI system design and this will determine the most effective system for a given user. We currently test users on the SMR- and P300-based BCI systems and then select the most appropriate system based on analyses of speed, accuracy, bit rate, usefulness, and likelihood of use (Nijboer et al. (2005)). This may prove to be the most efficient model as we move BCI systems into people's homes.

Acknowledgments

This work was supported in part by grants from the National Institutes of Health (HD30146 and EB00856), and the James S. McDonnell Foundation.

Notes

E-mail for correspondence: esellers@wadsworth.org

3   Brain-Computer Interfaces for Communication in Paralysis: A Clinical Experimental Approach

Thilo Hinterberger
Institute of Medical Psychology and
Behavioural Neurobiology
Eberhard-Karls-University Tübingen
Gartenstr. 29
72074 Tübingen, Germany

Division of Psychology
University of Northampton
Northampton, UK

Femke Nijboer, Andrea Kübler, Tamara Matuz, Adrian Furdea, Ursula Mochty, Miguel Jordan, and Jürgen Mellinger
Institute of Medical Psychology and Behavioural Neurobiology
Eberhard-Karls-University Tübingen, Gartenstr. 29
72074 Tübingen, Germany

Thomas Navin Lal, N. Jeremy Hill, and Bernhard Schölkopf
Max-Planck-Institute for Biological Cybernetics
Tübingen, Germany

Michael Bensch and Wolfgang Rosenstiel
Wilhelm-Schickard-Institute for Computer Science
University of Tübingen, Germany

Michael Tangermann
Fraunhofer–Institute FIRST
Intelligent Data Analysis Group (IDA)
Kekuléstr. 7, 12489 Berlin, Germany

Guido Widman and Christian E. Elger
Epilepsy Center
University of Bonn, Germany

Niels Birbaumer

Institute of Medical Psychology and
Behavioural Neurobiology
Eberhard-Karls-University Tübingen
Gartenstr. 29
72074 Tübingen, Germany

National Institute of Health (NIH)
NINDS
Human Cortical Physiology Unit
Bethesda, USA

3.1 Abstract

An overview of different approaches to brain-computer interfaces (BCIs) developed in our laboratory is given. An important clinical application of BCIs is to enable communication or environmental control in severely paralyzed patients. The BCI "Thought-Translation Device (TTD)" allows verbal communication through the voluntary self-regulation of brain signals (e.g., slow cortical potentials (SCPs)), which is achieved by operant feedback training. Humans' ability to self-regulate their SCPs is used to move a cursor toward a target that contains a selectable letter set. Two different approaches were followed to develop Web browsers that could be controlled with binary brain responses. Implementing more powerful classification methods including different signal parameters such as oscillatory features improved our BCI considerably. It was also tested on signals with implanted electrodes.

Most BCIs provide the user with a visual feedback interface. Visually impaired patients require an auditory feedback mode. A procedure using auditory (sonified) feedback of multiple EEG parameters was evaluated. Properties of the auditory systems are reported and the results of two experiments with auditory feedback are presented. Clinical data of eight ALS patients demonstrated that all patients were able to acquire efficient brain control of one of the three available BCI systems (SCP, μ-rhythm, and P300), most of them used the SCP-BCI. A controlled comparison of the three systems in a group of ALS patients, however, showed that P300-BCI and the μ-BCI are faster and more easily acquired than SCP-BCI, at least in patients with some rudimentary motor control left. Six patients who started BCI training after entering the completely locked-in state did not achieve reliable communication skills with any BCI system. One completely locked-in patient was able to communicate shortly with a ph-meter, but lost control afterward.

3.2 Introduction

Investigating the ability of humans to voluntarily regulate their own slow cortical potentials (SCPs) has been a major research focus in Tübingen since the eighties. The positive results obtained from initial experiments led to the development of clinical applications. An initial application was found in epilepsy therapy, training patients to voluntarily down-regulate their brain potentials toward a positive amplitude to reduce the amount of epileptic seizures (Kotchoubey et al. (1996)). The idea of developing a brain-computer interface

(BCI) for communication with patients suffering from "locked-in syndrome" was another challenging project, which started in 1996. A system was needed that allowed people to spell out letters with single trial responses given by the electroencephalographic (EEG) signals. This system was called the Thought-Translation Device (TTD), a BCI developed to enable severely paralyzed patients, for example, people diagnosed with amyotrophic lateral sclerosis (ALS), to communicate through self-regulation of SCPs (Birbaumer et al. (1999); Kübler et al. (1999); Hinterberger et al. (2003b)) (sections 3.3.3–3.3.4) and chapter 22.

In contrast to our method of using SCPs, other groups have mostly followed the approach of using brain oscillations, such as the μ-rhythm activity of 8 to 15 Hz, recorded over the motor areas for brain-computer communication (Wolpaw and McFarland (1994); Sterman (1977); Pfurtscheller et al. (1995)). When performing or imagining a movement, the μ-rhythm activity desynchronizes over the corresponding brain area (e.g., hand or tongue) (Sterman (1977)). Besides using SCPs to operate the TTD, our group developed an approach using oscillatory components as well. Instead of calculating an estimate of the spectral band power in a certain predefined frequency range, as most of the μ-rhythm-driven BCIs do, we attempted to classify the coefficients of an autoregressive model, which was sensitive to the predominant rhythmic activity. Using this approach, communication experiments were performed with signals from EEG, MEG, and ECoG derived from implanted electrodes (see sections 3.3.6–3.3.8) and chapter 14.

So far, the TTD and most of the other BCIs have been operated with visual feedback. Providing auditory feedback overcomes the limitations of visual feedback for patients in an advanced stage of ALS. Some of these patients have difficulties focusing their gaze; however, their audition remains intact, making auditory feedback the preferential feedback mode. Therefore, the TTD was modified to be entirely operated by brain signals as a voluntary response to auditory instructions and feedback. In section 3.3.4, we report the principles and experimental testing of a fully auditorily controlled BCI.

3.3   Methods

3.3.1   BCI Software

The Thought-Translation Device was first designed to train completely paralyzed patients to self-regulate their SCPs to enable verbal communication. The hardware of the device consists of an EEG amplifier, which is connected to a PC equipped with two monitors: one for the operator to supervise the brain-computer communication training, and one for the patient to receive feedback. For acquisition of the EEG, the TTD can be interfaced with a variety of EEG amplifiers that offer a high time constant (Tc$\geq$10 s) such as the EEG8 system (Contact Precision Instruments, Inc.) in connection with a 16 bit A/D converter (PCIM-DAS1602/16 from Measurement Computing, Inc.), the g.tec amplifiers, or the BrainAmp system (Brainproducts, Munich). Alternatively, interfaces exist for EEG amplifiers to be used in the MRI as well as MEG systems. For most of the BCI experiments, the EEG signal was sampled at 256 Hz and digitized with 16 bits/sample within an ampli-

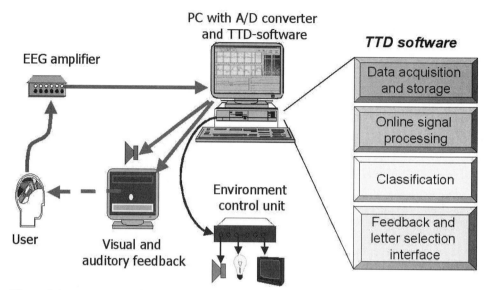

Figure 3.1   The TTD as a multimedia feedback and communication system. The EEG is amplified and sent to the PC with an A/D converter board. The TTD software performs online processing, storage, display, and analysis of the EEG. It provides feedback on a screen for self-regulation of various EEG components (e.g., SCPs) in a paced paradigm and enables a well-trained person to interface with a variety of tasks, e.g., a visual or auditory speller for writing messages or a Web browser for navigating through the World Wide Web using brain potentials only. All feedback information can be given auditorily to enable visually impaired patients to communicate with brain signals only.

tude range of at least ± 1 mV. The amplifier's low frequency cutoff was set to 0.01 Hz (i.e., a time constant of 16 s) and the high frequency cutoff to 40 to 70 Hz.

The current version of the TTD software derived from the BCI2000 standard (see chapter 21). The parameter handling, state information, and file format is identical to the definitions in the BCI2000 description. The available filters can be freely wired together and configured by the user during run-time and the data source is chosen at run-time as well. Spatial, temporal, and spectral filters are available for signal processing. Online artifact detection and correction can be performed. Classification can be done either by linear discriminant analysis (LDA), simple threshold classification, or by using a support vector machine (SVM) classifier. Several applications are available with the TTD: a two-dimensional feedback task, a spelling interface to write letters and messages (Perelmouter et al. (1999)), an interface to select Web pages from the Internet (Mellinger et al. (2003)), and interfaces to control external devices, such as switches, a robot, or orthosis. To economize the development of algorithms, a socket interface to MATLAB is available to exchange data at run-time that allows for performing calculations with MATLAB routines.

The paradigm of the SCP control for brain-computer communication is also implemented in the BCI2000 software (Schalk et al. (2004)). A detailed description of the BCI2000 is given in chapter 21.

3.3.2 Self-Regulation of Slow Cortical Potentials

SCPs are brain potential changes below 1 Hz, which up to several seconds and are generated in the upper cortical layers. Negative potential shifts (negativity) represent increased excitability of neurons (e.g., readiness) while a positive shift (positivity) is recorded during the consumption of cognitive resources or during rest. Healthy subjects, as well as locked-in patients, can learn to produce positive or negative SCP shifts when they are provided with visual feedback of their brain potentials and when potential changes in the desired direction are reinforced.

For SCP self-regulation training the recording site for the feedback signal was usually Cz (international 10-20 system) with the references at both mastoids. EEG was usually recorded from 3 to 7 Ag/AgCl-electrodes placed at Cz, C3, C4, Fz, and Pz and the mastoids. Additionally, one bipolar channel was used to record the vertical electrooculogram (vEOG) for online and offline artifact correction. For EOG correction, a fixed percentage (between 10 and 15 percent) of the vEOG signal was subtracted from the SCP signal at Cz. Furthermore, to prevent participants from controlling the cursor with their eye movements, the feedback signal was set to baseline in case the signal used for EOG correction exceeded the actual SCP changes (Kotchoubey et al. (1997)). Feedback was provided from Cz referenced to the mastoids and was updated sixteen times per second to provide a smooth cursor movement. SCPs were calculated by applying a 500 ms moving average to the EEG signal. The SCP value, taken immediately before the feedback started, served as the baseline, defining the center cursor position on the feedback screen. The baseline was subtracted from all SCP values. All trials with strong movement artifacts (SCP variations exceeding 200 mV within one trial and vEOG variations exceeding 800 mV) led to an invalid trial.

With the visual feedback modality, participants or patients viewed the course of their SCPs as the vertical movement of a feedback cursor on the screen. Vertical cursor movement corresponded to the SCP amplitude. Their task was to move the cursor toward the polarity indicated by a red rectangle at the top or bottom half of the screen.

Figure 3.2 (top) illustrates the different phases of the training process in a trial. The first 2–4 s of a trial consisted of a target presentation interval during which the target was illuminated in red, indicating the feedback task for this trial, and allowing the person to prepare for the corresponding SCP regulation. In the following selection interval, feedback was provided by the vertical position of a steady horizontally moving cursor. Cortical negativity moved the cursor up; positivity moved the cursor down. The center of the screen corresponded to the baseline level. The task was to move the cursor into the red area. A response was classified as correct if the average potential during the response interval carried the correct polarity or was inside the target boundaries of the required goal. Additionally, automatic classification algorithms, such as a linear discriminant classification or SVM, can be used for improvement of the correct response rate (Lal et al. (2004)). At the end of the selection interval the selected target was illustrated with blinking. Finally, during the response interval a smiley face combined with a sound of chimes rewarded a correct trial.

Performance was measured by the percentage of correct responses on valid trials. After a rate of 75 percent correct responses was reached, patients were trained to select letters and write messages using their self-regulative abilities for spelling (Birbaumer et al. (1999);

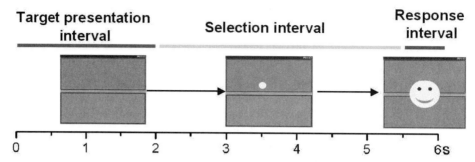

Figure 3.2   Illustration of the visual feedback information during SCP self-regulation training. Each trial is subdivided into intervals for target presentation, selection with feedback, and the report of the response.

Perelmouter et al. (1999)). Patients typically reach such levels of proficiency after one to five months of training, with one to two training days per week. A training day comprises seven to twelve runs, and a run comprises between 70 and 100 trials. With patients suffering from ALS, operant feedback training was conducted at the patients' homes with the users seated in wheelchairs or lying in bed.

The applications that will be described in the following paragraphs are a language support program including an advanced dictionary option, a fast communication program for basic desires, and an Internet browser. All these programs are driven by simple yes or no responses that serve as "select" or "reject" commands. These types of brain-computer communication also require three intervals in one trial: (1) the target presentation interval for presentation of the letter set, which was displayed in the target rectangle on the screen; (2) the selection interval, during which feedback was provided, and where self-regulation of SCP amplitudes was used to select or reject the letter set; and (3) a response interval indicating to the user the result of the selection. Selection errors require correction steps in the decision tree that were presented as "go back" options (see also figure 3.3).

3.3.3   Spelling by Brain-Computer Communication

The spelling device allows the user to select letters from a language alphabet, including punctuation marks, and to combine letters into words and sentences. Because the number of characters in an alphabet (typically about thirty) exceeds the number of brain response classes (two) that the user can produce, the selection of a letter must be broken down into a sequence of binary selections. This leads to the concept of presenting the alphabet's letters in a dichotomous decision tree, which the user navigates by giving brain responses (Perelmouter et al. (1999)). This concept was realized in a module called "language support program." Figure 3.3 shows the structure of the decision process.

The presentation of letters for spelling is realized with a binary letter selection procedure as illustrated in figure 3.3. Each box contains a letter set that can be selected or rejected. In each, trial a single letter or a set of letters can be selected or rejected by a binary brain response that corresponds to a cortical negative or positive potential shift. The letters are arranged in a way that facilitates the selection of the more frequent letters, whereas the less

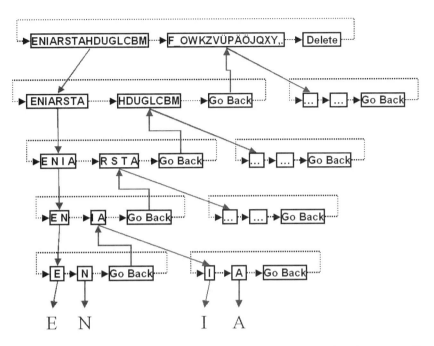

Figure 3.3   Schematic structure of the language support program. Boxes show letter sets offered during one trial; solid arrows show the subsequent presentation when a select response is produced; dotted arrows show the presentation following a reject response. When the level of single letters is reached, selection leads to the presentation of this letter at the top of the screen. Texts can thus be generated by adding letter to letter. At all except the uppermost level, failure to select one of the two choices results in the presentation of a "go back" option taking the user back to the previous level. At the top level, double rejection and selection of the delete function results in the deletion of the last written letter.

frequent letters require more steps to select. A selection will split the current letter set into two halves and present the first half for selection during the next trial (dotted arrows). A rejection response will present the second half for selection or proceed to the "go back" option (bold arrows). At the final level, the selection of a single letter will spell it. This paradigm can be used similarly for visual and auditory spelling.

In this system, writing the most conveniently situated letter, "E," takes five trials, that is, 20–25 s depending on the duration of a trial; whereas, writing the most remote sign takes nine trials, that is, 36–45 s. In an attempt to make free spelling less time-consuming, a simple personal dictionary has been introduced in which the experimenter may enter words that are frequently used by the patients (Hinterberger et al. (2001); Kübler et al. (2001b)). With the dictionary option, a complete word is suggested after at least two letters have been written and a corresponding word is available. This word can then be chosen with a single selection response.

3.3.4   Approaches for Brain-Controlled Web Surfing

3.3.4.1   Initial Approach: "Descartes"

The methods described above help the patients to express their ideas, thoughts, and needs. The Internet offers instantaneous access to desired information. Providing paralyzed patients with a BCI, which allows them to navigate through the World Wide Web by brain responses, would enable them to take part in the information exchange of the whole world. Therefore, a special Web browser named "Descartes" was developed (Hinterberger et al. (2001)).

Descartes can be controlled by binary decisions as they are created in the feedback procedure described in section 3.3.3. The browser functions are arranged in a decision tree, as previously described for the spelling of words. At the first level the patients can choose whether to write letters, to write an e-mail, or to surf the Web. When they decide to write an e-mail, the e-mail address is spelled in the first line using this language support program. When the patients decide to surf the Web, they first receive a number of predefined links arranged in the dichotomous decision tree. Each Web page that the patients have selected with their brain signals will be shown for a predefined time of one to two minutes. The wait-dialog indicates the remaining viewing time for the page, after which the feedback procedure will continue to select a related page. After the viewing time is over, the current page is analyzed for links on it. Then a dichotomous decision tree is dynamically produced, containing all links to related sites, and so the trials continue. The patients now have the option to select a link out of this tree in a similar manner to the spelling task. The links are sorted alphabetically so the desired link in the new tree can be found quickly. For example, they are first presented with the links between A and K, and then with the links between L and Z, and if both were ignored they receive a cancel option for returning to the prior level. The lowest level contains the name of the single links loaded after selection (figure 3.4).

3.3.4.2   An Improved Graphical Brain-Controllable Browser Approach: "Nessi"

The spelling concept was also used for a hypertext (Web) browser. Instead of selecting letters from a natural language alphabet, sequences of brain responses are used to select hyperlinks from Web pages. In the previous project (Descartes), links were extracted and presented on the feedback targets. The current approach uses graphical markers "in-place," that is, on the browser's Web page display (see figure 3.5) (Mellinger et al. (2003)). Colored frames are placed around user selectable items, circumventing any need to maintain a separate presentation of choices. The frame colors are assigned to the possible brain responses. By default, red frames are selected by producing cortical negativity and green frames are selected by the production of cortical positivity. As an aid, feedback is displayed at the left rim of the screen by depicting the vertical movement of a cursor that can be moved upward into a red area or downward into a green area. The user simply has to watch the current color of the desired link's frame that indicates the brain responses that have to be produced for its selection. By presenting a series of brain responses, as indicated by the changing color of the frame around that link, the link can be chosen with binary

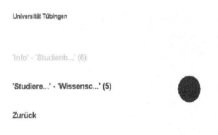

Universität Tübingen

'Info' - 'Studienb...' (6)

'Studiere...' - 'Wissensc...' (5)

Zurück

'Info' - 'Studienb...' (6)

Figure 3.4   After an Internet page is loaded, a dichotomous decision tree is dynamically produced, containing all links to related sites. During the ongoing selection procedure, the patient has the option to select a link out of this tree. The links are sorted alphabetically. In this figure, the patient can decide whether to choose one of the six links named from "Info" to "Studienb...," or one of the five links named from "Studiere..." to "Wissensc. ..."

decisions, neglecting any knowledge about its position in a selection tree. Besides links, other interactive elements on Web pages are accessible to the user, particularly text fields, for which a virtual keyboard is provided, opening up a wide range of hypertext-based applications. In addition, the user can read and write e-mails. Care was taken to keep the graphical e-mail interface very simple to speed up the communication process: Four sections of the e-mail window show user commands (reply, compose, next), incoming e-mail list, text of current e-mail, and a section for the user's reply text, respectively. E-mail addresses can be predefined for faster selection and text is entered on a virtual keyboard. To record the user's advances when browsing with the graphical brain-controllable browser, Nessi, a task-based browsing mode is available. The supervisor highlights a link and the user's task is to select that link as quickly as possible. Nessi records the number of correct choices made for later analysis by the supervisor. Similarly to the spelling task, the user must manage a dual task situation: figuring out the task and performing the corresponding brain response. Initial tests with this system revealed difficulties only when a Web page contains too many links. One of our almost completely locked-in patients managed to navigate to sites of his favorite soccer team in the first runs with the system.

3.3.5   An Auditory-Controlled BCI

A limitation was soon evident with the visual version of the TTD. For patients in an advanced stage of the disease, focusing gaze to sufficiently process the visual feedback or read the letters in the verbal communication paradigm is no longer possible. In this case, a nonvisual feedback modality such as auditory or tactile feedback had to be implemented. The implementation of auditory feedback is shown in the following section.

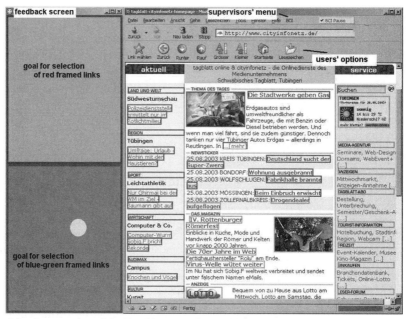

Figure 3.5   A screenshot of the Nessi browser. On the left, the feedback window is displayed with a red and a green field for the two brain responses. All links on the browser window have frames with one of the two colors that might change from trial to trial. By concentrating, viewing a specific link, and giving the corresponding brain response, the computer can identify the desired link and open it within only a few trials.

3.3.5.1   *Auditory Brain-Computer Communication Paradigms*

Figure 3.6 (bottom) describes the transformation of the visual feedback information to the auditory channel. For auditory feedback, the SCP amplitude shifts were coded in the pitch of MIDI sounds that were presented with sixteen notes, or "touches," per second. High-pitched tones indicated cortical negativity, low-pitched tones cortical positivity. The task was presented by a prerecorded voice spelling "up" or "down" to indicate that the patient has to increase or decrease the pitch of the feedback sound. If the result was correct, a harmonious jingle was presented at the end of the feedback period as positive reinforcement. In addition, the TTD can be operated providing combined visual and auditory feedback. For this purpose, the same instructions, feedback, and reinforcement as used for visual or auditory feedback were employed but presented simultaneously in both modalities. Successful regulation of an auditorily presented SCP or μ-feedback signal enables a locked-in patient to communicate verbally.

Figure 3.6 demonstrates four experimental paradigms that were tested with ALS patients: (1) the copy-spelling task in which a predefined word has to be spelled—the task is presented visually and visual feedback is provided; (2) training of self-regulation of SCPs in the auditory mode; (3) spelling in a completely auditory mode according to the selection paradigm; and (4) the question-answering paradigm for receiving yes/no answers in less skilled patients.

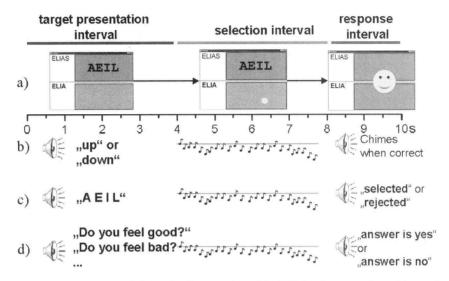

Figure 3.6   Visual feedback information for operation of the TTD has been transformed into voices and sounds to operate the TTD auditorily. Four communication paradigms are illustrated. For training a "locked-in" patient with the copy-spelling mode a predefined word has to be spelled. a) shows the visual stimuli for spelling. b) shows the stimuli for the auditory training of self-regulation of auditory displayed SCPs. c) depicts the stimuli in an auditory spelling system for brain-computer communication. In each trial a single letter or a set of letters can be selected or rejected by a binary brain response that corresponds to a cortical negative or positive potential shift. A voice informs the user at the end of a trial by saying "selected" or "rejected." In the auditory mode, a patient can spell words by responding to the suggested letter sets trial by trial. d) The question-answering paradigm allows for receiving yes/no answers even in less skilled patients.

In the auditory mode, the letter sequence to be selected is presented by a prerecorded, computer-generated voice at the beginning of the preparation interval. After the feedback period, the selection or rejection response is confirmed by a voice saying "selected" or "rejected," respectively. Words are spelled by responding to the suggested letter sets trial by trial until all letters of the word to be spelled have been selected. The auditory letter-selection communication paradigm was tested with a completely paralyzed patient without any other means of communication. Despite the fact that his performance for SCP self-regulation was at average only about 60 percent, he could spell words using a set of eight letters. To keep the patient motivated it was important to start spelling with personally meaningful words or ask personally relevant questions. However, to achieve a reliable answer from the less-skilled patients, a question-answering paradigm was developed that presented questions instead of letters (figure 3.6d). Repetitions of the same question allow detection of a statistically significant brain response and thus a reliable answer. The presentation of almost 500 questions to this patient showed that even with unreliable brain control (55 percent performance) a significant answer can be obtained after averaging the responses of all identical questions ($t(494) = 2.1$, $p < 0.05$) (Hinterberger et al. (2005a)). In other words, this equals an information transfer rate of 1 bit per 140 trials.

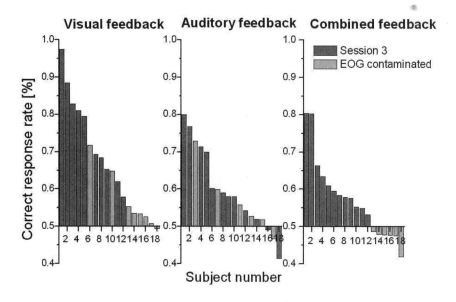

Figure 3.7   Comparison of performance of SCP self-regulation with visual, auditory, and combined visual and auditory feedback. The correct response rate (chance level 50 percent) is depicted for the third training day (session 3) for each of the 18 subjects per group. The grey bars indicate that the standardized mean differentiation of the two tasks of the EOG exceeds the differentiation of the SCP and could therefore be responsible for the SCP regulation effect as an artifact. The graph shows that visual feedback is superior in learning SCP self-regulation compared to auditory feedback, but successful SCP regulation can be achieved with auditory feedback as well.

3.3.5.2   *Comparison between Visual and Auditory Feedback*

An experiment was carried out to investigate the use of auditory feedback for controlling a brain-computer interface. The results of this study were reported in Hinterberger et al. (2004a) and Pham et al. (2005). Three groups of healthy subjects ($N = 3*18$) were trained over three sessions to learn SCP self-regulation by either visual, auditory, or combined visual and auditory feedback. The task to produce cortical positivity or negativity was randomly assigned. Each session comprised 10 runs with 50 trials each. Each trial of 6 s duration consists of a 2 s preparation interval and a 3.5 s selection interval followed by 0.5 s for presentation of the result and the reinforcing smiley associated with a jingle sound. As shown in figure 3.2, the task was presented either by an illuminated red or blue rectangle into which the feedback cursor should be moved, by a voice telling whether the feedback sound (the pitch reflected by the SCP-amplitude) should be high or low, or by the combination of both modalities. The performance of the third session was analyzed for each subject for each feedback condition. The results in terms of the correct response rate (chance level is 50 percent) are shown in figure 3.7.

All groups showed significant learning for their modality for the majority of the subjects. More than 70 percent correct responses in the third session were achieved by six (out of eighteen) subjects with visual feedback, by five subjects with auditory, and only by two with combined feedback. The average correct response rate in the third session was 67 percent in the visual condition, 59 percent in the auditory, and 57 percent in the combined condition. Overall, visual feedback is significantly superior to the auditory and combined feedback modality. The combined visual and auditory modality was not significantly worse than the auditory feedback alone (Hinterberger et al. (2004a)). The results suggest that the auditory feedback signal could disturb or negatively interfere with the strategy to control SCPs leading to a reduced performance when auditory feedback is provided.

3.3.6   Functional MRI and BCI

3.3.6.1   *Investigating Brain Areas Involved in SCP-Regulation*

To uncover the relevant areas of brain activation during regulation of SCPs, the BCI was combined with functional MRI. EEG was recorded inside the MRI scanner in twelve healthy participants who learned to regulate their SCP with feedback and reinforcement. The results demonstrated activation of specific brain areas during execution of the brain-regulation task allowing a person to activate an external device: successful positive SCP shift compared to a negative shift was closely related to an increase of the blood oxygen level dependent (BOLD) response in the anterior basal ganglia. Successful negativity was related to an increased BOLD in the thalamus compared to successful positivity. The negative SCP during the self-regulation task was accompanied by an increased blood flow mainly around central cortical areas as described by Nagai et al. (2004).

These results may indicate learned regulation of a cortico-striatal-thalamic loop modulating local excitation thresholds of cortical assemblies. The data support the assumption that human subjects learn the regulation of cortical excitation thresholds of large neuronal assemblies as a prerequisite for direct brain communication using an SCP-driven BCI. This skill depends critically on an intact and flexible interaction between the cortico-basal ganglia-thalamic-circuits.

The BOLD activation pattern during preparatory neuroelectric signals that was supposed to reflect the SCP was at the vertex (in line with Nagai et al. (2004)), in the midline medial prefrontal cortex, including the SMA, and cingulate cortex. Activations in our study were focused on the SMA, the precentral gyrus, and the inferior frontal gyrus and the thalamus. BOLD activation at vertex corresponded with the position of the electrode used for training where the strongest slow potential shifts were expected. These results demonstrated that the negative SCP reflects an anticipatory activation of premotor and motor areas independent of whether a motor act was required or not. In the present experiment, no overt motor response was observed; subjects prepared for a cognitive task only. The positioning of the electrodes at central regions of the scalp was therefore also supported by fMRI data.

3.3.6.2   *Real-Time Feedback of fMRI Data*

Real-time functional magnetic resonance imaging allows for feedback of the entire brain with a high spatial resolution. A noninvasive brain-computer interface (BCI) based on fMRI was developed by Weiskopf et al. (2003, 2004a). Data processing of the hemodynamic brain activity could be performed within 1.3 s to provide online feedback. In a differential feedback paradigm, self-regulation of the supplementary motor area (SMA) and parahippocampal place area (PPA) was realized using this technique. The methodology allowed for the study of behavioral effects and strategies of local self-regulation in healthy and diseased subjects.

3.3.7 Support-Vector-Machine Classification of Autoregressive Coefficients

In contrast to the SCPs that are defined by the frequency range below 1 Hz and classified according to their time-domain representation, EEG correlates of an imagined-movement are generally best represented by considering the amplitude of oscillatory components at higher frequencies in the 8–15 and 20–30 Hz ranges, which are modulated due to the desynchronization of the μ-rhythm over motor areas when imagining movements. For this, we use the coefficients of a fitted autoregressive (AR) model, which can capture the dominant peaks in the amplitude spectrum of a signal adaptively. While in the SCP training, the SCP constitutes one parameter whose behavior should be influenced in a predefined manner (producing positivity or negativity); the AR coefficients are a multidimensional feature representation whose numerical values are not related to fixed time- or frequency-domain features in a straightforward way. Therefore, a classifier must be trained to identify how the AR coefficients change during two or more tasks (e.g., imagination of finger movement versus tongue movement). We used a regularized linear support vector machine (SVM) classifier for classification of the AR coefficients.

Before these methods were included in the TTD, a real-time socket connection to MATLAB was established to let MATLAB do the job of calculating the AR model from the received EEG-data, classifying the coefficients and then sending the result back to the TTD that controls the application (e.g., spelling interface). Later, after the approach had been successfully tested, the AR module and SVM were included in the TTD so that the MATLAB environment was no longer needed (see figure 3.8).

This approach was applied successfully to signals from EEG (Lal (2005); Lal et al. (2005a)), ECoG (Lal et al. (2005a)), and MEG (Lal et al. (2005b)). A comparison of these datasets, and more details on the automatic classification approaches we have applied to them, is given in chapter 14 by Hill et al.

3.3.8 Brain-Computer Communication Using ECoG Signals

BCIs can be used for verbal communication without muscular assistance by voluntary regulation of brain signals such as the EEG. The limited signal-to-noise ratio in the EEG is one reason for the slow communication speed. One approach to improve the signal-to-noise ratio can be attempted by the use of subdural electrodes that detect the ECoG signal directly from the cortex. ECoG signals show an amplitude up to 10 times higher with a broader frequency range (0.016 to approximately 300 Hz, sampled at 1000 Hz) from a more focused area than EEG signals. The increased signal-to-noise ratio of invasive

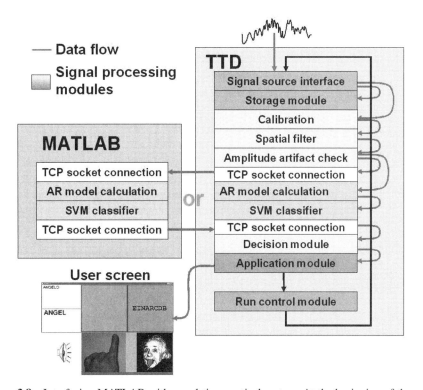

Figure 3.8 Interfacing MATLAB with a real-time cortical system: At the beginning of the experiments the calculation of the AR-coefficients as well as the SVM-classifier was not included in the TTD. A TCP/IP socket connection between the TTD and the MATLAB application allowed real-time data exchange and classification with MATLAB. After successful testings the algorithms were inserted into the TTD application. Online classification and training of the classifier now does no longer require MATLAB.

electrocorticographic signals (ECoG) is expected to provide a higher communication speed and shorter training periods.

Here, it is reported how three out of five epilepsy patients were able to spell their names within only one or two training sessions. The ECoG signals were derived from a 64-electrode grid placed over motor-related areas. Imagery of finger or tongue movements was classified with support-vector classification of autoregressive coefficients of the ECoG signal (see 3.3.7). In each trial, the task was presented to the patient for four seconds by an image of either Einstein's tongue or a finger (see figure 3.9).

The first stage of the session consisted of a training phase of at least 100 trials. The data between second 1.5 and 5 were used to calculate 3 AR-coefficients for each of the 64 channels. After training of the SVM classifier, the binary responses could be used for selection of letters. Before that, in the second stage, the classifier was tested by displaying the task images in the same way as in the training but with immediate feedback (correct or incorrect) after each trial. In the letter selection paradigm, two boxes were shown, one associated with the tongue picture and one associated with the finger picture. The sets of letters offered to be selected in a certain trial were displayed inside the box with the

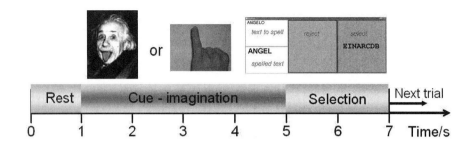

Figure 3.9 Overview of the trial structure during the data collection phase. Each trial started with a one second resting period. During the following four seconds imagination phase a picture of Einsteins tongue or a hand was shown as a cue to inform about the task. The period used for classification started 0.5 seconds after the cue onset. Each trial ended with a two seconds resting period.

Sub-ject	Sess-ions	Training		Testing with online classification		Spelling with online classification		
		Trials	CRR %	Trials	CRR %	Trials	CRR %	Letters spelled
1	1	210	*74*	120+8	**94**	-	-	
1	2	378	*87*	78+20	**80**	157	**64**	"ANGELO"
2	1	100	*63*	-	-	-	-	-
2	2	100	*60*	100	**56**	244	**73**	"MOMO"
4	1	200	*74*	-	-	164	**77**	"SUSANNE"
4	2	164	*88*	-	-	73	**88**	"THÖRNER"

Table 3.1 Bold: actual online performance. Italic: offline SVM cross-validation result.

finger picture. Therefore, patients had to imagine a finger movement in order to select a letter. The dichotomous letter selection procedure as described in section 3.3.3 was used. As the patients were not accustomed to the unusual order of the letters they were helped by indicating the imaginary task by highlighting the corresponding box. This assisted-spelling paradigm is referred to as copy spelling. Table 3.1 shows the correct response rate (CRR) for those patients who succeeded writing their names in the first two sessions.

Five epilepsy patients were trained in one or two sessions for only spelling with ECoG signals from their motor area. Three of them could write their name successfully within the first two sessions. The short training periods offer completely paralyzed patients the opportunity to regain communication using a BCI with invasive ECoG signals. However, this highly invasive method is suggested to be applied only to paralyzed patients without success in EEG-driven BCI training.

3.3.9 Comparison of Noninvasive Input Signals for a BCI

Although invasive brain-computer interfaces are thought to be able to deliver real-time control over complex movements of a neuroprosthesis, several studies have shown that noninvasive BCIs can provide communication and environmental control for severely paralyzed patients (Birbaumer et al. (1999); Wolpaw and McFarland (2004); Kübler et al. (2005a)). Most current noninvasive BCIs use sensorimotor rhythms (SMR), slow cortical potentials (SCPs), or the P300-evoked potential as input signals. Although these signals have been studied extensively in healthy participants and to a lesser extent in neurological patients, it remains unclear which signal is best suited for a BCI. For this reason, we compared BCIs based on slow cortical potentials (SCPs), sensorimotor rhythms (SMR), and the P300-evoked potential in a within-subject design in collaboration with the Wadsworth Center in Albany, New York (Schalk et al. (2004); Wolpaw et al. (2002)). A patient's best signal was chosen to serve as input signal for a BCI with which the patient could spell, so-called Free Spelling. Previous research has shown that a minimal performance of 70 percent correct is needed for communication (Kübler et al. (2001b)) (see also chapter 22).

Eight severely paralyzed patients (five men and three women) with amyotrophic lateral sclerosis were recruited. Background information of the patients can be found in figure 3.2. Eight patients participated in twenty sessions of SMR training. Six patients had ten sessions with the P300 BCI. In addition, five patients participated in twenty sessions of SCP training, whereas data from two other patients (D and G) were taken from previous studies (Kübler et al. (2004)). All patients but one were trained at home. For an overview of the design see figure 3.3. During each trial in SCP training, the patient was confronted with an active target at either the top or the bottom of a computer screen. A cursor moved steadily across the screen, with its vertical movement controlled by the SCP amplitude. The patient's task was to hit the target. Successful SCP regulation was reinforced by an animated smiling face and a chime. During each trial of SMR training, the patient was presented with a target consisting of a red vertical bar that occupied the top or bottom half of the right edge of the screen. The cursor moved steadily from left to right. Its vertical movement was controlled by SMR amplitude. During each trial of P300 training, the patient was presented with a matrix containing the alphabet (Farwell and Donchin (1988)). Rows and columns flashed randomly and sequentially, and the participant was asked to count the number of flashes of a certain target symbol (e.g., the letter "p"). Target flashes elicit a large P300 response while nontarget flashes do not.

Results show that although one patient (D) was able to learn successfully to self-regulate his SCP amplitude, performance was not sufficient for communication (Kübler et al. (2004)). None of the seven patients had a sufficient performance for communication after twenty sessions of SCP training. In contrast, half the patients ($n = 8$) learned to control their SMR amplitude with an accuracy ranging from 71 to 81 percent over the last three sessions (Kübler et al. (2005a)). Performance with the P300 ranged from 31.7 to 86.3 percent as an average over the last three sessions. Only two patients were able to achieve an online performance over 70 percent correct (patient A and G).

These data suggested that a brain-computer interface (BCI) based on sensorimotor rhythm (SMR) is the best choice for our sample of ALS patients. However, after evalu-

Patient	Age	Sex	ALS type	Time since diagnosis (months)	Artificial		Limb function	Speech
					Nutrition	Ventilation		
A	67	M	bulbar	17	yes	no	yes	no
B	47	F	spinal	24	yes	yes	none	slow
C	56	M	spinal	9	yes	yes	none	slow
D	53	M	spinal	48	no	no	weak	yes
E	49	F	spinal	12	no	no	weak	slow
F	39	M	spinal	36	yes	no	none	slow
G	36	F	spinal	96	no	no	minimal	slow
H	46	M	spinal	120	yes	yes	none	no

Table 3.2 Background information for all patients: patient code, age in years, sex, type of ALS, time since diagnosis in months, artificial nutrition and ventilation, limb function, and speech ability. Weak limb function refers to a patient who can still walk although very slowly and with risk of falling. Minimal limb function means that the patient already is in a wheelchair, but has some residual movement left in one foot or hand. Slow speech refers to a patient who speaks slowly and needs to repeat often what he or she says.

	SMR study	SCP study	P300 study	Free Spelling
Number of sessions	20	20	10	undefinded
Task	one-dimensional cursor control	one-dimensional cursor control	copy-spelling a 51-character sequence	Free Spelling
Patients	A,B,C,D,E,F,G,H	A,B,C,D,E,F,G	A,B,D,E,F,G	A,B,E,G

Table 3.3 Within-subject cross-over design of the comparison study. Undefined number of sessions means that the sessions are still ongoing.

ating the P300 data again with new classification methods (Sellers et al. (2006a)) it was found that performance could improve significantly by changing the configuration of the electrodes, the number of electrodes included into the online analysis, and the number of features of the signals.

The P300 matrix configuration was changed to a 7×7 format with more characters (i.e., the German letters ä, ö, ü, comma, and full stop). An "end" button was inserted to terminate the run. Four patients (A, B, E, and G) continued with the P300 sessions after completion of the study. These patients now achieve more than 70 percent correct and use the P300-BCI for Free Spelling, that is, they write words or short messages. For example, one patient (G) wrote: "Ich war am Samstag in Freiburg. Ich habe neue Klamotten gekauft" (translating to: I was in Freiburg last Saturday. I bought new clothes). These two sentences needed 76 selections (including correction of 4 errors). For this patient we reduced the number of sequences to 5, meaning that the columns and rows flashed 5 times leading to

10 flashes of the target character. The total time needed for writing these sentences was 13.3 minutes.

These results suggest that the P300-BCI might be the most efficient BCI for ALS patients, and it has the advantage of no training. However, most current BCIs require intact vision, which may be a problem for patients in the late stages of their diseases. For this reason, we are also investigating the feasibility of auditory BCIs.

3.3.10   Auditory BCI Systems Based on SMR and P300

Recently, we compared auditory and visual SMR feedback in a group of sixteen healthy subjects. They received auditory or visual feedback of SMR in three consecutive daily sessions comprising nine blocks of eight runs each (three blocks per daily session). High-SMR amplitude (relaxation, thinking of nothing in particular) was fed back by harp sound and low-SMR (movement imagery) by bongo sound. The intensity of the sounds was proportional to the alteration of SMR. Participants who received visual feedback were significantly better compared to those who received auditory feedback. Most interestingly, participants provided with visual feedback started in the first session with an accuracy of already 70 percent, whereas in the auditory group performance was at chance level. Later, training led to an improvement of performance in seven of eight participants in the auditory group, so that after three daily sessions no performance difference was found between the visual and the auditory group.

Taken together these results indicate that with visual feedback, participants have strategies immediately available to regulate SMR, whereas auditory feedback seems to retard learning. We speculate that this may be due to an increased demand for attentional resources in auditory feedback as compared to visual feedback. Learning to regulate SMR is possible, however, when provided with auditory feedback only.

We recently implemented an auditory P300 into the BCI2000 because patients in the locked-in state have difficulties looking at the entire P300 matrix and fixating on a target long enough to detect a P300. We provide such patients with an auditory P300 BCI, which will allow them to answer yes or no questions.

3.4   Summary and Conclusion

This chapter focussed on a number of different aspects that help develop BCI systems to be of use for paralyzed patients in a locked-in state. As illustrated in figure 3.10, different approaches aim at the improvement of the signal type, signal analysis, different designs of user applications, the patient-system interaction, and finally the understanding of the brain mechanisms underlying the successful regulation of SCPs. The major results of these five aspects of successful SCP-driven brain-computer communication are summarized.

(1)   BCI systems were tested with a variety of different types of data sources. Besides the standard applications in which ALS patients use EEG signals, BCI approaches using classification of oscillatory activity were also carried out in the MEG, and with

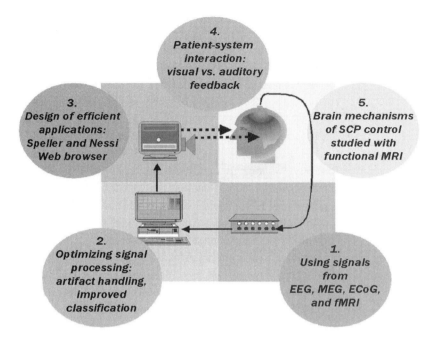

Figure 3.10   For successful brain-computer communication using SCPs, not only the properties of the system as a signal translation device must be investigated but also the interaction between the user and the system and finally the brain mechanisms themselves responsible for the systems' behavior.

ECoG in epilepsy patients implanted with electrode grids prior to surgery. In all these setups, users could operate a copy-spelling system by the use of motor-related μ-rhythm. FMRI feedback required a different software approach and was not used with a spelling application or environmental control.

(2) Signal processing and classification: In SCP self-regulation training, the computer does not adapt dynamically to the EEG response curve of a desired negative or positive potential shift. It requires the subjects' learning to produce reliable SCP shifts in both polarities. After the patient has reached a certain performance level without further improvement, the computer could optimize the number of correct responses by adapting to the response curve for example, by using additional classification algorithms. An improvement in the information transfer rate from 0.15 to 0.20 could be reached on average (Hinterberger et al. (2004b)). However, many of the highly successful SCP regulators adapt to the task without the need of further classification. Classification of autoregressive parameters using an SVM classifier was implemented as a method of classifying oscillatory activity of sensorimotor rhythm (SMR).

(3) Advanced applications from spelling to Web surfing: A wide range of applications have been developed that allow patients to communicate even in a locked-in state. A language support program with a dictionary enables paralyzed patients to communicate verbally. Patients can switch the system on and off without assistance from others, which provides the option to use the system twenty-four hours per day (Kaiser et al. (2001)). An environment-control unit allows the patients to control devices in their

environment. All applications are independent of muscular activity and are operated by self-control of slow cortical potentials only. A further improvement of the quality of life in locked-in patients can be provided by voluntary control of information available through the World Wide Web. Two types of binary controllable Web browsers were developed allowing the access to Web sites by a selection procedure using SCP feedback (Hinterberger et al. (2001)). In the "Nessi" browser based on the open source browser Mozilla, all links on a site were marked with a colored frame. Each color was associated with a brain response (e.g., green for cortical positivity and red for negativity). This program created a hidden internal binary selection tree and changed the colors of the links accordingly each trial. The task for the patient was simply to view the desired link and respond to the current color frame with the associated brain response (Mellinger et al. (2003)). Nessi was successfully tested in two ALS patients with remaining vision. The modular design of this system and its compatibility with both the TTD and the BCI2000 means that it can be used easily with more than two response conditions and with brain responses other than SCPs.

(4) Visual versus auditory feedback: As locked-in patients such as patients in end-stage ALS are sometimes no longer able to focus visually on a computer screen, a BCI should have the option to be controlled auditorily. Therefore, the TTD was modified to present all information necessary for brain-computer communication in the auditory channel. To investigate how well SCP regulation can be achieved with auditory feedback compared to visual feedback and combined visual and auditory feedback, a study with eighteen healthy subjects and each of the three modalities was carried out. The result showed that auditory feedback enabled most of the subjects to learn SCP self-regulation within three sessions. However, their performance was significantly worse than for participants who received visual feedback. Simultaneous visual and auditory feedback was significantly worse than visual feedback alone (Hinterberger et al. (2004a)).

(5) Brain mechanisms for successful SCP regulation: Two studies with functional MRI were carried out to investigate the blood oxygen level dependent (BOLD) activity during SCP control. In the first study, the patients were asked to apply the strategy they used for SCP regulation in the MRI scanner. In a second study, the EEG was measured and the SCP fed back in real time inside the scanner. A sparse sampling paradigm allowed simultaneous measurement of EEG and BOLD activity. An online pulse artifact correction algorithm in the TTD allowed undisturbed feedback of the SCP in the scanner (Hinterberger et al. (2004c)). Twelve trained subjects participated. Success in producing a positive SCP shift compared to a negative shift was related to an increase of the BOLD response in the basal ganglia. Successful negativity was related to an increased BOLD in the thalamus compared to successful positivity. These results may indicate the learned regulation of a cortico-striatal-thalamic loop modulating local excitation thresholds of cortical assemblies. The initial contingent negative variation (readiness potential) as a major component of the SCP was associated with an activation at the vertex where the feedback electrode was located. The data support the conclusion that human subjects learn the regulation of cortical excitation thresholds of

large neuronal assemblies as a prerequisite for direct brain communication using an SCP-driven BCI (Hinterberger et al. (2005b)).

Acknowledgments

This work was supported by the Deutsche Forschungsgemeinschaft (DFG, SFB 550 (B5)), the National Institutes of Health (NIH), the European Community IST Programme (IST-2002-506778 under the PASCAL Network of Excellence), the Studienstiftung des Deutschen Volkes (grant awarded to T.N.L.), and the Samueli Institute, CA (SIIB). We also thank Ingo Gunst, Tilman Gaber, Boris Kleber, Seung-Soo Lee, and Slavica von Hartlieb.

Notes

E-mail for correspondence: thilo.hinterberger@uni-tuebingen.de

4   Graz-Brain-Computer Interface: State of Research

Gert Pfurtscheller, Gernot R. Müller-Putz, Bernhard Graimann, Reinhold Scherer, Robert Leeb, Clemens Brunner, Claudia Keinrath, George Townsend, Muhammad Naeem, Felix Y. Lee, Doris Zimmermann, and Eva Höfler
Institute for Knowledge Discovery
Laboratory of Brain-Computer Interfaces
Graz University of Technology
Inffeldgasse 16a, 8010 Graz, Austria

Alois Schlögl
Institute of Human Computer Interfaces and
Laboratory of Brain-Computer Interfaces
Graz University of Technology
Krenngasse 37, 8010 Graz, Austria

Carmen Vidaurre
Department of Electrical Engineering and Electronics
State University of Navarra
Campus Arrosadia s/n
31006 Pamplona, Spain

Institute for Knowledge Discovery
Laboratory of Brain-Computer Interfaces
Graz University of Technology
Inffeldgasse 16a, 8010 Graz, Austria

Selina Wriessnegger and Christa Neuper
Department of Psychology
Section Applied Neuropsychology
University of Graz
Universitätsplatz 2, 8010 Graz, Austria

4.1   Abstract

A brain-computer interface (BCI) transforms signals originating from the human brain into commands that can control devices or applications. In this way, a BCI provides a new nonmuscular communication channel and control technology for those with severe neuro-muscular disorders. The immediate goal is to provide these users, who may be completely paralyzed, or "locked in," with basic communication capabilities so they can express their wishes to caregivers or even operate word processing programs or neuroprostheses. The Graz-BCI system uses electroencephalographic (EEG) signals associated with motor im-agery, such as oscillations of β or μ rhythms or visual and somatosensory steady-state evoked potentials (SSVEP, SSSEP) as input signal. Special effort is directed to the type of motor imagery (kinesthetic or visual-motor imagery), the use of complex band power features, the selection of important features, and the use of phase-coupling and adaptive au-toregressive parameter estimation to improve single-trial classification. A new approach is also the use of steady-state somatosensory evoked potentials to establish a communication with the help of tactile stimuli. In addition, different Graz-BCI applications are reported: control of neuroprostheses, control of a spelling system, and first steps toward an asyn-chronous (uncued) BCI for navigation in a virtual environment.

4.2   Background

Event-related desynchronization (ERD) was introduced for the first time in the seventies and used to quantify the dynamics of sensorimotor rhythms including μ and central β rhythms in a motor task (Pfurtscheller and Aranibar (1977)). In the following years, ERD became an important tool for studying the time-behavior of brain rhythms during motor, sensory, and cognitive processing (for review, see Pfurtscheller and Lopes da Silva (1999)). The area of brain-computer interface (BCI) research started at the Graz University of Technology with ERD classification in single electroencephalographic (EEG) trials during motor execution and motor imagery (Flotzinger et al. (1994); Kalcher et al. (1996); Pfurtscheller et al. (1996)). At the same time, a number of basic studies were conducted together with Dr. Wolpaw's BCI lab in Albany, New York (Pfurtscheller et al. (1995); Wolpaw et al. (1997, 1998)).

4.3   Components of Graz-BCI

When designing a BCI, several issues must be considered (figure 4.1): the mode of oper-ation, the type of input signal, the mental strategy, and feedback. Two distinct operating modes, cued (synchronous) and uncued (asynchronous), are possible. In the case of a syn-chronous BCI, the mental task must be performed in predefined time windows following visual, auditory or tactile cue stimuli. The time periods during which the user can affect control, for example, by producing a specific mental state, are determined by the system.

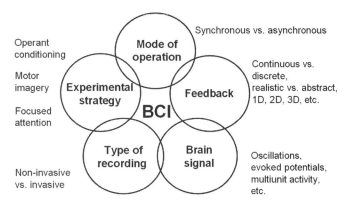

Figure 4.1 Components of a brain-computer interface.

Furthermore, the processing of the data is limited to these fixed periods. By contrast, an asynchronous BCI allows the user to determine an operation independently of any external cue stimulus. This implies that the time windows of the intended mental activities are unknown, and therefore the signal has to be analyzed continuously (Mason and Birch (2000); Millán and Mouriño (2003)). The majority of work on the Graz-BCIs is based on the synchronous mode (for review see Pfurtscheller et al. (2005a)), but systems operating in an asynchronous mode also have been implemented (Scherer et al. (2004a); Müller-Putz et al. (2005b)).

The electrical potentials (EEG) used for the Graz-BCI are recorded noninvasively from the scalp. In addition to EEG, studies on electrocorticographic (ECoG) signals recorded during self-paced movements have also been performed. The goal of these studies was to detect the motor action in single ECoG trials (Graimann et al. (2003)). In both studies (EEG and ECoG), the dynamics of oscillations, such as μ or β rhythms are analyzed and classified (Pfurtscheller et al. (2005b)). Additionally, two types of event-related potentials, the visual and somatosensory steady-state potentials (SSVEP, SSSEP) were used as input signal for the Graz-BCI (Müller-Putz et al. (2005a, 2006)).

Basically, three mental strategies can be distinguished: (1) operant conditioning, (2) pre defined mental task, and (3) attention to an externally paced stimulus. Operant conditioning, or self-regulation of slow cortical potentials (SCPs), in BCI research was intensively studied by Birbaumer's lab in Tübingen over the past twenty-five years (e.g., Birbaumer et al. (1990, 1999)). Using the strategy of a predefined mental task, specifically motor imagery and more recently attention to an externally paced visual stimulus, is characteristic for the Graz-BCI. In the case of motor imagery the user is previously instructed to imagine the movement of a specific body part, for example, left or right hand, both feet, or tongue. The basis of this strategy is that imagination of movement activates similar cortical areas and shows similar temporal characteristics to the execution of the same movement (e.g., Decety et al. (1994)); for details, see section 4.4.2. The use of steady-state evoked potentials (SSEPs) is based on direct recognition of a specific electrocortical response and generally does not require extensive training (for details, see section 4.4.8).

The feedback of performance is an important feature of each BCI system, since the users observe the executed commands (i.e., cursor movement or selected letters) almost simultaneously with the brain response produced. In the Graz-BCI, different types of feedback (FB) are used. Delayed (discrete) FB provides information of a correct versus incorrect response at the end of a trial, while continuous FB indicates immediately the discrimination ability of brain patterns. A recent study has shown that continuous visual FB can have benefits as well as detrimental effects on EEG control and that these effects vary across subjects (McFarland et al. (1998)). Recently, virtual reality has been employed in the Graz-BCI as a FB method (for details, see chapter 23).

4.4   Graz-BCI Basic Research

4.4.1   Graz-BCI Control with Motor Imagery

The Graz-BCI uses motor imagery and associated oscillatory EEG signals from the sensorimotor cortex for device control (Pfurtscheller and Neuper (2001)). The well-established desynchronization (i.e., ERD) of μ and β rhythms at the time of movement onset, and their reappearance (i.e., event-related synchronization, ERS) when the movement is complete, forms the basis of this sensorimotor-rhythm-controlled BCI. The major frequency bands of cortical oscillations considered here are μ (8–12 Hz), sensorimotor rhythm (12–15 Hz), and β (15–30 Hz).

Most relevant for BCI use is the fact that no actual movement is required to modulate the sensorimotor rhythms (Pfurtscheller and Neuper (1997)). There is increasing evidence that characteristic, movement-related oscillatory patterns may also be linked to motor imagery, defined as mental simulation of a movement (Jeannerod and Frak (1999)). By means of quantification of temporal-spatial ERD (amplitude decrease) and ERS (amplitude increase) patterns (Pfurtscheller and Lopes da Silva (1999)), it has been shown that motor imagery can induce different types of activation patterns, for example: (1) desynchronization (ERD) of sensorimotor rhythms (μ rhythm and central β oscillations) (Pfurtscheller and Neuper (1997)), (2) synchronization (ERS) of the μ rhythm (Neuper and Pfurtscheller (2001)), and (3) short-lasting synchronization (ERS) of central β oscillations after termination of motor imagery (Pfurtscheller et al. (2005b)).

To control an external device based on brain signals, it is essential that imagery related brain activity can be detected in real time from the ongoing EEG. Even though it has been documented that the imagination of simple movements elicits predictable temporally stable changes in the sensorimotor μ and β bands (i.e., small intrasubject variability; for a review, see Neuper and Pfurtscheller (1999)), there are also participants who do not show the expected imagination-related EEG changes. Moreover, a diversity of time-frequency patterns (i.e., high intersubject variability), especially with respect to the reactive frequency components, was found when studying the dynamics of oscillatory activity during movement imagination (cf. Wang et al. (2004); Pfurtscheller et al. (2005b)).

These differences in imagination-related EEG changes may be partly explained by varieties of motor imagery (Annett (1995); Curran and Stokes (2003)). In case there is

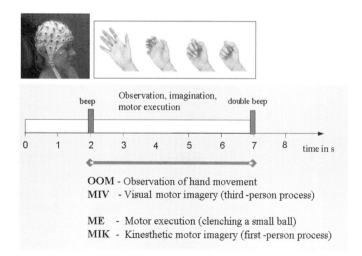

Figure 4.2 Experimental tasks and timing: The four tasks (OOM, MIV, ME, MIK) were presented in separate runs of fourty trials: Each started with the presentation of a fixation cross at the center of the monitor (0 s). A beep tone (2 s) indicated the beginning of the respective task: Subjects should either watch the movements of the animated hand, or perform movements themselves, or imagine hand movements until a double beep tone marked the end of the trial (7 s). A blank screen was shown during the intertrial period varying randomly between 0.5 and 2.5 s (modified from Neuper et al. (2005)).

no specific instruction, subjects may, for example, either imagine self-performed action with an "intrinsic view" or, alternatively, imagine themselves or another person performing actions in a "mental video" kind of experience. Whereas the first type of imagery is supposed to involve kinesthetic feelings, the second one may be based primarily on visual parameters. There is converging evidence that imagining is functionally equivalent to brain processes associated with real perception and action (Solodkin et al. (2004)). The different ways how subjects perform motor imagery are very likely associated with dissimilar electrophysiological activation patterns (i.e., in terms of time, frequency, and spatial domains).

In a recent study, we investigated the influence of the kind of imagery, involving kinesthetic and visual representations of actions (Neuper et al. (2005)). Participants were instructed either to create kinesthetic motor imagery (first-person process; MIK) or visual motor imagery (third-person process; MIV). In the so-called "first-person" process the subjects had to imagine a self-performed action whereas in the "third-person" process a mental image of a previously viewed "actor" had to be performed. Additionally, in a control condition, "real movements" were examined (i.e., the motor execution (ME) and visual observation (OOM) of physical hand movements, respectively); see figure 4.2.

The results of fourteen right-handed participants based on multichannel EEG recordings were applied to a learning classifier, the distinction-sensitive learning vector quantization (DSLVQ) (Pregenzer et al. (1996)), to identify relevant features (i.e., electrode locations and reactive frequency components) for recognition of the respective mental states. This method uses a weighted distance function and adjusts the influence of different input

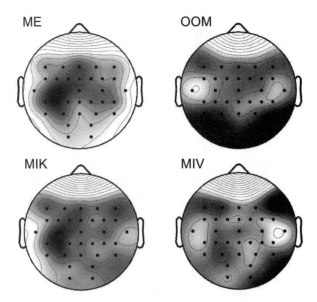

Figure 4.3 Topographical map of grand average classification accuracies (N=14) plotted at the corresponding electrode positions (linear interpolation), separately for the four experimental conditions (ME, OOM, MIK, MIV). Black areas indicate the most relevant electrode positions for the recognition of the respective task. Scaling was adjusted to minimum and maximum values obtained for each condition (ME (min/max%): 53/76; OOM (min/max%): 56/77; MIK (min/max%): 51/64; MIV(min/max%): 51/61); modified from Neuper et al. (2005).

features (e.g., frequency components) through supervised learning. This procedure was used to distinguish dynamic episodes of specific processing (motor execution, imagery, or observation) from hardly defined EEG patterns during rest.

The results revealed the highest classification accuracies, on average close to 80 percent, for real conditions (i.e., ME and OOM), both at the corresponding representation areas. Albeit a great variability among participants during the imagery tasks existed, the classification accuracies obtained for the kinesthetic type of imagery (MIK; 66%) were in average better than the results of the visual motor imagery (MIV; 56%). It is important to note that for the recognition of both, the execution (ME) and the kinesthetic motor imagery (MIK) of right-hand movement, electrodes close to position C3 provided the best input features (figure 4.3). Whereas the focus of activity during visual observation (OOM) was found close to parieto-occipital cortical areas, visual motor imagery (MIV) did not reveal a clear spatial pattern and could not be successfully detected in single-trial EEG classification.

These data confirm previous studies that motor imagery, specifically by creating kinesthetic feelings, can be used to "produce" movement-specific and locally restricted patterns of the oscillatory brain activity. Moreover, we can expect that specific instructions on how to imagine actions, along with careful user training, may contribute to enhance activation in primary sensorimotor cortical areas (Lotze et al. (1999b)) and furthermore improve BCI control. The potential that subjects may be able to learn to increase motor cortex activation during imagined movement has been demonstrated in a recent neurofeedback study using real-time functional magnetic resonance imaging (fMRI; DeCharms et al. (2004)). However, our data suggested a higher efficiency of kinesthetic imagery compared to the visual form; the parameters sensitive for certain mental states still should be optimized for each individual to accommodate for subject-specific variability.

4.4.2 μ-rhythm (De)synchronization and Single-Trial EEG Classification Accuracy

The (de)synchronization pattern displays a great inter- and intrasubject variability during motor imagery. Therefore, it is of interest whether μ-rhythm synchronization or μ ERS contribute to single-EEG trial classification and to discrimination between four different motor imagery tasks (left hand, right hand, both feet, and tongue). Time-frequency maps were calculated and used for selection of the α (μ) band rhythms (for details see Graimann et al. (2002)) with the most significant bandpower increase (ERS) or decrease (ERD) during motor imagery tasks at the central electrode positions C3, Cz, and C4.

Adaptive autoregressive (AAR) parameters were estimated for each of the sixty mono polar channels and every possible combination of bipolar channels. Accordingly, 1,830 single channel AAR estimates were obtained using the Kalman filtering algorithm. Next, the AAR estimates from each trial were divided into short segments. For each segment, a minimum Mahalanobis distance (MDA) classifier across all trials was calculated and applied to the same segment. Accordingly, an average measure for the classification accuracy of the four-class problem (four motor imagery tasks) was obtained for each segment. To measure distinctiveness the "kappa" coefficient (for details, see Schlögl et al. (2005)) was used:

$$\kappa = \frac{\text{acc} - n^{-1}}{1 - n^{-1}},$$

where acc is the accuracy and n is the number of classes (number of trials for each class is equal). Within the trial length of 7 s, the segment with the largest kappa value was used to set up the classifier. The classifier was cross-validated using the leave-one-out method and the maximal kappa value determined.

From all ERD/ERS numbers (three central electrode positions, four tasks) obtained in one subject, the standard deviation was calculated and termed "intertask variability" (ITV) (Pfurtscheller et al. (2006a)). A low ITV indicates an ERD on all central electrode positions during all motor tasks. In the case of a high ITV, the ERD was dominant during only hand motor imagery, whereas ERS was frequently found during foot and/or tongue motor imagery.

Figure 4.4 displays the relationship between ITV and best single-trial classification accuracy expressed by kappa in nine subjects. It shows that the power of single-trial discrimination among four different motor tasks increases when the ITV is high. This is not surprising because it is nearly impossible to discriminate among four motor imagery tasks when every task displays approximately similar central-localized ERD patterns.

During performance of different motor imagery tasks, a great intersubject variability and a considerable intrasubject variability concerning the reactivity of μ components was found. Such a diversity of ERD/ERS patterns during different imagery tasks is a prerequisite for an optimal distinctiveness among different motor imagery tasks when single trials

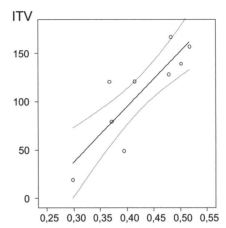

Figure 4.4   Relationship between ITV and kappa during motor imagery in nine able-bodied subjects (modified from Pfurtscheller et al. (2006a)).

are analyzed. That is, it is very hard to discriminate among more than two mental states and a small number of EEG channels when only imagery-induced ERD patterns are available because a number of psychophysiological variables related to perceptual and memory processes and task complexity also result in a desynchronization of alpha band rhythms.

4.4.3   Adaptive Autoregressive (AAR) Parameters

It is well known that the spectral properties of the EEG are a useful feature for BCI experiments. However, due to the use of fast fourier transform (FFT), the feature extraction was block-based and the feedback could not be presented continuously in time. Another method for spectral estimation is the autoregressive model. Besides stationary estimators (like Yule-Walker, Levinson-Durbin, Burg), adaptive estimation algorithms like the least-mean-squares (LMS), the recursive-least-squares (RLS), and Kalman filtering also are available. Adaptively estimated autoregressive model parameters (AAR parameters) are obtained with a time-resolution as high as the sampling rate. Accordingly, it was possible to provide continuous feedback in real time. The first online experiment is reported in the work of Schlögl et al. (1997b) using the LMS algorithm for AAR estimation. In parallel, the more advanced RLS method was also investigated in offline studies (Schlögl et al. (1997a); Pfurtscheller et al. (1998)) and the limitations due to the principle of uncertainty in nonstationary spectral analysis were investigated (Schlögl (2000a); Schlögl and Pfurtscheller (1998)). Based on these works, the estimation algorithms were also implemented in the new real-time platform using MATLAB/Simulink (Guger et al. (2001)), and the advantages of continuous feedback could be demonstrated (Neuper et al. (1999)).

With the advent of AAR parameters, the classifiers also have changed. Before, neural network classifiers commonly were applied, and with the introduction of AAR parameters linear discrimant analysis (LDA) was used mostly. Firstly, the use of LDA was motivated by pragmatic reasoning for its more simple and fast training procedure. However, LDA provided further advantages: It was robust, it provided a continuous discrimination function, and it needed less data for training. Thus, it became the standard classifier for AAR parameters. In particular, the continuous discrimination function was useful for providing a feedback that was continuous in magnitude. Thus, the combination of AAR and LDA provided an analysis system that was continuous in time and magnitude (Schlögl et al. (1997b); Schlögl (2000a)). Later, other feature extraction methods with continuous estimation also were used, for example, adaptive Hjorth and adaptive Barlow parameters, as well as bandpower estimates based on filtering, squaring, and smoothing (Guger et al. (2001)). Especially, the bandpower method in combination with subject-specific selection of the frequency bands has been widely applied.

More recently, AAR parameters have been used to compare different classifiers (Schlögl et al. (2005)). For this purpose, sixty channel EEG data during four different motor imagery movement tasks (left hand, right hand, foot, tongue) were used and the AAR parameters, using a model order of p=3, were estimated. The following classification systems have been applied to the AAR(3) parameters of all sixty monopolar channels: (1) a neural network based on k-nearest neighbor (kNN), (2) support vector machines (SVM), and (3) LDA. The best results were obtained with SVM, followed by LDA; kNN showed the worst results.

Another important spin-off is the application of adaptive concept for adaptive classifiers (see Vidaurre et al. (2005, 2006) and section 4.4.6).

4.4.4 Complex Band Power Features

Bandpower features have long been recognized as important for classification of brain patterns. In the past, phase information often has been incorporated indirectly as a consequence of other features, but not explicitly extracted and used directly as a feature. Traditionally, bandpower features are produced in the time domain by squaring the values of the samples and then smoothing the result. But it is also possible to produce these features directly in the frequency domain by performing a fast Fourier transform (FFT) of the EEG. Applying this technique produces complex results consisting of imaginary and real parts that capture not only bandpower (which may be derived from the magnitude) but also explicit phase information. Augmenting bandpower with explicit phase information has been shown to produce improved classification results. Given the nature of their derivation, these phase and amplitude features together have been named complex bandpower (CBP) features (Ramoser et al. (2000)).

To test the importance of phase, movement imagery data in a four-class paradigm was recorded from several subjects. Sixty electrodes were used with an interelectrode spacing of 2.5 cm. Signals from all electrodes were recorded to generate classification results using the method of common spatial patterns (CSP). Only fifteen electrodes most central to C3, C4, and Cz were used to generate CBP features.

The results discussed here were based on features generated by using a 250 ms sliding hamming window where the FFT of the signal was calculated. Thereafter, the results were smoothed using a one-second moving average filter. The phase information produced by the CBP method was differentiated to produce a result that captured the direction and amount of phase shift present in various frequency bands. Eight equally spaced frequency bands between 4 and 35 Hz were used to derive the CBP features for this study. A total of

480 CBP features were produced and a subset of eight were selected using the sequential floating forward selection (SFFS) feature selection method (Pudil et al. (1994); Graimann et al. (2005)).

The classification results generated from CBP features were compared to results generated by the CSP method and found to be comparable or superior. Additionally, another advantage of CBP over CSP is not only that it works well in the presence of artifacts, but that it requires far fewer electrodes than CSP. Furthermore, CBP requires far less training data than CSP to achieve good results. In tests it was found that CBP required approximately half the amount of training data compared with CSP to obtain similar or better results. Time courses showing average classification accuracy over the duration of the trials were generated to compare CBP and CSP and showed that superior results were generated by the use of CBP over CSP. The data was partitioned into all possible combinations of testing and training data in the way that all available runs preceding each test run were used as training data. On average, the "kappa" (details in Schlögl et al. (2005)) calculated for CBP was 0.11 higher than for CSP.

From the data available, various combinations of testing and training data were used. It was determined that the best general results were produced when all previously available data was used for training and the final experimental run was used as unseen data for testing. The results were computed for a group of four test subjects with and without the phase component of the signal to determine the importance of the phase information. It was found that the inclusion of phase information improved the classification accuracy expressed in kappa by 0.17 ± 0.1 (mean$\pm$SD). The conclusion was that phase information is an important and useful feature to consider in BCI research and incorporating such information leads to improved classification results (for details, see Townsend et al. (2006)).

4.4.5   Phase Synchronization Features

Currently, almost all BCIs ignore the relationships between EEG signals measured at different electrode recording sites. The vast majority of BCI systems rely on univariate feature vectors derived from, for example, logarithmic bandpower features or adaptive autoregressive parameters. However, there is evidence that additional information can be obtained by quantifying the relationships among the signals of single electrodes, which might provide innovative features for future BCI systems.

A method to quantify such relationships, the so-called phase locking value (PLV), already has been implemented and used to analyze ECoG signals in an offline study (Brunner et al. (2005)). The PLV measures the level of phase synchronization between pairs of EEG signals (Lachaux et al. (1999))

$$\text{PLV} = \frac{1}{N} \left| \sum_{n=1}^{N} \exp(j \{\phi_1(n) - \phi_2(n)\}) \right|.$$

Here, $\phi_i(n)$ is the instantaneous phase of the corresponding electrode $i = \{1, 2\}$ at time instant n calculated using either a Gabor wavelet or the Hilbert transform. The average can be calculated over different trials or, in case of a single-trial analysis, over several time

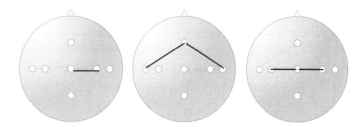

Figure 4.5   Most prominent phase couplings for three examplary subjects. Solid lines represent PLV features in a broad frequency range; dashed lines are narrow-band features (modified from Brunner et al. (in revision)).

samples. A PLV value of 1 means that the two channels are highly synchronized, whereas a value of 0 implies no phase synchronization at all. Basically, this method is similar to the cross-spectrum with the difference that PLV does not consider the signal amplitudes. This might be a more appropriate measure when studying synchronization phenomena in electrocorticographic signals since it directly captures the synchronization of the phases.

For single-trial classification in BCIs, offline analyses have been conducted by, for example, Gysels and Celka (2004) and also at our lab, which demonstrated that there is additional information in the PLV as opposed to classical univariate features already mentioned. More specifically, several PLV-based features were acquired from a number of subjects and the optimal feature set was selected for each subject individually by a feature selection algorithm. For example, we were using four monopolar EEG channels over C3, Cz, C4, and Fz—the PLV values were calculated within broad frequency ranges and computed for four different electrode pairs, namely, Fz-C3, Fz-C4, C3-Cz, and Cz-C4.

An interesting result of this feature selection process was the topographical position of the important synchronization features. Interhemispheric electrode pairs were rarely selected and couplings within one hemisphere were dominant in all subjects. Moreover, couplings involving the frontal electrode location occurred more often than the occipital region. Exemplarily, feature subsets showing the most important couplings for different subjects are illustrated in figure 4.5.

In a next step, an online model of the PLV was implemented and included in the Graz-BCI system. The three online sessions (each consisting of four to six runs, thirty trials per run) with three trained subjects were recorded. All subjects were able to control three mental states (motor imagery of left hand, right hand, and foot, respectively) with single-trial accuracies between 60 and 67 percent (33 percent would be expected by chance) throughout the whole session.

4.4.6   Adaptive Classifier

Usually, new classifiers or thresholds obtained from the data are applied and manually updated after a certain period of time, depending on the experience of the operator. The aim of our adaptive online classifier was to automatically adapt changes in the EEG patterns of the subject and to deal with their long-term variations (nonstationarities). In Graz, two different types of adaptive classifiers were tested in online experiments, ADIM and ALDA (Vidaurre et al. (2006)). ADIM is a classifier that estimates online the Information Matrix (Adaptive Information Matrix) to compute an adaptive version of the quadratic discriminant analysis (QDA). ALDA is an adaptive linear discriminant analysis based on Kalman filtering. Both classifiers were analyzed with different types of features using adaptive autoregressive (AAR) parameters, logarithmic bandpower, and the concatenation of both in one vector. The design of the experiments followed another idea different from the classical. The traditional scheme consisted of training sessions without feedback, the computation of a classifier using this nonfeedback data, and the performance of feedback sessions. The new adaptive system allowed starting immediately in the very first session with feedback by using a predefined subject-unspecific classifier. Afterward, it was updated online resulting in a subject-specific classifier. Thus, the subject could find a motor imagery strategy based only on the response of the system from the very first session.

Experiments were performed with eighteen naive subjects; six of them used AAR features and ADIM, another six used BP estimates, and the last six used the concatenation of AAR and BP combined with ALDA. This last group of subjects showed a clear reduction of the classification error from 28.0 ± 3.8 over session two (21.4 ± 4.0) to session three (16.0 ± 2.5). For further details, see chapter 18.

4.4.7   Importance of Feature Selection

Many feature extraction methods have been proposed for brain-computer communication. Some are known to be robust and have been applied successfully depending on the experimental strategy used. An example of such a robust method is bandpower, which extracts features for specific frequency ranges and is often used when motor imagery is performed. However, new feature extraction methods are continuously being investigated. For instance, features that do not represent only second order statistics from single channels are currently investigated in our lab (see below) and elsewhere. These methods often require parameters such as window length, frequency, and topography of channels. for which the ideal settings are unknown. Feature selection methods may be applied to find such settings by defining a subset of features out of a large pool of features calculated from different feature extraction methods with various parameter settings and different channels. In this way, feature selection can be employed to find suitable feature extraction methods and their parameter settings, and also to identify appropriate electrode positions. There are a large number of feature selection methods available, which can be subdivided into filter methods (e.g., Fisher distance, r2), wrapper methods (e.g., genetic algorithms, heuristic search strategies), and so-called embedded algorithms (e.g., linear programming). Distinction sensitive learning vector quantization (DSLVQ) is another example of an embedded algorithm, which was designed in the Graz-BCI for the selection of electrode positions (Pregenzer et al. (1994)) and frequency components (Pregenzer and Pfurtscheller (1999); Scherer et al. (2003)). Wrapper methods like genetic algorithms are very flexible and generally applicable, but they are usually also computationally demanding. We used genetic algorithms for finding suitable wavelet features in ECoG data (Graimann et al. (2004)) and for the design of an asynchronously controlled EEG-based virtual keyboard

(Scherer et al. (2004a)). Sequential floating forward selection (SFFS) suggested by Pudil et al. (1994) represents a good trade-off between selection performance and computational effort. Because of its simplicity (no parameters have to be selected) and good performance, SFFS has been used for various feature selection tasks in our lab (Townsend et al. (2006); Graimann et al. (2005)).

Often only a rather small amount of training data is available for offline analysis. In such cases, the generalization of offline results may be difficult. In fact, it can become even more difficult if feature selection is involved. Currently, we are investigating the generalization capability of various combinations of feature selection and classification methods and their small sample performance.

4.4.8 Steady-State Evoked Potentials

Repetitive visual or somatosensory stimulation can elicite steady-state visually evoked potentials (SSVEPs) or steady-state somatosensory evoked potentials (SSSEPs), respectively. Both sensory systems respond in individual so-called "resonance-like" frequency regions. The visual system can be subdivided into three parallel flicker visually evoked potential subsystems. The greatest SSVEP amplitudes are observed near 10 Hz (low frequency region) and followed by 16–18 Hz (peak of the medium frequency region). The high frequency subsystem has its resonance-like peak frequencies near 40–50 Hz and shows the smallest response. The somatosensory resonance-like frequency region is in the EEG β range having a peak frequency around 27 Hz (Müller et al. (2001)).

The SSVEP experiments were performed on ten subjects. A self-constructed stimulation unit (SU) was used for visual stimulation. It consisted of 32 LED bars whose flickering frequencies could be varied independently by a microcontroller. The LED bars were arranged in eight columns and four rows. The SU was mounted above the screen and the four LED bars of the SU's lower row were programmed to flicker with 6, 7, 8, and 13 Hz (Müller-Putz et al. (2005a)).

In a first experiment without feedback, the impact of harmonic components (first, second, and third) was studied. After computation of the spectral components by applying discrete Fourier transformation (DFT), six one versus one LDA classifiers were used to cover all combinations of classes in this four-class system. A class was then detected by applying majority voting. It was found that the average classification accuracy with the first harmonic was 53.1 percent, while the combination of three harmonics enhanced the accuracy significantly up to 63.8 percent.

Five subjects participated in online experiments with feedback with four flicker frequencies (6, 7, 8, and 13 Hz). After the training session (SS1), the classifier (SSVEP amplitudes obtained from a lock-in analyzer (Müller-Putz et al. (2005a))) was calculated out of the data. For the second session (SS2), feedback was delivered to the subjects while a cockpit of an aircraft was displayed on the screen. Every trial started with a beep tone. After 2 s, four bars were displayed at the upper part of the monitor (horizon). One of these bars was highlighted, indicating the LED bar the subject had to focus on. Simultaneously, a ball displaying the current classification result started to move from the bottom to the top of the screen. Three seconds later, a "hit" was indicated by a single beep tone. In the case of a

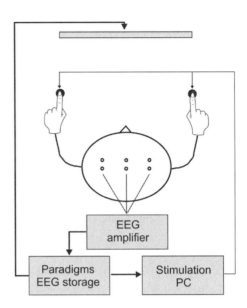

Figure 4.6 Stimulation units SSSEP-based BCI systems. Black discs symbolize the transducers that provide the stimulation with specific frequencies f_{T1} and f_{T2} (modified from Müller-Putz et al. (2006)).

miss, no tone was presented. The third session (SS3) was performed on a separate day using a new classifier (from SS2). Avoiding interference by complex visual input, the cockpit and the moving feedback ball were removed for SS4. In this last session, the background screen remained totally black. Only the four bars were displayed and the single feedback beep tone was delivered as described earlier.

Each subject performed four sessions totaling in 960 trials. Offline results from session SS1 (training session) ranged from 50.8 to 93.3 percent. In the feedback experiment (sessions SS2, SS3, and SS4), subjects reached a classificaton accuracy between 42.5 and 94.4 percent.

It can be summarized that the use of high harmonics as features for classification improves the classification accuracy of a four-class BCI and therefore can provide a system with a high information transfer rate (ITR). The highest ITR obtained was 31.5 bit/min (shortened trial length; for details, see Müller-Putz et al. (2005a)).

In another study we investigated the usability of SSSEPs for a brain-computer interface. Specifically, the following questions remain to be answered: Are SSSEP amplitudes constant and strong enough? Do they get mentally modulated and detected on a single-trial basis?

Transducers (12 mm, QMB-105 Star Inc., Edision, USA) have been used for the stimulation of both index fingers using tactile stimulation in the resonance-like frequency range of the somatosensory system (Müller et al. (2001)). A PC was set up to generate stimulation patterns (figure 4.6), with subject-specific frequencies (f_{T1}, f_{T2}) intensified with audio amplifiers.

Subjects were stimulated with their specific stimulation frequency (f_{T1}) on their right index fingers (Müller et al. (2001)). On their left index fingers a different stimulation frequency ($f_{T2} = f_{T1} - 5\,Hz$) was applied. Stimulation frequencies were in a range from 25 to 31 Hz (f_{T1}) and from 20 to 26 Hz (f_{T2}). The stimulator for f_{T1} was set to $\sim$90 μm stimulation amplitude and stimulation strength of f_{T2} was individually set so the subject found it equal to f_{T1}. For stimulation a sinusoidal character was used, producing a kind of weak tap stimulation. The subjects wore the finger parts of a rubber glove on their index fingers to prevent any electrical influences from the stimulators.

During the individual runs, acoustic noise was presented to the subjects to mask the stimulator noise. Subjects were asked to focus attention on the finger stimulation as indicated by the visual cue and to count appearing twitches at the desired index finger. The counting of the amplitude twitches should force the subjects to focus on the desired stimulation. After a training session, an LDA classifier was computed and used in feedback (discrete feedback in form of a tone at the end of a trial) sessions.

Four subjects participated in the BCI experiments. Two of them were unable to focus their attention during an entire session (usually 160 trials), which might have been due to concentration problems. Because of the simultaneous stimulation of both fingers, focusing on one specific finger was more difficult than, for example, gazing at one flickering light (out of two) as in the case of a SSVEP-based BCI. In the first case, the subjects must focus mentally on one target, whereas in the second case, the eye position primarily determines the target. However, a selection of runs with good performances leads to offline results of about 73 percent in this two-class problem.

The performance of the two remaining subjects was more promising. One subject could increase her performance from session to session. Her online accuracy of the last session was best with 71.7 percent (offline 75.0 percent). The other subject was even able to focus her attention from the beginning. Online performances ranged between 79.4 and 83.1 percent (offline accuracies between 83.8 and 88.1 percent) (Müller-Putz et al. (2006)).

It essentially was shown that it is possible to set up an SSSEP-based BCI. The main questions of amplitude stability and constancy of SSSEPs, the possibility of getting them modulated during focusing attention, and, not at least, the question of single-trial separability can be answered positively.

4.5 Graz-BCI Applications

4.5.1 Control of Neuroprostheses

The realization of a BCI that may help humans with paralyzed limbs to restore their grasp function is not unreachable anymore. It could be shown that during a number of training sessions subjects learn to establish separable brain patterns by the imagination of, for example, hand or foot movements. Furthermore, functional electrical stimulation (FES) can be used for the restoration of motor function. A small number of surface electrodes were placed near the motor point of the muscle or electrodes were implanted subcutaneously.

By applying stimulation pulses, action potentials are elicited leading to the contraction of the innervated muscle fibres.

At this time we have experience with an uncued (asynchronous) BCI in two male persons with high spinal cord injury (SCI). Both have been equipped with a neuroprosthesis. For one patient (30 years) suffering from a SCI at level C5 the hand grasp function of his left hand was restored with an FES using surface electrodes. During a long BCI-training period of four months in 1999, he learned to induce 17-Hz oscillations, which had been very dominant, and he retained this special skill over years so that a threshold detector could be used for the realization of a brain switch in 2003. The trigger signal generated was used to switch between grasp phases implemented into a stimulation unit. Three FES channels, provided by surface electrodes placed at the forearm and hand, were used for grasp restoration (in collaboration with the Orthopedic University Hospital II of Heidelberg). With this grasp he was able to hold, for example, a drinking glass (Pfurtscheller et al. (2003b)). The second patient (42 years, SCI sub C5) got a Freehand system implanted in his right hand and arm (Keith et al. (1989)) at the Orthopedic University Hospital II of Heidelberg in 2000. In 2004, he learned within a short training period of only three days to reliably produce a significant power decrease of EEG-amplitudes during left hand movement imagination. In this case, the BCI system emulated the shoulder joystick that is usually used. With the combination of the BCI-controlled Freehand system, he could successfully perform a part of a hand grasp performance test (Müller-Putz et al. (2005b)).

These results showed that in the future, BCI systems will be an option for the control of neuroprostheses in high SCI patients. Nevertheless, further research is necessary to minimize technical equipment and increase the number of degrees of freedom.

4.5.2   Control of a Spelling Application

Here we report the case of a 60-years-old male patient who suffered from amyotrophic lateral sclerosis (ALS) for more than five years. The goal of the study was to enable the patient to operate the cue-based two-class "virtual keyboard" (Obermaier et al. (2003)) spelling application. At the time the BCI-training started, the patient was already artificially ventilated, totally paralyzed, and almost had lost his ability to communicate. The training was undertaken at the patient's home in Vienna and supervised from Graz by tele-monitoring (figure 4.7a) (Müller et al. (2003b, 2004b); Lahrmann et al. (2005)).

Two bipolar EEG channels were recorded from four gold electrodes placed over the left and right sensorimotor area, according to the international 10-20 system. The electrodes were placed 2.5 cm anterior and posterior to position C3 and C4. Position Fz was used as ground. The EEG was amplified (sensitivity $50\mu V$), analog filtered between 5 and 30 Hz (filter order 2 with an attenuation of 40 dB) and sampled at a rate of 128 Hz.

To set up the online system, the training sessions were performed without feedback. The training consisted of a repetitive process of cue-based motor imagery trials. The duration of each trial varied randomly between 8 and 10 s and started with a blank screen. At second 2, a short warning tone was presented and a fixation cross appeared in the middle of the screen. From second 3 to 7 an arrow (cue) was shown indicating the mental task to be performed. Exemplarily, an arrow pointing to the left or to the right indicated the imagination of a left hand or right hand movement, respectively. The order of appearance of the arrows was randomized and at second 7 the screen was cleared. The feedback for online experiments was computed by applying LDA to logarithmic bandpower features extracted from the ongoing EEG. The BP estimate was computed sample-by-sample by digitally bandpass filtering the EEG, squaring the signal and averaging the samples over a 1-s period. The most reactive frequency components were selected by visually inspecting the ERD/ERS time-frequency maps (Graimann et al. (2002)). Two frequency bands were selected and extracted from each EEG channel. With the resulting four BP features, individual LDA classifiers were trained at different time points with the same latency within a trial (from second 0 to 8 every 0.5 s). For a better generalization, 10×10 cross-validation was used. For the online feedback, training the classifier at the time point with the best classification accuracy was chosen.

The basket paradigm (Krausz et al. (2003)) was selected to train the patient to reliably reproduce two different EEG patterns. The aim of the paradigm was to direct a ball, falling with a constant speed from the top of the screen, into the target (basket) positioned at the bottom of the screen (see figure 4.7b). The classification result was mapped to the horizontal position of the ball. After 82 feedback runs (one run consisted of 40 trials) recorded in 17 training days the classification accuracy increased from 49.3 percent (mean over 23 runs recorded during the first two days) to 82.6 percent (mean over 22 runs performed from day 11 to 17). The first of the two EEG patterns was characterized by a broad-banded ERD, the second by a narrow-banded ERS in the alpha band.

The BCI control achieved enabled the patient to use the two-class virtual keyboard (see figure 4.7c). After several copy spelling training runs, the patient also succeeded in free spelling. The patient voluntarily spelled "MARIAN," the name of his caregiver. The selection process is summarized in the table shown in the lower part of figure 4.7.

4.5.3 Uncued Navigation in a Virtual Environment

Three able-bodied subjects took part in these experiments. Before the asynchronous experiments could begin, subjects had to perform an intensive cue-based three-class feedback training in order to achieve reliable control of their own brain activity. The exercise was to move a "smiley" from the center of the screen toward the target located at one of the borders of the screen. Three bipolar EEG channels, filtered between 0.5 and 100 Hz, were recorded from hand and foot representation areas with a rate of 250 Hz. The discrimination among the three motor imagery tasks (CFR1) was performed by applying LDA to the spectral components (bandpower features). For more details on the three-class discrimination, see Scherer et al. (2004a). Since artifacts are crucial in BCI research, methods for muscle artifact detection, based on inverse filtering, and electrooculogram (EOG) reduction, based on regression analysis, were used during online experiments. Each time an artifact was detected a message was presented to the subject for a 1-s period.

To achieve asynchronous classification, a second classifier (CFR2) was calculated to discriminate between motor imagery (intentional control) and the noncontrol state. The latter was defined by extracting features from a recording where the subjects were sitting in front of a computer screen with eyes open and without performing motor imagery. Each

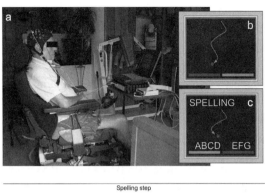

	Spelling step						
1	2	3	4	5	6	7	
ABCDEFGHIJKLMN	HIJKLMN	LMN	LM	**M**	Ok		
ABCDEFGHIJKLMN	ABCDEFG	ABCD	AB	**A**	Ok		
OPQRSTUVWXYZ_	OPQRSTU	OPQR	QR	**R**	Ok		
ABCDEFGHIJKLMN	HIJKLMN	HIJK	HI	**I**	Ok		
ABCDEFGHIJKLMN	ABCDEFG	ABCD	AB	**A**	Ok		
OPQRSTUVWXYZ_	OPQRSTU	STU	U	Modify	Back		
ABCDEFGHIJKLMN	HIJKLMN	LMN	LM	M	Modify	Back	
ABCDEFGHIJKLMN	HIJKLMN	LMN	N	Ok			

Figure 4.7 Upper part: a) ALS patient during BCI training at home. b) Basket paradigm. The task was to move the falling ball into the given target. c) Copy-spelling. By splitting iteratively the alphabet into two halves the selected letter can be isolated. Lower part: Abstract of the letter selection process that shows the spelling steps needed to write "MARIAN," the name of the patient's caregiver. The word was correctly spelled after canceling wrong selections (row 6 and 7).

time the classifier output of CFR2 exceeded a subject-specific threshold for a certain time, a change between control and noncontrol state did occur. In figure 4.8a, the Simulink model used for the online experiments is shown.

The task of the asynchronous paradigm, called "freeSpace," was to navigate through a virtual environment. Each user was placed into a virtual park composed of one tree and a number of hedges (figure 4.8b). The exercise was to pick up three items (coins) within three minutes. From a randomly selected starting point, the subjects could explore the park in the following way: Left or right-hand motor imagery resulted in a rotation to the left or right whereas foot or tongue motor imagery resulted in a forward motion. With this method, each part of the park could be reached. The subjects got instructions how to reach the targets. The selected path was solely dependent on the will of the subjects. Figure 4.8c shows pursued pathways for each subject from the same starting position. While two subjects were able to collect the three coins in 146 s and 153 s respectively, the third subject succeeded in picking up only two coins within the 3-minute period.

With these experiments we have shown for the first time that voluntary (free will, uncued) BCI-based control in virtual environment is possible when only the dynamics of 10-Hz and 20-Hz oscillations in three EEG derivations are analyzed. Further results about the use of virtual reality and feedback experiments can be found in Pfurtscheller et al. (2006b) and in chapter 23.

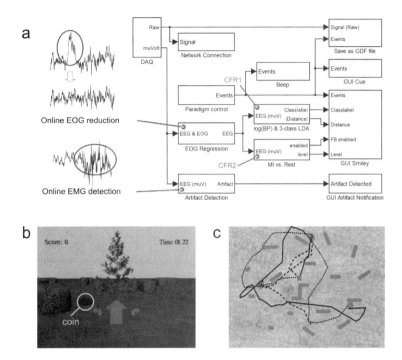

Figure 4.8 a) Simulink model used for online feedback experiments. One important feature of the system is online EOG reduction and muscle artifact detection. The combination of the two classifiers CFR1 (discrimination among motor imagery tasks) and CFR2 (discrimination between intended control and noncontrol state) allows an uncued (asynchronous) classification of the EEG. b) Feedback presented to the subjects. The screenshot shows a tree and hedges distributed in the virtual park. The size of the arrows indicates the detected mental activity and consequently the navigation command (turn left/right or move forward). If no motor imagery pattern is detected, the arrows have the same size and no navigation is performed. The dark round object on the left side represents a coin to collect. In the left upper corner is the number of collected coins and in the right upper corner is the time needed. c) Bird-view of the park showing the performance of a park walk from all three subjects with the same starting point (cross). The dark rectangles indicate the hedges and the circles the coins. Two subjects successfully collected all three coins (continuous and dotted line). The third subject (dashed line) picked up only two coins in three minutes.

4.6 Conclusion and Outlook

At present our work is partially focused to investigate the impact of different types of visual feedback on the classification accuracy (Pfurtscheller et al. (2006b)). In detail, moving virtual body parts and non-body parts are studied. It is expected that the observation of moving body parts can interfere with motor imagery and either improve or degrade the BCI performance.

Another point of research is to realize a so-called "brain-switch." This is a BCI system based on only one (or two) EEG recordings able to well discriminate between intentional control states and noncontrol or resting states. Here it is of importance to incorporate knowledge about the behavior of spatiotemporal ERD/ERS patterns during different mental strategies. Such a brain-switch can be combined with an SSVEP (SSSEP)-based BCI system to obtain a high information transfer rate. Last but not least we will realize an optical BCI prototype within the EU-project PRESENCCIA and validate this online system with a commercial multichannel Near Infrared Systems (NIRS).

Acknowledgments

This work was supported by the European PRESENCCIA project (IST-2006-27731), Austrian Science Fund (FWF) project P16326-BO2, Allgemeine Unfallversicherungsanstalt–AUVA, Lorenz-Böhler Gesellschaft, and the Land Steiermark.

Notes

E-mail for correspondence: pfurtscheller@tugraz.at

5 The Berlin Brain-Computer Interface: Machine Learning-Based Detection of User Specific Brain States

Benjamin Blankertz, Matthias Krauledat, and Klaus-Robert Müller
Fraunhofer–Institute FIRST
Intelligent Data Analysis Group (IDA)
Kekuléstr. 7, 12489 Berlin, Germany

Technical University Berlin
Str. des 17. Juni 135
10 623 Berlin, Germany

Guido Dornhege
Fraunhofer–Institute FIRST
Intelligent Data Analysis Group (IDA)
Kekuléstr. 7, 12489 Berlin, Germany

Volker Kunzmann, Florian Losch, and Gabriel Curio
Department of Neurology, Neurophysics Group
Campus Benjamin Franklin, Charité University Medicine Berlin
Hindenburgdamm 30, 12200 Berlin, Germany

5.1 Abstract

The Berlin Brain-Computer Interface (BBCI) project develops an EEG-based BCI system that uses machine learning techniques to adapt to the specific brain signatures of each user. This concept allows to achieve high quality feedback already in the very first session without subject training. Here we present the broad range of investigations and experiments that have been performed within the BBCI project. The first kind of experiments analyzes the predictability of performing limbs from the premovement (readiness) potentials including successful feedback experiments. The limits with respect to the spatial resolution of the somatotopy are explored by contrasting brain patterns of movements of (1) left vs. right foot, (2) index vs. little finger within one hand, and (3) finger vs. wrist vs. elbow vs. shoulder within one arm. A study of phantom movements of patients with traumatic amputations shows the potential applicability of this BCI approach. In a complementary approach, voluntary modulations of sensorimotor rhythms caused by motor imagery (left hand vs. right hand vs. foot) are translated into a proportional feedback signal. We report results of a recent feedback study with six healthy subjects with no or very little experience with BCI control: Half of the subjects achieved an information transfer rate above 35 bits per minute (bpm). Furthermore, one subject used the BBCI to operate a mental typewriter in free spelling mode. The overall spelling speed was 4.5 letters per minute including the time needed for the correction errors. These results are encouraging for an EEG-based BCI system in untrained subjects that is independent of peripheral nervous system activity and does not rely on evoked potentials.

5.2   Introduction

A brain-computer interface (BCI) is a man-to-machine communication channel operating solely on brain signatures of voluntary commands independent from muscular output; see Wolpaw et al. (2002); Kübler et al. (2001a); and Curran and Stokes (2003) for a broad overview. The Berlin Brain-Computer Interface (BBCI) is a noninvasive, EEG-based system whose key features are (1) the use of well-established motor competences as control paradigms, (2) high-dimensional features derived from 128-channel EEG, (3) advanced machine learning techniques, and—as a consequence—(4) no need for subject training. Point (3) contrasts with the operant conditioning variant of BCI, in which the subject learns by neurofeedback to control a specific EEG feature that is hard-wired in the BCI system (Elbert et al. (1980); Rockstroh et al. (1984); Birbaumer et al. (2000)). According to the motto "let the machines learn," our approach minimizes the need for subject training and copes with one of the major challenges in BCI research: the huge intersubject variability with respect to patterns and characteristics of brain signals.

We present two aspects of the main approach taken in the BBCI project. The first is based on the discriminability of premovement potentials in voluntary movements. Our initial studies (Blankertz et al. (2003)) show that high information transfer rates can be obtained from single-trial classification of fast-paced motor commands. Additional investigations point out ways of improving bit rates further, for example, by extending the class of detectable movement-related brain signals to the ones encountered, for example, when moving single fingers on one hand. A more recent study showed that it is indeed possible to transfer the results obtained with regard to movement intentions in healthy subjects to phantom movements in patients with traumatic amputations.

In a second step we established a BCI system based on motor imagery. A recent feedback study (Blankertz et al. (2006a)) demonstrated with six healthy subjects, with no or very little experience with BCI control, the power of the BBCI approach: Three subjects achieved an information transfer rate above 35 bits per minute (bpm) and two subjects above 24 and 15 bpm, while one subject could not achieve any BCI control. A more thorough neurophysiological analysis can be found in Blankertz et al. (2007). These results are encouraging for an EEG-based BCI system in untrained subjects that is independent of peripheral nervous system activity even when compared to results with very well-trained subjects operating other BCI systems.

In section 5.3, we present our single-trial investigations of premovement potentials, including online feedback (5.3.3), a study of "phantom movements" in amputees (5.3.4), and an exploration of the limits of discriminability of premovement potentials (5.3.5). In section 5.4 we present our BBCI feedback system based on motor imagery and the results of a systematic feedback study (5.4.3). Section 5.4.4 gives evidence that the control is solely dependent on central nervous system activity. In section 5.5 we point out lines of further improvement before the concluding discussion in 5.6.

5.3 Premovement Potentials in Executed and Phantom Movements

In our first approach we studied the premovement potentials in overlearned movements, like typewriting on a computer keyboard. Our aim here was to build a classifier based on the Bereitschaftspotenzial (readiness potential) that is capable of detecting movement intentions and predicting the type of intended movement (e.g., left vs. right hand) before EMG onset. The basic rationale behind letting healthy subjects actually perform the movements in contrast to movement imagination is that the latter poses a dual task (motor command preparation plus vetoing the actual movement). This suggests that movement imagination by healthy subjects might not guarantee an appropriate correspondence to paralyzed patients as the latter will emit the motor command without veto (but see Kübler et al. (2005a) for a study showing that ALS patients can indeed use modulations of sensorimotor rhythms for BCI control). To allow a safe transfer of the results in our setting to paralyzed patients it is essential to make predictions about imminent movements prior to any EMG activity to exclude a possible confound with afferent feedback from muscle and joint receptors contingent upon an executed movement. On the other hand, being able to predict movements in real time before EMG activity starts opens interesting perspectives for assistance of action control in time-critical behavioral contexts, an idea further pursued in Krauledat et al. (2004).

5.3.1 Left vs. Right Hand Finger Movements

Our goal is to predict in single-trials the laterality of imminent left vs. right finger movements at a time point prior to the start of EMG activity. The specific feature that we use is the readiness potential (RP or Bereitschaftspotenzial), which is a transient postsynaptic response of main pyramidal pericentral neurons (Kornhuber and Deecke (1965)). It leads to a pronounced cortical negativation that is focused in the corresponding motor area, that is, contralateral to the performing limb reflecting movement preparation; see figure 5.1. Neurophysiologically, the RP is well investigated and described (cf. Kornhuber and Deecke (1965); Lang et al. (1988); Cui et al. (1999)). New questions that arise in this context are (1) can the lateralization be discriminated on a single-trial basis, and (2) does the refractory behavior allow to observe the RP also in fast motor sequences? Our investigations provided positive answers to both questions.

In a series of experiments, healthy volunteers performing self-paced finger-movements on a computer keyboard with approximate tap-rates of 30, 45, 60, and 120 taps per

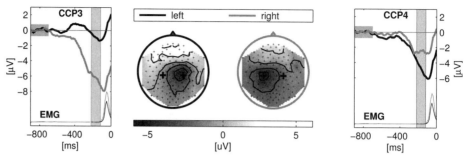

Figure 5.1 Response *averaged* event-related potentials (ERPs) of one right-handed subject in a left-hand vs. right-hand finger tapping experiment (N =275 resp. 283 trials per class). Finger movements were executed self-paced, i.e., without any external cue, in an approximate intertrial interval of 2 seconds. The two scalp plots show a topographical mapping of scalp potentials averaged within the interval -220 to -120 ms relative to keypress (time interval shaded in the ERP plots). Larger crosses indicate the position of the electrodes CCP3 and CCP4 for which the time course of the ERPs is shown in the subplots at both sides. For comparison, time courses of EMG activity for left and right finger movements are added. EMG activity starts after -120 ms and reaches a peak of 70 μV at -50 ms. The readiness potential is clearly visible, a predominantly contralateral negativation starting about 600 ms before movement and raising approximately until EMG onset.

minute (tpm). EEG was recorded from 128 Ag/AgCl scalp electrodes (except for some experiments summarized in figure 5.2 that were recorded with 32 channels). To relate the prediction accuracy with the timing of EMG activity we recorded electromyogram (EMG) from *M. flexor digitorum communis* from both sides. Also electrooculogram (EOG) was recorded to control for the influence of eye movements; compare figure 5.4. No trials have been discarded from analysis.

The first step toward RP-based feedback is evaluating the predictability of the laterality of upcoming movements. We determined the time point of EMG onset by inspecting classification performance based on EMG-signals (as in figure 5.4) and used it as an end point of the windows from which features for the EEG-based classification analysis were extracted. For the data set shown in figure 5.1 the chosen time point is -120 ms, which is in coincidence with the onset seen in averaged EMG activity. The choice of the relative position of the classification window with respect to the keypress makes sure that the prediction does not rely on brain signals from afferent nerves. For extracting the RP features and classification we used our approved BBCI method as described in the next section, 5.3.2. The result of EEG-based classification for all subjects is shown in figure 5.2 where the cross-validation performance is quantified in bits per minute (according to Shannon's formula) to trade-off accuracy versus decision speed. A discussion of the possible influence of noncentral nervous system activity on the classfication can be found in section 5.3.3, especially in figure 5.4.

The results indicate that the refractory period of the RP is short enough to effectively discriminate premovement potentials in finger movement sequences as fast as two taps per second. On the other hand, it turned out that the performance of RP-based premovement potential detection in a self-paced paradigm is highly subject-specific. Further investigation will study event-related desynchronization (ERD) effects in the μ and β frequency range

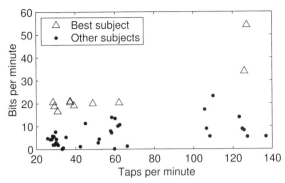

Figure 5.2   Tapping rates [taps per minute] vs. information transfer rate as calculated by Shannon's formula from the cross-validation error for different subjects peforming self-paced tapping at different average tapping rates with fingers of the left and the right hand. The results of the best subject (marked by triangles) were confirmed in several experiments.

(cf. Pfurtscheller and Lopes da Silva (1999)), compare systematically the discriminability of different features and combined RP+ERD features (cf. Dornhege et al. (2004a)), and search for modifications in the experimental setup in order to gain high performance for a broader range of subjects.

5.3.2   Preprocessing and Classification

The following feature extraction method is specifically tailored to extract information from the readiness potential. The method extracts the low-frequency content with an emphasis on the late part of the signal, where the information content can be expected to be largest in premovement trials. Starting points are epochs of 128 samples (i.e., 1280 ms) of raw EEG data as depicted in figure 5.3a for one channel. To emphasize the late signal content, the signal is convoluted with one-sided cosine window (figure 5.3b)

$$w(n) := 1 - \cos(n\pi/128) \quad \text{for } n = 0, \dots, 127,$$

before applying a Fourier transform (FT) filtering technique: From the complex-valued FT coefficients all are discarded but the ones in the pass-band (including the negative frequencies, which are not shown) (figure 5.3c). Transforming the selected bins back into the time domain gives the smoothed signal of which the last 200 ms are subsampled at 20 Hz, resulting in four feature components per channel (figure 5.3d). The full (RP) feature vector is the concatenation of those values from all channels for the given time window. For online operation those features are calculated every 40 ms from sliding windows.

Due to our observation that RP features under particular movement conditions are normally distributed with equal covariance matrices (Blankertz et al. (2003)), the classification problem meets the assumption of being optimally separated by a linear hyperplane. The data processing described above preserves gaussianity, hence we classify with regularized linear discriminant analysis (RLDA, see Friedman (1989)). Regularization is needed to

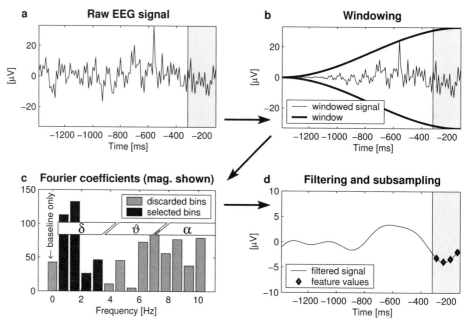

Figure 5.3 This example shows the feature calculation in one channel of a premovement trial $[-1400 - 120]$ ms with keypress at $t = 0$ ms. The pass-band for the FT filtering is 0.4–3.5 Hz and the subsampling rate is 20 Hz. Features are extracted only from the last 200 ms (shaded) where most information on the upcoming movement is expected.

avoid overfitting since we are dealing with a high-dimensional dataset with only few samples available. Details can be found in Blankertz et al. (2002, 2003).

5.3.3   RP-Based Feedback in Asynchronous Mode

The general setting is the following. An experimental session starts with a short period during which the subject performs self-paced finger movements. This session is called calibration session, and the data is used to train a classifier, which is then used to make instantaneous predictions on whether the subject intends a hand movement and what its laterality will be.

Although the results of the preceding section demonstrate that an effective *discrimination* of left-hand versus right-hand finger movements is possible well before keypress, it remains a challenge to build a system that predicts movement intentions from ongoing EEG. One point that made the previous classification task easier was that the single trials were taken from intervals in fixed-time relation to the keypress. For the implementation of a useful continuous feedback in an asynchronous mode (meaning without externally controlled timing), we need two more things: (1) the classifier must work reasonably well not only for one exact time point but for a broader interval of time, and (2) the system needs to detect the buildup of movement intentions such that it can trigger BCI commands without externally controlled timing.

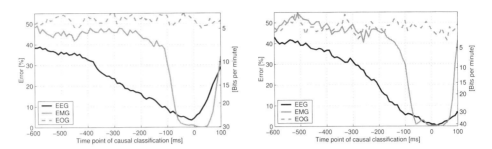

Figure 5.4   Comparison of EEG-, EMG-, and EOG-based classification with respect to the endpoint of the classification interval with $t = 0$ ms being the time point of keypress. For the left plot, classifiers were trained in a leave-one-out fashion and applied to a window sliding over the respective left-out trials on data of the calibration measurement. For the right plot, a classifier (for each type of signal) was trained on data of the calibration measurement and applied to a window sliding over all trials of a feedback session. Note that the scale of the information transfer rate [bits per minute] on the right is different due to a higher average tapping speed in the feedback session.

With respect to the first issue we found that a quite simple strategy (*jittering*) leads to satisfying results: Instead of taking only one window as training samples, ones extracts several with some time jitter between them. More specifically, we extracted two samples per keypress of the calibration measurement, one from a window ending at 150 the other at 50 ms before keypress. This method makes the resulting classifier somewhat invariant to time shifts of the samples to be classified, that is, better suited for the online application to sliding windows. Using more than two samples per keypress event did not improve classification performance further. Extracting samples from windows ending at 50 ms before keypress may seem critical since EMG activity start at about 120 ms before keypress. But what matters is that the trained classifier is able to make predictions before EMG activity starts no matter what signals it was trained on. That this is the case can be seen in figure 5.4 in which EEG-, EMG-, and EOG-based classification is compared in relation to the time point of classification. The left plot shows a leave-one-out validation of the calibration measurement, while the right plot shows the accuracy of a classifier trained on the calibration measurement applied to signals of the feedback session, both using jittered training.

To implement the *detection* of upcoming movements, we train a second classifier as outlined in Blankertz et al. (2002). Technically, the detector of movement intentions was implemented as a classifier that distinguishes between motor preparation intervals (for left and right taps) and "rest" intervals that were extracted from intervals between movements. To study the interplay of the two classifiers, we pursued exploratory feedback experiments with one subject, selected for his good offline results. Figure 5.5 shows a statistical evaluation of the two classifiers when applied in sliding windows to the continuous EEG.

The movement discriminator in the left plot of figure 5.5 shows a pronounced separation during the movement (preparation and execution) period. In other regions there is a considereable overlap. From this plot it becomes evident that the left/right classifier alone does not distinguish reliably between *movement intention* and *rest condition* by the magnitude of its output, which explains the need for a movement detector. The elevation for the left

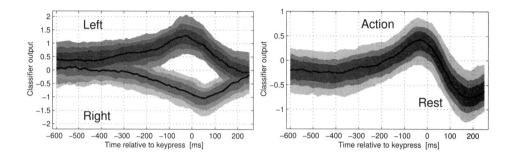

Figure 5.5 Classifiers were trained in a leave-one-out fashion and applied to windows sliding over unseen epochs yielding traces of graded classifier outputs. The tubes show the 10, 20, 30 resp. 90, 80, and 70 percentile values of those traces. On the left, the result is shown of the left vs. right classifier with tubes calculated separately for left and right finger tapping. The subplot on the right shows the result for the movement detection classifier.

class is a little less pronounced (e.g., the median is -1 at $t = 0$ ms compared to 1.25 for right events). The movement intention detector in the right plot of figure 5.5 brings up the movement phase while giving (mainly) negative output to the postmovement period.

These two classifiers were used for an exploratory feedback in which a cross was moving in two dimensions; see the left plot of figure 5.6. The position on the x-axis was controlled by the left/right movement discriminator, and the vertical position was determined by the movement intention detector. Obviously, this is *not* an independent control of two dimensions. Rather the cursor was expected to stay in the middle of the lower half during rest and it should move to the upper left or right field when a movement of the left resp. right hand was prepared. The red and green colored fields are the decision areas that only have a symbolic meaning in this application because no further actions are triggered. In a case study with one subject the expected behavior was indeed found. Although the full flavor of the feedback can be experienced only by watching it, we tried to demonstrate its dynamics by showing the traces of the first 100 trials of the feedback in the right plot of figure 5.6. Each trace displays an interval of the feedback signal -160 to -80 ms relative to keypress. The last 40 ms are intensified and the end point of each trace is marked by a dot.

5.3.4   Detection of 'Phantom Limb Commands'

One of the major goals of BCI research is to improve autonomy of people with severe motor disabilities by new communication and control options through interfacing the impaired connection from their intact command center, the brain, to its natural actuator organs, the muscles. Amputees might use BCIs, for example, to trigger movements of an electromechanical prosthesis. Accordingly, we elaborated on the BBCI paradigm to extend also to patients with traumatic amputations of one arm or hand. Specifically, we searched readiness potentials and event-related (de)synchronization (ERD/ERS) associated with real finger movements (intact side) and phantom (disabled side) finger movements. An ERD (ERS) is the attenuation (amplification) of pericentral μ and β rhythms in the

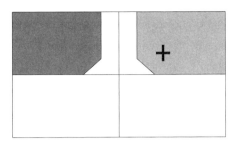 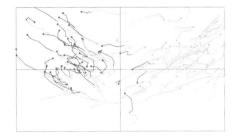

Figure 5.6 Left panel: In a BCI feedback experiment, a cursor was controlled by two classifiers. The output of a classifier trained to discriminate left-hand versus right-hand finger movements determined the x-coordinate, while a classifier trained to detect upcoming finger movements determined the y-coordinate. Accordingly, the cursor should stay in the lower center area when the subject is at rest while approaching one of the target fields upon movement intentions. This behavior was indeed achieved as can be seen in the right panel: Traces of feedback control. Each trace displays an interval of the feedback signal -160 to -80 ms relative to keypress. The last 40 ms are drawn with a thicker line and the end point of each trace is marked by a dot. Traces are shown in darker grey for subsequent left-hand finger taps.

corresponding motor areas. With respect to unilateral hand movements these blocking effects are visible bilaterally but with a clear predominance contralateral to the performing hand (cf. Pfurtscheller and Lopes da Silva (1999)).

One problem when trying to use the approach of section 5.3.1 is the lack of a time marker signal such as a keypress when acquiring premovement brain activity of phantom movements. For the sake of transfering the classifier from the calibration measurement to the detection of spontaneous motor intentions in an asynchronous feedback we refrained from using a cued reaction paradigm. Instead, we acquired calibration data in the following way: The patients listened to an electronic metronome with two tones of alternating pitch. While the deep sound indicated rest, concomitant with the higher sound they had to perform either a finger tap on a keyboard using the healthy hand or a phantom movement with a phantom finger. Accordingly the absence of a keypress around a high beat tone allows the post-hoc identification of a spontaneous phantom finger movement intention and its approximate timing (time of metronome beat).

We studied eight patients (1 women, 7 men; ages 37–74 years) with amputations between 16 and 54 years ago. Here, we report first results concerning the ERD. Remarkably, we found that all eight patients showed significant ($p < 0.05$ according to t-tests) "phantom-related" ERD/ERS of μ- and/or β-frequencies (interval: -600 to 0 ms relative to the beat) at the primary motor cortex. See examples in figure 5.7.

These preliminary results encouraged the ongoing further analyses on RP of phantom movements and on error rates of offline single-trial classifications, which eventually could form a basis for BCI-control of a prosthesis driven by phantom limb motor commands.

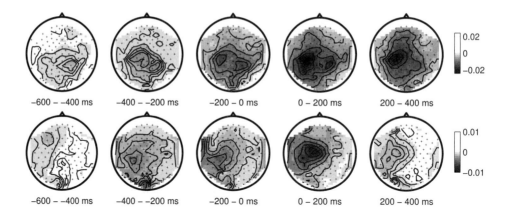

Figure 5.7   Scalp topographies of ERD. Signed r^2 values of the differences in ERD curves between phantom movement and rest. Upper row: an example for contralateral ERD of μ-activity (subject *bf* with right hand amputation). Lower row: an example for an ipsilateral ERD of β-activity (subject *bg* with left hand amputation). In these subjects, no ERS was observed.

5.3.5   Exploring the Limits of Single-Trial Classification with Fine Spatial Resolution

The information transmission rate of BCIs can be improved if single-trial analyses of movement-related scalp EEG parameters could reflect not only the gross somatotopic arrangement of, for example, hand versus foot, but also, for example, the finely graded representation of individual fingers, potentially enabling a kind of "mental typewriting." To examine the discriminability of BCI signals from close-by brain regions, we recorded 128-channel EEGs of healthy volunteers during self-paced movements of various limbs. The premovement potential topographies are shown in figure 5.8, analog to the maps in figure 5.1. The corresponding r^2-values are comparably low, but their consistent topographies suggests that the found differences indeed significantly reflect specific activations in sensorimotor cortices.

   The fact that it is in principle possible to distinguish the noninvasively recorded RPs associated with movements of limbs represented closely on the cortex in single-trial analysis encourages us in our efforts to improve the technical facilities necessary to gather these existing physiological informations properly and noninvasively.

5.4   BCI Control-Based on Imagined Movements

The RP feature presented in the previous section allows an early distinction among motor-related mental activities since it reflects movement intent. But even in repetitive movements, the discrimination decays already after about 1 s (cf. Dornhege (2006)). Accordingly, we take an alternative approach for the design of proportional BCI control, such as continuous cursor control. Here we focus on modulations of sensorimotor rhythms evoked by imagined movements. Our first feedback study (Blankertz et al. (2005)) demonstrates

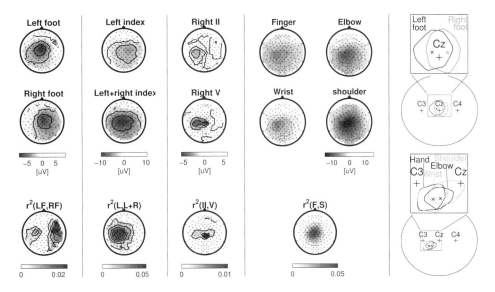

Figure 5.8   Upper two rows of topographies show averaged premovement potential patterns of one subject each in different self-paced limb moving tasks. The lower row visualizes r^2-values (squared biserial correlation coefficient) indicating significant differences at expected locations in all cases. The rightmost column shows the focal area and its peak of the RP for two experiments. Note that due to the slanted orientation, the contralateral foot areas project to ipsilateral scalp positions.

that it is possible to do so following our philosophy of minimal subject training while still obtaining high information transfer rates.

5.4.1   Experimental Setup

We designed a setup for a feedback study with six subjects who all had no or very little experience with BCI feedback. Brain signals were measured from 118 electrodes mounted on the scalp. To exclude the possibility of influence from non-central nervous system activity, EOG and EMG were recorded additionally; see section 5.4.4. Those channels were not used to generate the feedback signal.

Each experiment began with a calibration measurement (also called training session, but note that this refers to *machine* training) in which labeled trials of EEG data during motor imagery were gathered. This data is used by signal processing and machine learning techniques to estimate parameters of a brain-signal to control-signal translation algorithm. This algorithm can be applied online to continuously incoming signals to produce an instantaneous feedback.

In the training sessions, visual stimuli indicated for 3.5 s which of the following three motor imageries the subject should perform: (L) left hand, (R) right hand, or (F) right foot. The presentation of target cues was interrupted by periods of random length, 1.75 to 2.25 s, in which the subject could relax.

Then the experimenter investigated the data to adjust subject-specific parameters of the data processing methods and identified the two classes that gave best discrimination. See

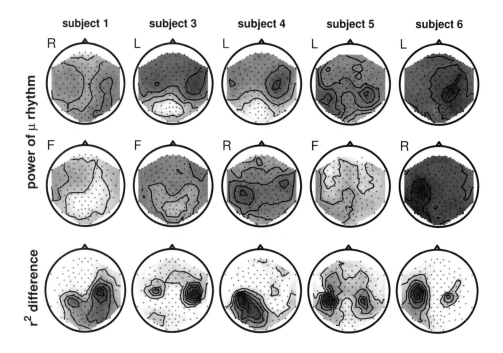

Figure 5.9 The upper two rows show a topographic display of the energy in the specific frequency band that was used for feedback (as baseline the energy in the interstimuli intervals was subtracted). Darker shades indicate lower energy resp. ERD. From the calibration measurement with three types of motor imagery, two were selected for feedback. Energy plots are shown only of those two selected conditions as indicated by the letters (L) left hand, (R) right hand, and (F) foot. The lower row shows the r^2 differences between the band energy values of the two classes demonstrating that distinctive information found over from (sensori-) motor cortices.

figure 5.9 for band-energy mappings of five successful subjects and r^2 maps showing that discriminative activity is found over (sensori-) motor cortices only. When the discrimination was satisfactory, a binary classifier was trained and three different kinds of feedback application followed. This was the case for five of six subjects who typically performed eight runs of twenty-five trials each for each type of feedback application.

During preliminary feedback experiments we realized that the initial classifier often was performing suboptimal, such that the bias and scaling of the linear classifier had to be adjusted. Later investigations have shown that this adaption is needed to account for the different experimental condition of the (exciting) feedback situation as compared to the calibration session. This issue will be discussed extensively in a forthcoming paper.

In the first feedback application (position-controlled cursor), the output of the classifier was directly translated to the horizontal position of a cursor. There were target fields at both sides, one of which was highlighted at the beginning of a trial. The cursor started in a deactivated mode (in which it could move but not trigger a target field) and became activated after the user has held the cursor in a central position for 500 ms. The trial ended when the activated cursor touched a target field that was then colored green or red, depending on whether it was the correct target or not. The cursor was deactivated and the next target appeared.

The second feedback application (rate-controlled cursor) was very similar, but the control of the cursor was relative to the actual position, that is, at each update step a fraction of the classifier output was added to the actual cursor position. Each trial started by setting the cursor to the middle of the screen and releasing it after 750 ms.

The last feedback application (basket game) operated in a synchronous mode and is similar to what is used in Graz (cf. Krausz et al. (2003)). A ball was falling down at constant speed while its horizontal position was controlled by the classifier output. At the bottom of the screen there were three target fields, the outer having half the width of the middle fields to account for the fact that outer positions were easier to hit.

5.4.2 Processing and Classification

The crucial point in the data processing is to extract some spatial filters that optimize the discriminability of multichannel brain signals based on ERD/ERS effects of the (sensori-) motor rhythms. Once these filters have been determined, features are calculated as the log of the variance in those surrogate channels. In our experience, those features can best be classified by linear methods; we use linear discriminant analysis (LDA). For online operation, features are calculated every 40 ms from sliding windows of 250 to 1000 ms (subject-specific). The spatial filters are calculated individually for each subject on the data of the calibration measurement by common spatial pattern (CSP) analysis (see Fukunaga (1990) and chapter 13). Details about the processing methods and the selection of parameters can be found in Blankertz et al. (2005).

5.4.3 Results

To compare the results of the different feedback sessions we use the information transfer rate (ITR, Wolpaw et al. (2002)) measured in bits per minute (bpm). We calculated this measure for each run according to the following formula:

$$\text{ITR} = \frac{\text{\# of decisions}}{\text{duration in minutes}} \cdot \left(p \log_2(p) + (1-p)\log(\frac{1-p}{N-1}) + \log_2(N) \right) \quad (5.1)$$

where p is the accuracy in decisions between N classes ($N = 2$ for cursor control and $N = 3$ for the basket game). Note that the *duration in minutes* refers to the total duration of the run including all intertrial intervals. In contrast to error rates or ROC curves, the ITR takes into account different duration of trials and different number of classes. The ITR of a random classifier is 0. Table 5.1 summarizes the information transfer rates that were obtained by the five subjects in the three feedback sessions. Highest ITRs were obtained in the "rate-controlled cursor" scenario, which has an asynchronous protocol.

One point that is, to our knowledge, special about the BBCI is that it can be operated at a high decision speed, not only theoretically, but also in practice. In the absolute cursor control the average trial length was 3 s, in rate-controlled cursor 2.5 s. In the basket feedback the trial length is constant (synchronous protocol) but was individually selected

Table 5.1 The first two columns compare the accuracy as calculated by cross-validation on the calibration data with the accuracy obtained online in the feedback application "rate-controlled cursor." Columns three to eight report the information transfer rates (ITR) measured in bits per minute as obtained by Shannon's formula, cf. (5.1). For each feedback application, the first column reports the average ITR of all runs (of 25 trials each), while the second column reports the peak ITR of all runs. Subject 2 did not achieve BCI control (64.6% accuracy in the calibration data).

	acc [%]		cursor pos. ctrl		cursor rate ctrl		basket	
	cal.	fb.	overall	peak	overall	peak	overall	peak
1	95.4	80.5	7.1	15.1	5.9	11.0	2.6	5.5
3	98.0	98.0	12.7	20.3	24.4	35.4	9.6	16.1
4	78.2	88.5	8.9	15.5	17.4	37.1	6.6	9.7
5	78.1	90.5	7.9	13.1	9.0	24.5	6.0	8.8
6	97.6	95.0	13.4	21.1	22.6	31.5	16.4	35.0
∅	89.5	90.5	10.0	17.0	15.9	27.9	8.2	15.0

for each subject, ranging from 2.1 to 3 s. The fastest subject was subject 4, who performed at an average speed of one decision every 1.7 s. The most reliable performance was achieved by subject 3: only 2 percent of the total 200 trials in the rate-controlled cursor were misclassified at an average speed of one decision per 2.1 s. Note that in our notion a trial is ranging from one target presentation to the next including the "noncontrol" period during which the selected field was highlighted.

In a later experiment subject 3 operated a mental typewriter based on the second feedback application. The alphabet (including a space and a deletion symbol) was split into two parts and those groups of characters were placed on the left resp. right side of the screen. The user selects one subgroup by moving the cursor to the respective side and the process is iterated until a "group" of one character is selected. The splitting was done alphabetically based on the probabilities of the German alphabet, but no elaborated language model was used. In a free-spelling mode, subject 3 spelled three German sentences with a total of 135 characters in 30 minutes, which is a typing speed of 4.5 letters per minute. Note that all errors have been corrected by using the deletion symbol. For details, see Dornhege (2006).

5.4.4   Investigating the Dependency of BCI Control

The fact that it is in principle possible to voluntarily modulate motorsensory rhythms without concurrent EMG activity was studied in Vaughan et al. (1998). Nevertheless, it must be checked for every BCI experiment involving healthy subjects. For this reason we always record EMG signals even though they are not used in the online system. On one hand, we investigated classwise averaged spectra, their statistical significant differences, and the scalp distributions and time courses of the power of the μ and β rhythm. The results substantiated that differences of the motor imagery classes indeed were located in sensorimotor cortices and had the typical time courses (except for subject 2 in whom no consistent differences were found) (cf. figure 5.9). On the other hand, we compared how

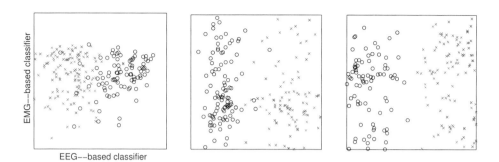

Figure 5.10   These plots show EEG- vs. EMG-control for three subjects. Classifiers were trained on
EEG- resp. on EMG-signals of the calibration measurement and applied to the data of the feedback
sessions. In each panel, the classifier output based on EEG is plotted (on the x-axis) against the output
of the EMG classifier (on the y-axis). These plots show that minimal EMG-activity occasionally
occurring in motor imagery does not correlate with the EEG-based classifier. This is also true for the
other subjects whose data are not shown here.

much variance of the classifier output and how much variance of the EMG signals can be
explained by the target class. Much in the spirit of Vaughan et al. (1998), we made the
following analysis using the squared biserial correlation coefficient r^2. The r^2-value was
calculated for the classifier output and for the bandpass filtered and rectified EMG signals
of the feedback sessions. Then the maximum of those time series was determined resulting
in one r^2-value per subject and feedback session for EMG resp. for the BCI-classifier
signal. The r^2 for EMG was in the range 0.01 to 0.08 (mean 0.04±0.03), which is very low
compared to the r^2 for the BCI-classifier signal that was in the range 0.36 to 0.79 (mean
0.52±0.15). Figure 5.10 shows for three subjects a scatter plot of the output of the EEG-
based classifier that was used in the feedback session and the output of an EMG-based
classifier providing evidence that the occurrence of minimal EMG activity in some trials
does not correlate with the EEG-based classifier. The fact that the BBCI works without
being dependent on eye movements or visual input was additionally verified by letting two
subjects control the BBCI with closed eyes, which resulted in a comparable performance
as in the closed loop feedback.

5.5   Lines of Further Improvement

5.5.1   CSSSP: CSP with Simultaneous Spectral Optimization

One drawback of the CSP algorithm is that its performance strongly depends on the choice
of the bandpass filter that needs to be applied to the EEG data in advance. Although Müller-
Gerking et al. (1999) found evidence that a broadband filter is the best general choice,
subject-specific choices can mostly enhance the results. Our common sparse spectral
spatial pattern (CSSSP) algorithm (Dornhege et al. (2006a)) eludes to the problem of
manually selecting the frequency band by simultaneously optimizing a temporal and a

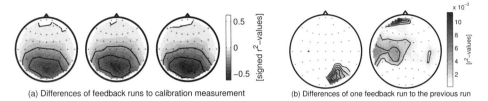

(a) Differences of feedback runs to calibration measurement   (b) Differences of one feedback run to the previous run

Figure 5.11 Subfigure (a) shows the differences in band energy from three feedback runs to the data of the calibration measurement as signed r^2-values. The decrease of occipital alpha is most likely due to the increase visual input during BCI feedback. Subfigure (b) shows the difference in band energy of one feedback run (2 and 3) to its predecessor run. The important obervation here is that the r^2-values for the differences between runs is 50 times smaller compared to (a).

spatial filter, that is, the method not only outputs optimized spatial filters, as the usual CSP technique, but also a temporal finite impulse reponse (FIR) filter that jointly enhance the discriminability of different brain states. Our investigation involving sixty BCI data sets recorded from twenty-two subjects show a significant superiority of the proposed CSSSP algorithm over classical CSP. Apart from the enhanced classification, the spatial and/or the spectral filter that are determined by the algorithm also can be used for further analysis of the data, for example, for source localization of the respective brain rhythms.

5.5.2   Investigating the Need for Adaptivity

Nonstationarities are ubiquitous in EEG signals. The questions that are relevant in BCI research are (1) how much of this nonstationarity is reflected in the EEG features, which are used for BCI control, (2) how strongly is the classifier output affected by this change in class distributions, and (3) how can this be remedied. We quantified the shifting of the statistical distributions in particular in view of band energy values and the features one gets from CSP analysis. In contrast to several studies, Millán (2004), Vidaurre et al. (2004a), andWolpaw and McFarland (2004) that found substantial nonstationarities that need to be accounted for by adaptive classification, our investigations lead to results of a somewhat different flavor. Notably, the most serious shift of the distributions of band energy features occurred between the initial calibration measurement and online operation. In contrast, the differences during online operation from one run to another were rather inconsequential in most subjects, see figure 5.11. In other subjects those shifts were largely compensated for by the CSP filters or the final classifier. The good news with respect to the observed shift of distributions is that a simple adaption of classification bias successfully cured the problem. A thorough description of this study including new techniques for visualization and a systematic comparison of different classification methods coping with shifting distributions can be found in Shenoy et al. (2006) and forthcoming papers.

5.6 Discussion and Outlook

The Berlin Brain-Computer Interface project makes use of a machine learning approach toward BCI. Working with high dimensional, complex features obtained from 128-channel EEG allows the system a distinguished flexibility for adapting to the specific individual characteristics of each user's brain. This way the BBCI system can provide feedback control even for untrained users typically after a twenty-minute calibration measurement that is used for the training of the machine learning algorithms.

In one line of investigation, we studied the detectability of premovement potentials in healthy subjects. It was shown that high bit rates in single-trial classifications can be achieved by fast-paced motor commands. An analysis of motor potentials during movements with different limbs, for example, finger II and V on one hand, exposed a possible way of further enhancement. A preliminary study involving patients with traumatic amputations showed that the results can in principle be expected to transfer to phantom movements. A restriction seems to be that the detection accuracy decreases with longer loss of the limb.

In a second approach, we investigated the possibility of establishing BCI control based on motor imagery without subject training. The result from a feedback study with six subjects impressively demonstrates that our system (1) robustly transfers the discrimination of mental states from the calibration to the feedback sessions, (2) allows a very fast switching between mental states, and (3) provides reliable feedback directly after a short calibration measurement and machine training without the need for the subject to adapt to the system, all at high information transfer rates; see table 5.1.

Recent BBCI activities comprise (1) mental typewriter experiments, with an integrated detector for the error potential, an idea that has be investigated offline in several studies (cf. Blankertz et al. (2003); Schalk et al. (2000); Parra et al. (2003); Ferrez and Millán (2005) and chapter 17), (b) the online use of combined feature and multiclass paradigms, and (3) real-time analysis of mental workload in subjects engaged in real-world cognitive tasks, for example, in driving situations.

Our future studies will strive for 2D cursor control and robot arm control, still maintaining our philosophy of minimal subject training.

Acknowledgments

We would like to thank Siamac Fazli, Steven Lemm, Florin Popescu, Christin Schäfer, and Andreas Ziehe for fruitful discussions.

This work was supported in part by grants of the *Bundesministerium für Bildung und Forschung* (BMBF), FKZ 01IBE01A/B, by the *Deutsche Forschungsgemeinschaft* (DFG), FOR 375/B1, and by the IST Programme of the European Community, under the PASCAL Network of Excellence, IST-2002-506778. This publication reflects only the authors' views.

Notes

E-mail for correspondence: benjamin.blankertz@first.fraunhofer.de

6   The IDIAP Brain-Computer Interface: An Asynchronous Multiclass Approach

José del R. Millán, Pierre W. Ferrez, and Anna Buttfield
IDIAP Research Institute
1920 Martigny, Switzerland

*Ecole Polytechnique Fédérale de
Lausanne (EPFL), Switzerland*

6.1   Abstract

In this chapter, we give an overview of our work on a self-paced asynchronous BCI that responds every 0.5 seconds. A statistical Gaussian classifier tries to recognize three different mental tasks; it may also respond "unknown" for uncertain samples as the classifier incorporates statistical rejection criteria. We report our experience with different subjects. We also describe three brain-actuated applications we have developed: a virtual keyboard, a brain game, and a mobile robot (emulating a motorized wheelchair). Finally, we discuss current research directions we are pursuing to improve the performance and robustness of our BCI system, especially for real-time control of brain-actuated robots.

6.2   Introduction

Over the past ten years we have developed a portable brain-computer interface (BCI) system based on the online analysis of spontaneous electroencephalogram (EEG) signals measured with scalp electrodes, which is able to recognize three mental tasks. Our approach relies on an asynchronous protocol where the subject decides voluntarily when to switch between mental tasks and uses a statistical Gaussian classifier to recognize, every 0.5 seconds, the mental task on which the subject is concentrating. Our subjects have been able to operate three brain-actuated devices: a virtual keyboard (Millán et al. (2004b); Millán (2003)), a video game (or brain game) (Millán (2003)), and a mobile robot (emulating a motorized wheelchair) (Millán et al. (2004a,b)) .

Like some of the other BCIs reported in the literature, our BCI is based on the analysis of EEG rhythms associated with spontaneous mental activity. In particular, we look at variations of EEG rhythms over several cortical areas related to different cognitive mental tasks such as imagination of movements, arithmetic operations, or language. The approach aims at discovering task-specific spatiofrequency patterns embedded in the continuous

EEG signal, that is, EEG rhythms over local cortical areas that differentiate the mental tasks (Anderson (1997); Millán et al. (2004b); Roberts and Penny (2000)).

In the next sections, we review the main components of our BCI system and report the main findings of our experience with different subjects. We also describe the three brain-actuated applications we have developed. Finally, we discuss current research directions we are pursuing to improve the performance and robustness of our BCI system, especially for real-time control of brain-actuated robots.

6.3   Operant Conditioning and Machine Learning

Birbaumer et al. (1999) as well as Wolpaw et al. (2000b) have demonstrated that some subjects can learn to control their brain activity through appropriate, but lengthy, training to generate fixed EEG patterns that the BCI transforms into external actions. In both cases, subjects are trained over several months to modify the amplitude of the EEG component they are learning to control. Other groups follow machine learning approaches to train the classifier embedded in the BCI (Anderson (1997); Blankertz et al. (2003); Millán (2003); Millán et al. (2004b); Pfurtscheller and Neuper (2001); Roberts and Penny (2000) and chapter 5). Most of these approaches, as ours, are based on a mutual learning process where the user and the brain interface are coupled together and adapt to each other. This should accelerate the training time. Thus, our approach allows subjects to achieve good performances in just a few hours of training in the presence of feedback (Millán (2003); Millán et al. (2004b)). In this case, analysis of learned EEG patterns confirms that for subjects to operate satisfactorily their personal BCIs, the BCI must fit the individual features of its owner (Millán et al. (2002a,c)).

Most of these works deal with the recognition of just two mental tasks (Babiloni et al. (2000); Birbaumer et al. (1999); Birch et al. (2002); Pfurtscheller and Neuper (2001); Roberts and Penny (2000) and chapter 5), or report classification errors higher than 15 percent for three or more tasks (Anderson (1997); Kalcher et al. (1996)). Some of the subjects who follow Wolpaw's approach are able to control their μ/β rhythm amplitude at four different levels and/or have simultaneous control of two rhythms (Wolpaw and McFarland (2004); Wolpaw et al. (2000b)). Our approach achieves error rates below 5 percent for three mental tasks, but correct recognition is 70 percent (Millán (2003); Millán et al. (2004b)). In the remaining cases (around 20–25%), the classifier doesn't respond, since it considers the EEG samples as uncertain.

The incorporation of rejection criteria to avoid making risky decisions, such as in the case of Millán's approach, is an important concern in BCI. The system of Roberts and Penny (2000) applies Bayesian techniques for rejection purposes, too. This is an alternative method of incorporating rejection rules into the classifier in a principled way. From a practical point of view, a low classification error is a critical performance criterion for a BCI; otherwise, users can become frustrated and stop utilizing the interface.

6.4   Synchronous vs. Asynchronous BCI

EEG-based BCIs are limited by a low channel capacity.[1] Most of the current systems have a channel capacity below 0.5 bits/s (Wolpaw et al. (2002)). One of the main reasons for such a low bandwidth is that current systems are based on *synchronous* protocols where EEG is time-locked to externally paced cues repeated every 4–10 s and the response of the BCI is the overall decision over this period (Birbaumer et al. (1999); Pfurtscheller and Neuper (2001); Roberts and Penny (2000); Wolpaw et al. (2000b)). Such synchronous protocols facilitate EEG analysis since the starting time of mental states are precisely known and differences with respect to background EEG activity can be amplified. Unfortunately, they are slow and BCI systems that use them normally recognize only two mental states.

On the contrary, other BCIs use more flexible *asynchronous* protocols where the subject makes self-paced decisions on when to stop doing a mental task and immediately start the next one (Birch et al. (2002); Millán (2003); Millán et al. (2004b,a); Scherer et al. (2004a)). In such asynchronous protocols, the subject can voluntarily change the mental task being executed at any moment without waiting for external cues. The time of response of an asynchronous BCI can be below 1 s. For instance, in our approach the system responds every 0.5 s. The rapid responses of asynchronous BCIs, together with their performance, give a theoretical channel capacity between 1 and 1.5 bits/s. However, this bit rate was rarely achieved in practice for long periods. The important point is that whenever the subject needs to operate the brain-actuated device at high speed, for instance, to steer a wheelchair in a difficult part of the environment, the BCI enables the subject to deliver a rapid and accurate sequence of mental commands.

It is worth noting that the use of statistical rejection criteria, discussed in section 6.3, also helps to deal with an important aspect of a BCI, namely "idle" states where the user is not involved in any particular mental task. In an asynchronous protocol, idle states appear during the operation of a brain-actuated device while the subject does not want the BCI to carry out any action. Although the classifier is not explicitly trained to recognize those idle states, the BCI can process them adequately by giving no response.

6.5   Spatial Filtering

EEG signals are characterized by a poor signal-to-noise ratio and spatial resolution. Their quality is greatly improved by means of a surface laplacian (SL) derivation, which requires a large number of electrodes (normally 64–128). The SL estimate yields new potentials that represent better the cortical activity originated in radial sources immediately below the electrodes. Alternatively, raw EEG potentials can be transformed to the common average reference (CAR), which consists of removing the average activity of all the electrodes. For other spatial filtering algorithms see chapter 13.

The superiority of SL- and/or CAR-transformed signals over raw potentials for the operation of a BCI has been demonstrated in different studies (Babiloni et al. (2000); McFarland et al. (1997a); Mouriño (2003)). SL filtering can be done either globally or locally. In the former case, the raw EEG potentials are first interpolated using spherical splines of order order and then the second spatial derivative is taken which is sensitive to localized sources of electrical activity (Perrin et al. (1989, 1990)). The second derivative is evaluated only at the locations of the desired electrodes. In the local method, the average activity of neighboring electrodes—normally four—is subtracted from the electrode of interest. Normally, the SL is estimated with a high number of electrodes. But Babiloni et al. (2001) have shown that, for the operation of a BCI, global SL waveforms with either a low or a high number of electrodes give statistically similar classification results. Millán et al. (2004b,a) compute SL derivations from a few electrodes using local methods. Mouriño et al. (2001) compare different ways to compute the SL based on a few electrodes.

6.6   Experimental Protocol

After a short evaluation, users select the three mental tasks that they find easier from the following set: "relax"; imagination of "left" and "right" hand (or arm) movements; "cube rotation"; "subtraction"; or "word association." More specifically, the tasks consist of relaxing, imagining repetitive self-paced movements of the limb, visualizing a spinning cube, performing successive elementary subtractions by a fixed number (e.g., $64 - 3 = 61$, $61 - 3 = 58$, etc.), and generating words that begin with the same letter.

In a given training session, a subject participates in several consecutive training trials (normally four), each lasting approximately 5 min, and separated by breaks of 5 to 10 min. The subject is seated and performs the selected task for 10 to 15 s. Then, the operator indicates the next mental task randomly. With this protocol, the nature of the acquisition is such that there is a time-shift between the moment the subject actually starts performing a task and the moment the operator introduces the label for the subsequent period. Thus, the acquired EEG data is not time-locked to any kind of event in accordance with the principle of asynchronous BCI. While operating a brain-actuated application, the subjects do essentially the same as during the training trial, the only difference being that now they switch to the next mental task as soon as the desired action has been carried out.

During the training trials, users receive feedback through three buttons on the computer screen, each a different color and associated with one of the mental tasks to be recognized. A button lights up when an arriving EEG sample is classified as belonging to the corresponding mental task. After each training session, the statistical classifier, see section 6.7, is optimized offline.

EEG potentials are recorded at a variable number of locations, from 8 to 64. The raw EEG potentials are first transformed by means of a surface Laplacian (SL). Then, we extract relevant features from a few EEG channels (from 8 to 15) and the corresponding vector is used as input to the statistical classifier. To compute the features, we use the Welch periodogram algorithm to estimate the power spectrum of each selected SL-transformed channel over the last second. We average three 0.5-s segments with 50 percent overlap, which gives a frequency resolution of 2 Hz. The values in the frequency band 8–30 Hz are normalized according to the total energy in that band. The periodogram, and hence an EEG sample, is computed every 62.5 ms (i.e., 16 times per second). The resulting EEG sample is analyzed by the statistical classifier. No artifact rejection algorithm (for removing or filtering out eye or muscular movements) is applied, and all samples are kept for analysis. Each session has 4,800 samples approximately.

6.7 Statistical Gaussian Classifier

This is a short summary of the classifier we use in our BCI. For more details, see Millán et al. (2004a) and also chapter 16. We use a Gaussian classifier to separate the signal into the different classes of mental task. Each class is represented by a number of Gaussian prototypes, typically less than four. That is, we assume that the class-conditional probability function of class C_k is a superposition of N_k Gaussian prototypes. We also assume that all classes have equal prior probability. All classes have the same number of prototypes N_p, and for each class each prototype has equal weight $1/N_p$. Thus, the activity a_k^i of the ith prototype of class C_k for a given sample x is the value of the Gaussian with centre μ_k^i and covariance matrix Σ_k^i. From this we calculate the posterior probability y_k of the class C_k: It is the sum of the activities of all the prototypes of class k divided by the sum of the activities of all the prototypes of all the classes.

The classifier output for input vector x is now the class with the highest probability provided that the probability is above a given threshold, otherwise the result is "unknown." This rejection criterion gives the BCI the flexibility to not make a decision at any point without explicitly modeling an idle state. The choice of this probability threshold was guided by a receiver operating characteristic (ROC) study (Hauser et al. (2002)); the actual value is selected based on the performance of the each subject during the initial period of training.

Usually each prototype of each class would have an individual covariance matrix Σ_k^i, but to reduce the number of parameters, the model has a single diagonal covariance matrix common to all the prototypes of the same class. During offline training of the classifier, the prototype centers are initialized by a clustering algorithm, generally self-organizing maps (Kohonen (1997)). This initial estimate is then improved by stochastic gradient descent to minimize the mean square error $E = \frac{1}{2} \sum_k (y_k - t_k)^2$, where t is the target vector in the form 1-of-C; that is, if the second of three classes was the desired output, the target vector is $(0, 1, 0)$. The covariance matrices are computed individually and are then averaged over the prototypes of each class to give Σ_k.

6.8 Brain-Actuated Prototypes

BCI systems are being used to operate a number of brain-actuated applications that augment people's communication capabilities, provide new forms of entertainment, and also enable the operation of physical devices.

Our asynchronous BCI can be used to select letters from a virtual keyboard on a computer screen and to write a message (Millán (2003); Millán et al. (2004b)). Initially, the whole keyboard (twenty-six English letters plus the space to separate words, for a total of twenty-seven symbols organized in a matrix of three rows by nine columns) is divided in three blocks, each associated to one of the mental tasks. The association between blocks and mental tasks is indicated by the same colors as during the training phase. Each block contains an equal number of symbols, namely nine at this first level (three rows by three columns). Then, once the statistical classifier recognizes the block on which the subject is concentrating, this block is split into three smaller blocks, each having three symbols this time (one row). As one of this second-level blocks is selected, it is again split into three parts. At this third and final level, each block contains a single symbol. Finally, to select the desired symbol, the user concentrates on the symbol's associated mental task as indicated by the color of the symbol. This symbol goes to the message and the whole process starts again. Thus, the process of writing a single letter requires three decision steps.

The actual selection of a block incorporates some additional reliability measures (in addition to the statistical rejection criteria). In particular, a part of the keyboard is selected only when the corresponding mental task is recognized three times in a row. Also, in the case of an eventual wrong selection, users can undo it by concentrating immediately on one of the mental tasks of their choice. Thus, the system waits a short time after every selection (3.5 s) before going down to the next level. The mental task used to undo the selection is that for which the user exhibits the best performance. For our trained subjects, it takes 22.0 s on average to select a letter. This time includes recovering from eventual errors.

Millán (2003) illustrates the operation of a simple computer game, but other educational software could have been selected instead. Other "brain games" have been developed by the Berlin team (Krepki et al. (2007)). In our case, the "brain game" is the classical Pac-man. For the control of Pac-man, two mental tasks are enough to make it turn left or right. Pac-man changes direction of movement whenever one of the mental tasks is recognized twice in a row. In the absence of further mental commands, Pac-man moves forward until it reaches a wall, where it stops and waits for instructions.

Finally, it is also possible to make a brain-controlled hand orthosis open and close (Pfurtscheller and Neuper (2001)). Wolpaw and McFarland (2004) have recently demonstrated how subjects can learn to control two independent EEG rhythms and move a computer cursor in two dimensions. Despite these achievements, EEG-based BCIs are still considered too slow for controlling rapid and complex sequences of movements. But recently, Millán et al. (2004b,a) have shown for the first time that asynchronous analysis of EEG signals is sufficient for humans to continuously control a mobile robot—emulating a motorized wheelchair—along nontrivial trajectories requiring fast and frequent switches between mental tasks. Two human subjects learned to mentally drive the robot between rooms in a house-like environment visiting three or four rooms in the desired order. Furthermore, mental control was only marginally worse than manual control on the same task. A key element of this brain-actuated robot is shared control between two intelligent agents—the human user and the robot—so the user only gives high-level mental commands that the robot performs autonomously. In particular, the user's mental states are associated with high-level commands (e.g., "turn right at the next occasion") and the robot executes these commands autonomously using the readings of its on-board sensors. Another critical feature is that a subject can issue high-level commands at any moment. This is possible because the operation of the BCI is asynchronous and, unlike synchronous approaches, does not require waiting for external cues. The robot relies on a behavior-based controller to implement the high-level commands to guarantee obstacle avoidance and smooth turns. In this kind of controller, on-board sensors are read constantly and determine the next action to take (Arkin (1998)). For details of the behavior-based controller embedded in the brain-actuated mobile robot, see Millán et al. (2004a).

6.9   Discussion

For brain-actuated robots, distinguished from augmented communication through BCI, fast decision-making is critical. In this sense, real-time control of brain-actuated devices, especially robots and neuroprostheses, is the most challenging application for BCI.

While brain-actuated robots have been demonstrated in the laboratory, this technology is not yet ready to be taken out and used in real-world situations. For this reason, we are working to improve our initial demonstrator, in collaboration with several European groups, along four lines. The first is the development of a more powerful adaptive shared autonomy framework for the cooperation of the human user and the robot in achieving the target. The second line is how to get a better picture of electrical activity all across the brain with high spatial accuracy without implanting electrodes but rather by a noninvasive estimation from scalp EEG signals. Local field potentials (LFP) are produced by the electrical activity of small groups of neurons. Recent developments in electrical neuroimaging allow the transformation of scalp-recorded EEG into estimated local field potentials (eLFP) as though they were directly recorded within the brain (Grave de Peralta Menendez et al. (2004)). Noninvasive eLFP has the potential to unravel scalp EEG signals, attributing to each brain area its own temporal (spectral) activity. Preliminary results have shown significant improvements in the classification of bimanual motor tasks using eLFP with respect to scalp EEG (Grave de Peralta Menendez et al. (2005b)). It is worth noting that through this technique we also could gain a better understanding of the nature of the brain activity driving the BCI. For more details on this research line, see chapter 16.

The third research line seek to improve the robustness of a BCI. Thus, a direction of research is online adaptation of the interface to the user to keep the BCI constantly tuned to its owner (Buttfield et al. (2006); Millán (2004)). The point here is that as subjects gain experience they develop new capabilities and change their brain activity patterns. In addition, brain signals change naturally over time. In particular, this is the case from one session to the next, where we train the classifier on the first session and apply it to the second. Thus, online learning can be used to adapt the classifier throughout its use and keep it tuned to drifts in the signals it is receiving in each session. Preliminary work shows the feasibility and benefits of this approach (Buttfield et al. (2006)). For more details on this research line, see chapter 18.

The fourth research line is the analysis of neural correlates of high-level cognitive states such as errors, alarms, attention, frustration, and confusion. Information about these states is embedded in the EEG with the mental commands intentionally generated by the user. The ability to detect and adapt to these states would enable the BCI to interact with the user in a much more meaningful way. One of these high-level states is the awareness of erroneous responses, whose neural correlate arises in the millisecond range. Thus, user's commands are executed only if no error is detected in this short time. Recent results have shown satisfactory single-trial recognition of errors that leads to significant improvement of the BCI performance (Ferrez and Millán (2005)). In addition, this new type of error potential—which is generated in response to errors made by the BCI rather than by the user—may provide feedback on the BCI performance that, in combination with online adaptation, could allow us to improve the BCI while it is being used. For more details on this research line, see chapter 17.

Acknowledgments

This work is supported by the Swiss National Science Foundation through the National Centre of Competence in Research on "Interactive Multimodal Information Management (IM2)," and also by the European IST Programme FET Project FP6-003758. This chapter reflects only the authors' views; funding agencies are not liable for any use that may be made of the information contained herein.

Notes

E-mail for correspondence: jose.millan@idiap.ch

(1) Channel capacity is the maximum possible information transfer rate, or bit rate, through a channel.

7   Brain Interface Design for Asynchronous Control

Jaimie F. Borisoff
Neil Squire Society
220 - 2250 Boundary Rd.
Burnaby, B.C., V5M 3Z3, Canada

International Collaboration on
Repair Discoveries
The University of British Columbia
6270 University Blvd., Vancouver
British Columbia, V6T 1Z4, Canada

Steve G. Mason
Neil Squire Society
220 - 2250 Boundary Rd.
Burnaby, B.C., V5M 3Z3, Canada

Gary E. Birch
Neil Squire Society
220 - 2250 Boundary Rd.
Burnaby, B.C., V5M 3Z3, Canada

International Collaboration on
Repair Discoveries
The University of British Columbia
6270 University Blvd., Vancouver
British Columbia, V6T 1Z4, Canada

Department of Electrical and
Computer Engineering
The University of British Columbia
2356 Main Mall, Vancouver
V6T 1Z4, Canada

7.1   Abstract

The concept of self-paced control has recently emerged from within the general field of brain-computer interface research. The use of assistive devices in real-world environments is best served by interfaces operated in an asynchronous manner. This self-paced or asynchronous mode of device control is more natural than the more commonly studied synchronized control mode whereby the system dictates the control of the user. The Neil Squire Society develops asynchronous, direct brain-switches for self-paced control applications.

Our latest switch design operated with a mean activation rate of 73 percent and false positive error rates of 2 percent. This report provides an introduction to asynchronous control, summarizes our results to date, and details some key issues that specifically relate to brain interface design for asynchronous control.

7.2 Introduction

Within the context of general brain interface (BI) technology research, The Neil Squire Brain Interface lab has focused on BI system design specifically for asynchronous control environments. This focus has arisen from our experience in the more general field of assistive technology research in which emphasis is placed on the use of assistive devices in real-world environments (Mason and Birch (2003); Mason et al. (2005b); Birch et al. (1995)). These environments are ones in which the most natural mode of device control is self-paced or asynchronous, in contrast to synchronized control environments where the system dictates the control of the user. Much of the BI research reported to date has been evaluated only during synchronized activities—thus, these results make it difficult to predict the usability of such systems in more typical control situations. The goal of our brain interface project is to develop a robust multistate, asynchronous brain-controlled switch for evaluation and operation in the most natural manner in real-world environments. This chapter intends to present an overview of asynchronous control, a summary of our efforts to develop asynchronous BI systems, as well as a discussion of several major issues that have arisen from asynchronous BI development.

7.3 Asynchronous Control

Asynchronous (and self-paced) control refers to the type of control where output signal levels are changed or commands are issued only when control is intended. We differentiate periods of intentional control (IC) from periods when there is no intention to control, a period which we refer to as the no control (NC) state. During the NC state, one would expect the system output to remain neutral or unchanged. Examples of NC periods are when a user is talking, daydreaming, thinking about a problem, or simply observing whatever application they are controlling. In many applications, people are more frequently in an NC state than actually intending control. Typical examples of this type of asynchronous control are turning on lights, changing television channels, and interacting with a computer. Asynchronous control is characteristic of most real-world control applications and is what most people expect from interface technology. For instance, when you remove your hand from your computer mouse, you enter an NC state and the mouse output remains stable and unchanged—that is, the mouse pointer does not continue to move on the computer screen. The mouse is then available for control simply by replacing your hand. In short, asynchronous control allows the user to define when things happen.

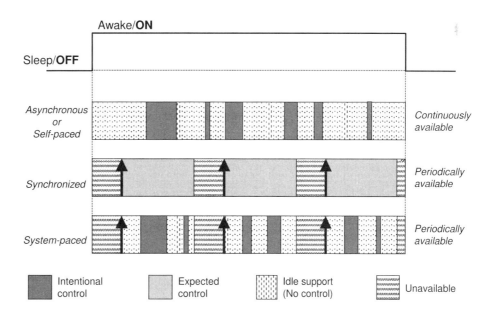

Figure 7.1 Schematic representation of different BI control paradigms. System operating paradigms in which intentional control and idle support are available are either asynchronous or system-paced paradigms. A synchronous paradigm assumes expected control during its periods of availability and does not support periods of no control. The arrows indicate system-driven cues, which need to be displayed to alert the user that a period of control availability is about to occur.

The neutral or unchanging system output response desired during periods of NC is what we call "system idling." Brain interface technology must support idling for effective and sophisticated control to be realized. This is analogous to a car engine in that when no gas is applied (the NC state), the engine idles at a stable rpm. If the car engine in this example was poor at idling, engine RPM would fluctuate, perhaps even stall. In the context of a discrete single-state BI switch, poor idling is indicated by false switch activations during periods of NC. Often how well BI transducers idle are measured by reporting the rate of false activations (or false positive (FP) error rates for examples of two-class discrete switches). However, BI transducer idling characteristics have not been reported in most BI research publications to date. Most publications report only true switch activations or true positives (TPs), the performance metric for measuring switch accuracy during the IC state. A more complete measure of asynchronous control would use both true and false activation rates as performance metrics.

In contrast to asynchronous operation, most BI transducers are only tested in synchronized (or synchronous) control environments. After a synchronized BI system is turned on, the user is regularly prompted for input and is allowed to control the assistive device only during specific periods explicitly defined by the system, as shown in figure 7.1. This is a system-driven control strategy, which is thought to be an awkward mode of interaction for most typical applications and can cause significant user frustration and fatigue. The differences between synchronous and asynchronous control are exemplified in a simple example of watching TV. An asynchronous TV controller allows users to simply change channels at any time they wish, and the channel selection is stable during the lengthy periods the users are watching TV (an NC state). In contrast, a synchronous TV controller would regularly poll the users to ask if they would like to change the channel. Synchronous TV control renders the changing of channels to specific periods of time set by the system, perhaps interrupting the users' viewing. This has the following two serious drawbacks: (1) the BI transducer will make a control decision regardless of whether the person is actually intending control, thus there is the possibility of accidentally changing channels; and 2) the fact that the users cannot change channels at their whim signifies that users would need to wait for the system polling period to occur in order to engage the BI transducer. Figure 7.1 provides a graphical representation of the various temporal control paradigms.

From our experience with assistive device development, two factors capture the essence of the temporal control paradigms used in BI technology (as well as other biometric-based interface technology): the previously mentioned idle support and system availability (Mason and Birch (2005)). Availability defines when the interface device allows user control and can be broadly categorized as continuously available (always on) or periodically available. Continuously available control is what we experience with standard computer interface devices: The device is always ready for the user to initiate control. Periodically available control is used (1) for initial trial-based technology development or (2) for restricting the signal processing complexity in real-world operation. It is assumed that for the periods between control periods, the interface device blocks a user's attempt to control, and outputs a value representing "no control is possible at this time."

As discussed, "idle support" indicates if the interface device will support idling. Control paradigms that do not support idling will produce an unintended action (i.e., an error) if and when the user enters the NC state. Given human nature, this will undoubtedly happen, although the frequency will depend on the user and the application. The problem with interface technology that does not support idling is referred to as the "Midas touch problem" by the eye-tracking community (Jacob (1990); Yamato et al. (2000)) since the system translates every "touch" (with the eyes/gaze) into some action, even if not intended.

Given these definitions, four primary control paradigms can be defined (Table 7.1) based on their idle support and availability. A more thorough discussion of these paradigms has been published (Mason and Birch (2005)). To summarize, they are asynchronous (or self-paced), synchronous, system-paced, and constantly engaged. The latter paradigm is an impractical mode of operation where the user is continuously controlling the interface without a break and any NC activity will cause an error; thus, it is not found in typical applications. Although four general operating paradigms have been identified, we feel that a BI system that operates in a true asynchronous mode would provide the most natural

Availability	Idle Support	
	No idle support	*Idle support*
Periodically	Synchronous (synchronized)	System-paced
Continuously	Constantly engaged	Asynchronous (self-paced)

Table 7.1 Control paradigms.

assistive device operation and greatly impact the independence of people with severe motor disabilities.

7.4 EEG-Based Asynchronous Brain-Switches

Asynchronous or self-paced control applications that require idle support and concomitant low FP rates need specific signal processing algorithms to handle the NC state. Not only must the TP rate of a BI system be optimized to accurately detect IC, focus must also be placed on the minimization of FP rates during periods when the user is not controlling the interface. As detailed in section 7.5, there is a trade-off between TP accuracy and FP rates; thus, the specific characteristics of an application need to be considered when optimizing asynchronous BI system performance.

The first asynchronous BI technology triggered from spontaneous electroencephalography (EEG) was our brain-switch based on the outlier processing method (OPM) signal processing (Birch et al. (1993)). The OPM used robust, statistical signal processing methods to extract single-trial voluntary movement-related potentials (VMRPs) from EEG related to finger movement. The accuracy of the OPM brain-switch was very high, with TP rates greater than 90 percent. However, the relatively poor performance during system idle periods with FP rates between 10 and 30 percent limits the usefulness of the OPM as an asynchronous switch. (Although we believe that the EEG feature extraction algorithms of the OPM will be useful in the development of a multiposition asynchronous brain-switch.)

A search for a set of EEG features more appropriate for asynchronous control was then conducted. This work also focused on attempted VMRPs because voluntary movement control is an existing and natural internal control system in humans that seems ideally suited as a neural mechanism for a BI transducer. We use the term "attempted" here to emphasize that individuals with spinal cord injury (SCI) attempt to move their fingers to control our transducers in the same manner that able-bodied people make real movements during our BI experiments. The only difference between the people with SCI and those without are the actual physical movements that may or may not occur during their attempted finger movement. It should also be noted that many labs use motor imagery instead of real or attempted movements, possibly a very different neural mechanism.

From a time-frequency analysis of EEG patterns elicited from NC states versus VMRP states, it was observed that the relative power in the 1–4 Hz band from ensemble VMRP data increased compared to data from the NC state (Mason and Birch (2000)). Thus, our attention was focused on this low frequency band. A wavelet analysis exposed a set of relatively stable spatiotemporal features from EEG channels over the supplementary motor area (SMA) and primary motor area (MI). Using this new feature set, the low-frequency asynchronous switch design, or LF-ASD, was developed as a new asynchronous brain-switch (Mason and Birch (2000)).

Our most recent online study using the LF-ASD demonstrated TP rates of 30 to 78 percent during IC states in combination with very low FP rates of 0.5 to 2 percent during NC, when used by both able-bodied and spinal cord injured subjects (Birch et al. (2002)). Note, as explained in section 7.5, the performance characteristics of a given asynchronous control design can vary over its receiver operating curve (ROC). In this study, we intentionally operated the system toward the lower end of FP activations because our subjects found the brain-switch frustrating to use if the FP rate was too high (usually over 2 percent from our experience).

Since the initial design, several offline studies have been performed that incorporated additional signal processing steps in order to improve the performance of the LF-ASD (Bashashati et al. (2005); Borisoff et al. (2004); Mason et al. (2004); Birch et al. (2003)). The addition of EEG signal normalization, switch output debounce, and feature set dimensionality reduction blocks produced design improvements that increased the TP rate by an average of 33 percent over the previous version (Borisoff et al. (2004)). Importantly, this performance gain was seen in both able-bodied subjects and subjects with high-level SCI (Borisoff et al. (2004)). We have also observed that there is valuable information in the temporal path with which the feature vectors navigate the feature space. We have created a new design using this information with preliminary results from four subjects of a mean TP rate of 73 percent for an FP rate of 2 percent (Bashashati et al. (2005)). These performance metrics represented a total system classification accuracy of more than 97 percent when the system is evaluated during continuous use. This brain-switch represents the state of the art in asynchronous BI switch technology, although more improvements are underway.

Despite the need for idle support in most real-world applications, few other BI laboratories have performed work on asynchronous transducers. The other notable players in this specific BI field are Levine and Huggins, who have been working in this area since the mid-1990s (Levine et al. (2000)); and Millán et al. (2004a), Yom-Tov and Inbar (2003), and Townsend et al. (2004), who have joined this effort more recently. Perhaps because of the relatively few long-term participants in asynchronous BI design, the terminology and evaluation methods used by these groups vary significantly. Fortunately, this is becoming more standardized as interest in this field grows, as seen at the Third International Meeting on Brain-Computer Interface Technology in Albany, New York, June 2005.

7.5   Asynchronous Control Design Issues

Our experience with asynchronous BI design and testing over the past several years has revealed many issues about the human-technology interface specific to asynchronous control that need to be addressed when studying this mode of control.

The first design issue is quite apparent: False positive rates during the NC state must be very low. From our experience, relatively high FP error rates cause undue user frustration with the interface. This invariably leads to poorer performance, concentration, and motivation over time. We have found that a subject would rather experience more trouble performing accurate hits (i.e., a low TP rate), which naturally forces more concentration and is challenging to the user, than have a high rate of seemingly haphazard false activations, which appear uncontrollable to the user.

One method of evaluating asynchronous control that considers both TP and FP rates is the use of receiver operating characteristic (ROC) curves. An example is shown in figure 7.2a with an expanded section highlighting low FP rates shown in figure 7.2b.

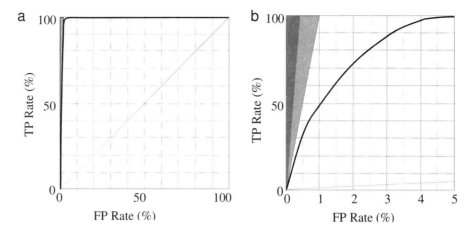

Figure 7.2 Asynchronous BI performance expressed with receiver operating characteristic (ROC) curves. The curve on the right is an exploded view of the 1–6% FP rate in the ROC curve on the left. The shaded regions depict targeted operating zones for various applications.

Because of the importance in operating BI transducers with low FP error rates, it may be beneficial to just focus on the right-most ROC curve shown. This focuses the design on performance metrics in which FP rates are relatively low (figure 7.2b). This also leads to another use for ROC curves: ROC curves reveal clues about "tuning" the performance of asynchronous controls. The ROC curve shows the entire scope of possible operating setups for a particular asynchronous BI device. By tuning various parameters in a BI design, one can force BI transducer operation to a desired operating point along the ROC curve. In the example of our two-state LF-ASD brain-switch (analogous to a toggle switch—either pulsed "on" or else in idle mode), the appropriate tuning is performed by scaling the relative magnitudes of NC state feature vectors versus intentional control state feature vectors in a subject's classification codebook (Borisoff et al. (2004)). In our online experiments, we tune our classifiers to operate the LF-ASD at an FP rate under 2 percent. Interestingly, with the LF-ASD, FP rates well under 1 percent seem necessary to keep average periods of time between FPs in the range of 30 seconds or more. These levels are depicted as shaded regions in figure 7.2.

Another possible caveat to this treatment of FP rates was revealed in our online experiments. We have shown that FPs typically clump together in a string of multiple, closely spaced false activations (Borisoff et al. (2004)). On a positive note, this clumping of FPs often leaves large periods of system idle time free of FPs. One simple method to deal with this performance issue is the use of switch-output jitter reduction methods. We recently added a switch debounce block to the signal processing stream in the LF-ASD to significantly improve error rates by reducing the FP jitter in the switch output (Borisoff et al. (2004)). The trade-off in this approach is transducer availability. Increasing the debounce time will decrease the time the transducer is available for classification (and thus control). An appropriate balance in these two effects would most likely be dependent on specific applications.

FP Rate (%)	Seconds	Minutes
2.00	3.1	0.05
1.00	6.3	0.10
0.50	12.5	0.21
0.25	25.0	0.42
0.10	62.5	1.04
0.01	625	10.4

Table 7.2 Intra-False Positive Rates: FP = false positive. Time is calculated from the average number of false positives when a BI transducer is outputting classifications at every 1/16th second. An FP rate below 0.25% is needed for periods of time between FPs that approach more than half a minute. The goal target zone for operation of the LF-ASD is shown in the shaded boxes.

As alluded to in the above paragraphs, another design issue regarding false positive rates is simply that not all reported FP rates are equal. The actual rate of error occurrences (in terms of a user's time) is completely dependent upon the output classification rate of a particular transducer. For example, the LF-ASD brain-switch produces a classification output every 1/16th of a second. At an operating FP rate of 1 percent, this rate corresponds to an FP every 6.3 seconds on average (assuming a uniform distribution of FPs). For another system that generates an output every 1 second, a 1 percent FP rate represents an FP every 100 seconds. A summary of how percentage FP rates translate to actual time between errors is shown in table 7.2 for a transducer that outputs every 1/16th of a second. Average time between errors greater than 30 seconds, which seems to be a reasonable design goal to aim for, require an FP rate of under 0.25 percent! Thus, false activation rates should probably be reported as time rates along with raw percentages.

Another issue related to FP rates and asynchronous control is the reporting methodology for experiments in which BI transducers are tested in synchronous environments. It is difficult, if not impossible, to determine if technology tested only in synchronized environments would be potentially useful for natural self-paced (asynchronous) control applications. As such, it would be beneficial to the community if researchers working with synchronized testing environments would report their transducer's response during NC states. Actually, it may be beneficial to report this regardless of potential asynchronous control use, as this characterizes the potential errors that would occur when a user is accidentally in an NC state (i.e., not paying attention) instead of an IC state when intentional control is expected.

The next asynchronous design issue follows from a simple application analysis that estimates the temporal characteristics of NC and IC states for specific applications. For instance, environmental controllers may have periods of time ranging from several seconds to tens of minutes between the issuance of IC commands (figure 7.3). In contrast, the neural control of a robotic device would typically have intercontrol times on the order of fractions of seconds during periods of intense usage (figure 7.3). These two applications with very different usage profiles could conceivably use the same BI transducer with different tuning characteristics (i.e., different TP and FP rates, or a different operating

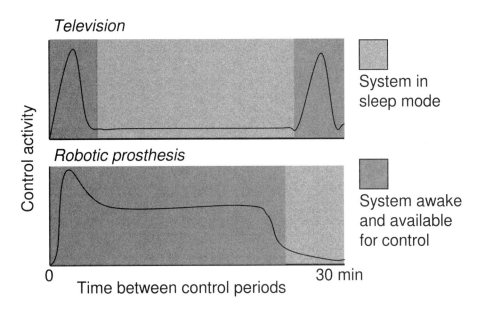

Figure 7.3 Usage profiles as represented by probability distributions of NC periods. Different applications have distinct usage profiles. Some applications have long periods of no control states, while other applications have a more constant level of control activity. Often it is beneficial to put the system into a sleep mode (lighter shades) during long periods of inactivity to minimize false positives.

point on an ROC curve). Thus, the usage profile of a specific application should drive the level of BI transducer performance needed.

A related issue is the ubiquitous ON/OFF problem in biometric-based assistive technology design. Developing an automated switch to turn a BI system ON is recognized as a difficult problem similar to the open microphone problem with speech recognition. For users that lack a means to do this physically, the technology requires a mechanism and method for users to turn the system on and off by themselves. Turning the system off is assumed to be one of the control options available to users once the system has been turned on. An automated BI-controlled mechanism to turn a system ON is actually one that must operate in awake versus sleep mode rather than on and off mode. Generally, such a controller has to differentiate between all possible innate brain states and the system awake state. Practically, the mechanism probably could be implemented as a sequence of commands, where each step in the sequence confirms user intent to turn the system to the awake mode. Developing this concept further in regards to application usage profiles, an application in which very long periods of NC states are inherent (such as watching television) could include an operating mode in which the BI device is put into sleep mode (figures 7.3 and 7.4). This would eliminate FPs during this period and only require a simple sequence of commands to step the transducer back to full awake mode whereby IC is again available (figures 7.3 and 7.4). Another factor to consider here is the ease (or difficulty) of correcting a mistake, and the cost of such a mistake. If an application has profound costs associated with an FP (an ex-

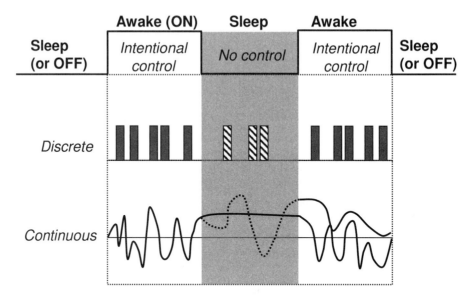

Figure 7.4 Control system operating modes. Once the device is physically turned ON (perhaps by an attendant), device operation may cycle between intentional control states and no control states. Device operation may also cycle between awake and sleep modes to minimize false positives (FPs). A discrete transducer is prone to false activations or FPs during the no control (NC) periods in awake mode, while a continuous transducer may be prone to unstable output during NC. To eliminate FPs or unstable output during long periods of NC, the device may be alternatively put into a sleep mode.

ample such as launching nuclear missiles is given here somewhat facetiously, however, it demonstrates this issue quite clearly), FPs could be greatly minimized by including multiple operating levels of the sleep mode. Stepping the system to full awake mode would require the system to sequence through successively higher modes, each of which has the characteristic of higher FP rates, and which requires intentional command sequences to access. Conversely, applications in which the costs of FPs are low and easily corrected may be operated with higher FP rates and less intricate sequences of sleep/awake levels. Thus, the seemingly simple observation of the differences in applications can lead to quite complex design criteria when optimizing BI systems.

The last design issue discussed here relates to the challenge inherent in the testing and evaluation of online, asynchronous systems designed for self-paced IC states and long periods of NC. The issue is one of how to structure tasks during customization, training, and testing phases in a manner that fulfills the needs of each specific phase. The initial customization of a BI transducer requires accurate time-stamping for system calibration and classifier training. This may necessitate the use of system-guided and system-paced tasks where the system knows exactly what the user intended and when. However, this may result in diminished transducer performance: For instance, a particular cuing mechanism used during the customization phase may cause visual and/or some other cognitively evoked potential. Thus, the brain signals recorded during customization may be different from the signals recorded during a true online asynchronous application run without the cueing mechanism. If possible, it would be beneficial to train and test on systems in very similar control environments. Another consideration is the apparatus necessary for data markup and synchronization. Online asynchronous evaluations using self-guided and self-paced tasks require the subject to self-report errors because the system is otherwise not aware of their intentions. In the past, we have employed a sip and puff mechanism for subject self-report of errors (i.e., false positives and false negatives). Since the subject is the only one aware of what has occurred, this method is a necessary one. The downside is that the data collected during periods of self-report are contaminated with various artifacts resulting from the act of reporting. Compared to synchronous BI system evaluations, an accurate assessment of asynchronous system performance is difficult with several considerations that may impact the evaluation.

7.6 Conclusion

Asynchronous brain interface design is a difficult, though rewarding, path as asynchronous control is the most natural and user-friendly mode of device control. A successful asynchronous BI design will enable sophisticated and effective control of many useful devices for a host of individuals with significant motor impairments. We have developed a two-state brain-switch prototype for asynchronous control applications that operates with total system classification accuracies of more than 97 percent when used by both able-bodied subjects and subjects with high-level spinal cord injuries. This typically represents a false positive activation rate of less than 2 percent during periods of no control, a performance that somewhat mitigates user frustration and enables rudimentary control. These brain-switches could be used with scanning menu systems in devices such as environmental controllers or virtual keyboards. However promising, these error rates are still too high for real-world use; thus, we continue to make improvements to our BI designs. We also strive to solve many of the other issues associated with asynchronous control design, especially those associated with system evaluations. We hope this approach provides a strong foundation for continued efforts to build a critically needed device for asynchronous control applications.

Acknowledgments

This work was supported by the Canadian Institutes of Health Research and the Natural Sciences and Engineering Research Council of Canada.

Notes

E-mail for correspondence: borisoff@gmail.com

II Invasive BCI Approaches

Introduction

Brain-computer interfaces, or brain-machine interfaces, can use neural activity recorded from the surface, such as EEG, or neural activity recorded from inside the skull or brain, such as ECoG or single- resp. multiunit activity. The chapters in this part consist of studies that use invasive recording methods to acquire BCI signals. As pointed out by Huggins et al. (see chapter 8), invasive techniques such as ECoG have several advantages relative to noninvasive methods such as EEG. These include the fact that they are permanently available and do not require application of electrodes prior to each recording session. ECoG provides a signal of broader bandwidth, which includes the interesting gamma frequency band. Invasive methods also provide more localized signals, which can translate into more distinct spatial input channels. Finally, invasive methods have a better signal-to-noise ratio since noise sources such as EMG or ocular artifacts are much less prominent. These advantages must, however, be weighed against the risk of surgery and the potential development of complications such as infection. In addition, problems that develop with the recording electrodes over time require either additional surgeries or a termination of device use. This is an ongoing discussion that is far from conclusive at this point (e.g., Lebedev and Nicolelis (2006); Berger and Glanzman (2005); Hochberg et al. (2006), see chapters 1 and 22). For example, Huggins et al. suggest that ECoG provides a good balance between the fidelity associated with more invasive techniques, such as implanted electrodes, and the safety associated with EEG.

In chapter 8, Huggins et al. provide empirical evidence that greater classification accuracy can be obtained with ECoG as compared to EEG. The data were collected in human patients being evaluated for surgery to treat epilepsy and were analyzed offline. This finding is important since many researchers claim that their methods are superior while not providing such explicit comparison.

Michael Black and John Donoghue (chapter 9) develop simple linear models for real-time control of cursor movement from a high-density microelectrode array implanted in monkey motor cortex. Black and Donoghue note that simple linear models are desirable because of ease of implementation and interpretability of results. In addition, the continuous output produced by a Kalman filter may be more appropriate for control of motor tasks than the output of discrete classifiers. His model is consistent with the known cosine tuning properties of motor cortex neurons. Since research has shown that motor units are tuned to several dimensions of movement, Black and Donoghue include position, velocity, and acceleration in this dynamic model and provide a proof of concept.

Dawn Taylor (chapter 10) discusses functional electrical stimulation for restoration of movement. The chapter describes random and systematic prediction errors that occur when units recorded from monkey motor cortex are used to predict arm movements with an open-loop paradigm. When animals receive visual feedback, the system becomes coadaptive. As a result, the animals are able to make use of the inherent ability of their nervous systems to make feedforward adjustments and to correct for consistent errors in the executed motor plan. In addition, feedback allows online corrections of random errors in the execution of the motor plan, and an increase in the information content of the recorded neural signals.

Nenadic et al. (chapter 11) also report on the offline analysis of field potentials recorded from human patients evaluated for epilepsy surgery. Depth recording electrodes were used in this case. Nenadic et al. used a novel feature extraction method, information discriminant analysis, to project a large number of features onto a smaller dimensional space, making the classification problem more computationally manageable. The authors conclude that local field potentials are suitable signals for neuroprosthetic use.

Shpigelman et al. (chapter 12) introduce kernel-based methods for predicting trajectories from spike data. An important point is the use of a novel kernel function—the spike kernel—that allows the combination of a nonlinear observation to state mapping with a linear state mapping. They refer to this model as a discriminative dynamic tracker (DDT). This model thus combines techniques from support vector regression and Kalman filtering.

The chapters in this part raise a number of interesting issues. Is the increased risk inherent with invasive recordings offset by improved performance? Do the demands of real-time performance with high-density recordings require simple models? Does the inherent closed-loop nature of communication and control impose additional requirements on system design? At present, the answers to these and many other questions about BCI system designs are not known. Many studies to date have provided proofs of principle. However, answering these fundamental questions about optimal system design will require further comparative studies that provide empirical support.

The relative advantage in signal quality of invasive recordings over noninvasive recordings will depend upon future developments in sensor technology in both of these areas. Currently, degradation of performance over time is a serious problem with chronic unit recording, although potential solutions to this problem are being investigated (e.g., Spataro et al. (2005)). Likewise research continues aimed at improving surface recording technology (e.g., Harland et al. (2002)), and new modalities may enter this field (e.g., Franceschini et al. (2003)). Computational demands imposed by more complex models for decoding continue to become less eminent with the development of faster computer hardware. However, different issues related to model complexity, such as the stability of dynamic coadapting systems, still remain and require dedicated research efforts.

The chapters in this part provide an interesting sample of approaches in the rapidly developing field of brain-machine communication and control. Though not exhaustive, they give some perspective on the diversity of approaches currently being explored. For further reading, we make reference to a number of important contributions to invasive BCI systems (e.g., Tillery and Taylor (2004); Carmena et al. (2003); Serruya et al. (2002); Nicolelis (2001); Shenoy et al. (2003); Hochberg et al. (2006); Kamitani and Tong (2005); Mehring et al. (2003); Leuthardt et al. (2004); Hill et al. (2006)) and recent reviews (e.g., Nicolelis (2001); Lebedev and Nicolelis (2006); Haynes and Rees (2006); Berger and Glanzman (2005)).

Dennis J. McFarland and Klaus-Robert Müller

8   Electrocorticogram as a Brain-Computer Interface Signal Source

Jane E. Huggins and Simon P. Levine
Departments of Physical Medicine and Rehabilitation and Biomedical Engineering
University of Michigan, Ann Arbor
1500 East Medical Center Drive, Ann Arbor
MI 48109-0032, USA

Bernhard Graimann
Laboratory of Brain Computer Interfaces
Graz University of Technology
Graz, Austria

Se Young Chun and Jeffrey A. Fessler
Department of Electrical Engineering and Computer Science
University of Michigan
Ann Arbor, USA

8.1   Abstract

The use of electrocorticogram (ECoG) as the signal source for brain-computer interfaces (BCIs) has advantages for both the potential BCI user and the BCI researcher. However, research using ECoG can be logistically challenging. Visualization of time- and frequency-based characteristics of movement-related potentials in ECoG illustrates the features available for detection by a BCI and their spatial distribution. A quantitative comparison of the detection possible with EEG and ECoG verifies the signal quality advantages of ECoG and the utility of spatial filtering for improving detection. A quadratic detector based on a two-covariance signal model is presented as the basis for a BCI using ECoG, and the detection achieved by the quadratic detector is compared to BCI methods based on cross-correlation and bandpower. The quadratic detector provides dramatically improved detection and response time over the cross-correlation-based method.

8.2 Introduction

Electrocorticogram (ECoG) is recorded by electrodes implanted inside the skull but not penetrating the brain, providing a unique balance between invasiveness and signal quality. Interest in ECoG as a control source for brain-computer interfaces (BCIs) has grown dramatically over the past decade. When the University of Michigan Direct Brain Interface (UM-DBI) project started in 1994, BCI research was focused almost entirely on electroencephalogram (EEG) in humans (Birch et al. (1993); Pfurtscheller et al. (1995); Wolpaw et al. (1991)), and intracerebral recordings in animals (Drake et al. (1988); Georgopoulos et al. (1988)). Apart from one report of an eye-gaze-controlled system in which intracranial electrodes were employed to avoid artifacts during daily interface use (Sutter (1992)), no other researchers were pursuing ECoG for development of an interface. In recent years, interest in ECoG as a signal source for BCIs has intensified. At the Third International Meeting on BCI Technology in 2005, 16 out of 120 abstracts included references to ECoG (Brain-Computer Interface Technology: Third International Meeting (2005)) compared to 1 abstract out of 23 at the First International BCI Meeting in 1999 (Brain-Computer Interface Technology: Theory and Practice—First International Meeting Program and Papers (1999)).

ECoG provides a number of practical benefits both to the BCI user and researcher. For a BCI user, the use of implanted electrodes (whether ECoG or intracerebral) provides the potential for the interface to be permanently available, eliminating both the need to have an assistant apply the electrodes whenever use of the interface is desired and variations in electrode placement that could affect performance. Implanted electrodes also reduce the visibility of the interface by minimizing or eliminating the need to wear external components. For the BCI researcher, there is the advantage of working with electrode technology that is in routine clinical use as well as many advantages in signal quality. Subdural ECoG electrodes have been shown to be anatomically and electrophysiologically stable (Margalit et al. (2003)), unlike intracerebral microelectrodes (Liu et al. (1999); Kipke et al. (2003)). ECoG avoids problems with muscular and ocular artifacts (Sutter (1992); Zaveri et al. (1992)) and offers greater localization of the origin of the signals (Salanova et al. (1993)) as well as a wider range of available frequencies (Leuthardt et al. (2004)) and higher signal-to-noise ratio as compared to EEG recordings (Margalit et al. (2003)). For both the BCI user and researcher, there is the potential benefit of shorter training times for BCI control with ECoG (Leuthardt et al. (2004)) in comparison to the prolonged training required by some EEG-based systems (Wolpaw et al. (2002)).

Disadvantages of ECoG electrodes for the subject include the risks of surgery, recovery time, and the necessity of a repeat surgery if replacement of the electrodes is required. For the researcher, the disadvantages of working with ECoG are the limited access to human subjects, the constraints on working in an acute care setting, and the lack of control over certain aspects of the experiment. Typically, human ECoG is available only when people have electrodes implanted as part of treatment for another condition such as intractable epilepsy. Clinical considerations for the treatment of this condition therefore take priority over research. While this is entirely appropriate, scheduling difficulties and the challenges of working in an acute hospital setting often limit time with the subject and introduce uncontrollable variability in experimental protocols.

ECoG subjects are selected based entirely on the availability of implanted electrodes. Variations in subject attention, concentration, and interest have the potential to affect subject performance. Some subjects are excited by the opportunity to participate in research, want to understand everything, and are highly motivated to succeed. Other subjects view participation as a minor variation in a generally boring day, but do not have a particular interest in the research or a desire to do well. All subjects are recovering from a recent surgery for electrode implantation and are experiencing varying degrees of pain and fatigue, and some may be recovering from a recent seizure. Some subjects have chronic memory problems or other impairments associated with their epilepsy. Further, access to the patients must be scheduled around clinically necessary procedures. Patient care activities such as taking pain medications may interrupt data collection sessions, though these can be done during breaks between data runs. Further, subjects in an epilepsy surgery program naturally will be anxious about their upcoming surgery and its potential benefit for their condition. Many subjects will have had changes to their normal medications for seizure suppression. In some cases, data collection sessions can be scheduled only at times when subjects have been sleep deprived in an attempt to precipitate a seizure for diagnostic purposes. Interruptions of experimental sessions that have psychological impact for the patient/subject are also possible. In one instance, a surgeon asked us to step out while he talked to the patient. When we resumed data collection, we found that the patient had been informed that he would not be able to be helped by the surgery. The patient chose to end the data collection session soon afterward.

The locations of ECoG electrodes implanted as part of the standard epilepsy surgery procedures are not under the control of the BCI researcher. Instead, electrode coverage is tailored to the epileptic symptoms of individual subjects with electrode placements being those that target typical regions of epileptic foci such as temporal lobe. Electrode coverage ranges from a few temporal strips accompanying temporal depth electrodes to bilateral grids over motor cortex.

These logistical constraints on experimental work emphasize factors for creating clinically accepted BCI systems that are frequently overlooked during the development process. The limited time with the ECoG subjects only allows for short training periods during a data collection session. Likewise, if any daily configuration was necessary in a clinical BCI, brevity would be an important factor. Epilepsy surgery subjects have many concerns and distractions apart from the BCI experiment. Likewise, in daily use, BCI operation must not require so much attention that the subject cannot think about the task for which the BCI is being used. As researchers, we attempt to reduce distractions and maximize time with the subjects. However, it is important to realize that many of the issues encountered during research in an acute care setting will reappear when BCIs move out of the experimental environment and into daily use. When developing a BCI for use in either an experimental or eventual clinical setting, practical considerations compel us to put a priority on not only reliable detection, but also on real-time system implementation, rapid interface response time, and short configuration and training periods.

8.3   Subjects and Experimental Setup

The subjects for this research were patients in an epilepsy surgery program either at the University of Michigan Health System, Ann Arbor, or Henry Ford Hospital, Detroit, who required implanted ECoG electrodes as part of surgical treatment for epilepsy. For these subjects, electrodes and electrode locations were chosen for clinical purposes without regard for research concerns. Subjects gave informed consent and the research protocols were approved by the appropriate institutional review boards. The electrodes were made of platinum or stainless steel and were 4 mm in diameter arranged in grids and strips with center-to-center distances of 10 mm in a flexible silicone substrate. Grid electrodes were implanted subdurally through a craniotomy while the patients were under general anesthesia. Some subjects also had cylindrical depth electrodes that penetrated the cortex. Depth electrodes had six to eight platinum contacts that were 2.3 mm wide and placed 10 mm apart on a closed plastic, 0.8 mm tube. Strip and depth electrodes could be placed through 14 mm burrholes under fluoroscopic guidance. Electrode location was documented using X-ray or CT and MRI scans before the patients were connected for clinical monitoring.

Recordings were made from up to 126 subdural electrodes implanted on the surface of the cerebral cortex. Subjects participated in one-two hour data collection sessions while seated in their hospital beds. Each subject performed sets of approximately fifty repetitions of a simple movement task. The recordings from all electrodes during one set of repetitions of a particular task by a particular subject is defined as one *dataset*. Some subjects performed up to four sets of the same task (four datasets) for a total of up to 200 repetitions. The task repetitions were self-paced and separated by approximately five seconds. Variability in electrode placement required selecting the task to be performed by the subject based on the available electrode locations. To maximize experimental uniformity, tasks were chosen from a standard set including tongue, lip, finger, pinch, and ankle tasks to correspond to electrode placements. Further customization of the task performed was sometimes necessary to accommodate electrode placement or a subject's physical limitations. Actual movements were used instead of imagined movements so that electromyography (EMG) from the self-paced tasks would produce a record of the time of each repetition of the task. Points of EMG onset (triggers) were determined using filtering, thresholding, and task repetitions with an unclear onset marked for exclusion from experimental trials. Most of the data were collected at a sampling rate of 200 Hz, with some at 400 Hz. During recording, the 20-Hz data was bandpass-filtered between 0.55 and 100 Hz while the 400-Hz data was bandpass-filtered between 0.5 and 150 Hz. The UM-DBI project has collected data from more than forty subjects in over 350 datasets with up to 126 ECoG electrode channels per dataset, which results in more than 15,000 channels of recorded ECoG. However, the selection of electrode locations solely for clinical purposes related to epilepsy means that the ECoG in these datasets may not include brain activity related to the task being performed.

8.4   Visualization of Movement-Related Patterns in ECoG

Visualization of the ECoG characteristics can be helpful in understanding the features available for detection by a BCI. Our initial approach to visualizing event-related activity in ECoG was to perform triggered averaging (Levine et al. (1999)). However, the event-related potentials (ERPs) revealed by triggered averaging include only activity phase-locked to the triggers (time domain features). Visualizing the oscillatory activity around the time of the triggers can reveal event-related changes in the frequency domain such as event-related desynchronization (ERD) and event-related synchronization (ERS) that otherwise might be overlooked. ERD/ERS maps arranged in the spatial configuration of the electrode arrays allow the visualization of statistically significant frequency changes around the events as well as their spatial distribution (Graimann et al. (2002)).

Figure 8.1 shows electrode locations and time and frequency domain features for subject C17, a 19-year-old female, performing middle finger extension (parts a and d) and tongue protrusion (parts b and e). The location of ERPs for the two tasks overlap (figure 8.1a and b), with the ERPs for the tongue protrusion task centered just above the sylvian fissure and the ERPs for the finger task superior to it, as would be expected. The ERD/ERS maps show the high frequency activity that is one of the key benefits of ECoG. Comparison of the ERP locations with the ERD/ERS for the two tasks shows a similar spatial distribution of the significant ERD/ERS activity. However, the locations of the strongest ERPs and the strongest ERD/ERS do not necessarily coincide. Indeed, both datasets include locations where there are minimal ERPs, but strong ERD/ERS. This implies that a brain-computer interface detection method designed around only ERPs or only ERD/ERS may be discarding useful data.

For the finger extension task, ERD/ERS activity begins well before movement onset (as documented by the onset of EMG activity). The early onset of spectral changes is also visible in individual trials (Fessler et al. (2005)). This proximity of the spectral changes to the trigger time could support a rapid interface response time.

In scalp EEG, self-paced movements are accompanied by three different types of ERD/ERS patterns: (1) contralateral dominant alpha and beta ERD prior to movement; (2) bilateral symmetrical alpha and beta ERD during execution of movement; and (3) contralateral dominant beta ERS after movement offset (Pfurtscheller and Lopes da Silva (1999)). In ECoG, ERD/ERS patterns can be found over a much broader frequency range. Short duration gamma bursts (gamma ERS) can be found in postcentral and parietal areas, which is most interesting since these patterns are usually not recorded by scalp EEG (Pfurtscheller et al. (2003a)). Figure 8.2 shows ERD/ERS maps of four postcentral channels from different subjects performing the same palmar pinch task. The same movement task induced different types of reactivity patterns. Figure 8.2a shows almost no alpha activity but gamma ERS embedded in beta ERD. Figure 8.2b displays much more prominent ERD/ERS patterns. Similar to figure 8.2a, there is hardly any postmovement beta ERS. In figure 8.2c, there is no gamma ERS. In contrast to figure 8.2a and b, figure 8.2c and d show very prominent postmovement ERS. Such a variety in activity patterns has important implications for the detection of these patterns. The detection system must find the set of the

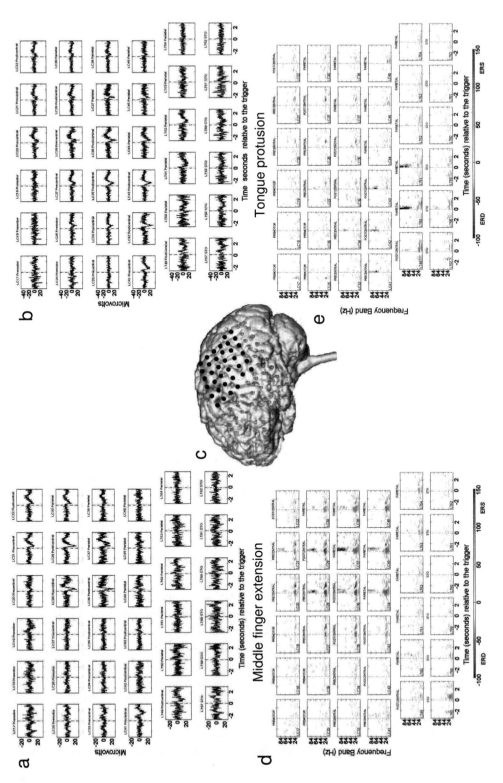

Figure 8.1   Time and frequency domain features from ECoG electrodes over sensorimotor cortex locations shown in c. ERPs for middle finger extension from 49 repetitions a and tongue protrusion from 46 repetitions b and ERD/ERS for finger from 47 repetitions d and tongue from 45 repetitions e.

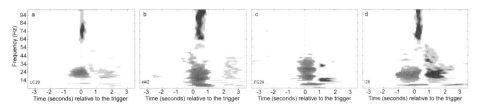

Figure 8.2   ERD/ERS maps for single electrodes over the postcentral gyrus in four different subjects performing a palmar pinch task.

most discriminating signal features for each subect-task combination individually. Or, in a model-based approach, the model parameters should be separately determined for each subject-task combination to obtain optimal results.

8.5   Quantitative Comparison of EEG and ECoG

EEG electrodes are seldom used in conjunction with ECoG; therefore, opportunities for direct comparison of EEG and ECoG are rare. Further, direct comparison would be contraindicated when the task performed was tongue or lip protrusion because of the susceptibility of EEG to contamination with EMG and/or movement artifact.

As an initial evaluation of the relative utility of EEG and ECoG, we performed a classification experiment (Graimann et al. (2005)) on segments of data from either event or idle (rest) periods in EEG and ECoG recorded under similar paradigms but with different subjects. Approximately 150 self-paced finger movements were performed by each of six subjects while EEG was recorded and by each of six epilepsy surgery patients while ECoG was recorded. EEG subjects were healthy and experienced in the movement task, and had a grid of 59 electrodes spaced approximately 2.5 cm apart. ECoG subjects were epilepsy surgery patients whose electrode locations were chosen for clinical purposes, resulting in variable electrode coverage. Artifact-free event periods from -1 to 0 s (AP00) and -0.5 and 0.5 s (AP05) relative to movement onset were extracted. Artifact-free idle periods were from 3.5 to 4.5 s after movement onset. Training was performed on the first 70 percent of the trials and testing on the remaining 30 percent. A 2×5 cross-validation was performed on the training data for feature selection. Classification between idle and AP00 or idle and AP05 was performed using a linear classifier calculated from Fisher linear discriminant analysis (FDA) with no spatial prefiltering (NSPF), using independent component analysis (ICA) and common spatial patterns (CSP). For the CSP conditions, spatial prefiltering was performed separately on delta, alpha/beta, and gamma activity prior to feature extraction. Spatial filters were calculated from the training data.

The actual classification results reported in table 8.1 were calculated from the test data (the 30 percent that was not used for feature selection). An outer cross-validation was not performed because the results on the test data were in line with the cross-validation results for feature selection. As shown in table 8.1, classification results on ECoG always exceeded the classification results on EEG. Spatial prefiltering brought the results on EEG to a level

	NSPF		with ICA		with CSP	
	AP00	AP05	AP00	AP05	AP00	AP05
EEG	0.63 ± 0.08	0.67 ± 0.12	0.72 ± 0.05	0.76 ± 0.10	0.71 ± 0.08	0.81 ± 0.11
ECoG	0.70 ± 0.07	0.83 ± 0.10	0.78 ± 0.04	0.90 ± 0.04	0.81 ± 0.06	0.94 ± 0.02

Table 8.1 The mean and standard deviation over all subjects of the percentage of event periods correctly classified for EEG and ECoG.

equivalent to that found on ECoG without spatial prefiltering. However, spatial prefiltering of the ECoG achieved a similar improvement in classification results. Therefore, in all cases, ECoG proved superior to EEG for classification of brain activity as event periods or idle periods. In fact, we expect that the differences between EEG and ECoG are even more pronounced, since in practice we would have artifacts in EEG and the ECoG electrodes would cover more appropriate electrode locations.

8.6   Shared Analysis and Evaluation Methods

The self-paced tasks performed by our subjects resulted in ECoG recordings labeled at only one instant per event (by the EMG triggers). We quantify the performance of a detection method by comparing the detections produced by the method to the event triggers labeling the ECoG data. A detection acceptance window relative to each trigger is used to define a valid detection (hit). All other detections are classified as false positives. The acceptance window typically includes time both before and after the trigger. The length of the acceptance window after each EMG trigger specifies the maximum-allowed delay between the actual occurrence of an event and its detection. Performance metrics are the hit percentage, which is the percentage of the triggers that were detected, and the false positive percentage, which is the percentage of the *detections* that were false. Calculating the false positive percentage as a percentage of the detections puts greater emphasis on the cost of false positives than would be the case in a sample-based calculation. For ease of comparison, the hit and false positive percentages were combined using an equally weighted cost function to create a statistic we called the "HF-difference," the difference between the hit percentage and the false positive percentage. The HF-difference varies between ±100 with 100 being perfect detection.

Although there are more than 350 datasets (containing recordings from all electrodes for one subject-task-repetition set), the lack of experimental control over electrode placement means that many of these datasets do not contain any channels that produce a good HF-difference for any detection method, nor would they be expected to, given the electrode locations. A representative subset of datasets (the test set) was therefore selected for method development and testing that produced a "good" HF-difference (defined for this purpose as > 50) on at least one channel for at least one detection method. Twenty datasets from ten subjects were selected for the test set that provided ECoG related to a variety of tasks both within and across subjects, relatively well-defined trigger channels, and examples of good and challenging channels for all the detection methods under development at the time. Each dataset contained ECoG channels from 30 to 126 electrodes for a total of 2,184 channels. The twenty datasets in the representative test set contain a total of 120 minutes of recording time (average 6.00 ± 2) and each dataset has an average of 49 ± 3 repetitions of a particular task.

The ECoG containing the first half of the repetitions in each channel is used for algorithm training, and the remaining half for testing. For the data of the test set, there were an average of 24 ± 2 repetitions in the training data for each channel with 25 ± 2 repetitions in the testing data. The test set contained a total of 62.1 minutes of recording time (average 3.1 ± 1). Each method discussed in sections 8.7–8.9 generates a specific decision feature (with a decision rate identical to the sampling rate) and detections are marked based on comparison of this decision feature to a hysteresis threshold. A detection is marked when the decision feature first rises above the upper threshold, whose value is optimized to maximize the HF-difference over the training data. No further detections are possible until the decision feature falls below the lower threshold, which is the mean of the decision feature over the entire course of the training data.

Although we have shown that analysis of multiple channels produces better detection than single-channel analysis for at least one method (Balbale et al. (1999)), for simplicity, the work presented here focuses on detecting event-related changes in ECoG recorded from individual electrodes.

8.7   Cross-Correlation Template Matching

Initially, our group used a cross-correlation template matching (CCTM) method for signal detection (Huggins et al. (1999)). For CCTM, we compute an ERP template using triggered averaging of the training data. Normalized cross-correlation between an ERP template with the ECoG of the test data forms the decision feature. Detections are determined and performance evaluated as described in the previous sections. Because a significant portion of the ERP template energy occurs after the trigger, the CCTM method typically uses templates that extend well after the trigger. However, this characteristic creates undesirable delay in the detection of events.

The CCTM approach is equivalent to a likelihood ratio test under a simple two-hypothesis statistical detection model. Let x denote one block of, say, 2 s of ECoG data, and suppose that x arises from one of the following pair of hypotheses:

$$
\begin{aligned}
H_0 &: \ x \sim \text{Normal}(0, \sigma^2 I) & \text{``rest''} \\
H_1 &: \ x \sim \text{Normal}(\mu, \sigma^2 I) & \text{``task/event,''}
\end{aligned}
\tag{8.1}
$$

where μ denotes the ERP template, σ^2 is the noise variance assuming white noise, and I denotes the identity matrix. For this model, the Neyman-Pearson optimal detector, formed from the likelihood ratio, is the inner product $x'\mu$. In practice, we must choose between rest and task not just once, but at each time point, so we slide the signal block x along the ECoG data, applying the template to each block. The resulting decision feature is the output of the CCTM method.

8.8   The Two-Covariance Signal Model and the Quadratic Detector

The "white noise" signal model (8.1) underlying CCTM ignores event-related changes in the signal power spectrum. As an alternative to (8.1) that accounts for power spectra changes, we have developed a quadratic detector based on a two-covariance signal model (Fessler et al. (2005)). We assume that each ECoG signal block x arises from one of the following two classes:

$$H_0 : \ x \sim \text{Normal}(0, K_0) \qquad \text{"rest"}$$
$$H_1 : \ x \sim \text{Normal}(0, K_1) \qquad \text{"task/event,"} \tag{8.2}$$

where K_0 and K_1 are the signal covariance matrices in the rest state and task state, respectively, and we ignore the ERP component μ for simplicity. By the Neyman-Pearson lemma, the most powerful test for such a detection problem is given by the likelihood ratio. Under model (8.2), the likelihood ratio simplifies (to within irrelevant constants) to the following quadratic form:

$$\Lambda(x) = x'(K_0^{-1} - K_1^{-1})x. \tag{8.3}$$

We slide the signal block along the ECoG data to form the decision feature, and then apply the detection and performance evaluation process described above.

8.8.1   Training

The covariance matrices K_0 and K_1 in (8.2) are unknown *a priori*, so one must estimate them from training data. If the length of the signal block is, say, 100 samples, corresponding to 0.5 s of ECoG data, then each covariance matrix is 100×100—too many parameters to estimate from limited training data. Therefore, we assume a pth order autoregressive (AR) parametric model for the signal power spectrum as follows:

$$x[n] = -\sum_{m=1}^{p} a_q[m]x[n-m] + u[n], \tag{8.4}$$

where n is the sample index, the square brackets $[n]$ denote discrete time signals, and $n > p$, $q = 0, 1$ (each hypothesis) and

$$u[n] \sim \text{Normal}(0, \sigma_q^2). \tag{8.5}$$

As usual, we assume that the $u[n]$ are independent and identically distributed (i.i.d.). Based on past work (Schlögl (2000b)), we currently use $p = 6$, although this has not been optimized. Thus, for a 6th order AR model, we must estimate 6 AR coefficients ($a_q[m]$) and a driving noise variance σ_q^2 for each of the two signal states, for a total of 14 unknown parameters. If each ECoG training data sample point were labeled as coming from a "rest" or "task" state, then it would be straightforward to find the maximum-likelihood (ML) estimates of the AR coefficients and driving noise variances using the

Yule-Walker equations (Kay (1988)). However, our ECoG experiments are unprompted with subjects performing self-paced tasks and our data is labeled by EMG onset at only a single time instant per event. This incomplete labeling complicates the training process. To label our training data for the purposes of estimating the AR model parameters, we must estimate which ECoG samples correspond to which state. We assume that the brain is in the "task" state for some (unknown) period before and after each EMG signal trigger. We parameterize these task-state intervals using a variable w that describes the width of the task interval around each EMG trigger and a variable c that describes the location of the center of each task-state interval relative to each EMG trigger time point. We assume that the remainder of the training data belongs to the "rest" state. (One could alternatively discard data in transition windows around the task-state intervals.) With this model we construct a joint probability density function for training data by adapting the procedure in Kay (1988):

$$
\log p(\boldsymbol{x}_{1,k}, \boldsymbol{x}_{0,k}, \forall k; \mathbf{a_1}, \sigma_1^2, \mathbf{a_0}, \sigma_0^2, c, w)
$$

$$
\approx -\frac{1}{2\sigma_1^2} \sum_{k=1}^{K-1} \sum_{n=p+1}^{N_{1,k}(c,w)} u_{1,k}^2[n; c, w] - \frac{1}{2\sigma_0^2} \sum_{k=1}^{K} \sum_{n=p+1}^{N_{0,k}(c,w)} u_{0,k}^2[n; c, w]
$$

$$
- \sum_{k=1}^{K-1} (N_{1,k}(c,w) - p) \log \sqrt{2\pi\sigma_1^2} - \sum_{k=1}^{K} (N_{0,k}(c,w) - p) \log \sqrt{2\pi\sigma_0^2}, \qquad (8.6)
$$

where $N_{q,k}(c, w)$ denotes the number of samples in the kth block under hypothesis q, and $x_{q,k}[n; c, w]$ indicates the nth data sample in the kth data block under hypothesis q. By construction, $N_{1,k}(c, w) = w$. For $q = 0, 1$:

$$
u_{q,k}[n; c, w] \triangleq x_{q,k}[n; c, w] + \sum_{m=1}^{p} a_q[m] x_{q,k}[n - m; c, w]. \qquad (8.7)
$$

The approximation in (8.6) is reasonable when $N_{q,k}(c, w)$ is large relative to p. Based on this model, we use a joint ML estimation procedure to estimate simultaneously the AR parameters and the center c and width w of the task-state interval as follows:

$$
(\hat{c}, \hat{w}) = \arg\max_{c,w} \max_{\mathbf{a_1}, \sigma_1^2, \mathbf{a_0}, \sigma_0^2}
$$
$$
\log \mathrm{Pr}(\boldsymbol{x}_{1,k}, \boldsymbol{x}_{0,k}, \forall k; \mathbf{a_1}, \sigma_1^2, \mathbf{a_0}, \sigma_0^2, c, w). \qquad (8.8)
$$

This joint labeling and training procedure requires an iterative search over the center c and width w parameters (outer maximization). The inner maximization has a simple analytical solution based on modified Yule-Walker equations to find the AR parameters.

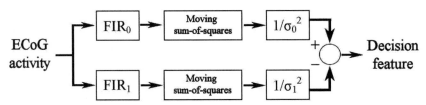

Figure 8.3   Quadratic detector implementation where FIR indicates the finite impulse response filter for each model.

8.8.2   Quadratic Detector Implementation

Implementing the quadratic detector (8.3) directly would be inefficient due to the large matrix sizes. Fortunately, for AR signal models one can implement (8.3) using simple FIR filters:

$$\Lambda(\boldsymbol{x}) = \Lambda_0(\boldsymbol{x}) - \Lambda_1(\boldsymbol{x}), \tag{8.9}$$

where

$$\Lambda_q(\boldsymbol{x}) \triangleq \frac{1}{\sigma_q^2} \sum_{n=p+1}^{N} u_q[n]^2, \qquad q = 0, 1 \tag{8.10}$$

where N denotes the number of samples in a signal block and the innovation signals are defined by

$$u_q[n] \triangleq x[n] + \sum_{m=1}^{p} a_q[m]x[n - m]. \tag{8.11}$$

The block diagram in figure 8.3 summarizes the implementation of the quadratic detector (8.9). The ECoG signal is passed through two FIR filters, each the inverse of the corresponding AR model. Then a moving sum-of-squares computes the power of the innovation signal, which is normalized by the ML estimates of the driving variances. The difference operation that produces the decision feature in essence compares "which model fits better."

Figure 8.4 illustrates how the variance of the innovations process works as a decision feature by plotting individually the normalized innovation variances $\Lambda_0(\boldsymbol{x})$ ("rest class") and $\Lambda_1(\boldsymbol{x})$ ("event class"). Near the trigger point the signal power spectrum becomes that of the event class, so the event-class innovations variance decreases whereas the rest-class innovations variance increases, leading to a large decision feature value.

8.9   Bandpower (BP) Method

While the quadratic detector was explicitly derived from a model of the signal and noise characteristics, many methods achieve good detection with a feature-based approach. A bandpower method was selected as a representative feature-based method for comparison

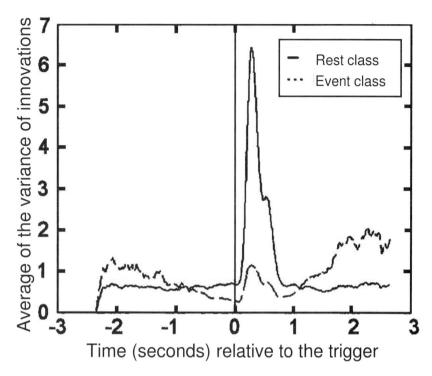

Figure 8.4   Average of variance of innovations process of each class around the trigger point.

with the quadratic detector because power values in specific frequency bands are one of the standard methods for extracting features describing oscillatory activity (Pfurtscheller et al. (2005a)). An additional advantage of using bandpower is that oscillatory activity in specific frequency bands are associated with specific cognitive or mental tasks in well-known brain areas (Pfurtscheller et al. (2003a)), although we do not present such a spatiotemporal analysis here.

Bandpower features were extracted by filtering the data with Butterworth filters of fourth order for the following frequency bands: 0–4, 4–8, 8–10, 10–12, 8–12, 10–14, 16–24, 20–34, 65–80, 80–100, 100–150, 150–200, 100–200 Hz. The last three bands were used only for datasets having a sampling rate of 400 Hz. The filtered signals were squared and smoothed by a 0.75 and 0.5 s moving average filter. The latter is used for frequency bands in the gamma range. To produce a one-dimensional decision feature for detection performance analysis, the signals were linearly combined by an evolutionary algorithm. An advantage of this approach is the fact that point-by-point class labels are not needed for training. The evolutionary algorithm uses the HF-difference directly to optimize the linear combination on the training set. (See Graimann et al. (2004) for details.)

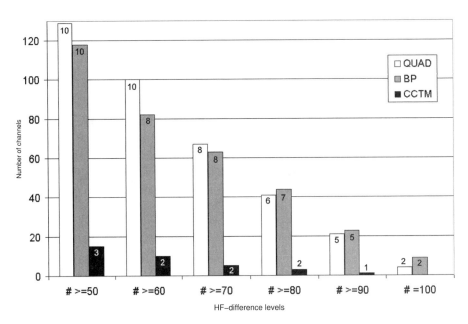

Figure 8.5   The number of channels for the quadratic, BP, and CCTM detection methods at each level of detection performance for a maximum allowed delay of 1 s. The average length of the test data for each channel is 3.1 $\pm$ 1 minutes. Columns are labeled with the number of subjects the channels represent.

8.10   Results

We compared the CCTM method, the BP method, and the quadratic detector using the test set of twenty datasets described in section 8.6 above. The results were evaluated for detection acceptance windows extending from 0.5 s before to 0.25, 0.5, or 1 s after each EMG trigger. These detection acceptance windows allowed us to examine the behavior of the methods under different delay constraints, since the reduction of delay in response time is a priority for use of these detection methods in real-time experiments. Figure 8.5 compares the HF-differences of the CCTM, BP, and quadratic detectors when the delay is constrained to be at most 1 s. The quadratic method and the BP method have many more viable channels and worked for all ten subjects, with the quadratic method reaching all subjects at a slightly higher performance level than the BP method. Figure 8.6 shows the maximum 0.5 s delay case. For this shortened delay, detection performance degrades considerably, yet there are still many viable channels for the quadratic and BP detectors, although not for all subjects. Figure 8.7 shows performance for the quadratic detector at all delays, showing that even with a maximum delay of 0.25 s there are still some viable channels for some subjects.

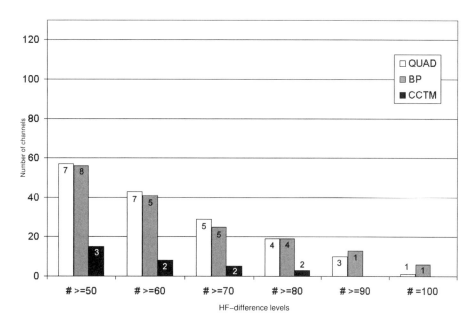

Figure 8.6 The number of channels for the quadratic, BP, and CCTM detection methods at each level of detection performance for a maximum allowed delay of 0.5 s. The average length of the test data for each channel is 3.1 ± 1 minutes. Columns are labeled with the number of subjects the channels represent.

8.11 Discussion

Appropriate metrics for reporting BCI performance are currently a topic of much discussion in the BCI community, especially for interfaces where the user operates the BCI in a self-paced manner. The incompletely labeled data resulting from self-paced experiments and the low probability of the event class makes classical metrics such as receiver operating characteristic (ROC) analysis (see chapter 19) and mutual information or bit-rate (see chapter 19) seem unfeasible. Further, for many assistive technology applications, the consequences of a false positive are difficult to reverse, making false positives very costly and therefore severely restricting the area of interest on an ROC curve. While the eventual range and capabilities of BCIs may be limited only by the imagination, it is important to realize that for some people even a simple binary output would break the barriers to communication that define their world. However, as the primary means of self expression, the reliability of the interface would be of vital interest. Thus, a reliable BCI with limited capabilities may be preferred to a multifunctional BCI with limited reliability.

The HF-difference is a novel metric for quantifying detection accuracy that is based on an underlying philosophy that the user of an interface is primarily interested in the reliability and trustworthiness of the interface. The HF-difference is independent of the sample rate and only indirectly related to the time between events. The hit percentage

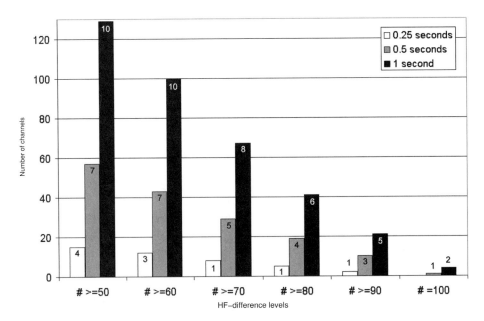

Figure 8.7 The number of channels at each level of detection performance for the quadratic detector at differing maximum allowed delays. The average length of the test data for each channel is 3.1 ± 1 minutes. Columns are labeled with the number of subjects the channels represent.

provides a measure of the reliability with which the interface can detect the events. The false positive percentage, which is calculated as a percentage of the *detections*, gives a measure of the trustworthiness of the interface output. This formula for the false positive percentage is intended to reflect the practical utility of the detection method better than a more traditional sample-by-sample measure. On the other hand, the HF-difference ignores several important characteristics of detection performance. The formula for the HF-difference does not include the time over which the measurement was made. So, while an HF-difference of 80 percent for five events over a 10-second period and over a 10-minute period are described by the same number, this level of performance over the longer period means a much larger number of correctly classified nonevent samples. Therefore, when using the HF-difference, it is important to report the time over which it was calculated.

We have described a quadratic detector for classifying ECoG signals. The quadratic detector is based on a two-covariance signal model that captures event-related changes in the power spectrum of the signal. The detector has a simple implementation that is suitable for real-time use. Empirical results on real ECoG data showed that the quadratic detector offers improved detection accuracy relative to the CCTM method and can provide reduced detection delay and therefore improved interface response time. The BP method also offers improved detection accuracy relative to the CCTM method, confirming that capturing spectral changes in the signal is important for detection. While the number of subjects for which good HF-differences were found with the different methods is an interesting result, it should not be considered predictive of the likelihood of good detection for subjects in general. The test set was selected to include datasets that produced good results on at least one channel and to include data to test the performance of various methods. However, appropriate anatomical location of electrodes was not considered, and instances of good detection in unlikely places and poor detection in likely places are sometimes seen.

We have recently implemented the quadratic detector in our real-time system, and studies with subject feedback and with imagined movements are forthcoming. There are several opportunities to improve the detection method further. Thus far, the quadratic detector ignores the ERP component. Determination of the AR order p is also an important issue. The optimality of the likelihood ratio is applicable to prompted experiments with a predetermined block of data, but is not necessarily optimal when applied with a sliding window. It would therefore be desirable to develop "optimal" detectors for unprompted experiments. Further, the use of a single event class may be an oversimplification. The power spectra shown in figures 8.1 and 8.2 suggest there are at least two distinct sets of spectral characteristics related to the event in addition to those related to the rest state. Separating these components rather than lumping them into single event and rest classes may improve performance. Alternatively, time-varying models (e.g., statespace or hidden Markov methods) might better capture how the spectral properties evolve over time (Foffani et al. (2004)). Finally, multichannel analysis is expected to produce improved detection accuracy, while simultaneously posing challenges to training in the context of a single experimental session.

Despite the challenges to doing research with ECoG, the high quality of the signals offers great potential for an accurate BCI for the operation of assistive technology. Methods incorporating both spectral and temporal changes related to voluntarily produced events will be key in producing reliable BCIs with rapid response times.

Acknowledgments

The authors gratefully acknowledge Alois Schlögl for discussions about spectral changes, Daniela Minecan, Lori Schuh, and Erasmo Passaro for assistance in collecting and interpreting ECoG data, and the many epilepsy surgery patients whose participation provided us with access to this data. The work was supported by R01EB002093 from the National Institute of Biomedical Imaging and Bioengineering, National Institutes of Health, USA.

Notes

E-mail for correspondence: janeh@umich.edu

9 Probabilistically Modeling and Decoding Neural Population Activity in Motor Cortex

Michael J. Black and John P. Donoghue
Departments of Computer Science and Neuroscience
Brown University
Providence RI 02912

9.1 Abstract

This chapter introduces and summarizes recent work on probabilistic models of motor cortical activity and methods for inferring, or decoding, hand movements from this activity. A simple generalization of previous encoding models is presented in which neural firing rates are represented as a linear function of hand movements. A Bayesian approach is taken to exploit this generative model of firing rates for the purpose of inferring hand kinematics. In particular, we consider approximations of the encoding problem that allow efficient inference of hand movement using a Kalman filter. Decoding results are presented and the use of these methods for neural prosthetic cursor control is discussed.

9.2 Introduction

One might think of the computer in this case as a prosthetic device. Just as a man who has his arm amputated can receive a mechanical equivalent of the lost arm, so a brain-damaged man can receive a mechanical aid to overcome the effects of brain damage. It makes the computer a high-class wooden leg.

Michael Crichton, *The Terminal Man* (1972)

Two fundamental shifts in neuroscience have recently led to a deeper understanding of the neural control of movement and are enabling the development of neural prosthesis that can assist the severely disabled by directly connecting their central nervous systems with assistive devices internal or external to the body. The first of these shifts is the result of new electrode array technology that allows the chronic implantation of hundreds of

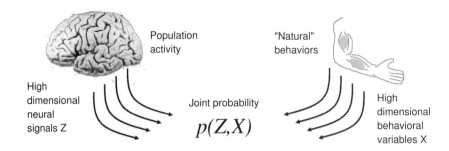

Figure 9.1 The problem of motor cortical modeling for prosthetic applications can be viewed as one of learning the joint probability of neural population activity and motor behavior. Neural data might correspond to spikes, firing rates, local field potentials, or electrocorticograms. Motor behaviors might correspond to joint angles, muscle activation, limb pose, or kinematic parameters. Here we focus on probabilistically modeling motor cortical firing rates and hand kinematics (position, velocity, and acceleration).

microelectrodes in the cortex that can sense and ultimately transmit outside the body the activity of populations of neurons. The second shift is part of a movement toward the study of more natural stimuli and behaviors. In contrast to previous work in neuroscience in which the activity of a single cell is correlated with a simple (e.g., one-dimensional) change in behavior, today neuroscientists can observe large populations of cortical cells and how they respond during rich behavioral tasks. With richness comes the cost of complexity that makes modeling and understanding the relationship between neural activity and behavior challenging. Neural population recordings can be thought of as a high dimensional time-varying signal while motor behavior can similarly be thought of as a high-dimensional time series corresponding to the biomechanical parameters of body pose and motion. We view the problem of modeling the neural code for prosthetic applications as one of learning a probabilistic model relating these high dimensional signals.

This approach is summarized in figure 9.1. We focus here on neural firing rates $\mathbf{z}_t = [z_{1,t} \ldots z_{n,t}]$ of a population of n cells recorded in primary motor cortex in monkeys and relate this activity to a vector of kinematics $\mathbf{x}_t$ representing the monkey's hand pose and movement at an instant in time t.[1] More generally, we want to know the relationship between an entire sequence of firing rates $Z_t = [\mathbf{z}_t \ldots \mathbf{z}_1]$ and hand movements $X_t = [\mathbf{x}_t \ldots \mathbf{x}_1]$ from time 1 to t. In general, we see the problem as one of modeling the joint probability $p(Z_t, X_t)$ of neural activity and hand motion. From such a general model a variety of quantities can be computed and statistical properties of the model analyzed. Here we focus on the problem of decoding, or inference, of hand kinematics from firing activity. The probabilistic approach allows us to exploit a variety of well understood and powerful tools for probabilistic inference.

The probabilistic modeling problem, however, is made challenging by the dimensionality of the neural population and the hand kinematics. Consequently, we will make a number of explicit approximations that will make modeling the probabilistic relationships tractable. In particular, we will exploit lower dimensional parametric models and assumptions of conditional independence. These will lead us to an efficient decoding algorithm that takes as input a sequence of neural firing rates and returns a sequence of probability distributions representing possible hand motions. This decoding algorithm is used in a neural motor prosthesis that directly connects the motor cortex of a monkey to a computer cursor and enables the monkey to move the cursor under brain control. Such a device provides the foundation for a new class of cortical brain-machine interfaces (BMIs) for the severely disabled and, in the near future, may be used to control other external devices such as robot arms or even the patient's own limbs through functional electrical stimulation (Lauer et al. (2000)).

This chapter introduces and summarizes recent work on probabilistically decoding motor cortical population activity. It briefly summarizes the major issues in the field: sensing neural activity, models of cortical coding, probabilistic decoding algorithms, and applications to neural prostheses. In particular, we start with the standard models of motor cortical tuning (e.g., directional tuning) and then show that these are narrow instantiations of a more general linear model relating hand motion and neural firing rates. From this generalization, we show that a well motivated decoding algorithm emerges based on Bayesian probability that provides a principled approach to decoding hand motions. One advantage of this Bayesian approach is that the assumptions made along the way are explicit in a way they are often not in competing approaches. Each of these assumptions provide an opportunity to improve the model and already there have been many such improvements that are beyond the scope of this introduction.

9.3   Sensing Neural Activity

Now listen to me closely, young gentlemen. That brain is thinking. Maybe it's thinking about music.

Maybe it has a great symphony all thought out or a mathematical formula that would change the

world or a book that would make people kinder or the germ of an idea that would save a hundred

million people from cancer. This is a very interesting problem, young gentlemen, because if this brain

does hold such secrets, how in the world are we ever going to find out?

Dalton Trumbo, *Johnny Got His Gun* (1982)

A variety of sensing technologies allow the recording of neural activity with varying levels of temporal and spatial resolution. To record the action potentials of individual cells, we use the Cyberkinetics/Bionic/Utah microelectrode array shown in figure 9.2a, which consists of a 10×10 grid of electrodes (Maynard et al. (1997)). The array is implanted in the arm area of the primary motor cortex (MI) in macaque monkeys as illustrated in figure 9.2b and data is transferred out of the brain through a percutaneous connector shown in figure 9.2c.

The implant area satisfies a number of constraints. First, our goal is to restore movement to people who have lost the ability to control their bodies directly. It long has been known that the activity of cells in this area of the brain is modulated by arm and hand movements (Georgopoulos et al. (1982, 1986)). While it may be possible to train people to use other brain regions to control movement, our working hypothesis is that it will be more "natural"

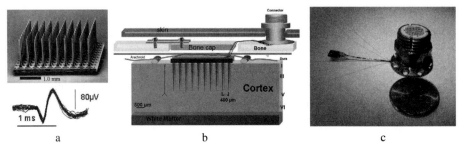

                   a   b   c

Figure 9.2 Implantable electrode array and connector. (a) Cyberkinetics/Bionic/Utah electrode
array and example waveforms recorded for one cell. (b) Sketch of the implanted array and connector.
(c) Size of array along with a percutaneous connector in reference to a U.S. penny.

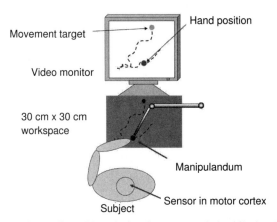

Figure 9.3 Experimental paradigm. Neural signals are recorded while hand motion controls a
computer cursor to hit targets presented at successive random locations on a computer monitor.

and hence easier to learn to control the movement of cursors or other devices using a
region of the brain already related to movement control. Second, this region is surgically
accessible and on the surface of cortex facilitating implantation.

Each electrode may record the activity of zero or more neurons. The activity on each
channel (electrode) is filtered and thresholded to detect action potentials. If the activity
of multiple cells (units) is detected on a single channel, the action potentials may be
sorted based on their waveform shape and other properties using manual or automatic spike
sorting techniques. A representative example of waveforms detected for an individual unit
using the device is shown in figure 9.2a. It is common to recorded from 40 to 50 distinct
cells from a single array. We have found however that, for neural prosthetic applications,
careful spike sorting may not be necessary and it may be sufficient to use the multiunit
activity of all cells recorded on a given channel (Wood et al. (2004)).

To model the relationship between neural firing rates and behavior we used neural
spiking activity recorded while a monkey performed a 2D cursor control task (Serruya et al.
(2002)). The monkey's hand motion and neural activity were recorded simultaneously and
were used to learn a probabilistic model as described in section 9.4. The task involved

moving a manipulandum on a 2D plane to control the motion of a feedback cursor displayed on a computer monitor (figure 9.3). In contrast to previous studies that focused on center-out reaching tasks (Carmena et al. (2003); Taylor et al. (2002)), this data was from a sequential random tracking task in which a target appeared on the screen and the monkey was free to move the feedback cursor as it liked to "hit" the target. When a target was acquired it disappeared and a new target appeared in a new random location. Target locations were drawn independently and identically from a uniform distribution over the 2D range of the 30 cm × 30 cm workspace. See Serruya et al. (2002) for more information on the sequential random tracking task.

9.4 Encoding

If spikes are the language of the brain, we would like to provide a dictionary ... perhaps even ... the analog of a thesaurus.

Rieke et al. (1999)

To model what aspects of movement are represented (encoded) by the brain, we adopt a probabilistic approach and learn a *generative model* of neural activity. In particular, we seek a function $f(\cdot)$ of the hand kinematics, $\mathbf{x}_t$ at time t, that "explains" the observed neural firing rates

$$\mathbf{z}_t = f(\mathbf{x}_t) + \mathbf{q}_t \tag{9.1}$$

where we expect the firing activity $\mathbf{z}_t$ to be noisy observations of a stochastic process and where $\mathbf{q}_t$ is a noise vector drawn from some distribution. Note that this generative model is descriptive rather than mechanistic—it does not say how the spatiotemporal dynamics of neural networks encode movement.

With the generative approach, the problem of modeling the neural code has four components:

(1) What neural data should be modeled (e.g., spikes, rates, local field potentials)?
(2) What behavioral variables are important (e.g., joint angles, torques, muscle activation, hand direction)?
(3) What functional relationship between behavior and neural activity is appropriate (e.g., linear or any number of nonlinear functions)?
(4) What model of "noise" should be used (noise may arise from the stochastic nature of the neurons as well as electrical noise, failures in spike detection/sorting, and more amorphous inadequacies of the functional model)?

In addressing the first question, here we focus on firing rates computed from spike counts in nonoverlapping 70 ms time bins. Firing rates of cells in MI long have been known to be modulated by hand motions and provide a reasonable input signal for neural decoding. While we could work with spike trains, this complicates the probabilistic modeling problem (Wood et al. (2006)).

The next choice pertains to the behavioral variables $\mathbf{x}_t$ we wish to model. Candidates here might include limb joint angles, torques, or muscle activity. While each of these has been shown to be correlated with neural firing rates, there is a simpler representation for the control of computer cursors: hand position, velocity, and acceleration. These kinematic parameters also have been shown to be related to modulation of firing rates. The choice here, however, is not completely independent of the next problem, which is the choice of the function f.

While f could be an arbitrary function (e.g., as embodied in an artificial neural network (ANN) (Wessberg et al. (2000))), we can impose some constraints on its choice. Low-dimensional parametric models, particularly linear ones, are desirable because they are easy to fit to relatively small amounts of data without overfitting. A second design criterion might be "interpretability," which ANN's lack.

In terms of interpretability, linear models have a distinct advantage in that they are a generalization of well known models of motor cortical coding. One of the hallmarks of cells in the arm area of MI is that they are "directionally tuned" (Georgopoulos et al. (1982); Schwartz et al. (1988)). This theory of motor cortical coding suggests that cells have a preferred direction, and when the hand moves in this direction a cell's firing rate is maximal. This is illustrated in figure 9.4 for a representative cell from our data. Mathematically, the firing rate z_t of a cell at time t can be expressed as the following function of hand direction θ_t:

$$z_t = h_0 + h\,\cos(\theta_t - \theta) = h_0 + h_x\cos(\theta_t) + h_y\sin(\theta_t) \tag{9.2}$$

where the h_i are scalar values that can be fitted to the data for a particular cell. Note that this equation is in the same form as our generative model above but that there is no explicit model of the noise.

The story does not end with directional tuning, however. Moran and Schwartz (1999), for example, noted that firing rates of MI cells increase with the *speed* at which a hand movement is performed; that is,

$$z_t = s_t(h_0 + h\,\cos(\theta_t - \theta)) = h_0^* + h_x^* v_{t,x} + h_y^* v_{t_y} \tag{9.3}$$

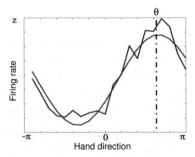

Figure 9.4 Cosine tuning. The firing rate of a cell (jagged curve) as a function of hand direction θ_t. This data is well fit by a so-called cosine tuning function (smooth curve). The direction of maximal firing, θ, is referred to as the preferred direction.

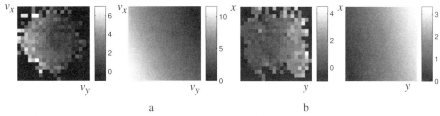

Figure 9.5 Linear tuning functions. (a) Firing rate as a function of hand *velocity* for one cell. Light colors correspond to higher firing rates than dark colors. Note that black corresponds to regions of velocity space that were never observed. On the left of (a) is a normalized histogram of the firing rates while on the right is the linear fit to this data. (b) A different cell shows approximately linear tuning with respect to hand *position* on a 2D plane.

where the h_i^* are, once again, scalar values and $v_{t,x}$ and $v_{t,y}$ represent the *velocity* of the hand in the x and y direction, respectively. Figure 9.5a illustrates this roughly linear velocity tuning for one motor cortical neuron.

Equation (9.3) then suggests that the firing rate of these cells is simply a linear function of hand velocity. Again, this is not the whole story. Firing rates of these cells also may be linearly tuned to hand position (Kettner et al. (1988)), hand acceleration, (Flament and Hore (1988)) and possibly even higher order derivatives of the hand motion (Wu et al. (2005)). Figure 9.5b shows the firing activity of a cell that is roughly linearly tuned to position. For a thorough treatment, see Paninski et al. (2004).

Taken together these findings suggest that firing rates may be approximated as a linear combination of simple hand kinematics (position, velocity, and acceleration); that is,

$$\mathbf{z}_t = H\mathbf{x}_t \qquad (9.4)$$

where, if $\mathbf{z}_t$ is a vector of n cells' firing rates and $\mathbf{x}_t = [x_t, y_t, v_{t,x}, v_{t,y}, a_{t,x}, a_{t,y}]^T$ contains the hand kinematics at time t, H is an $n \times 6$ matrix that relates hand pose/motion to firing rates. The inclusion of all these kinematic terms (position, velocity, and acceleration) in the model turns out to be important. It has been noted that not all cells in primary motor cortex are equally tuned to each of these variables; some cells are modulated more by one variable than another (Paninski et al. (2004)).

It is important to note that this model is a strict generalization of the traditional model of directional tuning. Previous decoding models such as the population vector method rely on tuning for direction or speed and direction (Schwartz et al. (1988, 2001)). These parameters are included in the linear model along with position and acceleration.

We now come to the final design choice in the generative framework; namely, what noise model should we use? Note first that firing rates are strictly positive and, over relatively small time windows, exhibit a roughly Poisson distribution. As a mathematical convenience, however, we would prefer to model the noise as Gaussian which will admit efficient inference algorithms as described in the following section 9.5. To facilitate such a model, we first center the firing rates by subtracting the vector of mean firing rates from all the data; the firing rates are no longer strictly positive. We do the same for the hand kinematics. We then approximate the noise as Gaussian; that is, $\mathbf{q}_t \sim N(0, Q)$.

Unlike previous approaches, this generative model explicitly (if only approximately) models the noise in the observations. In particular, we take Q to be a full error covariance matrix that models correlations in the noise among the cells. This is critical for accurate modeling since any model is going to be an approximation to the truth and there may be other hidden causes of firing rate modulation that may cause correlated errors in the observed firing rates.

9.5 Decoding

If I could find ... a code which translates the relation between the reading of the encephalograph and the mental image ... the brain could communicate with me.

Curt Siodmak, *Donovan's Brain* (1942).

The goal of motor-cortical decoding is to recover the intended movement, for example, hand kinematics $\mathbf{x}_t$, given a sequence of observed firing rates $Z_t = [\mathbf{z}_t \ldots \mathbf{z}_1]$. Probabilistically, we would like to represent the a posteriori probability of the hand motion $p(\mathbf{x}_t|Z_t)$. To represent this probability, we first make a few simplifying assumptions that prove quite reasonable in practice. For example, we assume that the hand kinematics at time t are independent of those at time $t-2$ and earlier conditioned on $\mathbf{x}_{t-1}$. This gives a simple form for the a priori probability of hand kinematics

$$p(\mathbf{x}_t|X_{t-1}) = p(\mathbf{x}_t|\mathbf{x}_{t-1}, \ldots, \mathbf{x}_1) = p(\mathbf{x}_t|\mathbf{x}_{t-1}). \tag{9.5}$$

We also assume that, given the kinematics $\mathbf{x}_t$ at time t, the firing rates at time t are conditionally independent of the hand kinematics at earlier times. This gives a simple form for the *likelihood* of firing rates conditioned on hand kinematics

$$p(\mathbf{z}_t|X_t) = p(\mathbf{z}_t|\mathbf{x}_t). \tag{9.6}$$

With these assumptions, Bayes' rule can be used to derive an expression for the posterior probability in terms of the likelihood and the prior

$$p(\mathbf{x}_t|Z_t) \propto p(\mathbf{z}_t|\mathbf{x}_t) \int p(\mathbf{x}_t|\mathbf{x}_{t-1}) p(\mathbf{x}_{t-1}|Z_{t-1}) d\mathbf{x}_{t-1}. \tag{9.7}$$

A "decoded" value for $\mathbf{x}_t$ can then be obtained by either computing the expected value or the maximum a posteriori value of $p(\mathbf{x}_t|Z_t)$.

This Bayesian formulation is very general and the likelihood and prior can be arbitrary. In the general case, the integral in (9.7) is problematic and must be computed using Monte Carlo sampling methods. For the recursive estimation of $p(\mathbf{x}_t|Z_t)$, this inference takes the form of a "particle filter" that has been applied to neural decoding (Brockwell et al. (2004); Gao et al. (2002, 2003a)). These methods, however, are computationally intensive and not yet appropriate for real-time decoding.

By making a few more simplifying assumptions, however, inference with this Bayesian formulation becomes straightforward. In particular, we observe that the prior probability of hand motions in our task is well approximated by a linear Gaussian model; that is,

$$\mathbf{x}_t = A\mathbf{x}_{t-1} + \mathbf{w}_t \tag{9.8}$$

where A is known as a state matrix that models the change in kinematics from one time to the next, and the noise, $\mathbf{w}_t \sim N(0, W)$, is normally distributed with mean zero and covariance W.

Assuming that the kinematics $\mathbf{x}_0$ is normally distributed at time 0, then $\mathbf{x}_t$ is normally distributed. This is convenient since it implies that firing rates $\mathbf{z}_t = H\mathbf{x}_t + \mathbf{q}_t$ conditioned on $\mathbf{x}_t$ are also normally distributed. While this assumption of Gaussian-distributed firing rates is only an approximation, performing a square-root transformation of the firing rates improves the approximation; for more details, see Gao et al. (2003a) and Wu et al. (2005).

With these assumptions, the likelihood term in (9.7) becomes

$$p(\mathbf{z}_t|\mathbf{x}_t) \propto \exp\left(-\frac{1}{2}(\mathbf{z}_t - H\mathbf{x}_t)^T Q^{-1}(\mathbf{z}_t - H\mathbf{x}_t)\right). \tag{9.9}$$

The assumptions tell us how firing rates are generated from intended hand movements. Bayes' rule tells us how to take such a generative model of firing rates and "turn it around" for the purpose of decoding hand kinematics from observed firing rates.

The linear and Gaussian assumptions mean that fitting the parameters H, Q, A, and W is straightforward via least-squares regression on training data (Wu et al. (2005)). Also, given linear Gaussian expressions for the likelihood and prior, the resulting posterior is also Gaussian. Estimating this Gaussian posterior can be done very easily and efficiently using the Kalman filter (Kalman (1960); Welch and Bishop (2001)) since the update of the posterior at each time instant can be performed in closed form. For details of the algorithm and its implementation for neural decoding, see Wu et al. (2005).

A few example reconstructions of hand trajectories are shown in figure 9.6 in which we display the expected hand kinematics, $\mathbf{x}_t$, at each time instant computed from test data not used to train the model. Reconstructed hand trajectories qualitatively match the true trajectories and quantitatively compare favorably to the state of the art (see Wu et al. (2005)). The Kalman filter provides a computationally efficient and accurate method for

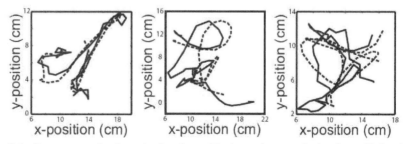

Figure 9.6   Reconstructed trajectories (portions of 1*min* test data – each plot shows 50 time instants (3.5*s*)): true target trajectory (dashed) and reconstruction using the Kalman filter (solid); from Wu et al. (2005).

neural decoding directly derived from our models of the neural code. Experiments in monkeys show that the method provides effective online cursor control (Wu et al. (2004b)). In particular, Wu et al. (2004b) showed a 50 percent improvement in the number of targets a monkey could hit in a given period of time using the Kalman filter as compared with a more traditional, non-generative, linear regression method (Carmena et al. (2003); Serruya et al. (2002)).

There is one additional detail that is relevant for accurate decoding: Changes in the firing rates of the cells tend to precede the observed activity. Consequently, it is appropriate to train the model with a built in lag j such that

$$\mathbf{z}_{t-j} = H\mathbf{x}_t + \mathbf{q}_t. \tag{9.10}$$

A fixed lag of approximately 140 ms improves decoding accuracy. The lag for each cell, however, may differ, and fitting individual lags improves decoding further but complicates learning the model parameters (Wu et al. (2005)). Wu et al. (2005) found that the Kalman filter with a 140 ms lag reconstructed hand trajectories for this data with a mean squared error (MSE) in hand position of 5.87 cm^2, while a nonuniform lag, optimized for each cell, reduced the MSE to 4.76 cm^2.

They also observed the value of representing a full error covariance matrix in the generative model. Using only a diagonal covariance matrix, which assumes conditional independence of the firing rates of different cells, resulted in an increase in the MSE from 5.87 cm^2 to 6.91 cm^2.

9.6   Interfaces

The big machine .... *Operated by remote control* .... *Operated by the electromagnetic impulses of individual Krell brains.*

W. J. Stuart, The Forbidden Planet (1956)

There have now been numerous demonstrations of neural control of devices using different recording technologies and different decoding algorithms (Carmena et al. (2003); Tillery et al. (2000); Schwartz et al. (2001); Serruya et al. (2002); Taylor et al. (2002); Wu et al. (2004b)). In the case of cortical implants, these methods can be classified according to two kinds of interfaces: discrete and continuous.

In the discrete task, a monkey has one of a fixed number of targets they must select by either direct arm motion or neural signals (Musallam et al. (2004); Shenoy et al. (2003)). Neural decoding in this case reduces to a discrete classification task. Furthermore, in the case that all the targets are equally likely (i.e., the prior is uninformative), Bayesian classification reduces to maximum-likelihood classification. Given a population of neurons in primary motor cortex or premotor areas, this classification task can be performed extremely accurately. In fact, monkeys can respond more rapidly under brain control than by making actual arm motions, and they quickly learn to perform target selection without moving their arm (Musallam et al. (2004); Shenoy et al. (2003)).

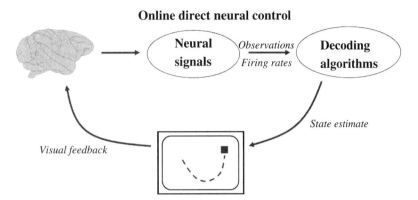

Figure 9.7 Closed-loop neural cursor control. Neural signals directly control cursor motion while subjects receive feedback about the cursor position through their visual systems. In our case, the neural signals are population firing rates and the decoding algorithm is the Kalman filter.

A variety of interfaces have been developed for disabled people using discrete selection such as this (though using EEG and not neural implants). Interfaces based on selection of a small number of states (e.g., binary) can be cumbersome to use. It is not yet known, however, how many discrete states can be recognized from a neural population of a given size.

The alternative we have pursued here is to recover a continuous control signal. The closed-loop control task is illustrated in figure 9.7 where the brain controls a 2D cursor position on a computer screen and a monkey (or human) receives visual feedback by viewing the cursor on a monitor. We suspect that for robot control tasks (e.g., moving a wheelchair or robot arm), continuous control will be preferable because it is inherently more flexible. It is also, however, more noise-prone, so there is a trade-off that gives higher spatial resolution with less accuracy. The trade-offs between discrete and continuous methods and their relevance for rehabilitation applications deserve further study.

One promising direction combines discrete and continuous control in a single interface (Wood et al. (2005)). The Bayesian decoding framework easily can accommodate a mixed state space with both continuous (2D) and discrete (task-oriented) parameters. The generative model then involves first selecting the task (continuous or discrete) and then generating the observations conditioned on the task. Decoding is slightly more complicated but can be achieved using a switching Kalman filter (Wu et al. (2004a)) or particle filter (Brockwell et al. (2004); Gao et al. (2002)). Recently, Wood et al. (2005) used such an approach to decode whether or not a monkey was performing a 2D control task and, if so, to decode the hand state with a linear Gaussian model. Such an approach holds promise for flexible brain-machine interfaces in which the user can switch between a variety of functions or control modes.

9.7   Discussion and Conclusions

The probabilistic modeling of the neural code presents many challenges. Beyond the simple linear Gaussian models explored here, there is likely an advantage in modeling the non-Gaussian and nonlinear nature of neural activity (Gao et al. (2003a); Kim et al. (2006); Wu et al. (2004a)). Beyond firing rates, we may wish to formulate probabilistic models of spike trains (Truccolo et al. (2005)). Efficient learning and decoding methods, however, do not currently exist for non-Gaussian, nonlinear models of point processes. There is an opportunity here to develop new machine learning methods for capturing the high-dimensional relationship between motor behavior and neural firing.

Moreover, here we consider only information from primary motor cortex. Additional information may be obtained from premotor and parietal areas. The Bayesian framework we have proposed provides a solid foundation to integrate sources of information from various brain areas in a principled way.

The approach does not, however, necessarily provide any new insight into how the brain controls movement. Like the approaches it generalizes (e.g., the population vector method), the relationships between firing rates and kinematics are purely descriptive. One cannot infer, for example, that the brain is somehow implementing a Kalman filter. Rather, all these methods describe attributes of the neural computation and not the computation itself.

This chapter only hints at the prosthetic applications of these methods. While Bayesian methods have been used for closed-loop neural control of cursors by monkeys (Wu et al. (2005)), the use of this or any decoding method in paralyzed humans remains to be explored. Particularly important in the case of paralyzed humans will be the issue of training and adaptation. Training data for the encoding model here, for example, will have to rely on imagined movement. Whether human users will be able to adapt their neural signals to improve control with a given decoder remains to be seen and may prove critical for practical motor-cortical control of devices.

While current methods provide a proof of concept that cortical implants can provide reliable control signals over extended periods of time, there is still much work to be done. Current continuous decoding results provide a somewhat "jerky" reconstruction—new decoding and control algorithms for damping the cursor reconstruction may enable a wider range of applications. The great challenge, however, is to move beyond simple 2D or 3D cursor control to ultimately give patients high-dimensional control of devices such as dexterous robot hands.

Acknowledgments

The research summarized here is the product of interdisciplinary research with a large number of collaborators we wish to thank. They include Elie Bienenstock, Matthew Fellows, Mijail Serruya, Yun Gao, Wei Wu, Frank Wood, Jessica Fisher, Shy Shoham, Carlos Vargas-Irwin, Ammar Shaikhouni, David Mumford, Arto Nurmikko, Beth Travers, Gerhard Friehs, and Liam Paninski.

This work was funded by the DARPA BioInfoMicro Program, NIH NINDS Neural Prosthesis Program and Grant NS25074, NIH-NINDS N01-NS-2-2345, NSF ITR award 0113679, NIH-NINDS R01 NS 50967-01 as part of the NSF/NIH Collaborative Research in Computational Neuroscience Program, the Veteran's Administration grant #A3772C, and the Office of Naval Research award N0014-04-1-082.

Notes

E-mail for correspondence: black@cs.brown.edu

(1) While here we focus on firing rates, the probabilistic modeling framework is more general and equally well applies to spike trains or other neural signals such as local field potentials. Focusing on rates, however, will simplify our probabilistic modeling problem. The same can be said for hand kinematics; for example, instead, we might model biomechanical properties of the arm dynamics.

10   The Importance of Online Error Correction and Feed-Forward Adjustments in Brain-Machine Interfaces for Restoration of Movement

Dawn M. Taylor
Department of Biomedical Engineering
Case Western Reserve University
Cleveland, OH, USA

Cleveland FES Center of Excellence
Louis Stokes Department of Veterans
Affairs Medical Center
Cleveland, OH, USA

10.1   Abstract

Intended movement can now be decoded in real time from neural activity recorded via intracortical microelectrodes implanted in motor areas of the brain. This opens up the possibility that severely paralyzed individuals may be able to use their extracted movement commands to control various assistive devices directly. Even direct control of one's own paralyzed limbs may be possible by combining brain recording and decoding technologies with functional electrical stimulation systems that generate movement in paralyzed limbs by applying low levels of current to the peripheral nerves. However, the microelectrode arrays can record only a small fraction of the neurons that normally are used to control movement, and we are unable to decode the user's desired movement without errors. This chapter discusses experiments in which a monkey used its cortical signals to control the movements of a 3D cursor and a robotic arm in real time. Both consistent errors and random errors were seen when decoding intended movement. However, the animal learned to compensate for consistent decoding errors by making feed-forward adjustments to its motor plan. The animal also learned to compensate for random decoding errors by using visual feedback to make online error corrections to the evolving movement trajectories. This ability to compensate for imperfect decoding suggests intracortical signals may be quite useful for assistive device control even if the current technology does not perfectly extract the users native movement commands.

10.2   Introduction

Brain-computer and brain-machine interfaces (BCIs and BMIs) detect neural activity from the brain and use those signals in real time to drive a computer or some other assistive device. These technologies have the potential to help people with severe motor disabilities by enabling them to control various devices directly with their neural activity. Creative researchers have used many different aspects of natural neural processing as a means to command assistive technologies. For example, some labs have used the involuntary neural responses that arise when people focus their attention on a desired letter, icon, or flashing cue on a screen (P300 (Donchin et al. (2000)), or visually evoked potentials (Gao et al. (2003b))). However, a large number of systems under development used neural signals involved with sensorimotor processing that accompany imagined or attempted movements of paralyzed limbs. These systems are most useful for individuals where: (1) the sensorimotor-related brain areas are still intact, and (2) the command signals needed by the assistive device are movement-related, such as the desired motion of a computer cursor or of an assistive robot. For movement-related devices, visual feedback plays a critical role in learning to use brain signals to control device functions.

One promising use of these brain-derived movement commands is in restoring control of arm and hand function to people with high-level spinal cord injuries. Implanted functional electrical stimulation (FES) technology has been around for decades and is used to activate paralyzed muscles in a coordinated fashion by applying controlled levels of electrical current to the peripheral nerves (Kilgore and Kirsch (2004)). These systems can restore a wide variety of functions in people with different levels of paralysis due to spinal cord injury. Commercial systems, such as the Freehand system, have restored hand grasp to hundreds of individuals with spinal cord injuries at the C5 to C6 level (Peckham et al. (2001)), and systems such as Vocare bladder system have restored bladder function to many others. FES systems are being developed to restore a paraplegic's ability to stand, transfer in and out of a bed or a wheelchair, and even walk using a walker. For people with high-level spinal cord injuries, FES now can restore independent breathing by activating the diaphragm muscles, thus freeing a person from dependence on a ventilator (for a review of clinical applications of FES, see Creasey et al. (2004); for consumer information, see FES, Neurotech Network of the Society to Increase Mobility).

However, the most likely FES technologies to be integrated with command signals from the brain are those that restore arm and hand function to individuals with spinal cord injuries at the C4 level or above. People with these high-level injuries are limited to generating command signals from the neck up. Their FES systems will need to activate many degrees of freedom to move and orient the arm and hand in a way that will generate useful function. Although a person could direct the complex movements of the full limb via non-brain-based commands generated from the face and neck, practical issues associated with this make using brain signals a more desirable option. Alternatives, such as mouth-operated joysticks, tongue-touch keypads, voice commands, facial movement commands, and eye-gaze commands, can be effective, but interfere with talking, eating, and normal social interaction. Accessing desired arm and hand movements directly from the brain will enable these individuals to direct the movements of their FES-activated arm and hand while still retaining normal use of their remaining head and neck functions.

Although the use of EEG signals to command the simple opening and closing of an FES hand-grasp system has been demonstrated (Pfurtscheller et al. (2003b)), work toward continuous control of the multidimensional movements needed for more complex arm and hand functions has been demonstrated only in other non-FES venues such as control of a robotic arm (Taylor et al. (2003); Carmena et al. (2003)) or of a computer cursor representing arm movements (Taylor and Schwartz (2001); Taylor et al. (2002); Serruya et al. (2002)). However, a closer look at these other studies provides evidence that the use of recorded brain activity is a viable option for command of these more complex upper-limb FES systems. This evidence comes in three forms, all of which have, so far, relied exclusively on visual feedback. First is the inherent ability of our nervous system to adjust and correct for consistent errors in the executed motor plan. Second is the ability to make online corrections to random errors in the execution of the motor plan, and the third is the ability of the brain to increase the useful information content of the recorded neural signals.

10.3   Decoder Limitations in BCIs/BMIs

With current technology, it is impossible to detect the firing activity of every neuron involved with executing a movement. In practice, implanted intracortical microelectrode arrays can detect the activity of, at most, only hundreds or even thousands of individual neurons; this is still only a very small fraction of the neurons actually involved with movement generation. With larger macroelectrodes used for electroencephalograms (EEGs) or electrocorticograms (ECoGs), the electrodes detect field potentials that reflect the average activity or net fields generated by all the neurons in the vicinity of these recording electrodes. These different recording options inevitably lead to gross under-sampling or else over-averaging of the true neural activity generated each time a person attempts to execute a movement command.

The true relationship between neural activity and intended movement is complex, stochastic in nature, and nonstationary over many different time scales. However, we are confronted with the task of developing practical decoding functions that extract intended movement from the limited recorded signals in a computationally efficient way. Fortunately, many standard engineering tools, such as linear filters and artificial neural networks, have been successful at approximating this complex input-output relationship to a level that has enabled some practical implementation of BCI and BMI technologies. However, these imperfect decoders still result in two types of errors: (1) relatively consistent errors that result in a similar deviation from the intended device movement path each time the movement is attempted; these errors stem from using an oversimplified and/or inaccurate decoding model to translate neural activity to desired device output; and (2) random errors that result from the stochastic nature of the neural firing processes as well as random errors resulting from the variability of the assistive device and/or in its interactions with the biological system. For BMI/BCI technologies to be effective, the user must learn to compensate for both consistent and random errors.

10.4 Feed-Forward Adjustment to Imperfect Decoders

Many motor control studies have shown that both humans and nonhuman primates rapidly learn to adjust their motor output if a *predictable* perturbation is applied during point-to-point reaching movements. This phenomenon has been demonstrated when real perturbations are physically applied to the arm in a predictable way (Gandolfo et al. (2000); Hwang et al. (2003); Singh and Scott (2003); Klassen et al. (2005)), and when perturbations are applied only to the visual feedback the subject receives about their movements (Cunnigham and Welch (1994); Kagerer et al. (1997); Wigmore et al. (2002); Bock et al. (2001); Miall et al. (2004)). In both cases, subjects learn to make feed-forward modifications to their motor output to correct for these errors even when the perturbations are complex functions of the actual hand movement, such as when cursor deviation is proportional and perpendicular to actual hand velocity.

In much the same way, inaccuracies in the decoding function in a BCI/BMI can result in consistent perturbations of the assistive device motion that the user observes. This is especially true in BMIs where an additional layer of errors is added to the observed movement due to inaccuracies of the device control system itself. However, visual feedback enables users to identify these consistent decoding and device errors and then compensate for the errors by modifying their motor plan. These principles of feed-forward adjustments are demonstrated in the following experiment where the activity of a few dozen neural units recorded via microwires in the arm area of the motor or premotor cortex was used to directly control the movements of a virtual cursor to eight different targets in a 3D center-out movement task (Taylor et al. (2002)).

Rhesus macaques were chronically implanted with stainless steel microwire arrays in motor and premotor cortical areas associated with proximal arm movements. An infrared position sensor (Optotrak, Northern Digital, Inc.) was placed on the animals' wrists and provided current wrist position information to the computer every 30 ms. A stereo monitor was used to project to the animal a 3D image of a moving cursor that was initially controlled by the animal's actual wrist position. The animal could not see its own arm, but instead saw the cursor that tracked its wrist position as the animal moved its arm throughout the workspace (figure 10.1a). The animal was trained to move this cursor (i.e., its wrist) from a center start position to one of eight different targets that would appear radially at the corners of a virtual cube (figure 10.1b). The animal received a liquid reward for successfully moving the cursor from the center start position to an outer target within a short 800 ms time limit.

Once the animal was trained to do this task, cursor movements were switched from being driven by the actual wrist position to being driven by the *predicted* wrist position, based on the real-time decoding of the firing rates of a few dozen neural units. Any random and/or consistent errors in our real-time decoder would result in deviations of the cursor from the actual trajectory of the wrist.

The decoding function used in this study was a simplistic "population vector"-type decoder where the change in cursor position $[\Delta X(t), \Delta Y(t), \Delta Z(t)]$ every 30 ms was based on a weighted sum of the normalized firing rates, $Ri(t)'$, of all units ($i = 1$ to n), as

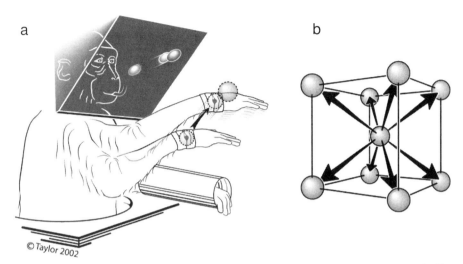

Figure 10.1   3D virtual testing environment used for the eight-target center-out movement task. The animal sees only a 3D stereo image of a cursor sphere and various targets—it cannot see its own arm. During training, the cursor sphere initially tracks the animal's arm movements, which are detected by a position sensor taped to the animal's wrist. However, once the animal is familiar with the task, the cursor sphere is moved based on the animal's neural activity, which is decoded into ΔX, ΔY, and ΔZ every 30 ms. In this center-out experiment, the animal is rewarded for moving the cursor sphere radially from a center start position to various targets that appear in the workspace. Part (a) shows the animal in the virtual training environment. Part (b) illustrates the 3D center-out task where movements start at a central target and go to one of eight outer targets located at the corners of an imaginary cube (used by permission, D. M. Taylor).

shown in (10.1). Normalization, as indicated by the prime notation, included subtracting each unit's mean firing rate and dividing by its standard deviation.

$$X(t) = \sum_{i=1}^{n} Ci_X Ri(t)'$$
$$Y(t) = \sum_{i=1}^{n} Ci_Y Ri(t)' \tag{10.1}$$
$$Z(t) = \sum_{i=1}^{n} Ci_Z Ri(t)'$$

It has been well documented that most arm area motor cortical cells have firing rates that are, at least in part, linearly related to intended movement direction. That is, neural firing rate $R(t)$ can be significantly fit to equation (10.2) below were $Mx(t)$, $My(t)$, and $Mz(t)$ make up a unit vector pointing in the desired movement direction at time t, and Bx, By, and Bz make up a vector pointing in the cells "preferred direction" (i.e., the direction of movement during which that cell's firing rate tends to be the highest) (Schwartz et al. (1988)).

$$R(t) = Bo + BxMx(t) + ByMy(t) + BzMz(t) \qquad (10.2)$$

The real-time decoding equation used in this experiment, (10.1), has been shown to be effective at predicting intended movement direction when neural firing patterns fit the linear relationship shown in (10.2), *and* enough neurons are used, *and* the preferred directions of those neurons are uniformly distributed throughout the workspace (Georgopoulos et al. (1988)). However, many other studies have shown neural firing activity has a much more complex relationship to intended movement than is captured by the decoding equation used here. Neural firing rates also have been shown to be related to position (Kettner et al. (1988); Caminiti et al. (1990); Paninski et al. (2004)), force (Evarts (1968); Ashe (1997)), joint kinematics (Fu et al. (1995)), and muscle activation (Morrow and Miller (2003)). Most important for this example is that neural firing rates also are related strongly to movement *speed* as well as direction (Moran and Schwartz (1999)). This relationship is more accurately captured by (10.3) where $||V||$ represents the magnitude of the movement velocity (i.e., speed) and Θ represents the angle between the movement direction and the cell's preferred direction (Moran and Schwartz (1999)).

$$R(t) = K_0 + K_1||V(t)|| + K_2||V(t)|| \cos(\Theta(t)) \qquad (10.3)$$

This aspect of neural firing was particularly important in this experiment because the short 800 ms time limit for the movement resulted in ballistic arm movements that spanned a large range of speeds throughout each movement trajectory. This, in effect, resulted in a speed-dependent perturbation of the brain-controlled cursor movements as the mismatch between decoding model, represented by (10.1) and (10.2), and the actual firing patterns, more accurately represented by (10.3), increased with the speed of the actual arm movements.

Figure 10.2a and 10.2b show examples of the animal's brain-controlled cursor movements to all eight targets in this ballistic control task where a simple population vector, (10.1), was used to translate neural activity into cursor movements in real time. Three-dimensional trajectories to all eight targets are shaded to match intended target (outer circles) and are plotted in two groups of four targets for easier 2D viewing. Figure 10.2c and 10.2d show the actual hand paths the animal made during the same brain-controlled cursor movements plotted in figure 10.2a and b.

Note the substantial difference in the actual hand trajectories in 10.2c and 10.2d compared with their associated brain-controlled cursor trajectories shown in 10.2a and 10.2b. The consistent deviations in the actual hand paths to each target in this ballistic movement task indicate that the animal learned to make feed-forward corrections in its motor output to compensate for the gross inadequacies of the simplistic decoding function used. Although the actual hand paths span only a limited section of the workspace, the distribution of trajectories intended for each target are still well differentiated within this limited area. This suggests the animal learned some very specific new motor output patterns that enabled it to move the brain-controlled cursor as needed in the larger 3D workspace.

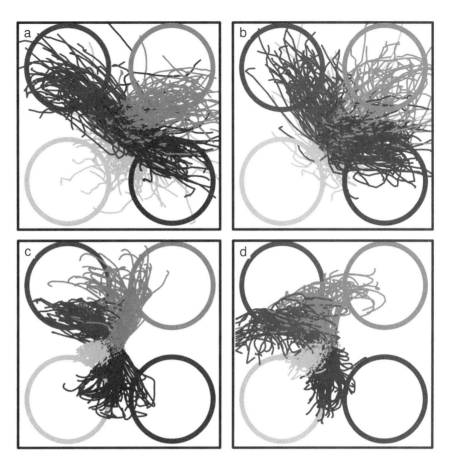

Figure 10.2   Cursor and hand paths during a ballistic 3D center-out movement task to eight different targets in a virtual environment. The animal's goal was to move the cursor from the center start position to one of eight radial targets within an 800 ms time limit. Brain-controlled cursor movements were generated in real-time from the recorded neural activity, which was decoded into intended movements using a simple population vector algorithm, (10.1). Trajectories are shaded to match their intended targets (outer circles). 3D trajectories to each of the eight different targets are plotted in two sets of four for easier 2D viewing. Plots (a) and (b) show the movement paths of the brain-controlled cursor. Plots (c) and (d) show the actual hand paths the animal made while making the brain-controlled cursor movements shown in (a) and (b).

This task was repeated over twenty days, and the animal showed significant improvement in the percentage of targets hit each day as a function of the number of days of practice (improvement of 0.9 percent per day, $p < 0.0009$). Although the animal effectively learned through trial and error how to move its actual arm in order to get the brain-controlled cursor to most of the targets within this short training time, the animal was unable to find an actual arm path that would be effective at consistently getting the cursor to the lower left targets (see figure 10.2a and 10.2b). This problem can arise when the decoding function requires a neural modulation pattern that does not normally occur with *any* generated arm movements, as in this monkey's case, or with any imagined or attempted movement, as would be the case in a paralyzed individual. In this situation, the decoding function would need to be modified to one that can extract a full range of movements using only the repertoire of firing patterns that the user can easily generate. Alternatively, it may be possible for the user to learn to generate these new neural patterns with more extensive training via learning-induced synaptic changes in the underlying network structure.

10.5 Real-Time Adjustments to Random Variability in the Motor System and in the Assistive Device

Although feed-forward adjustments can be made if consistent errors occur when inadequate decoding models are used to convert neural activity to desired device motions, random errors will still occur due to the stochastic nature of neural processing and our limited ability to access the firing activity of the full neural ensemble. Therefore, these errors cannot be predicted and cannot be preemptively corrected by the user. In this case, visual feedback can be used to correct the random decoding errors only *after* they occur. While devices such as a brain-controlled computer cursor will go exactly where the output of the neural decoder dictates, other technologies do not function quite so perfectly. The assistive device itself can add additional random movement errors on top of those due to the stochastic nature of the neural signals. Incorporating accurate sensors into the device control system would enable the device to automatically detect and correct its own movement errors. However, accurate sensors are not currently incorporated into many assistive technologies that are prone to this kind of variability. Therefore, the subject has to use visual feedback to make an online correction for both sources of random errors.

An FES system that generates arm and hand movements by stimulating the peripheral nerves is a prime example of a system that adds additional variability into the movement. Although stimulators can be programmed to reproducibly generate the same pattern of current pulses needed to generate a specific movement, the resulting limb movement many differ each time due to the unobservable differences in the state of the peripheral nerves and muscles at the cellular level at the time of stimulation. Currently, most upper limb FES systems do not use position sensors on the limbs to detect and correct mismatches between the generated movement and the movement command sent to the FES system controller. However, there is a move toward incorporating sensors and feedback control into newer FES systems. Until then, current FES users will have to rely on visual feedback to make real-time adjustments to their movements to correct for both random decoding errors and error in the generation of the limb movement via FES.

The ability to exclusively use visual feedback to correct for both random decoding errors and random device errors was demonstrated in a second study where monkeys controlled the 3D movements of a robotic arm in space. This was an extension of the monkey study described earlier. However, in this phase of the study, both of the animal's arms were restrained throughout the experiment, but the animal still controlled the 3D movements of a virtual cursor or robot with firing activity from its arm-related motor cortical areas. In this case, the decoding algorithm was adaptively determined as the animal attempted to move the virtual cursor to the targets by modulating its neural activity without making arm movements. The decoding function was similar to that shown in (10.1) with the coefficients $[Ci_X, Ci_X, Ci_X]$ iteratively refined based on decoding errors seen in recent movement attempts. This adaptive process rapidly converged to a new decoding function that enabled the animal to make long continuous sequences of highly accurate cursor movements to different targets distributed throughout the 3D workspace. Details of this adaptive algorithm have been reported elsewhere (Taylor et al. (2002)).

Once the animal was proficient in moving the virtual cursor to targets distributed throughout the workspace, we tested the animal's ability to similarly control the 3D endpoint of a six-degree-of-freedom robotic arm. To aid in this transition, the animal still viewed the movements through the same virtual interface it had been using in all previous experiments (figure 10.1). However, instead of controlling the cursor directly, the decoded neural activity was used to direct the movements of the robotic arm, and a position sensor on the end of the robot determined the position of the cursor in the animal's 3D virtual workspace. Whereas the cursor alone reflected consistent and random errors due only to errors in the decoding function, the robot added additional consistent and random errors that the animal had to compensate for via additional feed-forward modifications to the neural output and via online adjustments based only on real-time visual feedback. Although this robot had built-in sensors that enabled its internal control system to accurately move the endpoint to whatever position the command signal dictated, we implemented a control system that effectively added movement errors at each time step that would accumulate over the course of the movement. This was done by implementing an asynchronous "velocity mode" control algorithm for the robot.

In the plain cursor control task, the neural activity was decoded into the desired ΔX, ΔY, and ΔZ at each 30 ms time step, and those changes in cursor position were perfectly executed to build up a trajectory that precisely represented the time series of decoded signals. However, with the robot, the velocity command $[\Delta X/30\text{ms}, \Delta Y/30\text{ms}, \Delta Z/30\text{ms}]$ was passed to the robot approximately every 30 ms, but the inherent jitter and the inertial properties of the robot prevented it from instantaneously achieving the assigned velocity. Therefore, when the new velocity command was given after 30 ms, the robot did not always achieve the appropriate ΔX, ΔY, and ΔZ before the new velocity command took effect. Thus, the intended and actual $[\Delta X, \Delta Y, \Delta Z]$ differed at each time step, and movement errors accumulated as the trajectory evolved. This form of control reflected the random errors that could accumulate in a trajectory, such as when using an FES system without limb position sensors where there is no way to ensure the evolving limb trajectory matched the trajectory sent to it by the neural decoder.

In spite of the added variability to the movement output, the animal was able to use visual feedback to make real-time corrections to the random trajectory deviations. Figure 10.3a shows trajectories of the brain-controlled robot in the eight-target 3D center-out task (plotted here again in two sets of four for easier 2D viewing). Although the trajectories of the brain-controlled robot were noisier than those made when using neural signals to control the 3D cursor directly, the animal was equally successful at getting the robot trajectory to the desired target (plots of brain-controlled cursor movements using an equivalent adaptively determined decoding function can be found in Taylor et al. (2002), and comparisons of the brain-controlled trajectories with and without the robot can be found in Taylor et al. (2003)).

To assess the practical application of this brain-controlled robot system in a self-feeding task, we trained the animal to use the robot to acquire moving and stationary bits of food located throughout the workspace and then bring the food to its mouth. Our initial attempts to have the animal retrieve food by direct viewing of the robot and food were unsuccessful presumably because the animal didn't realize that he was able to remotely direct the movements of this unfamiliar machine. Therefore, to ease the transition, we first had the animal retrieve and deliver food to its mouth by viewing the activities in the familiar virtual environment of targets and cursors. Two position sensors were used in this task. One sensor was located on a spoon that was attached to the end of the robot arm. This sensor determined the cursor position in the animal's virtual display. Due to physical obstruction by the virtual reality support frame, the robot could not be placed within reach of the animal's mouth. Therefore, the spoon was attached to the robot by a long, approximately 30-cm, rod. Due to some play in the mounting hardware used to attach the rod to the robot, the spoon had excessive vertical jitter as the robot moved. This resulted in yet another source of random variability in the brain-controlled trajectory of the robot-driven spoon.

The second position sensor was attached to a pair of tongs that were used to hold the food in different locations throughout the workspace. This sensor location was displayed as the target during the first phase of each feeding movement. The monkey would have to move the robot (viewed as cursor) to the food (viewed as target). When the cursor hit the target, the person holding the food heard a beep and knew to release the food into the spoon. A second stationary target located directly in front of the animal's mouth then appeared in the virtual workspace. The animal then had to move the brain-controlled robot to the mouth target. If the spoon made it to the mouth target, the spoon automatically rotated; the food fell into a funnel and was pneumatically swept through a tube, around the virtual reality viewing screen, and into the animal's mouth. On some trials, the experimenter would move the food to new locations just before the robot got to it, thus requiring the animal to perform a sequential tracking task where it would chase the food throughout the workspace. Figure 10.3b illustrates the stationary food retrieval and delivery task. Figure 10.3c shows an example of the nonstationary food tracking task. Note the additional vertical oscillation in the trajectory due to vibrations of the spoon attached to the robot. In spite of the inaccuracies added to the movements by the robot, the animal easily retrieved bits of food throughout the workspace and delivered them to its mouth target. Further work

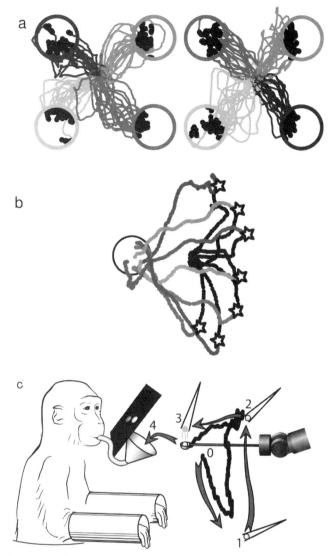

Figure 10.3   Movements of a brain-controlled robot viewed by the monkey through a virtual reality interface. Neural activity was used to direct the 3D movements of the robotic arm in real time. A position sensor on the end of the robot determined the movement of the virtual cursor. (a) Robot trajectories to eight targets in a 3D center-out task (plotted in two sets of four for easier 2D viewing). Trajectories are shaded to match their intended target. Black dots indicate when the virtual target was hit. (b) Robot trajectories from a stationary food retrieval task (overhead view). Trajectories (black) start from the center of the workspace and go to food targets located at various positions in the workspace (stars). Once the food is obtained, trajectories (grey) go to the "mouth" target located over a funnel (circle). Food is deposited into the funnel once this mouth target is reached. (c) Robot trajectory (black) from a moving food tracking and retrieval task. The spoon on the robot starts at point 0 and goes toward the food target at location 1. The food target is then moved to location 2 and then 3 as the robot follows. At point 3, the food is deposited into the spoon. Next a mouth target appears at point 4 and the animal moves the spoon to the mouth target. Once the spoon is over the funnel, the food is released into the funnel and pneumatically brought to the animal's mouth.(by permission, D.M.Taylor (2002))

by others in this area have now demonstrated that monkeys can retrieve food and bring it to their mouths by direct viewing of a brain-controlled robot without the use of the virtual reality interface (Spalding et al. (2005)).

10.6   Implications for Restoration of Arm and Hand Function

These and other studies illustrate the ability to use small numbers of neural signals recorded via intracortical microelectrodes to direct the continuous 2D (Serruya et al. (2002)) and 3D movements of computer cursors (Taylor and Schwartz (2001); Taylor et al. (2002)) and robotic devices (Taylor et al. (2003); Carmena et al. (2003)). Although our natural biological systems make use of somatosensory feedback to guide movement and correct errors, these studies suggest visual feedback alone enabled individuals to learn the consistent errors in decoding and device execution, thus allowing them to make appropriate feed-forward corrections in their neuromotor output. Therefore, it may not be necessary to generate complex decoders that accurately represent how intended movement is encoded in our recorded neural signals. Users can learn to modify their neural output to generate the desired movement via the imposed decoding scheme as long as the neural patterns needed to do so are within the subject's normal repertoire.

Visual feedback alone also was sufficient to enable subjects to correct for the type of random variability seen in the neural signals and in the execution of robot movements via an imperfect open-loop control system. Therefore, brain-based signals may be an effective means to command a wide range of assistive technologies including noisy physical systems, such as assistive robots, and FES systems that restore upper limb function.

It is likely that BMI function can be further improved by incorporating sensors on these assistive devices and feeding back that information to both the device control system directly and to the user via stimulation of the somatosensory cortex or through other neural pathways. This will be particularly useful for aspects of movement that are not easily visualized such as grip force or object slip. Work is underway by many groups to quantify the resolution and accuracy of the perceived somatosensory information that can be conveyed via microstimulation of the somatosensory cortex. Coarse movement information (e.g., left vs. right) has been successfully conveyed via cortical stimulation (Talwar et al. (2002)), but conveying finely graded continuous movement information is still an active area of research.

Current non-brain-based means of directing the movements of assistive devices (e.g., mouth-operated joysticks, tongue-touch keypads, sip-n-puff devices, voice recognition systems) also successfully rely primarily on visual feedback to enable the user to track and modify the resulting device movements. Somatosensory feedback is not currently part of most assistive devices for the severely paralyzed. Yet the available technologies, such as assistive robotic aids and FES systems, still can provide an increase in function and in the quality of life for the severely paralyzed individual. By using brain-based signals to command such devices in the future, people with high-level spinal cord injuries may regain the ability to reach and manipulate objects in a more natural way than with the other mouth- or face-based command options.

Our monkey experiments show that the individual neurons used for controlling the virtual or robotic movements became better at conveying the needed movement information to the decoder with regular practice (details reported elsewhere (Taylor et al. (2002))). The firing rates of the individual recorded units took on the imposed linear decoding function assigned to them by the decoder. They also increased their effective signal-to-noise ratio; that is, they increased their modulation ranges across movements in different directions while maintaining or reducing the variability in their firing rates during repeated movements to the same target directions. This improvement in the information conveyed by the neurons occurred with about an hour of practice a day only and with three to five days of practice a week only. Once practice was reduced to once every one to two weeks, these improvements started to decline. Reinstating practice three to five times a week resulted in a return of the improvement trend. It is likely that, once practical BCI/BMI systems are taken out of the lab and into the homes of paralyzed individuals, the improvements in the quality of the neurally controlled movements will be substantially greater than what has been shown so far in the animal studies, especially as these individuals learn to use and rely on these devices throughout their daily activities.

Acknowledgments

All monkey experiments were conducted at Arizona State University, Tempe, Arizona, and were approved by the university's Institutional Animal Care and Use Committee. Work was conducted in the lab of Andrew B. Schwartz, Ph.D., with robot assistance from Stephen I. Helms Tillery, Ph.D. Initial experiments were funded by the U.S. Public Health Service under contracts N01-NS-6-2347 and N01-NS-9-2321, a Philanthropic Educational Organization Scholarship, and a Whitaker Foundation Fellowship. Further analysis of the data was funded by the Veteran's Affairs Associate Investigator award, the Ron Shapiro Charitable Trust, and U.S. Public Health Service contract N01-NS-1-2333.

Notes

E-mail for correspondence: dxt42@case.edu

11   Advances in Cognitive Neural Prosthesis: Recognition of Neural Data with an Information-Theoretic Objective

Zoran Nenadic
Department of Biomedical Engineering
Department of Electical Engineering and Computer Science
University of California
Irvine, CA 92697

Daniel S. Rizzuto and Richard A. Andersen
Division of Biology
California Institute of Technology
Pasadena, CA 91125

Joel W. Burdick
Division of Engineering and Applied Science
California Institute of Technology
Pasadena, CA 91125

11.1   Abstract

We give an overview of recent advances in cognitive-based neural prostheses, and point out the major differences with respect to commonly used motor-based brain-machine interfaces. While encouraging results in neuroprosthetic research have demonstrated the proof of concept, the development of practical neural prostheses is still in the phase of infancy. To address complex issues arising in the development of practical neural prostheses we review several related studies ranging from the identification of new cognitive variables to the development of novel signal processing tools.

In the second part of this chapter, we discuss an information-theoretic approach to the extraction of low-dimensional features from high-dimensional neural data. We argue that this approach may be better suited for certain neuroprosthetic applications than the traditionally used features. An extensive analysis of electrical recordings from the human brain demonstrates that processing data in this manner yields more informative features than off-the-shelf techniques such as linear discriminant analysis. Finally, we show that the feature extraction is not only a useful dimensionality reduction technique, but also that the recognition of neural data may improve in the feature domain.

11.2   Introduction

The prospect of assisting disabled individuals by using neural activity from the brain to control prosthetic devices has been a field of intense research activity in recent years. The nature of neuroprosthetic research is highly interdisciplinary, with the brain-machine interfaces (BMIs) playing the central role. Although the development of BMIs can be viewed largely as a technological solution for a specific practical application, it also represents a valuable resource for studying brain mechanisms and testing new hypotheses about brain function.

Up to date, the majority of neuroprosthetic research studies have focused on deriving hand trajectories by recording their neural correlates, primarily, but not exclusively, from the motor cortex (Wessberg et al. (2000); Serruya et al. (2002); Taylor et al. (2002); Carmena et al. (2003); Mussa-Ivaldi and Miller (2003)). The trajectory information contained in the action potentials of individual neurons is decoded and the information is used to drive a robotic manipulator or a cursor on a computer screen. We refer to this neuroprosthetic approach as "motor-based." Additionally, progress has been made in interfacing electroencephalographic (EEG) signals and assistive devices for communication and control (Wolpaw et al. (2002)). These noninvasive techniques are commonly termed brain-computer interfaces (BCIs) (Wolpaw and McFarland (2004); Pfurtscheller et al. (2003c)).

While remarkable success in the development of BMIs has been achieved over the past decade, practical neural prostheses are not yet feasible. Building a fully operational neuroprosthetic system presents many challenges ranging from long-term stability of recording implants to development of efficient neural signal processing algorithms. Since the full scope of prosthetic applications is still unknown and it is unlikely that a single BMI will be optimal for all plausible scenarios, it is important to introduce new ideas about the types of signals that can be used. It is also important to address the many technological challenges that are currently impeding the progress toward operational neural prostheses. To this end, the neuroprosthetic research effort of our group spans several related directions including cognitive-based BMIs, decoding from local field potentials (LFPs), identification of alternative cognitive control signals, electrophysiologic recording advances, and development of new decoding algorithms.

In section 11.3, we give a brief overview of these research efforts. More details can be found in the relevant literature cited. In section 11.4, we discuss novel information-theoretic tools for extraction of useful features from high-dimensional neural data. Experimental results with electrically recorded signals from the human brain are presented in section 11.5, and the advantages of our technique over traditional ones are discussed. Concluding remarks are given in section 11.6.

11.3   Advances in Cognitive Neural Prosthesis

The motor-based approach, although predominantly used, is certainly not the only way of using brain data for neuroprosthetic applications. Shenoy et al. (2003) argue that neural activity present before or even without natural arm movement provides an important source of control signals. In nonhuman primates, these types of neural signals can be found, among other areas, in parietal reach region (PRR) of the posterior parietal cortex (PPC). PPC is an area located at an early stage in the sensory-motor pathway (Andersen et al. (1997)), and is involved in transforming sensory inputs into plans for actions, so-called "sensory-motor integration." In particular, PRR was shown to exhibit directional selectivity with respect to planned reaching movements (Snyder et al. (1997)). Moreover, these plans are encoded in visual coordinates (also called retinal or eye-centered coordinates) relative to the current direction of gaze (Batista et al. (1999)), thus providing extrinsic spatial information and underscoring the cognitive nature of these signals. We refer to this approach to neural prostheses as "cognitive-based." The human homologue of PRR has recently been identified in functional-magnetic-resonance imaging experiments (Connolly et al. (2003)).

11.3.1   Cognitive-Based Brain-Machine Interfaces

The cognitive-based approach to neural prostheses does not require the execution of arm movements; its true potential lies in assisting paralyzed individuals who are unable to reach but who are capable of making reaching plans. It has been shown through a series of experiments (Musallam et al. (2004)) that monkeys easily learn to control the location of a computer cursor by merely thinking about movements. Briefly, the monkeys were shown a transient visual cue (target) at different screen locations over multiple trials. After the target disappeared, the monkeys were required to plan a reach movement to the target location without making any arm or eye movements. This stage of the experiment is referred to as the "delay" or "memory period." The action potentials (spike trains) of individual neurons from PRR were collected during the memory period and were decoded in real time to predict the target location. If the correct location was decoded, a feedback was provided to the animals by illuminating the target location and the animals were rewarded. The trials were aborted if the animals made eye or arm movements during the memory period. This ensured that only cognitive and not motor-related signals were used for decoding, thus underscoring the potential of the cognitive-based approach for severely paralyzed patients.

With vision being the main sensory modality of the posterior parietal cortex (Blatt et al. (1990); Johnson et al. (1996)), PRR is likely to continue receiving appropriate error signals after paralysis. In the absence of proprioceptive and somatosensory feedback (typically lost due to paralysis), visual error signals become essential in motor learning. Musallam et al. (2004) have shown that the performance of a PRR-operated prosthesis improved over the course of several weeks. Presumably, the visual feedback allowed the monkeys to learn how to compensate for decoding errors.

After reaching goals are decoded, trajectories can be computed from low-level trajectory instructions managed by smart output devices, such as robots, computers, or vehicles, using supervisory control systems (Sheridan (1992)). For example, given the Cartesian coordinates of an intended object for grasping, a robotic motion planner can determine the detailed joint trajectories that will transport a prosthetic hand to the desired location (Andersen et al. (2004a)). Sensors embedded in the mechanical arm can ensure that the commanded trajectories are followed and obstacles are avoided, thereby replacing, at least to some degree, the role of proprioceptive and somatosensory feedback.

11.3.2   Local Field Potentials

LFPs represent the composite extracellular potential from perhaps hundreds or thousands of neurons around the electrode tip. In general, LFPs are less sensitive to relative movement of recording electrodes and tissues; therefore, LFP recordings can be maintained for longer periods of time than single cell recordings (Andersen et al. (2004b)). However, LFPs have not been widely used in BMIs, perhaps because of the assumption that they do not correlate with movements or movement intentions as well as single cell activity. Recent experiments in monkey PPC, in particular the lateral intraparietal (LIP) area and PRR, have demonstrated that valuable information related to the animal's intentions can be uncovered from LFPs. For example, it has been shown that the direction of planned saccades in macaques can be decoded based on LFPs recorded from area LIP (Pesaran et al. (2002)). Moreover, the performances of decoders based on spike trains and LFPs were found to be comparable. Interestingly, the decoding of behavioral state (planning vs. execution of saccades) was more accurate with LFPs than with spike trains. Similar studies have been conducted in PRR. It was found that the decoding of the direction of planned reaches was only slightly inferior with LFPs than with spike trains (Scherberger et al. (2005)). As with LIP studies, it has also been shown that LFPs in this area provide better behavioral state (planning vs. execution of reaching) decoding than do spike trains.

While the decoding of a target position or a hand trajectory provides information on *where* to reach, the decoding of a behavioral state provides the information on *when* to reach. In current experiments, the time of reach is controlled with experimental protocol by supplying a "go signal." Practical neural prostheses cannot rely on external cues to initiate the movement; instead this information should be decoded from the brain, and future BMIs are likely to incorporate the behavioral state information. Therefore, it is expected that LFPs will play a more prominent role in the design of future neuroprosthetic devices.

11.3.3   Alternative Cognitive Control Signals

The potential benefits of a cognitive-based approach to neural prosthesis were demonstrated first through offline analysis (Shenoy et al. (2003)) and subsequently through closed loop (online) experiments (Musallam et al. (2004)). Motivated by previous findings of reward prediction based on neural activity in various brain areas (Platt and Glimcher (1999); Schultz (2004)), Musallam et al. (2004) have demonstrated that similar cognitive variables can be inferred from the activity in the macaques' PRR. In particular, they have found significant differences in cell activity depending on whether a preferred or nonpreferred reward was expected at the end of a trial. The experiments included various preferred versus nonpreferred reward paradigms such as citrus juice versus water, large amount versus small amount of reward, and high probability versus low probability of reward. On each day, the animal learned to associate one cue with the expectation of preferred reward and another cue with nonpreferred reward. The cues were randomly interleaved on a trial-by-trial basis. This study demonstrated that the performance of brain-operated cursor control increases under preferred reward conditions, and that both the reach goals and the reward type can be simultaneously decoded in real time.

The ability to decode expected values from brain data is potentially useful for future BMIs. The information regarding subjects' preferences, motivation level, and mood could be easily communicated to others in a manner similar to expressing these variables using body language. It is also conceivable that other types of cognitive variables, such as the patient's emotional state, could be inferred by recording activity from appropriate brain areas.

11.3.4 Neurophysiologic Recording Advances

One of the major challenges in the development of practical BMIs is to acquire meaningful data from many recording channels over a long period of time. This task is especially challenging if the spike trains of single neurons are used, since typically only a fraction of the electrodes in an implanted electrode array will record signals from well-isolated individual cells (Andersen et al. (2004b)). It is also hard to maintain the activity of isolated units in the face of inherent tissue and/or array drifts. Reactive gliosis (Turner et al. (1999)) and inadequate biocompatibility of the electrode's surface material (Edell et al. (1992)) may also contribute to the loss of an implant's function over time.

Fixed-geometry implants, routinely used for chronic recordings in BMIs, are not well suited for addressing the above issues. Motivated by these shortcomings, part of our research effort has been directed toward the development of autonomously movable electrodes that are capable of finding and maintaining optimal recording positions. Based on recorded signals and a suitably defined signal quality metric, an algorithm has been developed that decides when and where to move the recording electrode (Nenadic and Burdick (2006)). It should be emphasized that the developed control algorithm and associated signal processing steps (Nenadic and Burdick (2005)) are fully unsupervised, that is, free of any human involvement, and as such are suitable for future BMIs. Successful applications of the autonomously movable electrode algorithm using a meso-scale electrode testbed have recently been reported in Cham et al. (2005) and Branchaud et al. (2005).

The successful implementation of autonomously movable electrodes in BMIs will be beneficial for several reasons. For example, electrodes can be moved to target specific neural populations that are likely to be missed during implantation surgery. Optimal recording quality could be maintained and the effects of cell migration can be compensated for by moving the electrodes. Finally, movable electrodes could break through encapsulation and seek out new neurons, which is likely to improve the longevity of recording.

Clearly, the integration of movable electrodes with BMIs hinges upon the development of appropriate micro-electro-mechanical systems (MEMS) technology. Research efforts to develop MEMS devices for movable electrodes are under way (Pang et al. (2005a,b)).

11.3.5   Novel Decoding Algorithms

In mathematical terms, the goal of decoding algorithms is to build a map between neural patterns and corresponding motor behavior or cognitive processes. Because of the randomness inherent in the neuro-motor systems, the appropriate model of this map is probabilistic. In practical terms, decoding for cognitive-based BMIs entails the selection of the intended reach target from a discrete set of possible targets. Consequently, the decoder is designed as a classifier, where observed neural data is used for classifier training.

Recent advances in electrophysiologic recordings have enabled scientists to gather increasingly large volumes of data over relatively short time spans. While neural data ultimately is important for decoding, not all data samples carry useful information for the task at hand. Ideally, relevant data samples should be combined into meaningful features, while irrelevant data should be discarded as noise. For example, representing a finely sampled time segment of neural data with a (low-dimensional) vector of firing rates, can be viewed as an heuristic way of extracting features from the data. Another example is the use of the spectral power of EEG signals in various frequency bands, for example, μ-band or β-band (McFarland et al. (1997a); Pfurtscheller et al. (1997)), for neuroprosthetic applications such as BCIs.

In the next section, we cast the extraction of neural features within an information-theoretic framework and we show that this approach may be better suited for certain applications than the traditionally used heuristic features.

11.4   Feature Extraction

Feature extraction is a common tool in the analysis of multivariate statistical data. Typically, a low-dimensional representation of data is sought so that features have some desired properties. An obvious benefit of this dimensionality reduction is that data becomes computationally more manageable. More importantly, since the number of experimental trials is typically much smaller than the dimension of data (so-called small-sample-size problem (Fukunaga (1990))), the statistical parameters of data can be estimated more accurately using the low-dimensional representation.

Two major applications of feature extraction are representation and classification. Feature extraction for representation aims at finding a low-dimensional approximation of data, subject to certain criteria. These criteria assume that data are sampled from a common probability distribution, and so these methods are often referred to as blind or unsupervised. Principal component analysis (PCA) (Jolliffe (1986)) and independent component analysis (ICA) (Jutten and Herault (1991)) are the best-known representatives of these techniques. In feature extraction for classification, on the other hand, each data point's class membership is known, and thus the method is considered supervised. Low-dimensional features are found that maximally preserve class differences measured by suitably defined criteria. Linear discriminant analysis (LDA) (Duda et al. (2001)) is the best known representative of these techniques. Once the features are extracted, a classifier of choice can be designed in the feature domain.[1]

A common heuristic approach to feature extraction is to rank individual (scalar) features according to some class separability criterion. For example, informative neural features are those that exhibit stimulus-related tuning, that is, they take significantly different values when conditioned upon different stimuli. The feature vector is then constructed by concatenating the several most informative features. While seemingly reasonable, this strategy is completely ignorant of the joint statistical properties of the features and may produce highly suboptimal feature vectors. More elaborate algorithms exist for the selection of scalar features (Kittler (1978)), but they are combinatorially complex (Cover and Campenhout (1977)) and their practical applicability is limited.

Another popular strategy for analyzing spatiotemporal neural signals is to separate the processing in the spatial and temporal domain. Data are first processed spatially, typically by applying off-the-shelf tools such as the Laplacian filter (McFarland et al. (1997a); Wolpaw and McFarland (2004)), followed by temporal processing, such as autoregressive frequency analysis (Wolpaw and McFarland (2004); Pfurtscheller et al. (1997)). However, the assumption of space-time separability is not justified and may be responsible for suboptimal performance. In addition, while spectral power features have clear physical interpretation, there is no reason to assume that they are optimal features for decoding. Rizzuto et al. (2005) have recently demonstrated that decoding accuracy with spectral power features could be up to 20 percent lower than a straightforward time domain decoding.

In the next two subsections, we introduce a novel information-theoretic criterion for feature extraction conveniently called "information-theoretic discriminant analysis" (ITDA). We show that informative features can be extracted from data in a linear fashion, that is, through a matrix manipulation.[2] For spatiotemporal signals, the feature extraction matrix plays the role of a spatiotemporal filter and does not require an assumption about the separability of time and space. Moreover, the features are extracted using their joint statistical properties, thereby avoiding heuristic feature selection strategies and computationally expensive search algorithms.

11.4.1   Linear Supervised Feature Extraction

In general, linear feature extraction is a two-step procedure: (1) an objective function is defined and (2) a full-rank feature extraction matrix is found that maximizes such an objective. More formally, let $R \in \mathbb{R}^n$ be a random data vector with the class-conditional probability density function (PDF) $f_{R|\Omega}(r \mid \omega_i)$, where the class random variable (RV) $\Omega = \{\omega_1, \omega_2, \cdots, \omega_c\}$ is drawn from a discrete distribution with the probability $P(\omega_i) \triangleq P(\Omega = \omega_i), \forall i = 1, 2, \cdots, c$. For example, R could be a matrix of EEG data from an array of electrodes sampled in time and written in a vector form. The class variable could be the location of a visual target, or some cognitive task such as imagination of left and right hand movements (Pfurtscheller et al. (1997)). The features $F \in \mathbb{R}^m$ are extracted as

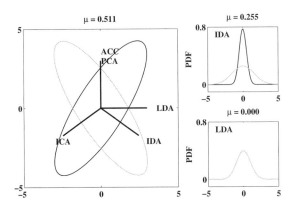

Figure 11.1   (Left) Two Gaussian class-conditional PDFs with $P(\omega_1) = P(\omega_2)$, represented by 3-Mahalanobis distance contours. The straight lines indicate optimal 1D subspace according to different feature extraction methods: PCA, ICA, LDA, ITDA and approximate Chernoff criterion (Loog and Duin (2004)) ACC. (Right) The PDFs of optimal 1D features extracted with ITDA and LDA.

$\mathsf{F} = \boldsymbol{T}\mathsf{R}$, where $\boldsymbol{T} \in \mathbb{R}^{m \times n}$ is a full-rank feature extraction matrix found by maximizing a suitably chosen class separability objective function $J(\boldsymbol{T})$.

Many objective functions have been used for supervised feature extraction purposes. In its most common form, LDA, also known as the Fisher criterion (Fisher (1936)) or canonical variate analysis, maximizes the generalized Rayleigh quotient (Duda et al. (2001)). Under fairly restrictive assumptions, it can be shown that LDA is an optimal[3] feature extraction method. In practice, however, these assumptions are known to be violated, and so the method suffers from suboptimal performance. A simple example where LDA fails completely is illustrated in figure 11.1. Another deficiency of LDA is that the dimension of the extracted subspace is at most $c - 1$, where c is the number of classes. This constraint may severely limit the practical applicability of LDA features, especially when the number of classes is relatively small.

Kumar and Andreou (1998) have developed a maximum-likelihood feature extraction method and showed that these features are better suited for speech recognition than the classical LDA features. Saon and Padmanabhan (2000) used both Kullback-Leibler (KL) and Bhattacharyya distance as an objective function. However, both of these metrics are defined pairwise, and their extension to multicategory cases is often heuristic. Loog and Duin (2004) have developed an approximation of the Chernoff distance, although their method seems to fail in some cases (see figure 11.1).

Mutual information is a natural measure of class separability. For a continuous RV R and a discrete RV Ω, the mutual information, denoted by $\mu I(\mathsf{R}; \Omega)$, is defined as

$$\mu I(\mathsf{R}; \Omega) \triangleq H(\mathsf{R}) - H(\mathsf{R} \mid \Omega) = H(\mathsf{R}) - \sum_{i=1}^{c} H(\mathsf{R} \mid \omega_i)\, P(\omega_i) \qquad (11.1)$$

where $H(\mathsf{R}) \triangleq -\int f_{\mathsf{R}}(\boldsymbol{r}) \log(f_{\mathsf{R}}(\boldsymbol{r}))\, d\boldsymbol{r}$ is Shannon's entropy. Generally, higher mutual information implies better class separability and smaller probability of misclassification. In particular, it was shown in Hellman and Raviv (1970) that $\varepsilon_{\mathsf{R}} \le 1/2\,[H(\Omega) - \mu I(\mathsf{R}; \Omega)]$, where $H(\Omega)$ is the entropy of Ω and ε_{R} is the Bayes error. On the other hand, the practical applicability of the mutual information is limited by its computational complexity, also known as the curse of dimensionality, which for multivariate data requires numerical integrations in high-dimensional spaces. Principe et al. (2000) explored the alternative definitions of entropy (Renyi (1961)), which, when coupled with Parzen window density estimation, led to a computationally feasible mutual information alternative that was applicable to multivariate data. Motivated by these findings, Torkkola developed an information-theoretic feature extraction algorithm (Torkkola (2003)), although his method is computationally demanding and seems to be limited by the curse of dimensionality. Next, we introduce a feature extraction objective function that is based on the mutual information, yet is easily computable.

11.4.2   Information-Theoretic Objective Function

Throughout the rest of the article we assume, that the class-conditional densities are Gaussian, that is, $\mathsf{R}\,|\,\omega_i \sim \mathcal{N}(\boldsymbol{m}_i, \boldsymbol{\Sigma}_i)$, with positive definite covariance matrices. The entropy of a Gaussian random variable is easily computed as

$$H(\mathsf{R}\,|\,\omega_i) = \frac{1}{2}\log((2\pi e)^n |\boldsymbol{\Sigma}_i|)$$

where $|\Sigma|$ denotes for the determinant of the matrix Σ. To complete the calculations required by (11.1), we need to evaluate the entropy of the mixture PDF $f_{\mathsf{R}}(\boldsymbol{r}) \triangleq \sum_i f_{\mathsf{R}|\Omega}(\boldsymbol{r}\,|\,\omega_i)P(\omega_i)$. It is easy to establish that $\mathsf{R} \sim (\boldsymbol{m}, \boldsymbol{\Sigma})$, where

$$\boldsymbol{m} = \sum_{i=1}^{c} \boldsymbol{m}_i P(\omega_i) \quad \text{and} \quad \boldsymbol{\Sigma} = \sum_{i=1}^{c} \left[\boldsymbol{\Sigma}_i + (\boldsymbol{m}_i - \boldsymbol{m})(\boldsymbol{m}_i - \boldsymbol{m})^{\mathsf{T}}\right] P(\omega_i). \quad (11.2)$$

Note that unless the class-conditional PDFs are completely overlapped, the RV R is non-Gaussian. However, we propose a metric similar to (11.1) by replacing $H(\mathsf{R})$ with the entropy of a Gaussian RV with the same covariance matrix $\boldsymbol{\Sigma}$:

$$\mu(\mathsf{R}; \Omega) \triangleq H_g(\mathsf{R}) - \sum_{i=1}^{c} H(\mathsf{R}\,|\,\omega_i)P(\omega_i) = \frac{1}{2}\left[\log(|\boldsymbol{\Sigma}|) - \sum_{i=1}^{c} \log(|\boldsymbol{\Sigma}_i|)P(\omega_i)\right] \quad (11.3)$$

where $H_g(\mathsf{R})$ is the Gaussian entropy. Throughout the rest of the article, we refer to this metric as a μ-metric.

We will explain briefly why the μ-metric is a valid class separability objective. For a thorough mathematical exposition, the reader is referred to Nenadic (in press). If the class-conditional PDFs are fully overlapped, that is, $\boldsymbol{m}_1 = \cdots = \boldsymbol{m}_c$ and $\boldsymbol{\Sigma}_1 = \cdots = \boldsymbol{\Sigma}_c$, it follows from (11.2) and (11.3) that $\mu(\mathsf{R}; \Omega) = 0$. Also note that in this case $\mathsf{R} \sim \mathcal{N}(\boldsymbol{m}, \boldsymbol{\Sigma})$, thus $\mu(\mathsf{R}; \Omega) = \mu I(\mathsf{R}; \Omega)$. On the other hand, if the class-conditional PDFs are different, R deviates from the Gaussian RV, so the μ-metric $\mu(\mathsf{R}; \Omega)$ can be viewed as a biased version of $\mu I(\mathsf{R};\Omega)$, where $\mu(\mathsf{R};\Omega) \geq \mu I(\mathsf{R};\Omega) \geq 0$ because for a fixed covariance matrix, Gaussian distribution maximizes the entropy $[H_g(\mathsf{R}) \geq H(\mathsf{R})]$. As the classes are more separated, the deviation of R from a Gaussian RV increases, and the μ-metric gets bigger. It turns out that this bias is precisely the negentropy defined as $\bar{H}(\mathsf{R}) \triangleq H_g(\mathsf{R}) - H(\mathsf{R})$, which has been used as an objective function for ICA applications (see Hyvärinen (1999) for survey). Therefore, ITDA can be viewed as a supervised version of ICA. Figure 11.1 confirms that ICA produces essentially the same result as our method (note the symmetry of the example), although the two methods are fundamentally different (unsupervised vs. supervised). Figure 11.1 also shows the μ-metric in the original space and subspaces extracted by ITDA and LDA.

The μ-metric has some interesting properties, many of which are reminiscent of the Bayes error ε_{R} and the mutual information (11.1). We give a brief overview of these properties next. For a detailed discussion, refer to Nenadic (in press). First, if the class-conditional covariances are equal, the μ-metric takes the form of the generalized Rayleigh quotient; therefore, under these so-called homoscedastic conditions, ITDA reduces to the classical LDA method. Second, for a two-class case with overlapping class-conditional means and equal class probabilities (e.g., figure 11.1), the μ-metric reduces to the well known Bhattacharyya distance. Like many other discriminant metrics, the μ-metric is independent of the choice of a coordinate system for data representation. Moreover, the search for the full-rank feature extraction matrix $\boldsymbol{T}$ can be restricted to the subspace of orthonormal projection matrices without compromising the objective function. Finally, the μ-metric of any subspace of the original data space is bounded above by the μ-metric of the original space. These properties guarantee that the following optimization problem is well posed. Given the response samples $\mathsf{R} \in \mathbb{R}^n$ and the dimension of the feature space m, we find an orthonormal matrix $\boldsymbol{T} \in \mathbb{R}^{m \times n}$ such that the μ–metric $\mu(\mathsf{F};\Omega)$ is maximized

$$\boldsymbol{T}^* = \arg \max_{\boldsymbol{T} \in \mathbb{R}^{m \times n}} \{\mu(\mathsf{F};\Omega) : \mathsf{F} = \boldsymbol{T}\mathsf{R}\} \quad \text{subject to} \quad \boldsymbol{T}\boldsymbol{T}^{\mathsf{T}} = \boldsymbol{I}. \quad (11.4)$$

Based on our discussion in section 11.4.2, it follows that such a transformation would find an m-dimensional subspace, where the class separability is maximal. Interestingly, both the gradient $\partial\mu(\mathsf{F};\Omega)/\partial\boldsymbol{T}$ and the Hessian $\partial^2\mu(\mathsf{F};\Omega)/\partial\boldsymbol{T}^2$ can be found analytically (Nenadic (in press)), so the problem (11.4) is amenable to Newton's optimization method.

11.5 Experimental Results

In this section, we compare the performances of LDA and ITDA on a dataset adopted from Rizzuto et al. (2005). The data represents intracranial encephalographic (iEEG) recordings from the human brain during a standard memory reach task (see figure 11.2). It should be noted that iEEG signals are essentially local field potentials (see section 11.3.2). At the start of each trial, a fixation stimulus is presented in the middle of a touchscreen and the participant initiates the trial by placing his right hand on the stimulus. After a short fixation period, a target is flashed on the screen, followed by a memory period. After the memory period, the fixation stimulus is extinguished, which signals the participant to reach to the

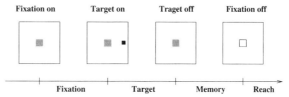

Figure 11.2 The timeline of experimental protocol.

memorized location (formerly indicated by the target). The duration of fixation, target, and memory periods varied uniformly between 1 and 1.3 s. The subject had 8 electrodes implanted into each of the following target brain areas: orbital frontal cortex (OF), amygdala (A), hippocampus (H), anterior cingulate cortex (AC), supplementary motor cortex (SM), and parietal cortex (P). The total number of electrodes in both hemispheres was 96. The targets were presented at 6 different locations: 0°, 60°, 120°, 180°, 240°, 300°; these locations respectively correspond to right, top right, top left, left, bottom left, and bottom right position with respect to the fixation stimulus. The number of trials per stimulus varied between 69 and 82, yielding a total of 438 trials. The electrode signals were amplified, sampled at 200 Hz and bandpass filtered. Only a few electrodes over a few brain areas showed stimulus-related tuning according to the location of the target. The goal of our analysis is to decode the target location and the behavioral state based on the brain data. Such a method could be used to decode a person's motor intentions in real time, supporting neuroprosthetic applications. All decoding results are based on a linear, quadratic, and support vector machine (SVM) classifier (Collobert and Bengio (2001)) with a Gaussian kernel.

11.5.1 Decoding the Target Position

To decode the target position, we focused on a subset of data involving only two target positions: left and right. While it is possible to decode all six target positions, the results are rather poor, partly because certain directions were consistently confused. The decoding was performed during the target, memory and reach periods (see figure 11.2). All decoding results are based on selected subsegments of data within 1 s of the stimulus that marks the beginning of the period. figure. 11.3 shows that only a couple of electrodes in both left and right parietal cortex exhibit directional tuning, mostly around 200 ms after the onset of the target stimulus. In addition, there is some tuning in the SM and OF regions. Similar plots (not shown) are used for the decoding during memory and reach periods.

For smoothing purposes and to further reduce the dimensionality of the problem, the electrode signals were binned using a 30 to 70 ms window. The performance (% error) of the classifier in the feature domain was evaluated through a leave-one-out cross-validation; the results are summarized in table 11.1. Note that the chance error is 50 percent for this particular task. For a given classifier, the performance of the better feature extraction method is shown in boldface, and the asterisk denotes the best performance per classification task. Except for a few cases (mostly with the quadratic classifier), the performance of the ITDA method is superior to that of LDA, regardless of the choice of classifier. More

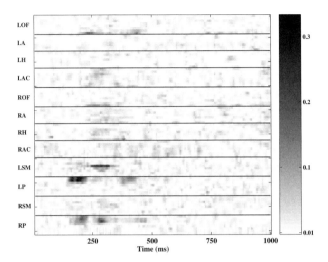

Figure 11.3   The distribution of the μ-metric over individual electrodes during the target period. The results are for two-class recognition task, and are based on 162 trials (82 left and 80 right). Different brain areas are: orbital frontal (OF), amygdala (A), hippocampus (H), anterior cingulate (AC), supplementary motor (SM), and parietal (P), with the prefixes L and R denoting the left and right hemisphere.

importantly, ITDA provides the lowest error rates in all but one case (target, SM), where the two methods are tied for the best performance. We note that all the error rates are significantly smaller ($p < 0.001$) than the chance error, including those during the memory period, which was not demonstrated previously (Rizzuto et al. (2005)). Also note that, in general, the SVM classifier is better combined with both ITDA and LDA features than are the linear and quadratic classifiers.

11.5.2   Decoding the Behavioral State

As discussed in section 11.3.2, for fully autonomous neuroprosthetic applications it is not only important to know *where* to reach, but also *when* to reach. Therefore, the goal is to decode what experimental state (fixation, target, memory, reach) the subject is experiencing, based on the brain data. To this end, we pooled the data for all six directions, with 438 trials per state, for a total of 1,752 trials. As with the target decoding, all the decoding results are based on selected subsegments of data within 1 s of the stimulus that marks the beginning of the period. Figure 11.4 shows that only a subset of electrodes exhibits state tuning (mostly the electrodes in the SM area during the second part of the trial state period). In addition, there is some tuning in the AC, H, and P areas. The data were further smoothed by applying a 40 to 50 ms window. The performance (% error) of the classifier in the feature space was evaluated through a stratified twenty-fold cross-validation (Kohavi (1995)), and the results are summarized in table 11.2.

Table 11.1 The average decoding errors and their standard deviations during the target, memory and reach periods. The columns represent the brain area, the number of electrodes N_e, the period (ms) used for decoding, the bin size (ms), the size of the data space (n), the type of the classifier (L-linear, Q-quadratic, S-SVM). The size of the optimal subspace (m) is given in the parentheses. Note that LDA is constrained to $m = 1$.

Period	Area	N_e	Time	Bin	n	Class.	LDA		(m)	ITDA		(m)
target	OF	4	160–510	70	20	L	6.17	± 0.24	(1)	**4.94***	± 0.22	(1)
						Q	**6.17**	± 0.24	(1)	8.02	± 0.27	(1)
						S	6.17	± 0.25	(1)	**4.94***	± 0.22	(1)
	P	2	150–450	50	12	L	7.41	± 0.26	(1)	**6.79***	± 0.25	(1)
						Q	8.02	± 0.27	(1)	**7.41**	± 0.26	(1)
						S	7.41	± 0.26	(1)	**6.79***	± 0.25	(2)
	SM	2	100–450	70	10	L	14.20	± 0.35	(1)	**13.58***	± 0.34	(3)
						Q	14.20	± 0.35	(1)	**13.58***	± 0.34	(2)
						S	**13.58***	± 0.34	(1)	**13.58***	± 0.34	(3)
	SM,P	2	120–520	40	20	L	5.56	± 0.23	(1)	**4.32***	± 0.20	(1)
						Q	**5.56**	± 0.23	(1)	**5.56**	± 0.23	(1)
						S	4.94	± 0.22	(1)	**4.32***	± 0.20	(1)
memory	OF	3	240–330	30	6	L	29.63	± 0.46	(1)	**28.40***	± 0.45	(1)
						Q	30.25	± 0.46	(1)	**28.40***	± 0.45	(2)
						S	31.48	± 0.47	(1)	**29.01**	± 0.46	(1)
	P	4	610–730	30	16	L	33.95	± 0.48	(1)	**32.72**	± 0.47	(1)
						Q	**33.33**	± 0.47	(1)	35.80	± 0.48	(1)
						S	31.48	± 0.47	(1)	**29.63***	± 0.46	(4)
	SM	2	250–370	30	8	L	29.63	± 0.45	(1)	**29.01**	± 0.46	(6)
						Q	29.63	± 0.46	(1)	**25.93**	± 0.44	(3)
						S	29.63	± 0.46	(1)	**24.69***	± 0.43	(4)
	SM, P,A	3	620–680	30	6	L	28.40	± 0.45	(1)	**26.54***	± 0.44	(1)
						Q	**27.16**	± 0.45	(1)	28.40	± 0.45	(1)
						S	27.16	± 0.45	(1)	**26.54***	± 0.44	(1)
reach	OF	2	270–420	50	6	L	10.49	± 0.31	(1)	**9.26**	± 0.29	(1)
						Q	10.49	± 0.31	(1)	**9.88**	± 0.30	(1)
						S	9.88	± 0.30	(1)	**8.64***	± 0.28	(1)
	OF	4	250–550	50	24	L	6.79	± 0.25	(1)	**6.17**	± 0.24	(1)
						Q	**6.79**	± 0.25	(1)	**6.79**	± 0.25	(1)
						S	6.17	± 0.24	(1)	**4.94***	± 0.22	(22)

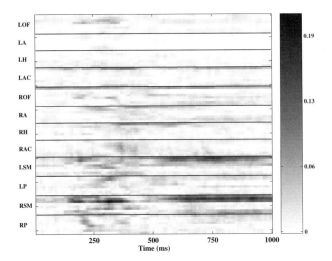

Figure 11.4 The distribution of the μ-metric over individual electrodes. The results are for four-class recognition task based on 1,752 trials (438 trials per state).

Table 11.2 The average behavioral state decoding errors and their standard deviations with pooled data (6 directions, 4 trial states). Note that LDA is constrained to $m \leq 3$.

Area	N_e	Time	Bin	n	Class.	LDA		(m)	ITDA		(m)
SM	4	500–1000	50	40	L	24.70	±0.04	(3)	**24.17**	±0.04	(4)
					Q	24.82	±0.04	(3)	**24.58**	±0.04	(5)
					S	24.76	±0.04	(3)	**23.99***	±0.04	(4)
SM	3	120–400	40	21	L	35.36	±0.06	(3)	**35.06**	±0.05	(9)
					Q	36.25	±0.05	(3)	**31.31***	±0.05	(12)
					S	35.42	±0.06	(3)	**31.43**	±0.06	(14)
SM, AC,H	4	250–500	50	20	L	29.23	±0.06	(3)	**28.75**	±0.06	(3)
					Q	28.99	±0.06	(3)	**27.74***	±0.06	(5)
					S	28.93	±0.06	(3)	**27.74***	±0.06	(5)
P	4	200–350	50	12	L	48.69	±0.06	(3)	**47.86**	±0.05	(10)
					Q	**48.99**	±0.07	(3)	50.89	±0.05	(10)
					S	49.70	±0.05	(3)	**47.68***	±0.04	(10)

Note that the chance error is 75 percent for this particular task. Except for one case, the classification accuracy with ITDA features is superior to LDA features, regardless of the classifier choice. Additionally, the best single performance always is achieved with the ITDA method. Note that the best decoding results are obtained from the SM area in the interval [500–1000] ms. Interestingly, we were able to decode the trial states from the parietal area, although the accuracy was considerably lower (just above 50 percent).

11.5.3   Discussion

Based on the analyzed data, we conclude that the classification with ITDA features is more accurate than the classification with LDA features, with an improvement as high as 5 percent. In rare cases where LDA provides better performance, the quadratic classifier was used. This could mean that LDA features fit the quadratic classifier assumptions (Gaussian classes, different covariance matrices) better than do ITDA features. Nevertheless, ITDA features are in general better coupled to the quadratic classifier than are LDA features. The advantages are even more apparent when ITDA is used in conjunction with the linear and SVM classifier. Similar behavior was observed when ITDA was tested on a variety of data sets from the UCI machine learning repository (Hettich et al. (1998)). Details can be found in Nenadic (in press).

In all cases, the best performance is achieved in a subspace of considerably lower dimension than the dimension of the original data space, n. Therefore, not only is the classification easier to implement in the feature space, but the overall classification accuracy is improved. While theoretical analysis shows that dimensionality reduction cannot improve classification accuracy (Duda et al. (2001)), the exact opposite effect is often seen in dealing with finitely sampled data.

Like many other second-order techniques, for example, LDA or ACC, ITDA assumes that the class-conditional data distribution is Gaussian. Although this assumption is likely to be violated in practice, it seems that the ITDA method performs reasonably well. For example, the performance in the original space with the SVM classifier is Gaussian-assumption free, yet it is inferior to the SVM classifier performance in the ITDA feature space. Likewise, it was found in Nenadic (in press) that unless data is coarsely discretized and the Gaussian assumption is severely violated, the performance of ITDA does not critically depend on the Gaussian assumption.

11.6   Summary

We have reviewed recent advances in cognitive-based neural prosthesis. The major differences between the cognitive-based and the more common motor-based approach to BMIs have been discussed. To maximize information encoded by neurons, better understanding of multiple brain areas and the types of signals the brain uses are needed. Part of our research effort is to identify sources of information potentially useful for neuroprosthetic applications. Other research efforts are focused on technological issues such as the stability of recording, the development of unsupervised signal analysis tools, or the design of complex decoding algorithms.

The decoding of neural signals in cognitive-based BMIs reduces to the problem of classification. High-dimensional neural data typically contains relatively low-dimensional useful signals (features) embedded in noise. To meet computational constraints associated with BMIs, it may be beneficial to implement the classifier in the feature domain. We have applied a novel information-theoretic method to uncover useful low-dimensional features in neural data. We have demonstrated that this problem can be posed within an optimization framework, thereby avoiding unjustified assumptions and heuristic feature selection strategies. Experimental results using iEEG signals from the human brain show that our method may be better suited for certain applications than are the traditional feature extraction tools. The study also demonstrates that iEEG signals may be a valuable alternative to spike trains commonly used in neuroprosthetic research.

Acknowledgments

This work is partially supported by the National Science Foundation (NSF) under grant 9402726 and by the Defense Advanced Research Projects Agency (DARPA) under grant MDA972-00-1-0029. Z. Nenadic also acknowledges the support from the University of California Irvine (UCI) set-up funds. The authors would like to thank the anonymous reviewers for their constructive criticism. The authors would also like to acknowledge the editors for their timely processing of this manuscript.

Notes

E-mail for correspondence: znenadic@uci.edu

(1) Consistent with engineering literature (Fukunaga (1990)), we consider the feature extraction as a preprocessing step for classification. Some authors, especially those using artificial neural networks, consider feature extraction an integral part of classification.

(2) Recently, a couple of nonlinear feature extraction methods have been proposed (Roweis and Saul (2000); Tenenbaum et al. (2000)) where features reside on a low-dimensional manifold embedded in the original data space. However, linear feature extraction methods continue to play an important role in many applications, primarily due to their computational effectiveness.

(3) Optimality is in the sense of Bayes.

12

A Temporal Kernel-Based Model for Tracking Hand Movements from Neural Activities

Lavi Shpigelman
School of Computer Science
and Engineering
The Hebrew University Jerusalem
91904, Israel

Interdisciplinary Center for
Neural Computation
The Hebrew University Jerusalem
91904, Israel

Koby Crammer and Yoram Singer
School of Computer Science and Engineering
The Hebrew University Jerusalem
91904, Israel

Rony Paz and Eilon Vaadia
Interdisciplinary Center for
Neural Computation
The Hebrew University Jerusalem
91904, Israel

Department of Physiology
Hadassah Medical School
The Hebrew University Jerusalem
91904, Israel

12.1 Abstract

We devise and experiment with a dynamical kernel-based system for tracking hand movements from neural activity. The state of the system corresponds to the hand location, velocity, and acceleration, while the system's input are the instantaneous spike rates. The system's state dynamics is defined as a combination of a linear mapping from the previous *estimated* state and a kernel-based mapping tailored for modeling neural activities. In contrast to generative models, the activity-to-state mapping is learned using discriminative methods by minimizing a noise-robust loss function. We use this approach to predict hand trajectories on the basis of neural activity in the motor cortex of behaving monkeys and find that the proposed approach is more accurate than a static approach based on support vector regression and the Kalman filter.

12.2 Introduction

This chapter focuses on the problem of tracking hand movements, which constitute smooth spatial trajectories, from spike trains of a neural population. We do so by devising a dynamical system that employs a tailored kernel for spike rate patterns along with a linear mapping corresponding to the states' dynamics. Consider a situation where a subject performs free hand movements during a task that requires high precision. In the lab, it may be a constrained reaching task while in real life it may be an everyday task such as eating. We wish to track the hand position given only spike trains from a recorded neural population. The rationale of such an undertaking is twofold. First, this task can be viewed as a step toward the development of a brain-machine interface (BMI), which is gradually becoming a solution for motor-disabled patients. Recent studies of BMIs (Tillery et al. (2003); Carmena et al. (2003); Serruya et al. (2002)) (being online and feedback-enabled) show that a relatively small number of cortical units can be used to move a cursor or a robot effectively, even without the generation of hand movements, and that training of the subjects improves the overall success of the BMIs. Second, an open-loop (offline) movement decoding (e.g., Isaacs et al. (2000); Brockwell et al. (2004); Wessberg et al. (2000); Shpigelman et al. (2003); Mehring et al. (2003)), while inappropriate for BMIs, is computationally less expensive, and easier to implement, and it allows repeated analysis, providing a handle to understand neural computations in the brain.

Early studies (Georgopoulos et al. (1983)) show that the direction of arm movement is reflected by the population vector of preferred directions weighted by current firing rates, suggesting that intended movement is encoded in the firing rate, which, in turn, is modulated by the angle between a unit's preferred direction (PD) and the intended direction. This linear regression approach is still prevalent and is applied, with some variation of the learning methods, in closed and open-loop settings. There is relatively little work on the development of dedicated nonlinear methods.

Both movement and neural activity are dynamic and therefore can be modeled naturally by dynamical systems. Filtering methods often employ generative probabilistic models such as the well known Kalman filter (Wu et al. (2005)) or more neurally specialized models (Brockwell et al. (2004)) in which a cortical unit's spike count is generated by a probability function of its underlying firing rate that is tuned to movement parameters. The movement, being a smooth trajectory, is modeled as a linear transition with (typically additive Gaussian) noise. These methods have the advantage of using the smooth nature of movement and provide models of what neurons are tuned to. However, the requirement of describing a neural population's firing probability as a function of movement state is hard to satisfy without making costly assumptions. The most prominent are the assumptions of conditional independence of cells given their movement and of their relation being linear with Gaussian noise.

Kernel-based methods have been shown to achieve state-of-the-art results in many application domains. Discriminative kernel methods such as support vector regression (SVR) forgo the task of modeling neuronal tuning functions. Furthermore, the construction of kernel-induced feature spaces lends itself to efficient implementation of distance measures over spike trains that are better suited to comparing two neural population trajectories than to the Euclidean distance in the original space of spike counts per bins (Shpigelman et al. (2003); Eichhorn et al. (2004)). However, SVR is a "static" method that does not take into account the smooth dynamics of the predicted movement trajectory, which imposes a statistical dependency between consecutive examples (resulting in nonsmooth predictions).

This chapter introduces a kernel-based regression method that incorporates linear dynamics of the predicted trajectories. In section 12.3, we formally describe the problem setting. We introduce the movement tracking model and the associated learning framework in section 12.4. The resulting learning problem yields a new kernel for linear dynamical systems. We provide an efficient calculation of this kernel and describe our dual space optimization method for solving the learning problem. The experimental method is presented in section 12.5. Results, underscoring the merits of our algorithm are provided in section 12.6, and conclusions are given in section 12.7.

12.3   Problem Setting

Our training set contains m trials. Each trial (typically indexed by i or j) consists of a pair of movement and neural recordings designated by $\left\{ \mathbf{Y}^i, \mathbf{O}^i \right\}$. $\mathbf{Y}^i = \left\{ \mathbf{y}_t^i \right\}_{t=1}^{t_{end}^i}$ is a time series of movement state values and $\mathbf{y}_t^i \in \mathrm{R}^d$ is the movement state vector at time t in trial i. We are interested in reconstructing position; however, for better modeling, $\mathbf{y}_t^i$ may be a vector of position, velocity, and acceleration (as is the case in section 12.5). This trajectory is observed during model learning and is the inference target. $\mathbf{O}^i = \left\{ \mathbf{o}_t \right\}_{t=1}^{t_{end}^i}$ is a time series of neural spike counts and $\mathbf{o}_t^i \in \mathrm{R}^q$ is a vector of spike counts from q cortical units at time t. We wish to learn a function $\mathbf{z}_t^i = f\left(\mathbf{O}_{1:t}^i \right)$ that is a good estimate (in a sense formalized in the sequel) of the movement $\mathbf{y}_t^i$. Thus, f is a causal filtering method.

We confine ourselves to a causal setting since we plan to apply the proposed method in a closed loop scenario where real-time output is required. In tasks that involve no hitting of objects, hand movements are typically smooth. Endpoint movement in small time steps is loosely approximated as having constant acceleration. On the other hand, neural spike counts (which are typically measured in bins of 50–100 ms) vary greatly from one time step to the next. In summary, our goal is to devise a dynamic mapping from sequences of neural activities ending at a given time to the instantaneous hand movement characterization (location, velocity, and acceleration).

12.4   Movement Tracking Algorithm

Our regression method is defined as follows: given a series $\mathbf{O} \in \mathrm{R}^{q \times t_{end}}$ of observations and, possibly, an initial state $\mathbf{y}_0$, the predicted trajectory $\mathbf{Z} \in \mathrm{R}^{d \times t_{end}}$ is

$$\mathbf{z}_t = \mathbf{A} \mathbf{z}_{t-1} + \mathbf{W} \phi\left(\mathbf{o}_t \right) \quad , t_{end} \geq t > 0 \,, \tag{12.1}$$

where $\mathbf{z}_0 = \mathbf{y}_0$ (and $\mathbf{z}_t$ is an *estimate* of $\mathbf{y}_t$), $\mathbf{A} \in \mathbf{R}^{d \times d}$ is a matrix describing linear movement dynamics, and $\mathbf{W} \in \mathbf{R}^{d \times q}$ is a weight matrix. $\phi(\mathbf{o}_t)$ is a feature vector of the observed spike trains at time t and is later replaced by a kernel operator (in the dual formulation to follow). Thus, the state transition is a linear transformation of the previous state with the addition of a nonlinear effect of the observation. Note that unfolding the recursion in (12.1) yields

$$\mathbf{z}_t = \mathbf{A}^t \mathbf{y}_0 + \sum_{k=1}^{t} \left(\mathbf{A}^{t-k} \mathbf{W} \phi(\mathbf{o}_k) \right) .$$

Assuming that $\mathbf{A}$ describes stable dynamics (the eigenvalues of $\mathbf{A}$ are within a unit circle), then the current prediction depends, in a decaying manner, on the previous observations. We further assume that $\mathbf{A}$ is fixed and wish to learn $\mathbf{W}$ (we describe our choice of $\mathbf{A}$ in section 12.5). In addition, $\mathbf{o}_t$ may also encompass a series of previous spike counts in a window ending at time t (as is the case in section 12.5). Also, note that this model (in its non-kernelized version) has an algebraic form that is similar to the Kalman filter (to which we compare our results later).

12.4.1 Primal Learning Problem

The optimization problem presented here is identical to the standard SVR learning problem (e.g., Smola and Schölkopf (1998)) with the exception that $\mathbf{z}_t^i$ is defined as in (12.1), while in standard SVR, $\mathbf{z}_t = \mathbf{W} \phi(\mathbf{o}_t)$ (i.e., without the linear dynamics). Given a training set of fully observed trials $\left\{ \mathbf{Y}^i, \mathbf{O}^i \right\}_{i=1}^{m}$, we define the learning problem to be

$$\min_{\mathbf{W}} \frac{1}{2} \|\mathbf{W}\|^2 + c \sum_{i=1}^{m} \sum_{t=1}^{t_{end}^i} \sum_{s=1}^{d} \left| \left(\mathbf{z}_t^i \right)_s - \left(\mathbf{y}_t^i \right)_s \right|_\varepsilon , \tag{12.2}$$

where $\|\mathbf{W}\|^2 = \sum_{a,b} (\mathbf{W})_{ab}^2$ (the Frobenius norm). The second term is a sum of training errors (in all trials, times, and movement dimensions). $| \cdot |_\varepsilon$ is the ε insensitive loss and is defined as $|v|_\varepsilon = \max \{0, |v| - \varepsilon\}$. The first term is a regularization term that promotes small weights and c is a fixed constant providing a trade-off between the regularization term and the training error. Note that to compensate for different units and scales of the movement dimensions one could either define a different ε_s and c_s for each dimension of the movement or, conversely, scale the sth movement dimension. The tracking method combined with the optimization specified here defines the complete algorithm. We name this method the discriminative dynamic tracker (DDT).

12.4.2 A Dual Solution

The derivation of the dual of the learning problem defined in (12.2) is rather mundane (e.g., Smola and Schölkopf (1998)) and is thus omitted. Briefly, we replace the ε-loss with pairs of slack variables. We then write a Lagrangian of the primal problem and replace $\mathbf{z}_t^i$ with its definition from (12.1). We then differentiate the Lagrangian with respect to the slack variables and $\mathbf{W}$ and obtain a dual optimization problem. We present the dual problem in a top-down manner, starting with the general form and finishing with a kernel definition. The form of the dual is

$$\max_{\boldsymbol{\alpha},\boldsymbol{\alpha}^*} -\frac{1}{2}\left(\boldsymbol{\alpha}^*-\boldsymbol{\alpha}\right)^T \mathcal{G}\left(\boldsymbol{\alpha}^*-\boldsymbol{\alpha}\right)+\left(\boldsymbol{\alpha}^*-\boldsymbol{\alpha}\right)^T\mathbf{y}-\left(\boldsymbol{\alpha}^*+\boldsymbol{\alpha}\right)^T\varepsilon$$
$$s.t.\ \boldsymbol{\alpha},\boldsymbol{\alpha}^* \in [\mathbf{0},\mathbf{c}]. \tag{12.3}$$

Note that the above expression conforms to the dual form of SVR. Let ℓ equal the size of the movement space (d), multiplied by the total number of time steps in all the training trajectories. $\boldsymbol{\alpha},\boldsymbol{\alpha}^* \in \mathbf{R}^\ell$ are vectors of Lagrange multipliers, $\mathbf{y} \in \mathbf{R}^\ell$ is a column concatenation of all the training set movement trajectories $\left[\left(\mathbf{y}_1^1\right)^T \cdots \left(\mathbf{y}_{t_{end}^m}^m\right)^T\right]^T$, $\varepsilon = [\varepsilon,\dots,\varepsilon]^T \in \mathbf{R}^\ell$, and $\mathcal{G} \in \mathbf{R}^{\ell \times \ell}$ is a Gram matrix ($\mathbf{v}^T$ denotes transposition). One difference between our setting and the standard SVR lies within the size of the vectors and Gram matrix. In addition, a major difference is the definition of $\mathcal{G}$. We define $\mathcal{G}$ here in a hierarchical manner. Let $i,j \in \{1,\dots,m\}$ be trajectory (trial) indexes. $\mathcal{G}$ is built from blocks indexed by $\mathbf{G}^{ij}$, which are in turn made from basic blocks, indexed by $\mathbf{K}_{tq}^{ij}$ as follows

$$\mathcal{G} = \begin{pmatrix} \mathbf{G}^{11} & \cdots & \mathbf{G}^{1m} \\ \vdots & \ddots & \vdots \\ \mathbf{G}^{m1} & \cdots & \mathbf{G}^{mm} \end{pmatrix}, \quad \mathbf{G}^{ij} = \begin{pmatrix} \mathbf{K}_{11}^{ij} & \cdots & \mathbf{K}_{1t_{end}^j}^{ij} \\ \vdots & \ddots & \vdots \\ \mathbf{K}_{t_{end}^i 1}^{ij} & \cdots & \mathbf{K}_{t_{end}^i t_{end}^j}^{ij} \end{pmatrix},$$

where block $\mathbf{G}^{ij}$ refers to a pair of trials (i and j). Finally, each basic block $\mathbf{K}_{tq}^{ij}$ refers to a pair of time steps t and q in trajectories i and j respectively. t_{end}^i, t_{end}^j are the time lengths of trials i and j. Basic blocks are defined as

$$\mathbf{K}_{tq}^{ij} = \sum_{r=1}^{t}\sum_{s=1}^{q}\left(\mathbf{A}^{t-r}\right)k_{rs}^{ij}\left(\mathbf{A}^{q-s}\right)^T, \tag{12.4}$$

where $k_{rs}^{ij} = k\left(\mathbf{o}_r^i,\mathbf{o}_s^j\right)$ is a (freely chosen) basic kernel between the two neural observations $\mathbf{o}_r^i$ and $\mathbf{o}_s^j$ at times r and s in trials i and j, respectively. For an explanation of kernel operators, we refer the reader to Vapnik (1995) and mention that the kernel operator can be viewed as computing $\phi\left(\mathbf{o}_r^i\right)\cdot\phi\left(\mathbf{o}_s^j\right)$ where ϕ is a fixed mapping to some inner product space. The choice of kernel (being the choice of feature space) reflects a modeling decision that specifies how similarities among neural patterns are measured. The resulting dual form of the tracker is $\mathbf{z}_t = \sum_k \boldsymbol{\alpha}_k \mathcal{G}_{tk}$ where $\mathcal{G}_t$ is the Gram matrix row of the new example.

It is therefore clear from (12.4) that the linear dynamic characteristics of DDT result in a Gram matrix whose entries depend on previous observations. This dependency is exponentially decaying as the time difference between events in the trajectories grow. Note that the solution of the dual optimization problem in (12.3) can be calculated by any standard quadratic programming optimization tool. Also, note that direct calculation of $\mathcal{G}$ is inefficient. We describe an efficient method in the sequel.

12.4.3   Efficient Calculation of the Gram Matrix

Simple, straightforward calculation of the Gram matrix is time consuming. To illustrate this, suppose each trial is of length $t_{end}^i = n$; calculation of each basic block would take $\Theta(n^2)$ summation steps. We now describe a procedure based on a dynamic programming method for calculating the Gram matrix in a constant number of operations for each basic block.

Omitting the indexing over trials to ease notation, we are interested in calculating the basic block $\mathbf{K}_{tq}$. First, define $\mathbf{B}_{tq} = \sum_{k=1}^{t} k_{kq} \mathbf{A}^{t-k}$. The basic block $\mathbf{K}_{tq}$ can be recursively calculated in three different ways from (12.4):

$$\mathbf{K}_{tq} = \mathbf{K}_{t(q-1)} \mathbf{A}^T + \mathbf{B}_{tq} \tag{12.5}$$

$$\mathbf{K}_{tq} = \mathbf{A} \mathbf{K}_{(t-1)q} + \left(\mathbf{B}_{qt}\right)^T \tag{12.6}$$

$$\mathbf{K}_{tq} = \mathbf{A} \mathbf{K}_{(t-1)(q-1)} \mathbf{A}^T + \left(\mathbf{B}_{qt}\right)^T + \mathbf{B}_{tq} - k_{tq} \ . \tag{12.7}$$

Thus, by adding (12.5) to (12.6) and subtracting (12.7) we get

$$\mathbf{K}_{tq} = \mathbf{A} \mathbf{K}_{(t-1)q} + \mathbf{K}_{t(q-1)} \mathbf{A}^T - \mathbf{A} \mathbf{K}_{(t-1)(q-1)} \mathbf{A}^T + k_{tq} I \ .$$

$\mathbf{B}_{tq}$ (and the entailed summation) is eliminated in exchange for a 2D dynamic program with initial conditions

$$\mathbf{K}_{1,1} = k_{11} I \quad , \quad \mathbf{K}_{1,q} = \mathbf{K}_{1(q-1)} \mathbf{A}^T + k_{1q} I \quad , \quad \mathbf{K}_{t,1} = \mathbf{A} \mathbf{K}_{(t-1)1} + k_{t1} I$$

12.4.4   Suggested Optimization Method

One possible way to solve the optimization problem (essentially, a modification of the method described in Crammer and Singer (2001) for classification) is to sequentially solve a reduced problem with respect to a single constraint at a time. Define

$$\delta_i = \left| \sum_j \left(\boldsymbol{\alpha}_j^* - \boldsymbol{\alpha}_j \right) \mathcal{G}_{ij} - y_i \right|_\varepsilon - \min_{\boldsymbol{\alpha}_i, \boldsymbol{\alpha}_i^* \in [0,c]} \left| \sum_j \left(\boldsymbol{\alpha}_j^* - \boldsymbol{\alpha}_j \right) \mathcal{G}_{ij} - y_i \right|_\varepsilon \ .$$

Then δ_i is the amount of ε-insensitive error that can be corrected for example i by keeping all $\boldsymbol{\alpha}_{j \neq i}^{(*)}$ constant and changing $\boldsymbol{\alpha}_i^{(*)}$. Optimality is reached by iteratively choosing the example with the largest δ_i and changing its $\alpha_i^{(*)}$ within the $[0, c]$ limits to minimize the error for this example.

12.5   Experimental Setting

The data used in this work was recorded from the primary motor cortex of a rhesus (Macaca Mulatta) monkey (~4.5 kg). The monkey sat in a dark chamber and up to eight electrodes were introduced into the MI area of each hemisphere. The electrode signals were amplified, filtered, and sorted. The data used in this report were recorded on eight different days and include hand positions (sampled at 500 Hz), and spike times of single units (isolated by signal fit to a series of windows) and multiunits (detection by threshold crossing) sampled at 1 ms precision. The monkey used two planar-movement manipulanda to control two cursors on the screen to perform a center-out reaching task. Each trial began when the monkey centered both cursors on a central circle. Either cursor could turn green, indicating the hand to be used in the trial. Then, one of eight targets appeared (go signal), the center circle disappeared, and the monkey had to move and reach the target to receive liquid reward. The number of multiunit channels ranged from 5 to 15, the number of single units was 20 to 27, and the average total was 34 units per dataset. The average spike rate per channel was 8.2 spikes/s. More information on the recordings can be found in Paz et al. (2003).

The results we present here refer to prediction of instantaneous hand movements during the period from "go signal" to "target reached" times of both hands in successful trials. Note that some of the trials required movement of the left hand while keeping the right hand steady, and vice versa. Therefore, although we considered only movement periods of the trials, we had to predict both movement and nonmovement for each hand. The cumulative time length of all the datasets was about 67 minutes. Since the correlation between the movements of the two hands tend toward zero, we predicted movement for each hand separately, choosing the movement space to be $[x, y, v_x, v_y, a_x, a_y]^T$ for each of the hands (preliminary results using only $[x, y, v_x, v_y]^T$ were less accurate).

We preprocessed the spike trains into spike counts in a running window of 100 ms (choice of window size is based on previous experience (Shpigelman et al. (2003))). Hand position, velocity, and acceleration were calculated using the 500 Hz recordings. Both spike counts and hand movement were then sampled at steps of 100 ms (preliminary results with a step size of 50 ms were negligibly different for all algorithms). A labeled example $\{\mathbf{y}_t^i, \mathbf{o}_t^i\}$ for time t in trial i consisted of the previous 10 bins of population spike counts and the state, as a 6D vector for the left or right hand. Two such consecutive examples would than have 9 time bins of spike count overlap. For example, the number of cortical units q in the first dataset was 43 (27 single and 16 multiple) and the total length of all the trials that were used in that dataset is 529 s. Hence, in that session there are 5,290 consecutive examples where each is a 43×10 matrix of spike counts along with two 6D vectors of endpoint movement.

To run our algorithm we had to choose base kernels, their parameters, $\mathbf{A}$ and c (and θ, to be introduced below). We used the Spikernel (Shpigelman et al. (2003)), a kernel designed to be used with spike rate patterns, and the simple dot product (i.e., linear regression). Kernel parameters and c were chosen (and subsequently held fixed) by fivefold cross-validation over half of the first dataset only. We compared DDT with the Spikernel and with the linear kernel to standard SVR using the Spikernel and the Kalman filter. We also obtained tracking results using both DDT and SVR with the standard exponential kernel. These results were slightly less accurate on average than with the Spikernel and are therefore omitted here. The Kalman filter was learned assuming the standard state space model ($\mathbf{y}_t = \mathbf{A}\mathbf{y}_{t-1} + \eta$, $\mathbf{o}_t = \mathbf{H}\mathbf{y}_t + \xi$, where η, ξ are white Gaussian noise with appropriate correlation matrices) such as in Wu et al. (2005). $\mathbf{y}$ belonged to the same 6D state space as described in section 12.3. To ease the comparison, the same matrix $\mathbf{A}$ that

Table 12.1 Mean R^2, MAE_ε and MSE (across datasets, folds, hands, and directions) for each algorithm.

Algorithm	R^2			MAE_ε			MSE		
	pos.	vel.	accl.	pos.	vel.	accl.	pos.	vel.	accl.
Kalman filter	0.64	0.58	0.30	0.40	0.15	0.37	0.78	0.27	1.16
DDT-linear	0.59	0.49	0.17	0.63	0.41	0.58	0.97	0.50	1.23
SVR-Spikernel	0.61	0.64	0.37	0.44	**0.14**	**0.34**	0.76	0.20	0.98
DDT-Spikernal	**0.73**	**0.67**	**0.40**	**0.37**	**0.14**	**0.34**	**0.50**	**0.16**	**0.91**

was learned for the Kalman filter was used in our algorithm (though we show that it is not optimal for DDT), multiplied by a scaling parameter θ. This parameter was selected to produce best *position* results on the training set. The selected θ value is 0.8.

The figures that we show in section 12.6 are of test results in fivefold cross-validation on the rest of the data. Each of the eight remaining datasets was divided into five folds. Four fifths were used for training (with the parameters obtained previously and the remaining one fifth as a test set). This process was repeated five times for each hand. Altogether we had $8_{\text{sets}} \times 5_{\text{folds}} \times 2_{\text{hands}} = 80$ folds.

12.6   Results

We begin by showing average results across all datasets, folds, hands, and X/Y directions for the four algorithms that are compared. Table. 12.1 shows mean correlation coefficients (R^2, between recorded and predicted movement values), mean ε insensitive absolute errors (MAE_ε), and mean squared errors (MSE). R^2 is a standard performance measure, MAE_ε is the error minimized by DDT (subject to the regularization term), and MSE is minimized by the Kalman filter. Under all the above measures the DDT-Spikernel outperforms the rest with the SVR-Spikernel and the Kalman Filter alternating in second place.

To understand whether the performance differences are significant we look at the distribution of position (X and Y) R^2 values at each of the separate tests (160 altogether). Figure 12.1 shows scatter plots of R^2 results for position predictions. Each plot compares the DDT-Spikernel (on the Y axis) with one of the other three algorithms (on the X axes). In spite of the large differences in accuracy across datasets, the algorithm pairs achieve similar success, with the DDT-Spikernel achieving a better R^2 score in almost all cases.

To summarize the significance of R^2 differences, we computed the number of tests in which one algorithm achieved a higher R^2 value than another algorithm (for all pairs, and in each of the position, velocity, and acceleration categories). The results of this tournament among the algorithms are presented in figure 12.2 as winning percentages. The graphs produce a ranking of the algorithms, and the percentages are the significances of the ranking between pairs. The DDT-Spikernel is significantly better than the rest in tracking position.

The matrix $\mathbf{A}$ in use is not optimal for our algorithm. The choice of θ scales its effect. When $\theta = 0$, we get the standard SVR algorithm (without state dynamics). To illustrate the

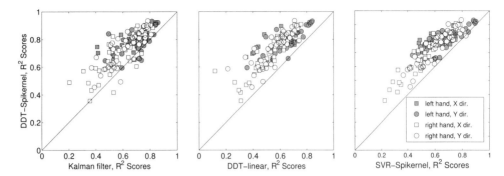

Figure 12.1 Correlation coefficients (R^2, of predicted and observed hand positions) comparisons of the DDT-Spikernel versus the Kalman filter (left), DDT-linear (center), and SVR-Spikernel (right). Each data point is the R^2 value obtained by the DDT-Spikernel and by another method in one fold of one of the datasets for one of the two axes of movement (circle/square) and one of the hands (filled/nonfilled). Results above the diagonals are cases were the DDT-Spikernel outperforms.

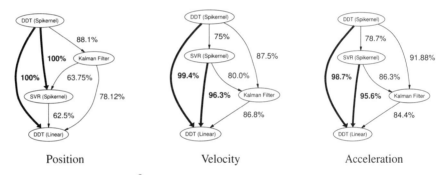

Figure 12.2 Comparison of R^2-performance among algorithms. Each algorithm is represented by a vertex. The weight of an edge between two algorithms is the fraction of tests in which the algorithm on top achieves a higher R^2 score than the other. A bold edge indicates a fraction higher than 95%. Graphs from left to right are for position, velocity, and acceleration, respectively.

effect of θ, we present in figure 12.3 the mean (over five folds, X/Y direction, and hand) R^2 results on the first dataset as a function of θ. The value chosen to minimize position error is not optimal for minimizing velocity and acceleration errors. Another important effect of θ is the number of the support patterns in the learned model, which drops considerably (by about one third) when the effect of the dynamics is increased. This means that more training points fall strictly within the ε-tube in training, suggesting the kernel that tacitly results from the dynamical model is better suited for the problem. Lastly, we show a sample of test tracking results for the DDT-Spikernel and SVR-Spikernel in figure 12.4. Note that the acceleration values are not smooth and, therefore, are least aided by the dynamics of the model. However, adding acceleration to the model improves the prediction of position.

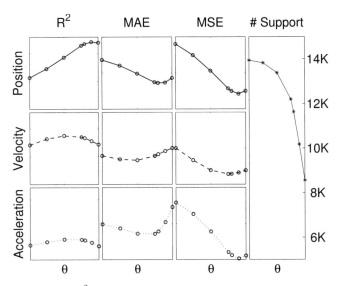

Figure 12.3   Effect of θ on R^2, MAE_ε, MSE, and the number of support vectors.

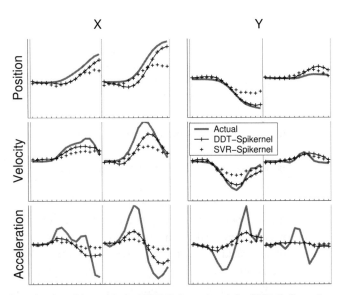

Figure 12.4   Sample of tracking with the DDT-Spikernel and the SVR-Spikernel.

12.7 Conclusion

We described and reported experiments with a dynamical system that combines a linear state mapping with a nonlinear observation-to-state mapping. The estimation of the system's parameters is transformed to a dual representation and yields a novel kernel for temporal modeling. When a linear kernel is used, the DDT system has a similar form to the Kalman filter as $t \to \infty$. However, the system's parameters are set to minimize the regularized ε-insensitive ℓ_1 loss between state trajectories. DDT also bares similarity to SVR, which employs the same loss yet without the state dynamics. Our experiments indicate that by combining a kernel-induced feature space, and linear state dynamics with using a robust loss we are able to leverage the trajectory prediction accuracy and outperform common approaches. Our next step toward an accurate brain-machine interface for predicting hand movements is the development of a learning procedure for the state dynamic mapping $\mathbf{A}$ and further developments of neurally motivated and compact representations.

Acknowledgments

This study was partly supported by GIF grant I-773-8.6/2003, by a center of excellence grant (8006/00) administered by the ISF, BMBF-DIP, and by the U.S. Israel BSF.

Notes

E-mail for correspondence: shpigi@cs.huji.ac.il

III BCI Techniques

Introduction

The goal of brain-computer interface research is the development of suitable techniques to map the high-dimensional brain signal into a control signal for a feedback application. Generally, one can distinguish two ways to achieve this goal. In the operant conditioning approach (e.g., Birbaumer et al. (1999)), a fixed translation algorithm is used. The user has to learn how to control the application based on the observed feedback. Unfortunately, this process requires extensive training for weeks or even months. On the other hand, in the machine learning approach, a learning machine is adapted to the specific brain signals of the user based on a calibration measurement in which the subject performs well-defined mental tasks such as imagined movements (e.g., Blankertz et al. (2006a)). Although not specifically required to, the subject inevitably also adapts to the system. This process is often called coadaptation and usually gives rise to further improvement after some time. Note that in most current BCI systems, elements of both strategies, that is, operant conditioning and machine learning, can be found.

In this part of the book, we focus on techniques mainly for machine learning that allow us to improve the decoding of the brain signal into a control signal. Here typically EEG is used to examplify this process. It should be noted, however, that the data analysis approaches outlined also can be used for invasive data or even data analysis beyond the field of BCI.

In chapter 13, we start by presenting several techniques from signal processing and machine learning that are of use for BCI analysis. Furthermore, we address the topic of generalization, that is, the question whether the performance of an algorithm evaluated on some offline data will be representative also for future data, say, of a feedback experiment.

Chapter 14 discusses the question of which spatial filtering can be used profitably. The problem is illuminated for different recording methods (ECoG, EEG, and MEG). Finally the question of how many trials are needed to successfully train a classifier is addressed.

In the following chapters, two techniques for feature extraction will be introduced. First, Anderson et al (chapter 15) describe their short-time PCA approach to process EEG signal. In a second chapter by Menendez et al (chapter 16), local field potentials for feature extraction are discussed.

In chapter 17, we introduce a method to process error potentials.

One major challenge in brain-computer interface research is to deal with the nonstationarity of the recorded brain signals caused, for example, by different mental states or different levels of fatigue. One solution to this problem is the choice of features that are invariant to nonstationarities. Another choice, which we discuss in chapter 18, is to continuously adapt the classifier during the experiment to compensate for the changed statistics. In this chapter, three views by the groups in Martigny, Graz, and Berlin are presented.

Finally, we illuminate in chapter 19 the question of how we can compare different BCI systems. To this end, different evaluation criteria such as information transfer rate and kappa-value are introduced and compared.

Note that this part is intended to present an overview of existing data analysis methods for BCI; it will inevitably remain somewhat biased and incomplete. For more details, the reader is provided with many pointers to the literature.

Guido Dornhege and Klaus-Robert Müller

13 General Signal Processing and Machine Learning Tools for BCI Analysis

Guido Dornhege
Fraunhofer–Institute FIRST
Intelligent Data Analysis Group (IDA)
Kekuléstr. 7, 12489 Berlin, Germany

Matthias Krauledat, Klaus-Robert Müller, and Benjamin Blankertz
Fraunhofer–Institute FIRST   *Technical University Berlin*
Intelligent Data Analysis Group (IDA)   *Str. des 17. Juni 135*
Kekuléstr. 7, 12489 Berlin, Germany   *10 623 Berlin, Germany*

13.1 Abstract

This chapter discusses signal processing and machine learning techniques and their application to brain-computer interfacing. A broader overview of the general signal processing and classification methods as used in single-trial EEG analysis is given. For more specialized algorithms, the reader is referred to the original publications. Furthermore, validation techniques and robustification are discussed briefly.

13.2 Introduction

Brain-computer interface research essentially involves the development of suitable techniques to map the high-dimensional EEG signal into a (typically one- to three-dimensional) control signal for a feedback application. The operant conditioning approach (Birbaumer et al. (1999); Elbert et al. (1980); Rockstroh et al. (1984)) uses a fixed translation algorithm to generate a feedback signal from EEG. Users are instructed to watch a feedback signal and to find out how to voluntarily control it. Successful operation is reinforced by a reward stimulus. In such BCI systems the adaption of the user is crucial and typically requires extensive training. On the other hand, machine learning oriented groups construct user adapted systems to relieve a good amount of the learning load from the subject. Using machine learning techniques, we adapt many parameters of a general translation algorithm to the specific characteristics of the user's brain signals (Blankertz et al. (2002, 2006a); Müller and Blankertz (2006); Millán et al. (2004a) and chapters 5 and 14). This is done by a statistical analysis of a calibration measurement in which the subject performs well-defined mental acts such as imagined movements. Here, in principle, no adaption of the user is required, but it can be expected that users will adapt their behavior during feedback operation. Most BCI systems are somewhere between those extremes. Some of them are continuously adapting the parameters of feature extraction or classification (see chapter 18).

Starting with the unprocessed EEG data, one has to reduce the dimensionality of the data without losing relevant information. Prominent techniques for this feature extraction are presented in sections 13.3 and 13.4. These features then must be translated into a control signal (see section 13.6). This can be done, for example, by a classifier, a regression, or a filter. Here we do not distinguish between those types and we call them classifier. Linear discriminant analysis (see section 13.6.2), for example, is derived as a classifier. But it is equivalent to a least square regression (see section 13.6.4) on the class labels and could be interpreted also as a kind of filter. The problem of how to estimate the performance of a classifier on new data—the estimation of the generalization error—is discussed in section 13.8. It should be mentioned that EEG data are usually distorted by artifacts whose detrimental influence on the classifier may need to be reduced. We briefly discuss this problem, called robustification, in section 13.9. Finally, because the EEG signal is highly nonstationary, one needs either to process data in such a way that the output of a static classifier is invariant to these changes or the classifier should adapt to the specific changes over time. Adaptation methods are discussed in detail in chapter 18.

An alternative overview of possible machine learning techniques in the context of BCI is given in Müller et al. (2004a).

13.2.1   Why Machine Learning for Brain-Computer Interfacing?

Traditional neurophysiology investigates the "average(d)" brain. As a simple example, an investigation of the neural correlates of motor preparation of index finger movements would involve a number of subjects repeatedly doing such movements. A grand average over all trials and all subjects would then reveal the general result, a pronounced cortical negativation focused in the corresponding (contralateral) motor area. On the other hand, comparing intrasubject averages (cf. figure 13.1) shows a huge subject-to-subject variability, which causes a large amount of variance in the grand average. Now let us go one step further by restricting the investigation to one subject. Comparing the session-wide averages in two (motor imagery) tasks between the sessions recorded on different days, we encounter again a huge variability (session-to-session variability) (cf. figure 13.2). This suggests that an optimal system needs to be adapted to each new session and each individual user. When it comes to real-time feedback as in brain-computer interfaces, we still have to go one step further. The system needs to be able to identify the mental state of a subject based on one single trial (duration ≤ 1 s) of brain signals. Figure 13.3 demonstrates the strong trial-to-trial variance in one subject in one session (the experiment being the same as above). Nevertheless, our BBCI system (see chapter 5) was able to classify all those tri-

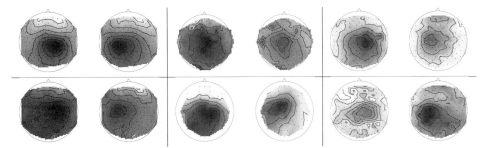

Figure 13.1   Six subjects performed left- vs. right-hand index finger tapping. Even though the kind of movement was very much the same in each subject and the task involves a highly overlearned motor competence, the premovement potential maps (−200 to −100 ms before keypress; dark means negative, light means positive potential) exhibit a great diversity among subjects.

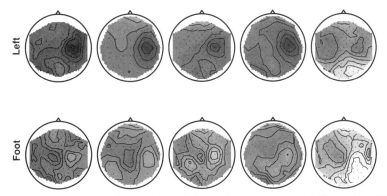

Figure 13.2   One subject imagined left- vs. right-hand movements on different days. The maps show spectral power in the alpha frequency band. Even though the maps represent averages across 140 trials each, they exhibit an apparent diversity.

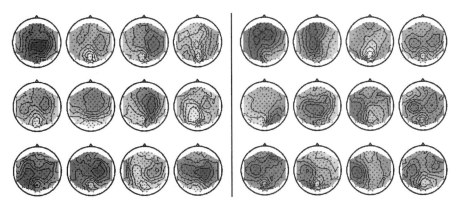

Figure 13.3   One subject imagined left- vs. right-hand movements. The topographies show spectral power in the alpha frequency range during single trials of 3.5-s duration. These patterns exhibit an extreme diversity although recorded from one subject on one day.

als correctly. The tackling of the enormous trial-to-trial variability is a major challenge in BCI research. Given the high subject-to-subject and session-to-session variability, it seems appropriate to have a system that adapts to the specific brain signatures of each user in each session. We believe that advanced techniques for machine learning are an essential tool in coping with all kinds of variabilities demonstrated in this section.

13.2.2   Why Preprocessing?

Usually it is difficult for classification algorithms to extract relevant information if the dimensionality of the data (feature vector) compared to the number of existing examples is high. This problem is called "Curse of Dimensionality" in the machine learning world. Accordingly, the dimensionality has to be reduced suitably in the sense that *undiscriminative* information is eliminated whereas *discriminative* information remains. As a numeric example, say that a BCI system should calculate a control signal from a 1-second window of a 32-channel EEG sampled at 100 Hz. Then the number of dimensions of the raw features is 3,200. Many classification algorithms are based on the estimation of a feature covariance matrix, which has in this case more than 5,118,400 parameters. Traditional statistical estimation methods need several times more samples than parameters to estimate, which here would require an impossible amount of calibration data. Regularization techniques can be used in cases where the number of training samples is less than the number of feature dimensions, but given the low signal-to-noise ratio in EEG, the gap for classifying directly on raw data is suboptimal (see Blankertz et al. (2003) for quantitative results). Accordingly preprocessing steps that decrease the dimensionality of the features are needed. While some processing methods rely on neurophysiological a priori knowledge (e.g., spatial Laplace filtering at predefined scalp locations; see section 13.4.3), other methods are automatic (e.g., spatial filters determined by a common spatial pattern analysis; see section 13.4.6).

13.3   Spectral Filtering

13.3.1   Finite and Infinite Impulse Response Filter

If restrictions to some frequency band are reasonable, due to the chosen paradigm, one can choose between several filter methods. A common approach is the use of a digital frequency filter. Regarding the desired frequency range, two sequences a and b with length n_a and n_b are required, which can be calculated in several ways, for example, butterworth or elliptic (cf. Oppenheim and Schafer (1989)). Afterward the source signal x is filtered to y by

$$a(1)y(t) = \quad b(1)x(t) + b(2)x(t-1) + \ldots + b(n_b)x(t-n_b-1)$$
$$- a(2)y(t-1) - \ldots - a(n_a)y(t-n_a-1)$$

for all t.

The special case where n_a and a are constrained to be 1 is called the finite impulse response (FIR) filter. The advantage of IIR filters is that they can produce steeper slopes (between pass- and stop-bands), but it is more intricate to design them because they can become unstable, while FIR filters are always stable.

13.3.2   Fourier-Based Filter

Another alternative for temporal filtering is Fourier-based filtering. By calculating the short-time Fourier transformation (STFT) (see Oppenheim and Schafer (1989)) of a signal one switches from the temporal to the spectral domain. The filtered signal is obtained by choosing a suitable weighting of the relevant frequency components and applying the inverse Fourier transformation (IFT). The length of the short time window determines the frequency resolution. To filter longer signals, the overlap-and-add technique (Crochiere (1980)) is used. The spectral leakage effect that can hamper Fourier-based techniques can be reduced by the right choice of the window (cf. Harris (1978)).

13.4   Spatial Filtering

Raw EEG scalp potentials are known to be associated with a large spatial scale owing to volume conduction. In a simulation in Nunez et al. (1997), only half the contribution to one scalp electrode comes from sources within a 3 cm radius. This is in particular a problem if the signal of interest is weak, for example, sensorimotor rhythms, while other sources produce strong signals in the same frequency range like the α rhythm of the visual system. Several spatial filtering techniques are used to get more localized signals, or signals corresponding to single sources. Some of the prominent techniques are presented in this section. As a demonstration of the importance of spatial filters, figure 13.4 shows spectra of left vs. right hand motor imagery at the right hemispherical sensorimotor cortex. All plots are calculated from the same data but using different spatial filters. While the raw channel shows only a peak around 9 Hz but almost no discrimination between the two conditions, the bipolar and the common average reference filter can improve a little. However, the Laplace and much more so the CSP filter reveal a second spectral peak around 12 Hz with strong discriminative power.

13.4.1   Bipolar Filtering

While in EEG recordings often all channels are measured as voltage potential relative to a standard reference (referential recording), it also is possible to record all channels as voltage differences between electrode pairs (bipolar recording). From referential EEG, one can easily get bipolar channels by subtracting the respective channels, for example,

$$\text{FC4} - \text{CP4} = (\text{FC4} - \text{Ref}) - (\text{CP4} - \text{Ref}) = \text{FC4}_{\text{Ref}} - \text{CP4}_{\text{Ref}}.$$

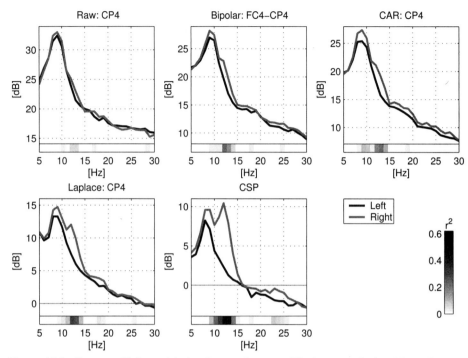

Figure 13.4 Spectra of left vs. right hand motor imagery. All plots are calculated from the same dataset but using different spatial filters. The discrimination between the two conditions is quantified by the r^2-value (see section 13.5).

Bipolar filtering reduces the effect of spatial smearing by calculating the local voltage gradient. This puts an emphasis on local activity while contributions of more distant sources are attenuated.

13.4.2   Common Average Reference (CAR)

To obtain common average reference signals, the mean of all EEG channels is subtracted from each individual channel. While the influence of far field sources is reduced, CAR may introduce some undesired spatial smearing. For example, artifacts from one channel can be spread into all other channels.

13.4.3   Laplace Filtering

More localized signals can be obtained by a Laplace filter. In a simple approximation, Laplace signals are obtained by subtracting the average of surrounding electrodes from each individual channel, for example,

$$C4_{Lap} = C4_{Ref} - \frac{1}{4} \left(C2_{Ref} + C6_{Ref} + FC4_{Ref} + CP4_{Ref} \right).$$

Data   PCA–filtered data

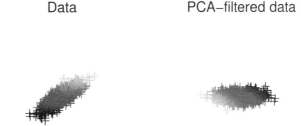

Figure 13.5 On the left, Gaussian-distributed data are visualized. After applying PCA the source signals on the right are retained. Each data point has the same grey level in both plots.

The choice of the set of surrounding electrodes determines the charateristics of the spatial filters. Mostly used are small Laplacians (as in the example) and large Laplacians using neighbors at 20 percent distance with distance as defined in the international 10-20 system. See also the discussion in McFarland et al. (1997a).

13.4.4 Principal Component Analysis

Given some data $x_k \in \mathbb{R}^m$ for $k = 1, ..., n$, PCA tries to reduce the dimensionality of the feature space to p dimensions by finding an optimal approximation of the data x_k by $x_k \approx b + W a_k$ with $b \in \mathbb{R}^m$, $a_k \in \mathbb{R}^p, p \leq m$, and $W \in \mathbb{R}^{m,p}$. If this optimization is done by minimizing the squared error $\sum_{k=1,...,n} \|x_k - (b + W a_k)\|_2$ and simultaneously fixing the diagonal of $W^\top W$ to 1, one finds the solution by choosing $b = \frac{1}{n} \sum_{k=1,...n} x_k$, W by the eigenvectors of the highest p eigenvalues (suitably scaled) of the so-called scatter matrix $\sum_{k=1,...,n} (x_k - b)(x_k - b)^\top$ and $a_k = W^\top (x_k - b)$. Consequently, W consists of orthogonal vectors, describing the p-dimensional subspace of $\mathbb{R}^m$, which shows the best approximation to the data. For normal distributed data, one finds the subspace by examining the covariance matrix, which indicates the direction with the largest variation in the data. In figure 13.5 the principal components of a two-dimensional Gaussian distribution are visualized. In this case the data were only rotated.

In Schölkopf et al. (1998) this idea is extended to nonlinear structures by kernelization and is called kernel PCA (kPCA) and applied to denoising in Mika et al. (1999, 2003).

13.4.5 Independent Component Analysis

Suppose n recorded signals $x(t) = (x_1(t), ..., x_n(t))$ for $t = 1, ..., T$ are given. The basis assumption of ICA is that these n signals are modeled as stationary, instantaneous linear combinations of n unknown source signals $s(t) = (s_1(t), ..., s_n(t))$ with $x_i(t) = \sum_{j=1}^n a_{i,j} s_j(t)$ for $i = 1, ..., n$ and $t = 1, ..., T$. This can be reformulated to $x(t) = As(t)$ with the so-called mixing matrix $A = (a_{i,j})_{i,j=1,...,n}$, which is assumed to be square and invertible. One needs further assumptions to be able to reconstruct A and s if both are unknown. The key assumption of ICA is the independence of the source signals, that is, that the time course of $s_i(t)$ does not provide any information about the time course of

Source signals   Mixed signals   Demixed signals

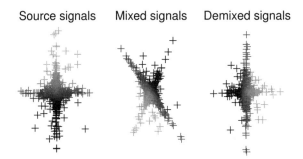

Figure 13.6 On the left, two independent source signals (Gaussian to the power of 3) are shown. After multiplication of a mixing matrix the mixed signal in the middle is achieved. After applying JADE the signals on the right are revealed. Each data point has the same grey level in both plots.

$s_j(t)$ for $j \neq i$. Thus, ICA tries to find a separating matrix B such that the resulting signals $\hat{s}(t) = Wx(t)$ are maximally independent.

Driven by this goal, one can find a solution (unique except for permutation and scaling) if at most one source has a Gaussian distribution, the source signals have different spectra, or the source signals have different variances. Tools from information geometry and the maximum likelihood principle have been proposed to get an objective function for an optimization approach (see Hyvarinen et al. (2001) for an overview).

Several algorithms exist that assume non-Gaussianity, for example, JADE (joint-approximate diagonalization of eigenmatrices) (cf. Cardoso and Souloumiac (1993)), FastICA (cf. Hyvärinen (1999)), or Infomax (cf. Bell and Sejnowski (1995)). If one assumes time structure (like different spectra or variances), the prominent algorithms are TDSEP (cf. Ziehe and Müller (1998)) and SOBI (cf. Belouchrani et al. (1997)). If one assumes independent data (i.e., no time structure) but nonstationarity in the data, SEPA-GAUS (cf. Pham (1996)) is also an interesting tool. All these algorithms use the linear assumption $x(t) = As(t)$.

In NGCA (cf. Blanchard et al. (2006)), a non-Gaussian subspace is estimated by linearly projecting the noninformative, that is, Gaussian subspace that may even contain more than one Gaussian source. For nonlinear extensions of the TDSEP algorithm by kernelization, we refer to, for example, Harmeling et al. (2002, 2003).

The typical ICA situation is visualized in figure 13.6. Here two independent source signals (Gaussian to the power of three) were mixed by a random nonorthogonal matrix to get the mixed signals. Now the JADE algorithm was applied to the data so that the demixed signals remain. After suitable reordering and scaling, they are very similar to the source signal. PCA would fail here since the mixed signals are not orthogonal in general, which is the key assumption for PCA.

13.4.6   Common Spatial Patterns

The CSP technique (see Fukunaga (1990)) allows us to determine spatial filters that maximize the variance of signals of one condition (e.g., imagining a left-hand movement) and at the same time minimize the variance of signals of another condition (e.g., imagining a right-hand movement). Since variance of bandpass filtered signals is equal to bandpower, CSP filters are well suited to discriminate mental states that are characterized by ERD/ERS effects (Koles and Soong (1998)). As such it has been well used in BCI systems (Guger et al. (2000); Blankertz et al. (2006a)) where CSP filters are calculated individually for each subject on the data of a calibration measurement.

Technically, CSP analysis goes as follows: Let X_1 and X_2 be the (time $\times$ channel) data matrices of the bandpass filtered EEG signals (concatenated trials) under the two conditions, and Σ_1 and Σ_2 be the corresponding estimates of the covariance matrices $\Sigma_i = X_i^\top X_i$. These latter two matrices are simultaneously diagonalized in a way that the eigenvalues of Σ_1 and Σ_2 sum to 1. Practically, this can be done by calculating the generalized eigenvectors V:

$$V^\top \Sigma_1 V = D \quad \text{and} \quad V^\top (\Sigma_1 + \Sigma_2) V = I \tag{13.1}$$

where I is the identity matrix and the diagonal matrix D contains the eigenvalues of Σ_1. The column vectors of V (eigenvectors) are the filters of the common spatial patterns. Looking at one filter V_j (j-th row V), the variance of the projected signals of condition 1 is $\text{var}(X_1 V_j) = V_j^\top \Sigma_1 V_j = d_j$ (d_j being the jth diagonal element of D, i.e., the eigenvalue of V_j). From (13.1) we get

$$V^\top \Sigma_2 V = I - V^\top \Sigma_1 V = I - D \tag{13.2}$$

so the variance of the projected signals of condition two is $\text{var}(X_2 V_j) = 1 - d_j$. This means that the best contrast is provided by filters with high Σ_1-eigenvalues (large variance for condition one and small variance for condition two) and by filters with low Σ_1-eigenvalues (and vice versa). Accordingly, taking the six filters corresponding to the three largest and the three smallest eigenvalues would be a reasonable choice. But when a large amount of calibration data is not available it is advisable to use a more refined technique to select the patterns or manually choose them by visual inspection.

Several extensions to the CSP algorithm have been proposed, for which we refer the interested reader to the original publications. Extensions to multiclass algorithms are discussed in Dornhege et al. (2004a,b). Separate CSPs in different frequency bands were used in Blanchard and Blankertz (2004) to win the BCI Competition II for data set IIa. Algorithms for the simultaneous optimization of spectral and spatial filters are proposed in Lemm et al. (2005), Dornhege et al. (2006b), and Tomioka et al. (2006).

13.5 Discriminability of Features

When analyzing a new experimental paradigm, usually a larger variety of features is derived. Measures of discriminability of the features may help to choose a subset of those features for the actual BCI system in a semiautomatic manner. For techniques for automatic feature selection, the reader is referred to Guyon et al. (2006b), Lal et al. (2004), Schröder et al. (2005), and Müller et al. (2004a).

One example for a measure of discriminability is the Fisher score. Given the labels, the Fisher score for data $(x_k)_{k=1,\dots,N}$ with labels $(y_k)_{k=1,\dots,N}$ is defined for all dimensions i by

$$s_i = \frac{|\mu_1^{(i)} - \mu_{-1}^{(i)}|}{\sigma_1^{(i)} + \sigma_{-1}^{(i)}}$$

with $\mu_y^{(i)} := \frac{1}{\#\{k:y_k=-y\}} \sum_{k:y_k=-y} x_{k,i}$ and $\sigma_y^{(i)} = \frac{1}{\#\{k:y_k=y\}} \sum_{k:y_k=y} (x_{k,i} - \mu_y^{(i)})^2$ for $y = \pm 1$. Alternatively, one could also choose students' t-statistics or biserial correlation coefficients (r- resp. r^2-values, see Müller et al. (2004a)). See Guyon et al. (2006a) for more scoring functions.

13.6   Classification

We start with n labeled trials in the form (x_i, y_i) for $i = 1, \dots, n$ with $x_i \in \mathbb{R}^m$ as data points in some Euclidean space and $y_i \in \{1, \dots, N\}$ as class labels for $N > 2$ different classes or $y_i \in \{\pm 1\}$ as class labels for a binary problem. The goal of classification is to find a function $f : \mathbb{R}^m \to \mathbb{R}^N$ resp. $f : \mathbb{R}^m \to \mathbb{R}$ such that for an $x \in \mathbb{R}^m$ the function $\operatorname{argmax} f(x)$ resp. $\operatorname{sign} f(x)$ is a good estimate for the true label. For example, if the data can be described by a probability distribution X (for the data) and Y (for the label), one would try to minimize the misclassification risk $P(\operatorname{argmax} f(X) \neq Y)$ or $P(\operatorname{sign} f(X) \neq Y)$. Unfortunately, the probability distributions are usually not given; only a finite number of samples coming from these distributions are presented. Thus, in this case the probability distribution must be estimated.

It should be mentioned that in the following we use the one-dimensional classifier $f : \mathbb{R}^m \to \mathbb{R}$ instead of the two-dimensional classifier $f : \mathbb{R}^m \to \mathbb{R}^2$ for binary problems. Note that both formulations are equivalent since finding the maximum of two values can be decided by the sign of the difference.

We first introduce quadratic discriminant analysis (QDA) (see section 13.6.1) and its specialization linear discriminant analysis (LDA) (see section 13.6.2), which both start with some assumptions concerning the probability distribution of the data and estimate all model parameters. The classifier is then determined by the minimization of the misclassification risk. For practical cases, an important variant exists that takes care of overfitting effects by suitable regularization called regularized (linear) discriminant analysis (RDA or RLDA) (see section 13.6.3).

Afterward we discuss least qquare regression (LSR) (see section 13.6.4), Fisher discriminant analysis (see section 13.6.5), support vector machines (see section 13.6.6), and linear programming machines (LPM) (see section 13.6.7). Further methods can be found in the literature, for example, Adaboost (Meir and Rätsch (2003)), Neural Networks (Bishop (1995); Orr and Müller (1998)), or decision trees (Breiman et al. (1984); Friedman (1991)).

For nonlinear problems, kernel-based methods (Vapnik (1995); Schölkopf and Smola (2002); Müller et al. (2001)) have proven to be very successful. However, nonlinear methods need to estimate more parameters, so a larger training set is needed. Although the linear case is a special case of "nonlinear" classifiers, for data allowing approximately a linear separation, linear classifiers are typically more robust (cf. Müller et al. (2003a)).

A further overview of existing classification methods for BCI can be found in Anderson (2005).

13.6.1 Quadratic Discriminant Analysis

Let us consider the following situation, namely that the given data are normal distributed:

Theorem 13.6.1
Let $X \in I\!\!R^m, Y \in \{1, ..., N\}$ or $Y \in \{\pm 1\}$ random variables with $m, N \in I\!\!N, N \geq 2$ fixed and $(X|Y = y) \sim \mathcal{N}(\mu_y, \Sigma_y)$ normal distributed for $y = 1, ..., N$ or $y = \pm 1$ with $\mu_y \in I\!\!R^m$ and $\Sigma_y \in I\!\!R^{m,m}$ positive definite. Furthermore, define $\hat{f} : I\!\!R^m \to I\!\!R^N$,

$$x \mapsto \left(-\frac{1}{2} x^\top \Sigma_y^{-1} x + \mu_y^\top \Sigma_y^{-1} x - \frac{1}{2} \mu_y^\top \Sigma_y^{-1} \mu_y + \log(P(Y = y)) - \frac{1}{2} \log(\det(\Sigma_y)) \right)_{y=1,...,N}$$

resp. $\hat{f} : I\!\!R^m \to I\!\!R$

$$x \mapsto \left(-\frac{1}{2} x^\top \Sigma_1^{-1} x + \mu_1^\top \Sigma_1^{-1} x - \frac{1}{2} \mu_1^\top \Sigma_1^{-1} \mu_1 + \log(P(Y = 1)) - \frac{1}{2} \log(\det(\Sigma_1)) \right)$$
$$- \left(-\frac{1}{2} x^\top \Sigma_{-1}^{-1} x + \mu_{-1}^\top \Sigma_{-1}^{-1} x - \frac{1}{2} \mu_{-1}^\top \Sigma_{-1}^{-1} \mu_{-1} + \log(P(Y = -1)) - \frac{1}{2} \log(\det(\Sigma_{-1})) \right).$$

Then for all functions $f : I\!\!R^m \to \{1, ..., N\}$ or $f : I\!\!R^m \to \{\pm 1\}$ with $\bar{f} := \mathrm{argmax}(f)$ or $\bar{f} := \mathrm{sign}(f)$ it holds true that

$$E(f(X) = Y) \leq E(\bar{f}(X) = Y).$$

In other words, $\bar{f}$ is the Bayes optimal classifier for this problem.

See Duda et al. (2001) for the proof. These results can be further simplified if equal class priors are assumed. This optimal classifier for normal-distributed data is called Quadratic Discriminant Analysis (QDA). To use it, one must estimate the class covariance matrices and the class means. This is usually done by $\mu_y = \frac{1}{\#\{j:y_j=y\}} \sum_{j:y_j=y} x_j$ and $\Sigma_y = \frac{1}{\#\{j:y_j=y\}-1} \sum_{j:y_j=y} (x_j - \mu_y)(x_j - \mu_y)^\top$ if the data are given as column vectors. Note that the optimality of the classifier can be granted only if the parameters of the distribution are known. But if the distribution has to be estimated, which is usually the case, the required classifier is typically not optimal anymore.

13.6.2 Linear Discriminant Analysis

Under specific assumptions, theorem 13.6.1 can be simplified as follows:

Corollary 13.6.2

In the situation of theorem 13.6.1 with $\Sigma = \Sigma_y$ for all $y \in \{1, ..., N\}$ resp. $y \in \{\pm 1\}$ the optimal function $\hat{f}$ is given by

$$\hat{f}(x) = \left(\mu_y^\top \Sigma^{-1} x - \frac{1}{2} \mu_y^\top \Sigma^{-1} \mu_y + \log(P(Y = y)) \right)_{y=1,...,N}$$

resp.

$$\hat{f}(x) = \left((\mu_1 - \mu_{-1})^\top \Sigma^{-1} x - \frac{1}{2}(\mu_1 - \mu_{-1})^\top \Sigma^{-1}(\mu_1 + \mu_{-1}) + \log\left(\frac{P(Y = 1)}{P(Y = -1)} \right) \right).$$

This classifier is called linear discriminant analysis (LDA). Again one can simplify this problem by assuming equal class priors. The parameters can be estimated as above where Σ is estimated by the mean of the Σ_i, weighted by the class priors.

13.6.3   Regularized (Linear) Discriminant Analysis

In LDA and QDA one has to estimate mean and covariance of the data. Especially for high-dimensional data with few trials this estimation is very imprecise, since the number of unknown parameters is quadratic in the number of dimensions. Thus, overfitting and loss of generalization can result from the wrong estimation. To improve the performance, Friedman (1989) suggests the introduction of two parameters λ and γ into QDA. Both parameters modify the covariance matrices because the risk of overfitting for the covariance matrix is higher than for the means.

The first parameter λ tries to robustify the estimation of the covariances for each class by taking the covariances for the other classes into account. If Σ_y denotes the estimated covariance for class $y = 1, ..., N$ resp. $y = \pm 1$, the overall covariance Σ can be defined by $\Sigma = \frac{1}{N} \sum_{y=1}^{N} \Sigma_y$ resp. $\Sigma = 0.5(\Sigma_1 + \Sigma_{-1})$. Then λ is used to interpolate between Σ_y and Σ in the following way:

$$\hat{\Sigma}_y = (1 - \lambda)\Sigma_y + \lambda \Sigma$$

with $\lambda \in [0, 1]$. With $\lambda = 0$ RDA complies normal QDA and with $\lambda = 1$ normal LDA.

The second parameter $\gamma \in [0, 1]$ works on the single covariances $\hat{\Sigma}_y$. First of all, one should note that it is more probable for Gaussian distributions to overestimate the directions coming from eigenvectors with high eigenvalues of Σ_y. Thus, one introduces the parameter γ, which decreases the higher eigenvalues and increases the lower eigenvalues of the estimated covariance matrix until with $\gamma = 1$ a sphere remains. One derives this *shrunken* covariance matrix by

$$\bar{\Sigma}_y = (1 - \gamma)\hat{\Sigma}_y + \frac{\gamma}{m}\text{trace}\left(\hat{\Sigma}_y\right) I$$

with m as the dimensionality of the data. If $\hat{\Sigma}_y = V^\top D V$ is the spectral decomposition of $\hat{\Sigma}_y$ with $V^\top V = I$ one gets

$$\bar{\Sigma}_y = (1 - \gamma)V^\top D V + \frac{\gamma}{m}\text{trace}\left(\hat{\Sigma}_y\right) V^\top V = V^\top [(1 - \gamma)D + \frac{\gamma}{m}\text{trace}\,(D)\,I]V.$$

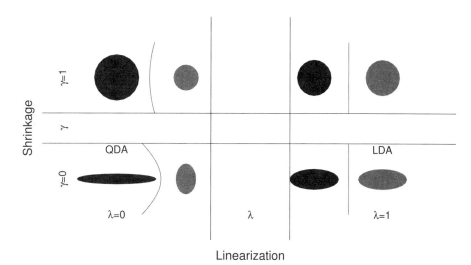

Figure 13.7   Starting with two estimated covariances and parameters $\lambda = \gamma = 0$ (the QDA situation) shown in the lower left plot, one is able to modify this estimation by two parameters. With increasing λ the matrices are made more similar until with $\lambda = 1$ the same covariances are achieved (LDA) (lower right). The second parameter γ shrinks each individual covariance matrix until with $\gamma = 1$ a sphere remains (upper left). In the extreme case $\lambda = \gamma = 1$ two equal spheres are achieved (upper right). If $\lambda = 1$ (right column) this algorithm is called RLDA, since a linear classifier remains. In all cases the resulting classification hyperplane is visualized.

Thus, $\bar{\Sigma}_y$ has the same eigenvectors with modified eigenvalues in the required form. The above formal approach of introducing hyperparameters to avoid overfitting is called regularization (see Schölkopf and Smola (2002)). QDA is applied with $\bar{\Sigma}_y$ instead of Σ_y. This modification is called **regularized discriminant analysis**. In the special case where $\lambda = 1$ one calls this method **regularized linear discriminant analysis**. Figure 13.7 shows the influence of the parameters λ and γ for a binary problem.

13.6.4   Least Square Regression

Although multiclass extensions exist for the following classifiers, we only introduce the binary algorithms here.

Suppose an unknown function f projects elements of $\mathbb{R}^m$ to $\mathbb{R}$ (possibly with some noise). The idea of regression is to find a function g based on some given examples x_i and $f(x_i)$ that optimally matches the unknown function f. Usually g is chosen based on some function class, for example, linear functions. One can use this approach for classification, too. Here the function f describes the mapping from the data to their class label. In least square regression (cf. Duda et al. (2001)) one tries to minimize the squared error made between the realization and the estimation by the function g. If a linear function class is assumed, one consequently minimizes $g(w) = \sum_i (w^\top x_i + b - y_i)^2$ (or simplified $g(w) = \sum_i (w^\top x_i - y_i)^2$ by appending ones to x_i ($[x_i, 1]^\top$) and the b to w ($[w, b]^\top$)). If one defines $x = [x_1, ..., x_n]$ and $y = [y_1, ..., y_n]^\top$, this can be written as $\min g(w) = \min \|x^\top w - y\|_2^2$. Taking the derivative with respect to w and setting it equal to zero one gets $xx^\top w = xy$, and if $xx^\top$ is invertible $w = (xx^\top)^{-1}xy$. If it is not invertible, one can introduce a small value ε and use $xx^\top + \varepsilon$ instead of $xx^\top$. Finally, one can introduce regularization, too. To do so g is exchanged by $g(w) = w^\top w + C\|x^\top - y\|_2^2$ with some $C > 0$ where the unregularized solution is achieved if $C \to \infty$.

One can prove that the w calculated by this approach is equal to the w calculated by LDA, but the bias b can differ. Furthermore, the regularization works similarly except that range and scaling are different.

13.6.5 Fisher Discriminant Analysis

For some arbitrary w we define $\mu_y = \frac{1}{\#\{i|y_i=y\}} \sum_{i|y_i=y} x_i$, $\tilde{\mu}_y(w) = w^\top \mu_y$ and $\tilde{s}_y^2(w) = \sum_{i|y_i=y}(w^\top x_i - \tilde{\mu}_y)^2$. Note that one can easily add a bias term such as LSR, too. The idea of the Fisher discriminant analysis (cf. Duda et al. (2001)) is to maximize the difference between the projected class means whereas the variance of the projected data is minimized. In other words, one looks for the maximum of

$$g(w) := \frac{(\tilde{\mu}_1(w) - \tilde{\mu}_{-1}(w))^2}{\tilde{s}_1^2(w) + \tilde{s}_{-1}^2(w)}.$$

One can calculate that $(\tilde{\mu}_1(w) - \tilde{\mu}_{-1}(w))^2 = w^\top S_B w$ with $S_B = (\mu_1 - \mu_{-1})(\mu_1 - \mu_{-1})^\top$ and $\tilde{s}_y^2(w) = w^\top S_y w$ with $S_y = \sum_{i|y_i=y}(x_i - \mu_y)(x_i - \mu_y)^\top$, and thus $\tilde{s}_1^2(w) + \tilde{s}_{-1}^2(w) = w^\top S_W w$ with $S_W = S_1 + S_{-1}$. S_W is called the within-class scatter matrix and S_B the between-class scatter matrix. Consequently, $g(w) = \frac{w^\top S_B w}{w^\top S_W w}$. This quotient is the well known Rayleigh quotient. One can determine the maximum of g by calculating the generalized eigenvalues λ_i and eigenvectors w_i between S_B and S_W (i.e., $S_B w_i = \lambda_i S_W w_i$) and choosing the highest one $\lambda_{\max}$ with corresponding eigenvector w (i.e., $S_B w = \lambda_{\max} S_W w$). An easier analytical solution can be obtained if S_W is invertible. Since $S_B w = c(\mu_1 - \mu_{-1})$ with some real-valued constant c (S_B has rank one), one gets $cS_W^{-1}(\mu_1 - \mu_{-1}) = \lambda_{\max} w$. Since the value of $g(w)$ does not depend on the scaling of w, one can fix $w = S_W^{-1}(\mu_1 - \mu_{-1})$ as a solution. Finally, one should note that the Fisher discriminant can be regularized, too. Here one would exchange S_W by $S_W + CI$ with some constant $C \geq 0$. Unregularized Fisher discriminant is then a special case of regularized Fisher Discriminant for $C = 0$.

One can prove that the w calculated by this approach is the same as calculated by LDA, but the bias b can differ.

Mika et al. (2001) presents a mathematical programming approach to calculate Fisher's discriminant. Although this method is computationally more demanding, the approach allows one to derive several different variants, like sparse Fisher and kernelizations (see section 13.6.8) thereof.

13.6.6 Support Vector Machine

Suppose the given data can be separated by a hyperplane perfectly, that is, a projection w and a bias b can be found such that $y_i(w^\top x_i + b) > 0$ for all i. Without loss of generality, one can scale w and b such that $\min_{i|y_i=y} y(w^\top x_i + b) = 1$ for $y = \pm 1$. In this case the classifier is said to be in canonical form (Vapnik (1995)). With these values the distance from the discriminating hyperplane to the closest point (which is called the margin) can be determined to be $\frac{1}{\|w\|_2}$. For different hyperplanes in canonical form, those with smaller w and thus with higher margin should be preferred. Consequently, this can be formulated mathematically in the following optimization problem:

$$\min \frac{1}{2}\|w\|_2^2 \qquad \text{s.t. } y_i(w^\top x_i + b) \geq 1 \quad \text{for all } i. \tag{13.3}$$

Unfortunately, perfect separation is usually not possible. Thus, one modifies this approach and allows errors by modifying the constraint to $y_i(w^\top x_i + b) \geq 1 - \xi_i$ for all i with $\xi_i \geq 0$ (*soft margin*) and additionally punishes the error made in the objective by adding $\frac{C}{n}\sum_i \xi_i$ with some constant $C > 0$. This machine is called C-SVM. By analyzing the dual problem, one finds that w can be determined by $w = \sum_i \alpha_i y_i x_i$ with some real numbers α_i. For data points x_i with $y_i(w^\top x_i + b) > 1$, one additionally gets that $\alpha_i = 0$. Thus, only a few data points (called support vectors) are required for calculating w. But note that usually all points are required to get this set of support vectors.

A slightly different formulation of the C-SVM is given by the ν-SVM

$$\min_{w,\rho,b,\xi} \frac{1}{2}\|w\|_2^2 - \nu\rho + \sum_i \xi_i \qquad \text{s.t. } \rho > 0, \, y_i(w^\top x_i + b) \geq \rho - \xi_i, \, \xi_i \geq 0 \quad \text{for all } i \tag{13.4}$$

with some $0 \leq \nu < 1$. One can prove that the solution to the ν-SVM is equal to the solution of the C-SVM with $C = \frac{1}{\rho}$.

The advantage of the ν-SVM consists of the fact that the parameter ν informs us about the number of support vectors, namely that the fraction of margin errors (data points with $\xi_i > 0$) is smaller than ν, which in turn is smaller than the fraction of support vectors.

A more detailed overview about support vector machines can be found in Vapnik (1995), Schölkopf and Smola (2002), and Müller et al. (2001).

13.6.7 Linear Programming Machine (LPM)

In a support vector machine the trained hyperplane normal vector w usually has only nonzero entries. To get a sparse solution for w, that is, with many entries equal to zeros, a slight modification of the SVM approach is made in the following way:

$$\min \frac{1}{m}\|w\|_1 + \frac{C}{n}\sum_i \xi_i \qquad \text{s.t. } y_i(w^\top x_i + b) \geq 1 - \xi_i, \, \xi_i \geq 0 \quad \text{for all } i.$$

Here the 1-Norm for w is used instead of the 2-Norm. One can prove that with higher C the number of zero entries in w increases. The sparsity of the hyperplane can be used, for example, for feature extraction, that is, for excluding nonrelevant features.

As an example, we use an EEG dataset (see Dornhege et al. (2004a, 2006b)). Here a subject was asked to imagine left hand movements or foot movements several times. The spectrum between 6 and 30 Hz of this EEG data was calculated by usual FFT for all channels for all trials. Then an LPM classifier was trained on these data. The weights of this classifier are visualized in figure 13.8 on the left. As the feature extraction method, one

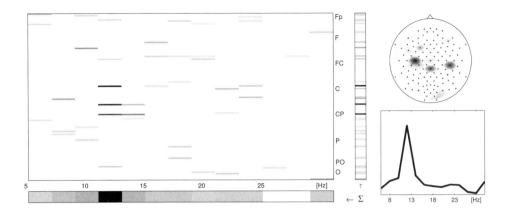

Figure 13.8   On the left, the weights of an LPM during classification of imagined left hand and foot movements on FFT features for all channels. On the top right, the sums of these weights for each channel are shown as spatial distribution. In both figures dark points correspond to high weights, whereas white points correspond to zero, i.e., less important features. On the bottom right, the sums of the classifier weights for each frequency bin are shown. High values correspond to important frequencies.

should use all nonzero entries, which would decrease the number of features from 1,534 to 55 in this case. The sums of weights for each channel and each frequency bin also are visualized in figure 13.8. The spatial distribution is plotted on the top right and shows the expected neurophysiological structure, namely that the channels about motor cortex are most important. On the bottom right the sums of the frequency bins are visualized, which show that the activity around 11–12 Hz is most important. This can be suitably interpreted by neurophysiology since an ERD in the μ rhythm can be expected during imagination of movements.

Note that analogously to the ν-SVM, a ν-LPM can be formulated. More information about linear programming machines are found in Bennett and Mangasarian (1992) and Campbell and Bennett (2001).

13.6.8   The Kernel Trick

The space of linear functions is very limited and cannot solve all existing classification problems. Thus an interesting idea is to map all trials by a function ϕ from the data space to some (maybe infinite-dimensional) feature space and apply a linear method there (see Boser et al. (1992); Vapnik (1995); Schölkopf and Smola (2002); Müller et al. (2001)). The mapping is realized by

$$\Phi : \mathbb{R}^N \to \mathcal{F}, \mathbf{x} \mapsto \Phi(\mathbf{x}),$$

that is, the data $x_1, \ldots, x_n \in \mathbb{R}^N$ is mapped into a potentially much higher dimensional feature space $\mathcal{F}$.

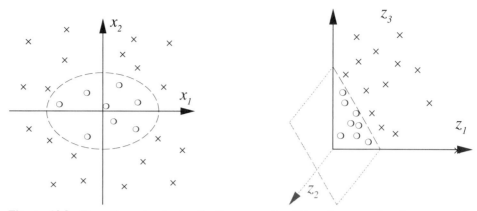

Figure 13.9 Two dimensional classification example. Using the second order monomials x_1^2, $\sqrt{2}x_1 x_2$, and x_2^2 as features, a separation in feature space can be found using a *linear* hyperplane (right). In input space this construction corresponds to a *nonlinear* ellipsoidal decision boundary (left). From Müller et al. (2001).

Although this sounds very complex, for some classification algorithms like SVM (cf. Müller et al. (2001)), LPM (cf. Campbell and Bennett (2001)), or Fisher Discriminant (cf. Mika (2002)) only the scalar product in feature space is required to set up a classifier and be able to apply it. This scalar product in feature space is called the kernel function $K : I\!\!R^m \times I\!\!R^m \to I\!\!R, (x, y) \mapsto \langle \phi(x), \phi(y) \rangle$. A large number of kernels exist like the RBF kernel ($K(x, y) = \exp(-\frac{\|x - y\|_2^2}{2\sigma^2})$) or the polynomial kernel ($K(x, y) = (\langle x, y \rangle + c)^k$) with some further parameters. Kernels can be engineered and adapted to the problem at hand; for the first engineered SVM kernel see Zien et al. (2000). Furthermore, there are theorems about the existence for a feature mapping if a kernel function $I\!\!R^m \times I\!\!R^m \to I\!\!R$ is given (see Müller et al. (2001)). Thus, with the help of the kernel trick, more complex (nonlinear) structures can be learned in an optimal manner.

As an example, we use two-dimensional data from two classes (see figure 13.9 on the left). After suitable mapping the data can be classified linearly (see figure 13.9 on the right).

Note that the kernelization trick can also be applied to any scalar product-based linear algorithm (cf. Schölkopf et al. (1998)), for example, to feature extraction methods like PCA (cf. Schölkopf et al. (1998)) called kPCA, and ICA (cf. Harmeling (2005)).

A discussion of linear versus nonlinear classification methods in BCI context is found in Müller et al. (2003a).

13.7   Technique to Combine Different Features

In the case of BCI analysis, one can potentially extract different features, for example, slow cortical potentials and attenuation of oscillatory features for imagined or real movements. If more than one feature can be used and evidence is given that they are independent of each other, then the following algorithm PROB can be used effectively for classification. This algorithm is presented in Dornhege et al. (2003b, 2004a). The question of whether slow cortical potentials and attenuation of oscillatory features during imagined movements are uncorrelated is also discussed there.

We start with a set of N feature vectors $x_j \in \mathcal{F}_j$ (n number of trials) described by random variables X_j for $j = 1, \dots, N$ with class labels $Y \in \{1, \dots, M\}$ (M number of different classes). Furthermore, let us assume that functions $f_j : \mathcal{F}_j \to I\!R^M$ are given for all j such that the function $\operatorname{argmax} f_j$ is the Bayes optimal classifier[1] for each j, which minimizes the misclassification risk. We denote by $X = (X_1, \dots, X_N)$ the combined random vector, by $g_{j,y}$ the densities of $f_j(X_j)|Y = y$, by f the optimal classifier on the combined feature vector space $\mathcal{F} = (\mathcal{F}_1, \dots, \mathcal{F}_N)$, and by g_y the density of $f(X)|Y = y$.

For all $j = 1, \dots, N$ and all possible features $z = (z_1, \dots, z_N)$ we get

$$\operatorname{argmax}(f_j(z_j)) = \operatorname{argmax}_y g_{j,y}(z_j)$$
$$\operatorname{argmax}(f(z)) = \operatorname{argmax}_y g_y(z).$$

Let us assume that the features are independent. This assumption allows us to factorize the combined density, that is, to compute $g_y(x) = \prod_{j=1}^{N} g_{j,y}(x_j)$ for the class labels $y = \{1, \dots, M\}$. This leads to the optimal decision function

$$f(z) = \operatorname{argmax} \sum_{j=1}^{N} f_j(z_j).$$

If we additionally assume that all feature vectors X_j's are Gaussian distributed with equal covariance matrices, that is, $P(X_j|Y = y) = \mathcal{N}(\mu_{j,y}, \Sigma_j)$, the following classifier

$$\operatorname{argmax} f(x) = \operatorname{argmax}_y \left(\sum_{j=1}^{N} [w_j^\top x_j - \frac{1}{2}(\mu_{j,y})^\top w_j] \right)$$

with $w_j := \Sigma_j^{-1} \mu_{j,y}$ is achieved.

In terms of LDA, this corresponds to forcing to zero the elements of the estimated covariance matrix that belong to different feature vectors. Consequently, since less parameters have to be estimated, distortions by accidental correlations of independent variables are avoided. It should be noted that analogously to quadratic discriminant analysis (QDA) (see Friedman (1989)), one can formulate a nonlinear version of PROB with Gaussian assumption but different covariance matrices for each class.

To avoid overfitting, PROB can be regularized, too. There are two possible ways: fitting one parameter to all features or fitting one parameter for each feature.

13.8   Caveats in the Validation

The objective when evaluating offline classifications is to estimate the future performance of the investigated methods, or in other words the generalization ability of the learning machine. Note that the most objective report of BCI performance is the results of actual feedback sessions. But in the development and enhancement of BCI systems it is essential to make offline investigations. Making BCI feedback experiments is costly and time-consuming. So, when exploring new ways for processing or classifying brain signals, one would first validate and tune the new methods before integrating them into an online system and pursuing feedback experiments. Yet there are many ways that lead to an (unintentional) overestimation of the generalization ability. In this section, we discuss what must be noted when analyzing the methods presented in this chapter. A much more thorough discussion of the evaluation methods for BCI classifications will be the subject of a forthcoming paper.

13.8.1   The Fundamental Problem

The essence in estimating the generalization error is to split the available labeled data into training and test set, to determine all free hyperparameters and parameters on the training set, and then to evaluate the method on the test data. To ensure that the estimation of the error is unbiased, the test data must not have been used in any way before all parameters have been calculated, all hyperparameters have been selected, and all other selections have been made. In a cross-validation or a leave-one-out validation the data set is split in many different ways into training and test set, the procedure as outlined above is performed for each split, and finally the mean of all errors obtained for the test data is taken as estimate for the generalization error. A common error in the evaluation of machine learning techniques—not only in a BCI context—is that some preprocessing steps or some parameter selections are performed on the whole data set before the cross-validation. If the preprocessing acts *locally* on each sample, there is no problem, but if the preprocessing of one sample depends somehow on the distribution of all samples, the basic principle that the test set must remain unseen until all free parameters have been fixed, is violated. This violation will very likely lead to a severe underestimation of the generalization error; of course the degree of violation cannot be stated generally as it depends on many factors.

When enough data samples are available, the problem can be solved by having a threefold split of the data into training, test, and validation set. All parameter settings from which we intend to select would be trained on the training and applied to the validation set. The setting with the best performance on the validation set is chosen and applied to the test set. In a cross-validation, one has many of such threefold splits and the mean error on the test set is taken as an estimate of the generalization error.

While this procedure is conceptually sound, it is often not a viable way in BCI context where available labeled samples are very limited compared to the complexity of the data. In such a setting, doing model selection on one fixed split is not robust. One can circumvent this problem when sufficient computing resources (computing power or time) are available by doing a *nested* cross-validation. While the outer cross-validation is used to get the estimation of the generalization error, there is an inner cross-validation performed on each training set of the outer validation to do the model selection (see Müller et al. (2001)).

13.8.2   Evaluating Classifiers with Hyperparameters

Machine learning classifiers have parameters whose values are adapted to given labeled data (training data) by some optimization criterion, such as w, b, or ξ in SVMs (13.3). Some classifiers also have some so-called hyperparameters, such as ν in the ν-SVM

(13.4). These are parameters that also have to be adapted to the data, but for which no direct optimization criterion exists. Typically, hyperparameters control the capacity of the classifier or the raggedness of the separation surface. In the classifier presented in section 13.6.7, the hyperparameter C controls the sparsity of the classifier (sparser classifiers have less capacity). To validate the generalization ability of a classifier with hyperparameters, one has to perform a nested cross-validation, as explained above. On each training set of the outer cross-validation, an inner cross-validation is performed for different values of the hyperparameters. The one with minimum (inner) cross-validation error is selected and evaluated on the test set of the outer cross-validation.

13.8.3   Evaluating Preprocessing Methods

The fundamental problem discussed in section 13.8.1 appears when a preprocessing method (such as CSP) is applied to the whole dataset before the cross-validation, such a procedure would be "cheating." Even a preprocessing that is not label-dependent can be problematic when it operates nonlocally in the above sense. To make an unbiased validation nonlocal processings have to be performed *within* the cross-validation, whereby all parameters have to be estimated from the training data. For example, a correct evaluation of a method that uses ICA as preprocessing must calculate the projection matrix *within* the cross-validation on each training set. Data of the test set are projected using that matrix. While the bias introduced by applying ICA before the cross-validation can be expected to be marginal, it is critical for the label-dependent method CSP.

13.8.4   Evaluating Feature Selection Methods

It is very tempting to evaluate feature selection methods by running the feature selection on the whole dataset and then doing a cross-validation on the dataset of reduced features, but again this would be cheating. Unfortunately, such a procedure is found in a number of publications, but it is conceptually wrong and may very well lead to a severe underestimation of the generalization error. As argued in section 13.8.3, a preprocessing such as feature selection must be performed *within* the cross-validation. When the method has hyperparameters (like the number of features to extract) the selection of these hyperparameters has to be done by an *inner* cross-validation (see section 13.8.2).

13.9   Robustification

Robustness is the ability of a system to cope with distorted or invalid input. Biomedical signals such as EEG typically are contaminated by measurement artifacts and noise from nonneurophysiological sources. Also, sources from the central nervous system that do not contribute to the signal of interest typically are regarded as noise. Data points particularly affected by those kinds of noise do not fit the model assumptions. In terminology of machine learning, such data points are called outliers, see, for example, Barnett and Lewis (1994); Huber (1981); Hampel et al. (1986); Birch et al. (1993); Schölkopf et al. (2001);

Tax and Duin (2001); and Laskov et al. (2004). An effective discriminability of different brain states requires an effective estimation of some properties of the data, such as mean or covariance matrix. If outliers impede this estimation, a suboptimal or even highly distorted classifier can be the consequence.

In the literature, many different methods can be found for how to identify outliers. A common method is the definition of a distance function in connection with a threshold criterion. The distance of each point from a common reference then can be interpreted as a measure of "normality," that is, points with an unusually high distance (e.g., exceeding the predefined threshold) are then marked as outliers. As an example, the Mahalanobis distance of the data point x from the mean μ is defined as

$$r^2(x) = (x - \mu)^t \Sigma^{-1}(x - \mu),$$

where Σ denotes the covariance matrix.

A different distance, not relying on the estimation of parameters of the distribution, has been suggested in Harmeling et al. (2006). The outlier index δ of the point x is defined as the length of the mean of the vectors pointing from x to its k nearest neighbors, that is,

$$\delta(x) = \|\frac{1}{k} \sum_{j=1}^{k} (x - z_j(x))\|,$$

where $z_1(x), \ldots, z_k(x) \in \{x_1, \ldots, x_n\}$ are the k nearest neighbors of x.

Apart from the general issue of choosing an outlier detection method, it is also an inherent property of multidimensional time series data like EEG that the dimensions of the feature space may have different qualities: Usually, data points are given with a certain number of repetitions (trials), and they contain channel information and the temporal evolution of the signal. A natural approach is to specifically use this information to find outliers within a certain dimension, that is, removing channels with an increased noise level (due to high impedances at the specific electrode) or removing trials that are contaminated by artifacts from muscular or ocular activity. In Krauledat et al. (2005), different methods of dealing with outliers have been shown to improve classification performances on a large number of datasets.

13.10   Practical Example

To end this chapter, we provide one worked-through example of applying signal processing and machine learning methods composed of three parts to BCI data. First, we design processing and classification methods for event-related potential shifts and then for power modulations of brain rhythms. Both analyses are performed on the very same dataset so we can, in a third step, fuse both approaches with a feature combination technique that results in a very powerful classification as demonstrated in the BCI Competitions (see section 13.10.5).

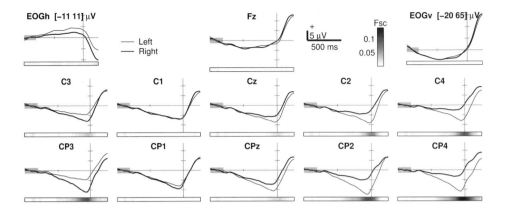

Figure 13.10   Classwise averaged time course of event-related potentials related to left- vs. right-hand finger movements (selected channels over motor cortex). The shaded rectangulars indicate the period of baseline correction. The Fisher score quantifies the discriminability between the two classes and is indicated below each channel in grey scale code.

13.10.1   Experimental Setup for the Worked-Through Example

A healthy subject performed self-paced finger movements on a computer keyboard with an approximate tap-rate of 45 taps per minute. EEG was recorded from 52 Ag/AgCl scalp electrodes during 677 finger movements. The goal of our analysis is to predict in single trials the laterality of imminent left- versus right-hand finger movements at a time point prior to the start of EMG activity. An analysis of simultaneously recorded EMG from both forearms (*M. flexor digitorum communis*) found no significant EMG activity before -120 ms relative to keypress (see section 5.3.1). Therefore, we design classification methods that classify windows ending 120 ms before keypress.

13.10.2   Classifying on Event-Related Potential Shifts

Our first approach to the given dataset is to look at the event-related potentials. As we are interested in the premovement potentials that *precede* the actual movement execution, we divide to epochs the data in time intervals from -1000 to 250 ms. (That is, each epoch is a multichannel time course running from -1000 to 250 ms relative to one keypress.) To obtain smoother curves, we apply a moving average low-pass filter with a window length of 100 ms. This is a simple form of a FIR filter (see section 13.3). Furthermore, we subtract from each epoch the average of the time interval -1000 to -800 ms (baseline correction). To quantify the discriminative information, we calculate for each channel and each time point the Fisher score (see section 13.5). Figure 13.10 shows the classwise (left-hand and right-hand finger movements) averaged epochs with the Fisher score indicated in grey scale code below each channel. The figure shows a pronounced negativation that grows stronger contralateral to the performing limb when approaching the time point of keypress. For more information on this readiness potential, see section 5.3 and references therein. A

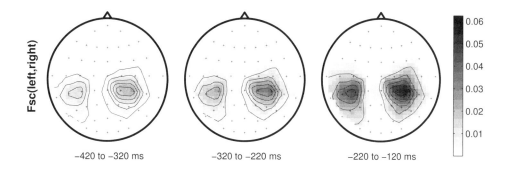

Figure 13.11 The Fisher scores that are calculated for each time point and each channel are averaged across the indicated three time intervals and displayed as scalp patterns. The discrimination between the brain potentials corresponding to the preparation of left vs. right hand movements originates in the corresponding motor cortices. No contribution from task-related eye movements is visible in the investigated time intervals.

further outcome of this analysis is that the difference of scalp potentials is not induced by eye movements since the Fisher scores in the EOG channels are very small, especially in the time interval of interest that ends 120 ms before keypress. Figure 13.11 visualizes the Fisher score as scalp topographies. Here the Fisher score values for all channels are averaged in the time intervals [-420 -320], [-320 -220], and [-220 -120] and are displayed as scalp patterns. The foci in these patterns show that the difference in brain potentials originates, as expected, in the respective motor areas.

After this visual inspection of the data, we design the feature extraction and the classification method. The patterns in figure 13.11 suggest that we can safely discard channels that are very frontal (Fpz, AF3, AF4) and very occipital (O1, Oz, O2). Then, to classify on the potential shifts it is desireable to get rid of the higher frequencies that are noise in this respect. Since we see from figure 13.10 that the discrimination increases with time, we use an STFT to accomplish the low-pass filtering (see section 13.3.2) using a window that puts emphasis on the late part of the signal, namely a one-sided cosine window

$$w(n) := 1 - \cos(n\pi/100) \quad \text{for } n = 0, \ldots, 99$$

(see section 5.3.2 for details). This filter is applied to raw EEG epochs that are taken in the one-second interval from -1120 to -120 ms relative to keypress. After applying the STFT, the coefficients corresponding to the frequencies 1 to 4 Hz only are retained while the rest is set to 0 and transformed back by IFT (see section 13.3.2). From these smoothed signals, the last 200 ms are subsampled at 20 Hz resulting in four feature components per channel (see the illustration in section 5.3.2). This results in a 184-dimensional feature vector (4 points in time times 46 channels) for which we need to choose a classifier. In our experience this readiness potential feature can very well be separated linearly (see Blankertz et al. (2003)). Since the dimensionality of the features is relatively high compared to the number of available training samples, we use a regularized linear discrimnant analysis[2] classifier (see section 13.6.3). For the evaluation of this processing/classification method, we perform

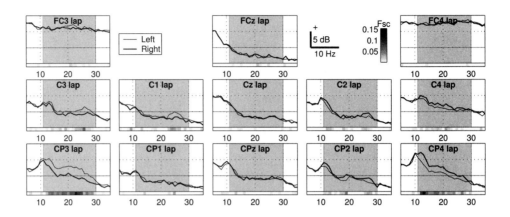

Figure 13.12 Classwise averaged spectra of brain potentials during the preparation of left- vs. right-hand finger movements (time interval -1120 to -120 ms). The Fisher score quantifies the discriminability between the two classes and is indicated below each channel in grey scale code. The shaded frequency band shows the best discrimination and is therefore used for further analysis and classification.

a 10×10-fold cross-validation with an inner cross-validation loop on each training set of the outer cross-validation to select the regularization parameter of the RLDA classifier (see section 13.8.2). This way we obtained an estimated generalization error of 11 percent. The usage of spatial filters (see sections 13.4.1, 13.4.3, and 13.4.2) did not result in better performance.

13.10.3 Classifying on Modulations of Brain Rhythms

It is known that executed movements are not only preceded by movement-related readiness potentials but also by event-related modulations of the sensorimotor rhythms (Pfurtscheller and Lopes da Silva (1999). Here we investigate those modulations and design a classification method based on this phenomenon. The first step is to look at the class-specific spectra to find the frequency bands that show the best discrimination. To this end, we segment the data into epochs of 1 s ending 120 ms before keypress (see section 13.10.1). Then we apply a spatial Laplace filter (see section 13.4.3) to obtain more localized signals that better reveal the discriminative frequency bands (see figure 13.4). Analogous to section 13.5, we calculate Fisher scores for each frequency bin and channel. Figure 13.12 shows the classwise averaged spectra with Fisher scores indicated by grey scale code. The large shaded rectangles indicate the frequency band 11–30 Hz that shows the best discrimination according to the Fisher scores. The next step is to investigate the time course of instantaneous power in this frequency band. To this end, we take a butterworth IIR filter of order five with bandpass 11–30 Hz (see section 13.3.1) and apply this filter to the raw EEG signals. We epoch the signals in the time interval -1500 to 500 ms, apply a spatial Laplace filter and calculate the envelope of the bandpass-filtered signals by a Hilbert transform. Finally, we smooth the obtained time courses by a moving average filter with a 100 ms window. For baseline correction we subtract in each channel the average across all epochs and the

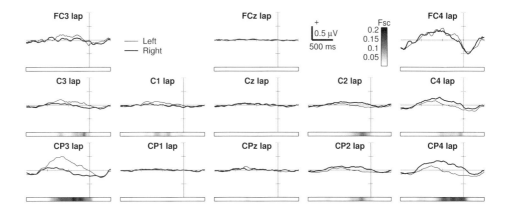

Figure 13.13   Classwise averaged instantaneous spectral power in the frequency band 11–30 Hz related to left- vs. right-hand finger movements (selected channels over motor cortex). The Fisher score quantifies the discriminability between the two classes and is indicated below each channel in grey scale code.

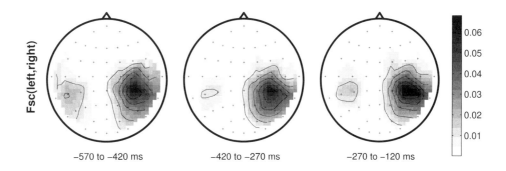

Figure 13.14   The Fisher scores that are calculated for each time point and each channel of the curves shown in figure 13.13 are averaged across the indicated three time intervals and displayed as scalp patterns. The discrimination between the time courses of bandpower during the preparation of left vs. right hand movements originates in the corresponding motor cortices. No contribution from task-related eye movements is visible in the investigated time intervals.

whole time interval. Again we calculate the Fisher score for each time point and channel of the resulting time series. The obtained curves in figure 13.13 show a bilateral but mainly ipsilateral increase of band energy (event-related synchronization, ERS) starting at about -1000 ms and a contralateral decrease of band energy (event-related desynchronization, ERD) starting about 500 ms. The visualization of Fisher scores as scalp topographies in figure 13.14 show a similar picture as for the event-related potentials (figure 13.11) but with less symmetric foci that are more pronounced on the right hemisphere and the location is more lateral. Again substantial contributions to the discrimination are located over motor cortices.

After a visual inspection of the data, we design the feature extraction and the classification method. The patterns in figure 13.14 suggest that we can safely discard channels that are very frontal (Fpz, AF3, AF4). For classification we apply the IIR bandpass filter as we did to the raw EEG signals. The Fisher scores in figure 13.13 indicate that the discrimination becomes good after 570 ms prior to movement. Accordingly, we collect epochs corresponding to the time interval -570 to -120 ms. These are the features that are used by a CSP/LDA classification method: Using a CSP analysis the data is reduced to the 6 CSP channels corresponding to the three largest eigenvalues of each class (see section 13.4.6). For these time series the variance is calculated in three equally sized subintervals (corresponding to the same intervals that are displayed in figure 13.14). This gives an estimate of the instantaneous bandpower at those three time intervals within each epoch. To make the distribution of the resulting vectors more Gaussian (distribution assumption of LDA, see section 13.6.2), we apply the logarithm. The dimensionality of the obtained vectors is eighteen (three bandpower values in time for six CSP channels), that is, small enough that we can classify them by LDA here even without regularization. The cross-validation that we perform to estimate the generalization error needs to take into account that the CSP analysis uses label information. So the calculation of CSP needs to be performed *within* the cross-validation loop on each training set (see section 13.8.3). This way we obtained an estimated generalization error of 21 percent.

13.10.4   Combination of Different Kinds of Features

In the two previous sections we derived two different kinds of features that both gave good classification performance. The two features rely on different neurophysiological phenomena, the readiness potential (RP feature), and event-related (de-)synchronization (ERD feature). One further step in improving the classification accuracy is to combine those two features. The straightforward way to accomplish this is to concatenate the two feature vectors and classify as before. But neurophysiological studies suggest that the RP and the ERD features reflect different aspects of sensorimotor cortical processes. In the light of this a priori knowledge, the combination method presented in section 13.7 seems promising. Indeed, the cross-validation of the feature combination classifier PROB obtained with 7.5 percent error has the best result. Here we used regularized PROB with one single regularization parameter. For the cross-validation, the selection of this parameter was done within the inner cross-validation loop.

13.10.5   A Final Remark

Concerning the generalization errors that have been estimated in the previous sections, although the cross-validation that was used to estimate them was designed such that it is not biased, the whole analysis still could be biased to underestimate the generalization error. The visual inspection that was performed to design the feature extraction method and some of its parameters (as the frequency band) used the whole dataset. Typically the bias is not so severe when the twiddling in the manual tuning is not too heavy (provided the estimation of the generalization error is technically sound; see section 13.8.3).

A performance assessment that has no such bias can be obtained in BCI Competitions (Blankertz (2005b)). Until submission deadline the labels of the test set are kept secret.[3] The combination method of the previous section proved to be effective in the first BCI Competition by winning the contest for dataset II (EEG-synchronized imagined-movement task) (see Sajda et al. (2003)). Note that also in subsequent BCI Competitions, for several datasets the winning teams use techniques that combined RP- and ERD-type features (BCI Competition II, dataset V, see Zhang et al. (2004); Blankertz (2003); and BCI Competition III, datasets I, IIIb, and IVa, see Blankertz et al. (2006c); Blankertz (2005a)).

13.11   Conclusion

The purpose of this chapter is to provide a broad overview of ML and SP methods for BCI data analysis. When setting up a new paradigm, care has to be exercised, to use as much medical prior knowledge for defining appropriate features. This modeling holds the key to further processing. If possible, outliers need to be removed. Once the features are specified, a regularized classifier is mandatory to control against overfitting and thus to enhance the robustness of the BCI. Model selection and feature selection should be done in a "clean" manner using nested cross-validation or hold-out sets, since "cheating" will in practice inevitably lead to overoptimistic results.

Acknowledgments

The studies were supported by a grant of the *Bundesministerium für Bildung und Forschung* (BMBF), FKZ 01IBE01A/B. This work was supported in part by the IST Programme of the European Community, under the PASCAL Network of Excellence, IST-2002-506778. This publication reflects only the authors' views.

Notes

E-mail for correspondence: guido.dornhege@first.fhg.de

(1)   At this point no assumptions about the distribution of the data are made.
(2)   A model selection with a full RDA model (see section 13.6.3) resulted in choosing $\lambda = 1$, that is, the linear case RLDA.
(3)   Evaluations done after the publication of the test labels, however, are not safe from the overfitting bias.

14   Classifying Event-Related Desynchronization in EEG, ECoG, and MEG Signals

N. Jeremy Hill, Thomas Navin Lal, and Bernhard Schölkopf
Max Planck Institute for Biological Cybernetics
Tübingen, Germany

Michael Tangermann
Fraunhofer–Institute FIRST
Intelligent Data Analysis Group (IDA)
Kekuléstr. 7, 12489 Berlin, Germany

Thilo Hinterberger
Institute of Medical Psychology and   *Division of Psychology*
Behavioural Neurobiology   *University of Northampton*
Eberhard-Karls-University Tübingen   *Northampton, UK*
Gartenstr. 29
72074 Tübingen, Germany

Guido Widman and Christian E. Elger
Epilepsy Center
University of Bonn, Germany

Niels Birbaumer
Institute of Medical Psychology and   *National Institute of Health (NIH)*
Behavioural Neurobiology   *NINDS*
Eberhard-Karls-University Tübingen   *Human Cortical Physiology Unit*
Gartenstr. 29   *Bethesda, USA*
72074 Tübingen, Germany

14.1   Abstract

We present the results from three motor imagery-based brain-computer interface experiments. Brain signals were recorded from eight untrained subjects using EEG, four using

ECoG, and ten using MEG. In all cases, we aim to develop a system that could be used for fast, reliable preliminary screening in the clinical application of a BCI, so we aim to obtain the best possible classification performance in a short time. Accordingly, the burden of adaptation is on the side of the computer rather than the user, so we must adopt a machine learning approach to the analysis. We introduce the required machine-learning vocabulary and concepts, and then present quantitative results that focus on two main issues. The first is the effect of the number of trials—how long does the recording session need to be? We find that good performance could be achieved, on average, after the first 200 trials in EEG, 75–100 trials in MEG, and 25–50 trials in ECoG. The second issue is the effect of spatial filtering—we compare the performance of the original sensor signals with that of the outputs of independent component Analysis and the common spatial pattern algorithm, in each of the three sensor types. We find that spatial filtering does not help in MEG, helps a little in ECoG, and improves performance a great deal in EEG. The unsupervised ICA algorithm performed at least as well as the supervised CSP algorithm in all cases—the latter suffered from poor generalization performance due to overfitting in ECoG and MEG, although this could be alleviated by reducing the number of sensors used as input to the algorithm.

14.2 Introduction

Many different recording technologies exist today for measuring brain activity. In addition to electroencephalography (EEG) and invasive microelectrode recording techniques that have been known for some time, research institutes and clinics now have access to electrocorticography (ECoG), magnetoencephalography (MEG), near-infrared spectrophotometry (NIRS), positron emission tomography (PET), and functional magnetic resonance imaging (fMRI), any of which might be potentially useful in the design and implementation of brain-computer interface systems. Each technology has its own particular set of advantages and limitations with regard to spatial and temporal resolution as well as cost, portability, and risk to the user. Comparative studies are required in order to guide development, and to explore the trade-offs between these factors.

Bulky, expensive systems (PET, fMRI, MEG) cannot be deployed as day-to-day BCI systems in users' homes, but they may offer advantages in the early stages of BCI use. For example, they may be valuable for conducting *screening* procedures, in which a potential user is scanned for one or two sessions to ascertain what patterns of brain activity can be most clearly measured and most easily modulated by voluntary intention. An ideal screening would give clinicians the best possible basis on which to decide which task/stimulus setting the user should invest time training with, and (if invasive methods are being considered) where electrodes should be implanted. Regular periodic visits to the scanner might also be a valuable part of early BCI training. However, to justify the cost of screening and training in this way, we would need to know whether the technology yields advantages, for example, in terms of signal quality, efficiency, or precision of source localization, that could not otherwise be obtained with cheaper methods.

Here we present a comparative study of motor-imagery BCI experiments based on EEG, ECoG, and MEG. In all three, our goal is to develop techniques of analysis that could be used for efficient screening using a simple binary synchronous (trial-based) paradigm, to determine whether subsequent lengthy training in motor imagery might be worthwhile. This requires that we obtain good classification performance as quickly as possible, ideally within the duration of a single recording session. In longer-term user training regimes, it might be desirable to fix the mapping between brain activity and output a priori, with users learning to adjust their brain activity such that the mapped recordings meet the desired output. However, in this shorter-term setting, users arrive untrained and do not necessarily know how to control their brain activity in the optimal manner: the most effective mental strategy may differ from person to person, and its subjective character may not be easily describable in any case. Users have relatively little time to adjust and optimize their performance, yet we must still achieve the best results we can. Therefore, for current purposes the burden of adaptation in brain-computer communication lies on the side of the computer—we follow the same principle of "letting the machines learn" that guides the Berlin Brain-Computer Interface project (Krauledat et al. (2004)). We envisage screening as consisting of multiple discrete trials in which the user is repeatedly asked to produce brain-states of different classes. The mapping from brain states to the desired output is not known and must be inferred from this limited set of example mappings—a problem of *empirical inference* for which a machine learning approach is well suited.

After briefly describing the neurological basis of our studies, the recording technologies and experimental setup, we introduce some of the machine learning concepts, terms, and tools we need. We then describe our analysis procedure, present results, and conclude. In particular, we are interested in the question of how many trials are necessary to yield good classification performance—in other words, how soon could we have broken off the testing session, and still have obtained comparable results?

14.3   Neurological Phenomena of Imagined Movement

When a person is neither moving nor about to move, the electrical activity of the motor cortex is dominated by frequencies in the 8–12 Hz (α-band) and 18–22 Hz (β-band) ranges. These signal components are often referred to as μ rhythms, or more generally as sensorimotor rhythms (SMR).

At the beginning of the planning phase, about 1–1.5 s before a movement is executed, the SMR gradually diminishes, an effect known as event-related desynchronization (ERD). Slower shifts and deflections in electrical signal, known as movement-related potentials (MRP), also can be observed at roughly the same time. Both neurological phenomena can be recorded best over the motor cortex contralateral to the movement.

It is known that ERD is also present when movements are only imagined (e.g., Pfurtscheller et al. (1998)) or attempted (Kauhanen et al. (2004)). Unfortunately, not all users show ERD in motor imagery, although it is possible to train healthy subjects (Guger et al. (2003)) as well as patients with ALS (Kübler et al. (2005a)) to control their SMR such that the recorded activity becomes more classifiable. When present, ERD can be detected relatively easily and is therefore used in the majority of BCI studies.

Using both aspects—MRP and ERD—of the recorded signal leads to improved classification performance (Dornhege et al. (2003b)), a result supported by the work of Babiloni et al. (1999) who argue that MRP and ERD represent different aspects of cortical processing. In the current study, however, only a very small minority of our subjects showed useable MRPs in our imagined movement task—for simplicity, we therefore focus our attention on ERD.

14.4   Recording Technology

Since our focus is on ERD, we can consider only recording methods that have sufficient temporal resolution to capture changes in the α and β bands. This rules out technologies such as PET, fMRI, and NIRS that rely on the detection of regional changes in cerebral blood oxygenation levels. We briefly introduce the three recording systems we have used: EEG, ECoG, and MEG.

14.4.1   EEG

Extracranial electroencephalography is a well-studied recording technique for cerebral activity that has been practiced since its invention by Hans Berger in 1929. It measures electrical activity, mainly from the cortex, noninvasively: Electrical signals of the order of 10^{-4} volts are measured by passive electrodes (anything from a single electrode to about 300) placed on the subject's head, contact being made between the skin and the electrode by a conducting gel. EEG shows a very high temporal resolution of tens of milliseconds but is limited in its spatial resolution, the signals being spatially blurred due to volume conduction in the intervening tissue.

EEG experiments account for the large majority of BCI studies due to the hardware's low cost, risk, and portability. For a selection of EEG motor imagery studies, see Wolpaw et al. (1997); Birch et al. (2003); McFarland et al. (1997a); Guger et al. (1999); Dornhege et al. (2004a); Lal et al. (2004).

14.4.2   ECoG

Electrocorticography or intracranial EEG is an invasive recording technique in which an array of electrodes, for example an 8×8 grid, is placed surgically beneath the skull, either outside or underneath the dura. Strips containing smaller numbers of electrodes also may be inserted into deeper regions of the brain. Unlike invasive microelectrode recording techniques, ECoG measures activity generated by large cell populations—ECoG measurements are thus more comparable to extracranial EEG, but the electrode's close proximity to the cortex and the lack of intervening tissue allows for a higher signal-to-noise ratio, a better response at higher frequencies, and a drastic reduction in spatial blurring between neighboring electrode signals and contamination by artifacts.

Naturally, intracranial surgery is performed at some risk to the patient. Today, ECoG implantation is not widespread, but is mostly carried out as a short-term procedure for the localization of epileptic foci, prior to neurosurgical treatment of severe epilepsy. Patients typically have electrodes implanted for one or two weeks for this purpose, a window of opportunity that is being exploited to perform a variety of brain research including motor imagery BCI (Graimann et al. (2004); Leuthardt et al. (2004); Lal et al. (2005a)).

14.4.3 MEG

Magnetoencephalography is a noninvasive recording technique for measuring the tiny magnetic field fluctuations, of the order of 10^{-14} tesla, induced by the electrical activity of populations of cerebral neurons—mainly those in the cortex, although it has been reported that it is also possible to measure activity from deeper subcortical structures (Llinas et al. (1999); Tesche and Karhu (1997); Baillet et al. (2001)). Relative to fMRI, the spatial resolution of MEG is rather low due to the smaller number of sensors (100–300), but it has a high temporal resolution comparable to that of EEG, in the tens of milliseconds.

Due to the extremely low amplitude of the magnetic signals of interest, MEG scanners must be installed in a magnetically shielded room to avoid the signals being swamped by the earth's magnetic field, and the sensors must be cooled, usually by a large liquid helium cooling unit. MEG scanners are consequently rather expensive and nonportable.

Kauhanen et al. (2004) presented an MEG study of sensorimotor rhythms during attempted finger movements by tetraplegic patients. Very recently we introduced an online motor imagery-based BCI using MEG signals (Lal et al. (2005b)).

14.5 Experimental Setup

Three experiments form the basis for this chapter: one using EEG (described in more detail by Lal et al. (2004)), one using ECoG (Lal et al. (2005a)), and one based on MEG recordings (Lal et al. (2005b)).

There were eight healthy subjects in the EEG experiment, seated in an armchair in front of a computer monitor. Ten healthy subjects participated in the MEG experiment, seated in the MEG scanner in front of a projector screen. In the ECoG experiment, four patients with epilepsy took part, seated in their hospital beds facing a monitor.

Table 14.1 contains an overview of the three experimental setups. Depending on the setup, subjects performed up to 400 trials. Each trial began with a small fixation cross displayed at the center of the screen, indicating that the subject should not move and should blink as little as possible. One second later the randomly chosen task cue was displayed for 500 ms, instructing the subject to imagine performing one of two movements: These were left hand and right hand movement[1] for the EEG study, and movement of either the left little finger or the tongue[2] for the MEG and the ECoG studies (ECoG grids were implanted on the right cerebral hemisphere). The imagined movement phase lasted at least 3 s and then the fixation point was extinguished, marking the end of the trial. Between trials was a short relaxation phase of randomized length between 2 and 4 s.

Table 14.1 Overview of the three experiments.

	EEG	ECoG	MEG
Subjects	8	4	10
Trials per subject	400	100–200	200
Sensors	39	64–84	150
Sampling rate (Hz)	256	1000	625

14.6   Machine Learning Concepts and Tools

The problem is one of binary classification, a very familiar setting in machine learning. Here we introduce some of the vocabulary of machine learning, in the context of BCI, to explain the tools we use. For a more thorough introduction to machine learning in BCI, see Müller et al. (2004a).

For each subject, we have a number of *data points*, each associated with one of two *target labels*—this is just an abstract way of stating that we have a number of distinct trials, each of which is an attempt by the subject to communicate one of two internal brain states. Each data point is a numerical description of a trial, and its target label denotes whether the subject performed, for example, imagined finger movement or imagined tongue movement on that trial. Classification is the attempt to extract the relevant information from one subset of the data points (the training subset, for which labels are given) to be able to predict as accurately as possible the labels of another subset (the test subset, for which label information is withheld until the time comes to evaluate final classification accuracy). Extraction of the relevant information for prediction on unseen data is termed *generalization* to the new data.

Each data point can be described by a large number of *features*, each feature being (for the current purposes) a real number. The features are the dimensions of the space in which the data points lie. We can choose the feature representation by selecting our preprocessing: a single trial, measured and digitized as t time samples from each of s sensors, may, for example, be fully described by the s times t discrete sample values, and this feature representation may or may not be useful for classification. An alternative feature representation might be the values that make up the amplitude spectra of the s sensor readings—the same data points have now been mapped into a different *feature space*, which may or may not entail an improvement in the ease of classification.

Note that both these feature representations specify the positions of data points in very high-dimensional spaces. Successful generalization using a small number of data points in a relatively high-dimensional space is a considerable challenge (Friedman (1988)).

14.6.1   Support Vector Machines

For classification, we choose a support vector machine (SVM), which has proven its worth in a very diverse range of classification problems from medical applications (Lee et al. (2000)) and image classifications (Chapelle et al. (1999)) to text categorization (Joachims

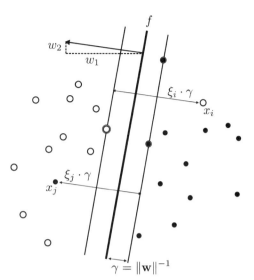

Figure 14.1   Linear SVM. The data are separated by a hyperplane with the largest possible margin γ. For the separable case (ignoring misclassified points x_i and x_j), the three-ringed points lying exactly on the margin would be the support vectors (SVs). For nonseparable datasets, slack variables ξ_k are introduced—depending on the scaling of these, more points will become SVs.

(1998)) and bioinformatics (Zien et al. (2000); Sonnenburg et al. (2005)). Its approach is to choose a *decision boundary* between classes such that the *margin*, that is, the distance in feature space between the boundary and the nearest data point, is maximized—intuitively, one can see that this might result in a minimized probability that a point, its position perturbed by random noise, will stray over onto the wrong side of the boundary. Figure 14.1 shows a two-dimensional (i.e., two-feature) example.

When one has more features to work on than data points, it is often all too easy to find a decision boundary that separates the training data perfectly into two classes, but *overfits*. This means that the *capacity* of the classifier (loosely, its allowable complexity; see Vapnik (1998) for the theoretical background) is too large for the data, with the result that the classifier then models too precisely the specific training data points it has seen, and does not generalize well to new test data. Rather than attempt to separate all the data points perfectly, we may obtain better generalization performance if we allow for the possibility that some of the data points, due to noise in the measurement or other random factors, are simply on the wrong side of the decision boundary. For the SVM, this leads to the *soft-margin* formulation

$$f : \mathbb{R}^d \to \{-1, 1\}, \qquad \mathbf{x} \mapsto sign(\mathbf{w}^* \cdot \mathbf{x} + b^*)$$

$$(\mathbf{w}^*, b^*) = \operatorname*{argmin}_{\mathbf{w} \in \mathbb{R}^d,\ b \in \mathbb{R}} \|\mathbf{w}\|_2^2 + C \sum_{k=1}^{n} \xi_k^2 \ \text{ subject to } \ y_k(\mathbf{w} \cdot \mathbf{x}_k + b) \geq 1 - \xi_k, \ \ (k = 1, ..., n)$$

where $\mathbf{x}_k$ is the d-dimensional vector of features describing the kth data point and y_k is the corresponding label, either -1 or $+1$. The classifying function f, whose parameters $\mathbf{w}$ (the normal vector to the separating hyperplane) and b (a scalar bias term) must be optimized. The constraint $y_k(\mathbf{w} \cdot \mathbf{x}_k + b) \geq 1$ would result in a hard-margin SVM—the closest point would then have distance $\|\mathbf{w}\|^{-1}$ to the hyperplane, so minimizing $\|\mathbf{w}\|$ under this constraint maximizes the margin. The solution for the hyperplane can be written in terms of the support vectors, which, in the hard-margin case, are the points lying exactly on the margin (highlighted points in figure 14.1). A soft margin is implemented by incorporating a penalty term ξ_k for each data point that lies on the wrong side of the margin, and a regularization parameter C, which specifies the scaling of these penalty terms relative to the original criterion of margin maximization. Depending on C, the optimal margin will widen and more points will become support vectors.

For a given C there is a unique SVM solution, but a suitable value for C must somehow be chosen. This a question of model selection which often is addressed by cross-validation: the available training data points are divided randomly into, for example, ten nonoverlapping subsets of equal size. For each of these ten subsets (or test folds, the model is trained on the other 90 percent (the training fold) and tested on the test fold. The average proportion of mistakes made across the ten test folds is taken as the cross-validation error, and the model (in this case, the choice of C) with the smallest cross-validation error wins.

One of the SVM's noteworthy features is that it is a *kernel algorithm* (see Schölkopf et al. (1998); Schölkopf and Smola (2002)), that is, one that does not require an explicit representation of the features, but can work instead using only a *kernel matrix*, a symmetric square matrix K with each element K_{ij} equal to some suitable measure of similarity between data point i and data point j. This has two advantages. The first is that the time and memory requirements for computation depend more on the number of data points than on the number of features—a desirable property in a trial-based BCI setting since recording a few hundred trials is relatively time-consuming, whereas each trial may be described by a relatively large number of features. The second advantage is that one may use nonlinear similarity measures to construct K, which is equivalent to performing linear classification on data points that have been mapped into a higher-dimensional feature space and which can consequently yield a more powerful classifier, *without* the requirement that the feature-space mapping be known explicitly (the so-called kernel trick). However, it has generally been observed in BCI classification applications (e.g., see Müller et al. (2003a)) that, given a well-chosen sequence of preprocessing steps (an explicit feature mapping), a further implicit mapping is usually unnecessary: thus, a linear classifier, in which K_{ij} is equal to the dot product between the feature representations of data points i and j, performs about as well as any nonlinear classifier one might attempt. This is often the case in situations in which the number of data points is low, and indeed we find it to be the case in the current application.

Thus, we use a linear SVM for the current study, and this has the advantage of interpretability: The decision boundary is a hyperplane, so its orientation may be described by its normal vector $\mathbf{w}$, which is directly interpretable in the explicitly chosen feature space (e.g., in the space of multichannel amplitude spectra). This vector gives us a measure of the relative importance of our features[3] and as such is useful in feature selection. In figure 14.1, where we have just two features, the horizontal component of the hyperplane normal vector $\mathbf{w}$ is larger than the vertical, which tells us what we can already see from the layout of the points, namely that horizontal position (feature one) is more important than vertical position (feature two) in separating the two classes. Some features may be entirely irrelevant to classification (so the corresponding element of **w** should be close to 0). Although the SVM can be formulated as a kernel algorithm and thus does not require explicit feature representation, the number of relevant features relative to the number of irrelevant features is still critical: We would prefer each dot product K_{ij} to be dominated by the sum of the products of relevant features, rather than this information being swamped by the products of irrelevant (noise) features. When one has a large number of features, good feature selection can make a large difference to classification performance.

See Burges (1998), Müller et al. (2001), and Schölkopf and Smola (2002) for a more comprehensive introduction to SVMs.

14.6.2 Receiver Operating Characteristic Curves and the AUC Measure

A receiver operating characteristic (ROC) curve is a plot of a one-dimensional classifier's "hit" rate (e.g., probability of the correct identification of a finger-movement trial) against its "false alarm" rate (e.g., probability of misidentification of a tongue trial as a finger trial). As one varies the threshold of the classifier, one moves along a curve in this two-dimensional space (a lower threshold for classifying trials as finger trials results in more "hits," but also more "false alarms"). The area under the curve (AUC) is a very informative statistic for the evaluation of performance of classification and ranking algorithms, as well as for the analysis of the usefulness of features. For example, we might order all our data points according to their value on a particular single feature axis (say, the amount of bandpower in a band centerd on 10 Hz, measured by a particular sensor at a particular time after the start of the trial) and compute the AUC score of this ordering. An AUC of 1 indicates perfect separability: All the finger trials lie above the highest of the tongue trials on this axis. An AUC of 0 also indicates perfect separability: All the finger trials lie below the lowest of the tongue trials. Thus, a value close to 0 or 1 is desirable,[4] whereas a value of 0.5 would indicate that the chosen feature axis is entirely uninformative for the purposes of separating the two classes.

ROC analysis gives rise to many attractive statistical results (for details and references see Flach (2004)). One attractive property of the AUC score as a measure of feature usefulness is that it is a bounded scale, on which the three values 0, 0.5, and 1 have very clear intuitive interpretations. Another is that it is entirely insensitive to monotonic transformations of the feature axis, relying only on the ordering of the points, and is thus free of any parametric assumptions about the shapes of the class distributions.

Note, however, that we use AUC scores to evaluate features in isolation from each other, which may not give the full picture: It is easy to construct situations in which two highly correlated features each have AUC scores close to 0.5, but in which the sum of the two features separates classes perfectly. Therefore, analysis of individual feature scores should go hand-in-hand with the examination of optimal directions of separation in feature space, by examining the weight vector of a suitably trained classifier. For the current datasets, we find that the two views are very similar, so we plot only the AUC picture.

14.7   Preprocessing and Classification

Starting 500 ms after offset of the visual task cue, we extract a window of length 2 s. For each trial and each sensor, the resulting timeseries is low-pass-filtered by a zero-phase-distortion method with a smooth falloff between 45 and 50 Hz, downsampled at 100 Hz, and then linearly detrended.

Due to the downsampling, signal components at frequencies higher than 50 Hz are no longer represented in the data. This is no great loss in EEG, since EEG cannot in general be expected to yield much useful information at frequencies higher than this, but it might have been possible to obtain good higher-frequency information in ECoG and MEG. However, based on an examination of the AUC scores of individual frequency features in each subject's data set, and also of the weight vector of a linear classifier trained on the data, we did not find any indication that this information helped in separating classes in the current task. Figure 14.2 shows typical patterns of AUC scores *before* filtering and downsampling (one representative subject for each of the three sensor types). For all frequencies, there is some "noise" in the AUC values—depending on the number of trials available, values between about 0.4 and 0.6 will be obtained by chance. For all three sensor types, it is only below about 40–50 Hz that we see meaningful patterns in which AUC scores differ significantly from 0.5. While the AUC representation considers each feature only in isolation, an almost identical pattern was observed (for all subjects) in the weights of the linear classifier, which takes linear combinations of features into account.

Therefore, our analysis is restricted to a comparison of the extent to which class-relevant information in the 0–50 Hz range can be recovered using the different recording techniques. It would certainly be interesting to examine the potential use of higher-frequency information—perhaps class-relevant nonlinear combinations of high-frequency features might be discovered using nonlinear classification techniques, or perhaps the higher frequencies might be useful for classification when represented in different ways, other than as amplitude spectra. However, such a study is likely to require considerably larger datasets for individual subjects than those we currently have available, and is beyond the scope of this chapter.

For each number of trials n from 25, in steps of 25, up to the maximum available, we attempt to classify the first n trials performed by the subject. Classification performance is assessed using tenfold cross-validation, conducted twice with different random seeds. On each of these twenty folds, only the training fold (roughly 90 percent of the n trials) is used for training and for feature and model selection—the label information from the remaining $n/10$ trials is used only to compute a final test accuracy estimate for the fold. Where necessary, model and feature selection was performed by a second level of tenfold cross-validation, *within* the training fold of the outer cross-validation, as described by Müller et al. (2004a), Lal et al. (2005a), and Lal et al. (2005b). Final performance is estimated by averaging the proportion of correctly classified test trials across the twenty outer folds.

Before classification, a spatial filter is computed (see section 14.7.1) and applied to both the training and test trials. Then, amplitude spectra are computed by the short-time Fourier transform (STFT) method of Welch (1967): A time series is split into five segments

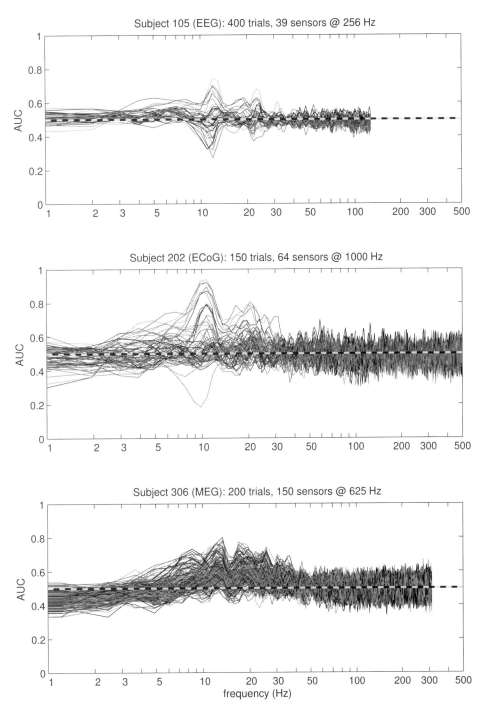

Figure 14.2   AUC scores for multichannel amplitude spectra: representative examples from EEG, ECoG, and MEG. Each curve shows the AUC scores corresponding to the frequency-domain features from one of the available sensor outputs.

each overlapping the next by 50 percent, a temporal Hanning window is applied to each, and the absolute values of the discrete Fourier transforms of the five windowed segments are averaged. For each trial, this gives us a vector of 65 values per sensor (or rather, per spatially filtered linear combination of sensors, which we will call a "channel") as inputs to the classifier.

We use a linear support vector machine as the classifier. First, the regularization parameter is optimized using tenfold cross-validation within the training trial subset. Then we employ the technique of recursive channel elimination (RCE) first described by Lal et al. (2004). This is a variant of recursive feature elimination (RFE), an embedded feature-selection method proposed by Guyon et al. (2002) in which an SVM is trained, its resulting weight vector is examined, and the subset of features with the lowest sum squared weight is eliminated (the features being grouped, in our case, into subsets corresponding to channels). Then the procedure is repeated, retraining and re-eliminating for ever-decreasing numbers of features. We run RCE once on the complete training subset, the reverse order of elimination giving us a rank order of channel importance. Then we perform tenfold cross-validated RCE within the training subset, testing every trained SVM on the inner test fold to obtain an estimate of performance as a function of the number of features. Based on the rank order and the error estimates, we reduce the number of channels: We choose the minimum number of channels for which the estimated error is within two standard errors of the minimum (across all numbers of features). This procedure is described in more detail in Lal et al. (2005b), and embedded feature selection methods are treated in more depth by Lal et al. (in press). Finally, the regularization parameter is reoptimized on the dataset after channel rejection and the classifier is ready to be trained on the training subset of the outer fold in order to make predictions on the test subset.

We summarize the procedure in algorithm 14.1.

14.7.1 Spatial Filtering

A spatial filter is a vector of weights specifying a linear combination of sensor outputs. We can represent our signals as an s-by-t matrix X, consisting of s time series, each of length t, recorded from s different sensors. Spatial filtering amounts to a premultiplication $X' = WX$, where W is an r-by-s matrix consisting of r different spatial filters. If an appropriate spatial filter is applied before any nonlinear processing occurs (such as the nonlinear step of taking the absolute values of a Fourier transform to obtain an amplitude spectrum), then classification performance on the resulting features will often improve. This is illustrated in figure 14.3, where the AUC scores of the amplitude spectra from one subject in the EEG experiment are considerably better on both training and test folds if the correct spatial filters have been applied. We compare three spatial filtering conditions: no spatial filtering (where W is effectively the identity matrix, so we operate on the amplitude spectra of the raw sensor outputs), independent components analysis (described in section 14.7.1.1) and common spatial pattern filtering (described in section 14.7.1.2).

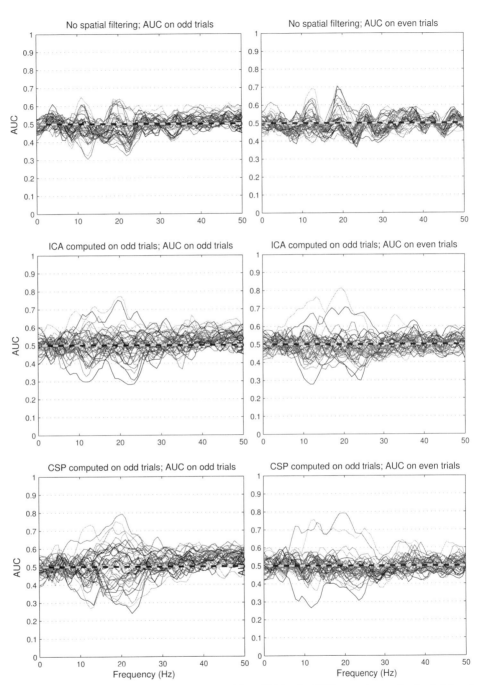

Figure 14.3 Effects of spatial filtering on subject 104 in the EEG experiment. In the left-hand column, we see AUC scores for the amplitude spectra of the odd-numbered trials (a total of 200), and on the right we see AUCs on the even-numbered trials (also 200). In the top row there is no spatial filtering, in the middle we have applied a square filter matrix W obtained by ICA (section 14.7.1.1) on the odd-numbered trials, and in the bottom row we have applied a square W obtained by CSP (section 14.7.1.2) on the odd-numbered trials.

Algorithm 14.1 Summary of error estimation procedure using nested cross-validation.

Require: preprocessed data of one subject
1: **for** ($n = 25$ to maximum available in steps of 25) **do**
2:      take first n trials performed by the subject
3:      **for** (outer fold $= 1$ to 20) **do**
4:          split data: 90% training set, 10% test set
5:          with training set do:
6:              compute spatial filter W
7:              10-fold inner CV: train SVMs to find regularization parameter C
8:              10-fold inner CV: RCE to estimate error as a function of number of channels
9:              RCE on whole training set to obtain channel rank order
10:              reduce number of channels
11:              10-fold inner CV: train SVMs to find regularization parameter C
12:              train SVM S using best C
13:          with test set do:
14:              apply spatial filter W
15:              reject unwanted channels
16:              test S on test set
17:              save error
18:      **end for**
19: **end for**
Output: estimated generalization error (mean and standard error across outer folds)

14.7.1.1 Independent Component Analysis (ICA)

Concatenating the n available trials to form s long time series, we then compute a (usually square) separating matrix W that maximizes the independence of the r outputs. This technique is popular in the analysis of EEG signals because it is an effective means of linear blind source separation, in which differently weighted linear mixtures of the signals of interest ("sources") are measured, and must be "demixed" to estimate the sources themselves: Since EEG electrodes measure the activity of cortical sources through several layers of bone and tissue, the signals are spatially quite "blurred" and the electrodes measure highly correlated (roughly linear) mixtures of the signals of interest. To find a suitable W, we use an ICA algorithm based on the Infomax criterion (as implemented in EEGLAB—see Delorme and Makeig (2004)), which we find to be comparable to most other available first-order ICA algorithms in terms of resulting classification performance, while at the same time having the advantage of supplying more consistent spatial filters than many others. Note that, due to the large amount of computation required in the current study, we compute W based on all n trials rather than performing a separate ICA for each outer training/test fold. Target label information is not used by ICA, so there is no overfitting as such, but it could potentially be argued that the setting has become unrealistically "semisupervised" since the (computationally expensive) algorithm training cannot start until the novel input to be classified has been measured. However, by performing a smaller set of pilot experiments (two values of n for each subject, and only ten outer folds instead of twenty) in which ICA *was* recomputed on each outer fold, we were able to verify that this did not lead to any appreciable difference in performance, either for individual subjects or on average.

14.7.1.2   Common Spatial Pattern (CSP) Analysis

This technique (due to Koles et al. (1990)) and related algorithms (Wang et al. (1999); Dornhege et al. (2003a); Lemm et al. (2005); Dornhege et al. (2004b)) are supervised methods for computing spatial filters whose outputs have maximal between-class differences in variance. For this to be useful, the input to the algorithm must be represented in such a way that class-dependent changes in the signal are reflected in a change in signal variance: For event-related desynchronization in motor imagery, this can be achieved by applying a zero-phase-distortion bandpass filter that captures the part of the spectrum in which sensorimotor rhythms are expressed. The variance of the filtered signal, which has zero mean, is a measure of amplitude in the chosen band. Here we use a bandpass filter between 7 and 30 Hz (we generally found that this broad band performed approximately as well as any specifically chosen narrow band). Often, the variances of the spatially filtered channels themselves (forming a feature vector $\mathbf{v} = [v_1 \ldots v_r]$) are used as features for classification. This makes sense given that the algorithm aims specifically to maximize class differences in this statistic, and it is a convenient way of reducing the dimensionality of the classification problem. In section 14.8.3, we adopt this approach, discarding the subsequent channel selection stage to save processing time. However, we were able to obtain slightly better performance on the EEG datasets if we computed CSP spatial filters on the temporally filtered timeseries, applied these the whole (temporally *unfiltered*) timeseries, computed Welch spectra and classified them as described above. Therefore, we report the latter results in section 14.8.1.

Since CSP uses label information, it *must* be performed once for each outer training/test fold, using the training subset only. The drawback to CSP is its tendency to overfit, as illustrated in figure 14.4 where we have taken 200 trials from one subject in the 39-channel EEG experiment (upper panel), and 200 trials from the same subject in the 150-channel MEG experiment (lower panel). In each case we have trained the CSP algorithm on half of the available data, and applied the resulting spatial filters W to the other half. We retain the maximum number of spatial patterns, $r = s$, and plot the AUC scores of the features $v_1 \ldots v_r$, lighter bars denoting separation of the training trials and darker bars denoting separation of the test trials. In the lower panel we see that, when the algorithm is given a larger number of channels to work with, it finds many linear combinations of channels whose amplitude in the 7–30 Hz band separates the classes nearly perfectly (AUC scores close to 0 or 1). However, the large majority of these patterns tells us nothing about the test trials—only the last two spatial patterns separate the test trials well. In the EEG context, we see that overfitting occurs, but to a lesser extent.[5]

The lines of crosses indicate the eigenvalues returned by the CSP algorithm's diagonalization of the whitened class covariance matrix (for an accessible account of the algorithm details, see Müller-Gerking et al. (1999); Lemm et al. (2005)). These are in the range $[0, 1]$ and are an indicator of the amount of between-class difference in variance that each spatial pattern is able to account for. Values close to 0.5 indicate the smallest differences and val-

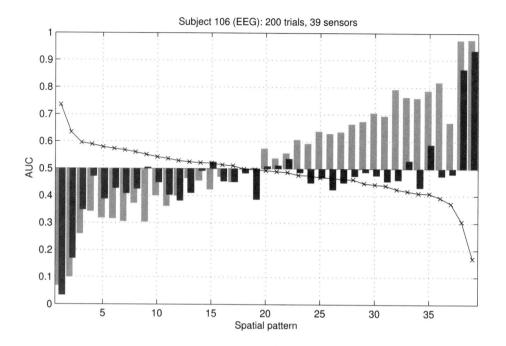

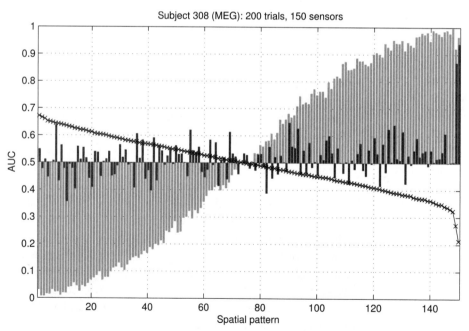

Figure 14.4　Large differences in performance of the CSP algorithm on training data (grey bars) and test data (black bars), as indicated by an AUC measure of class separability computed separately for the projected variance on each spatial pattern. This overfitting effect is extremely pronounced in 150-channel MEG (lower panel), and less so in 39-channel EEG (upper panel). Crosses show the eigenvalues corresponding to each spatial pattern in the CSP decomposition.

ues close to 0 or 1 denote the largest differences and therefore potentially the most useful
spatial patterns. The eigenvalues tell us something related, but not identical, to the AUC
scores. In the end, we are interested in the classifiability of single trials in as-yet-unseen
data. The eigenvalues are only an indirect measure of single-trial classifiability, since they
tell us about the fractions of variance accounted for across many trials. Variance is not
a robust measure, so a large eigenvalue *could* arise from very high SMR-modulation in
just a small minority of the trials, with the majority of the trials being effectively inseparable according to the spatial pattern in question. AUC scores, on the other hand, are a
direct measure of trial separability according to individual features. Hence, AUC scores on
the data that the CSP algorithm has not seen (black bars in figure 14.4) are our standard
for evaluating the generalization performance of each spatial pattern. By contrast, AUC
scores computed from the training trials alone (grey bars) show a grossly inflated estimate
of performance, which illustrates the overfitting effect. The eigenvalues show a somewhat
intermediate picture. On one hand, they are computed only on the training trials, and accordingly their magnitude is better predicted by looking at the AUC on training trials than
at the AUC on test trials. On the other hand, they also contain information that, in the current examples, allows us to identify which components are really useful according to our
standard (tallest black bars). First, by sorting the spatial patterns by eigenvalue, we have
correctly sorted the useful components to the extreme ends of the plot. Second, the useful
patterns are identifiable by an acceleration in the eigenvalue spectrum toward the ends (c.f.
Wang et al. (1999)).

In practice, the eigenvalues are a fairly good and often-used predictor of the generalization performance of each spatial pattern. Some such predictor is necessary, since CSP's
overfitting will often lead to poor generalization performance. Standard remedies for this
employ a feature selection stage after CSP, with the aim of retaining only those spatial patterns that are likely to be useful. Selection strategies may vary: One common approach is
to take only the first k in patterns, in the order of preference indicated by the eigenvalues,
number k being either fixed or determined by cross-validation of the CSP algorithm within
the training set. The results reported in section 14.8.1 employ this strategy with k fixed at
five, which we found to produce results roughly as good as a cross-validation strategy.[6]

In section 14.8.3, we employ an additional tactic: Since the degree of overfitting is
determined largely by the number of free parameters in the optimization, and the algorithm
finds one scaling parameter per sensor in each spatial pattern, it makes sense to attempt to
reduce the number of sensors used as input to the CSP algorithm. We do this using a
preliminary step in which Welch spectra of the raw sensor outputs are computed, an SVM
is trained (cross-validating to find the best regularization parameter), and the weight vector
is used to provide a measure of relative channel importance, as in RCE. Going back to
the time-domain representation, the top 10, 25, 39, and (in ECoG and MEG) 55 sensors
found by this method were then passed into CSP. Spatial patterns were then chosen by
a cross-validation method: CSP was run on each of 10 inner training folds and variances
$v_1 \ldots v_r$ were computed on the corresponding test fold and saved. At the end of cross
validation, each trial then had a new representation $\mathbf{v}$, and AUC scores corresponding to
each of these features could be computed on the whole outer training fold, and these are
useful for selection since they generally correlate well with the AUC scores on unseen

data. The significance of the AUC values was expressed in terms of the standard deviation expected from random orderings of a data set of the same size. Eigenvalue positions with AUC scores more than two standard deviations away from 0.5 were retained in the outer CSP.

14.8   Results

14.8.1   Performance of Spatial Filters Using All Available Sensors

In figure 14.5, classification accuracy is plotted as a function of n for each subject, along with average performance in each of the three experiments (EEG, ECoG, and MEG). We plot the time-course of the *overall* effectiveness of the experimental setup, subject, and classifier taken all together: Our curves are obtained by computing performance on the first 25 trials performed by the subject, then recomputing based on the first 50 trials, and so on (instead of on a random 25 trials, then a random 50 trials). As a result, the observed changes in performance with increasing n reflect not only the effect of the amount of input on classifier performance, but also changes in the subjects' performance, whether due to practice, fatigue, or transient random influences.

Note that, for two out of eight subjects in the EEG condition (subjects 101 and 102), and 1 out of 10 in MEG (subject 303), we were never able to classify at significantly better than chance level. These subjects were omitted from the averaging process and from the further analysis of section 14.8.3. The strength of sensorimotor rhythms and the degree to which their modulation with imagined movement is measurable varies from person to person. One must expect that some subjects will be unable to use a motor imagery-based BCI at all, and that performance of the remainder will vary between individuals. Given the necessarily small size of our three subject groups, we are unable to draw strong conclusions as to the effect of recording technology on absolute performance level, to say, for example, whether MEG is a significantly better option than EEG. Another effect of between-subject variation is that, though we find certain individual subjects in all three groups who are able to attain high performance levels (say, > 90%), average performance is poor. However, it should be borne in mind that, with one exception,[7] the subjects had never taken part in a motor imagery BCI experiment before, and that performance is therefore based on a maximum of three hours' experience with the paradigm, and without feedback.

In the EEG experiment, both ICA (grey asterisks) and CSP (open diamonds) allow very large improvements in performance relative to the condition in which no spatial filtering was used (filled circles). This effect is clear in the averaged data as well as in the individual subject plots. In ECoG, the difference between ICA and no spatial filtering is slight, although ICA is at least as good as no spatial filtering for all four subjects; CSP is consistently a little worse than both. In MEG, there is no consistent benefit or disadvantage to ICA over the raw sensor outputs, and again CSP is worse, this time by a larger margin.

The failure of CSP in ECoG and MEG is likely to be related to the overfitting effect already discussed. This is clearest for subject 310 when 200 trials are used: Although spatial filters exist (and have been found by ICA) that can improve classification performance,

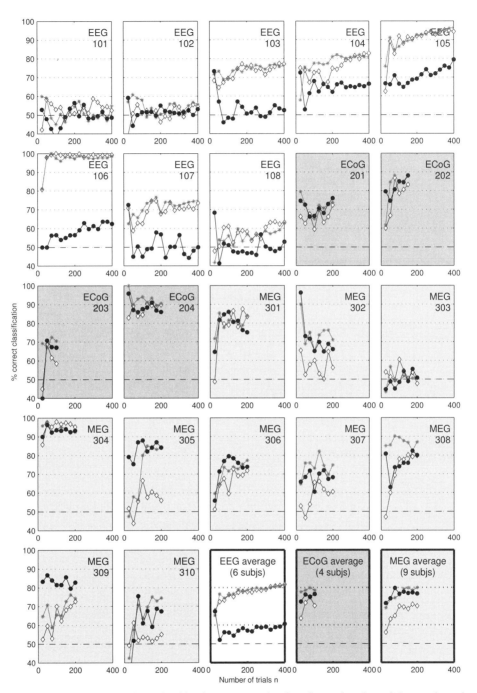

Figure 14.5   For each subject, classification accuracy is plotted as a function of the number of trials performed and the spatial filtering method employed: Filled circles denote no spatial filtering, asterisks denote ICA, and open diamonds denote CSP. The last three plots show averages for the EEG, ECoG, and MEG experiments, respectively, across all subjects for whom classification had been possible at all.

CSP fails to find any patterns that help to classify the data because useless (overfitted) spatial patterns dominate the decomposition of the class covariance matrices.

Overall, maximum performance can be achieved using about 200 trials in EEG and 75–100 trials in MEG. For ECoG, though it is harder to draw strong conclusions due to the smaller number of subjects and trials, it generally appears that the curves are even flatter: The best results already can be obtained with only 25–50 trials.

One curious feature of the results is the strikingly good performance without spatial filtering for some subjects (103, 104, 107, 108, 302, and 308) when only the first 25 trials are tested, quickly dropping to much poorer performance when more trials are taken. A possible explanation for this is the test trials on each outer fold were drawn uniformly and randomly from the first n trials—when n is very small, this means that the test trials were performed, on average, closer in time to the training trials than when n is larger. If the subjects' signals exhibit properties that are nonstationary over time, this may lead to an advantage when the training and test trials are closer together. Such effects merit a more in-depth analysis, which is beyond the scope of this report.

14.8.2 Topographic Interpretation of Results

Figure 14.6 shows topographic maps of the features selected by our analysis for seven of our subjects. Sensor ranking scores were obtained by recursive channel elimination on data that had not been spatially filtered; each of the twenty outer training/test folds of the analysis returned a channel ranking, and these ranks were averaged across folds and then divided by their standard deviation across folds. The result indicates which channels were ranked highly most consistently (darker colors indicating channels ranked as more influential). We also plot spatially interpolated projected amplitudes[8] for the top two independent components (selected by recursive channel elimination in the first outer training/test fold) and the first two spatial patterns (indicated by the best two eigenvalues in the first outer fold).

In general, we see that ICA and CSP recover very similar patterns of activation that are consistent with the modulation of activity in motor and premotor cortical areas. In EEG, both algorithms recover patterns centerd on C4/CP4 in the right hemisphere (where we would expect modulation associated with imagined left hand movement) and C3/CP3 in the left (imagined right hand movement). In MEG, we see patterns consistent with parietal-central and central-frontal dipoles in the right hemisphere where we would expect to see modulation associated with imagined left hand movement. Subject 308 appears to use sources in both hemispheres. In the ECoG, the top two independent components and the top spatial pattern are all highly localized, activation in each case being focused on just three or fewer electrodes located above the motor cortex.

For subjects 202, 304, and 306, the second spatial pattern shows a more complicated topography. Given that CSP generally performs less well than ICA for these subjects, we may suspect that this is a reflection of overfitting. Presented with a large number of sensors, the algorithm can account for class differences in signal variance by combining sensors in spatial configurations that are more complicated than necessary, which in turn results in poorer generalization performance.

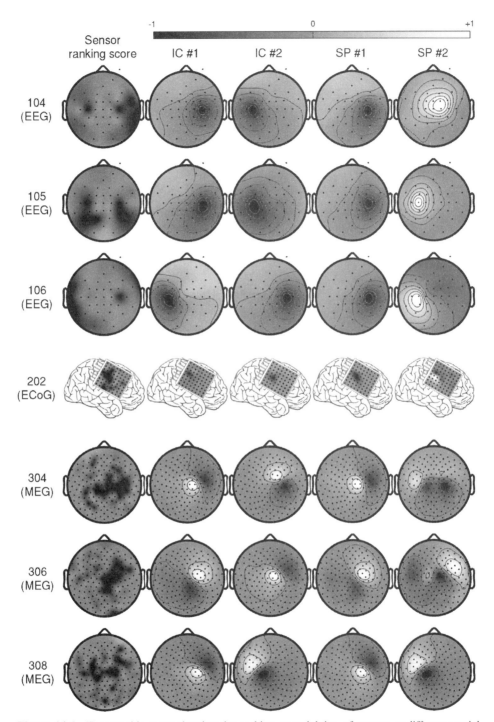

Figure 14.6 Topographic maps showing the ranking or weighting of sensors at different spatial locations for three EEG subjects, one ECoG subject, and three MEG subjects. Sensor ranking scores (first column) are obtained by recursive channel elimination on the data when no spatial filtering is used. The top two independent components (columns 2–3) are selected by recursive channel elimination after independent component analysis. The top two spatial patterns (columns 4–5) are selected using the eigenvalues returned by the CSP algorithm. Topographic maps are scaled from -1 (black) through 0 (grey) to 1 (white) according to the maximum absolute value in each map.

Finally, we note that the ranking scores of the raw sensors, while presenting a somewhat less tidy picture, generally show a similar pattern of sensor importance to that indicated by the ICA and CSP maps (note that the ranking score patterns may reflect information from influential sources beyond just the first two components we have shown). The sensors most consistently ranked highly are to be found in lateralized central and precentral regions, bilaterally for the EEG experiment and for subject 308, and with a right-hemisphere bias for the others. For further examination of the performance of recursive channel elimination in the identification of relevant source locations, see Lal et al. (2004, 2005a,b).

14.8.3   Effect of Sensor Subsetting

In figure 14.7 we show average classification accuracy at $n = 25, 50, 100$, and 200 (respectively in the four rows from top to bottom) for EEG, ECoG, and MEG (left to right). Classification performance of CSP is shown as a function of the number of sensors the algorithm is permitted to work with ("more" denoting the maximum available: 64, 74, or 84 in ECoG, and 150 in MEG).

First we note that, in our EEG data, performance is better the more sensors are used, up to the maximum of 39 available in the current study. For ECoG and MEG, this trend is reversed when the number of available trials is small. This is in line with our intuition about overfitting: We suffer when attempting to recombine too many channels based on a small number of data points. For $n = 25$, $s = 10$ is the best number of sensors to choose, and CSP performance may then equal (and even exceed, although the difference is not significant) the best classification previously possible with ICA (in ECoG) or with the raw sensors outputs (in MEG). As the number of trials n increases to 50 and beyond, the peak shifts to the left (it is useful to have more sensors available as the number of trials increases) and the slope becomes shallower as the difference between CSP and the raw sensors diminishes (overfitting becomes less of an issue).

14.9   Summary

We have compared the classifiability of signals obtained by EEG, ECoG, and MEG in a binary, synchronous motor imagery-based brain-computer interface. We held the time interval, and (after failing to find any information useful for the classification in frequencies above 50 Hz) also the sampling frequency constant across sensor types, and classified event-related desynchronization effects in the signals' amplitude spectra using regularized support vector machines and automatic feature selection.

We varied the number of trials used in order to see how quickly we might reach maximum classification performance with our unpracticed subjects. Maximum performance, averaged across subjects, was roughly equal across sensor types at around 80 percent, although subject groups were small and between-subject variation was large, so we attach no particular weight to this observation. Maximum performance was attained after about 200 trials in EEG, 75–100 trials in MEG, and 25–50 trials in ECoG.

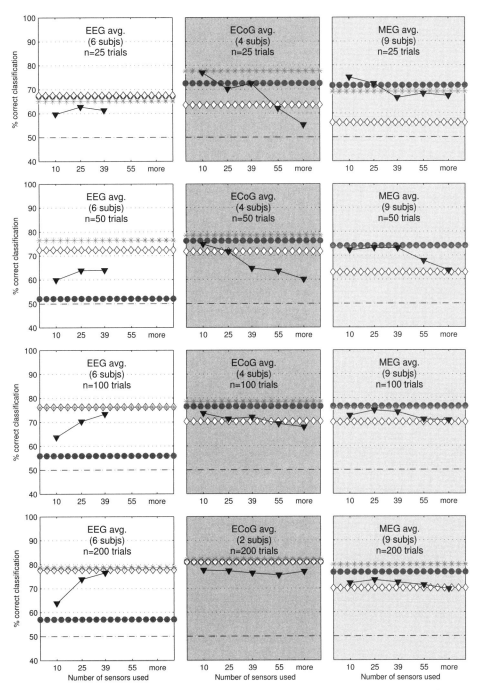

Figure 14.7   Filled triangles indicate average classification accuracy of the CSP algorithm for each sensor type (EEG, ECoG, and MEG, respectively, in the three columns from left to right), as a function of the number of sensors used as input to the algorithm, and the number of trials (25, 50, 100, and 200, respectively, in the four rows from top to bottom). For comparison, horizontal chains of symbols denote the average performance levels reported in the previous analysis of figure 14.5: filled circles for no spatial filtering, asterisks for ICA, and open diamonds for CSP with a fixed number of patterns $k = 5$.

Performance was affected by spatial filtering strategy in a way that depended on the recording hardware. For EEG, where signals are highly spatially blurred, spatial filtering is crucial; large gains in classification accuracy were possible using either first-order independent component analysis or the common spatial pattern algorithm, the performance of these two approaches being roughly equal. For ECoG and MEG, as one might expect from systems that experience less cross-talk between channels, spatial filtering was less critical; the MEG signals were the "cleanest" in this regard, in that there was no appreciable difference in performance between classification of the raw sensor outputs and classification of any of the linear combinations of sensors we attempted. First-order spatial filtering would appear to be become largely redundant for the detection of event-related desynchronization as the volume conduction problem diminishes (down to the level at which it is still present in ECoG and MEG).

Across all three conditions, ICA was the best (or roughly equal to best) spatial filtering strategy. CSP suffered badly from overfitting in the ECoG and MEG conditions when large numbers of sensors (> 40) were used, resulting in poor generalization performance. This could be remedied by sparsification of the spatial filters, where a subset of the sensors was selected and the rest discarded—a strategy that was particularly effective when the number of trials was very small, but which never resulted in a significant overall win for optimized spatial filters over raw sensor outputs. We did not find a convincing advantage, with any of the three sensor types, of supervised optimization of the spatial filters over blind source separation.

Acknowledgments

We would like to thank Hubert Preissl, Jürgen Mellinger, Martin Bogdan, Wolfgang Rosenstiel, and Jason Weston for their help with this work, as well as the two anonymous reviewers whose careful reading of the chapter and helpful comments enabled us to make significant improvements to the manuscript.

The authors gratefully acknowledge the financial support of the *Max-Planck-Gesellschaft*, the *Deutsche Forschungsgemeinschaft* (SFB550/B5 and RO1030/12), the European Community IST Programme (IST-2002-506778 under the PASCAL Network of Excellence), and the *Studienstiftung des deutschen Volkes* (grant awarded to T. N. L.).

Notes

E-mail for correspondence: jez@tuebingen.mpg.de

(1)   Visual cues: a small left- or right-pointing arrow, near the center of the screen.

(2)   Visual cues: small pictures of either a hand with little finger extended or of Einstein sticking his tongue out.

(3)   Many authors use linear discriminant analysis for this purpose—we choose to use weight vector from the SVM itself, appropriately regularized, since in theory the

SVM's good performance relies less on parametric assumptions about the distribution of data points, and in practice this results in a better track record as a classifier.

(4)   In most classical formulations, AUC scores are rectified about 0.5, there being no sense in reporting that a classifier performs "worse than chance" with a score lower than 0.5. However, since here it is entirely arbitrary to designate a "hit" as the correct detection of a finger trial rather than a tongue trial, a value of 0 can be considered just as good as a value of 1, and retaining the unrectified score in the range $[0, 1]$ aids us in interpreting the role of a given feature.

(5)   The overfitting effect in EEG can also be seen by comparing the left and right panels in the bottom row of figure 14.3, paying particular attention to the center of the desired 7–30 Hz band.

(6)   One may also attempt to perform channel selection after CSP *without* using the eigenvalues or cross-validating the CSP algorithm itself, but this is hampered by the fact that the training data have been transformed by an algorithm that overfits on them: Cross-validation error rates in subsequent model and feature selection tend to be uninformatively close to 0, and classifiers end up underregularized. To investigate a possible workaround for this, we tried splitting each training set into two partitions: one to be used as input to CSP to obtain spatial filters W, and the other to be transformed by W and then used in channel selection and classifier training as described above. We experimented with a 25:75 percent partition, as well as 50:50 and 75:25, of which 50:50 was found to be the best for nearly all values of n. However, the resulting performance was worse than in the simpler strategy of performing CSP on the whole training set and taking the best five eigenvalues—the reduction in the number of trials available for CSP exacerbates the overfitting problem to an extent that is not balanced by the improvement in feature and model selection. The results of the partition experiments are not shown.

(7)   The exception is subject 308 in the MEG condition, who had previously taken part in the EEG condition—106 and 308 are the same person.

(8)   Each map is spline-interpolated from a single column of the mixing matrix W^{-1}, the inverse of the spatial filter matrix. The column corresponding to a given source tells us the measured amplitude of that source as a function of sensor location.

15 Classification of Time-Embedded EEG Using Short-Time Principal Component Analysis

Charles W. Anderson and James N. Knight
Department of Computer Science
Colorado State University
Fort Collins, CO 80523

Michael J. Kirby
Department of Mathematics
Colorado State University
Fort Collins, CO 80523

Douglas R. Hundley
Department of Mathematics
Whitman College
Walla Walla, WA 99362

15.1 Abstract

Principal component analysis (PCA) is often used to project high-dimensional signals to lower dimensional subspaces defined by basis vectors that maximize the variance of the projected signals. The projected values can be used as features for classification problems. Data containing variations of relatively short duration and small magnitude, such as those seen in EEG signals, may not be captured by PCA when applied to time series of long duration. Instead, PCA can be applied independently to short segments of data and the basis vectors themselves can be used as features for classification. Here this is called the short-time principal component analysis (STPCA). In addition, the time-embedding of EEG samples is investigated prior to STPCA, resulting in a representation that captures EEG variations in space and time. The resulting features of the analysis are then classified via a standard linear discriminant analysis (LDA). Results are shown for two datasets of EEG, one recorded from subjects performing five mental tasks, and one from the third BCI Competition recorded from subjects performing one mental task and two imagined movement tasks.

15.2   Introduction

Principal component analysis (PCA) is commonly used to project data samples to a lower-dimensional subspace that maximizes the variance of the projected data. For many datasets, PCA is also used to isolate the information in the data into meaningful components, such as "eigenfaces" (Turk and Pentland (1991)) and "eigenlips" (Kirby et al. (1993)) in applications involving analysis of face images.

For classification problems, PCA is usually applied to a collection of samples from all classes with the hope that the projection of new samples onto the PCA basis form components whose amplitudes are related to the class. This approach may fail to capture variations that appear in the data over short time intervals. Such variations contribute little to the overall variance of the data, but may be critical in classifying samples into the correct classes.

Features of short duration can be captured by applying PCA to short time windows of data. This results in multiple bases, one for each window. To project data samples using these multiple bases, they must somehow be combined into a single basis. An alternative approach is used here. Rather than projecting the data to form features on which classification is performed, the bases themselves are taken as the features. Our hypothesis is that the directions of significant variation within each window will capture the information needed to correctly classify the data in the window. We refer to this method as short-time PCA, or STPCA.

A unique aspect of the representations studied here is that the EEG samples are augmented by samples delayed in time, forming a time-embedded representation described in the next section and in Kirby and Anderson (2003). With this modification, PCA becomes a tool for simultaneously analyzing spatial and temporal aspects of the data, where the resulting features are classified using linear discriminant analysis (LDA). A related approach using common spatial patterns was recently described in Lemm et al. (2005).

Results are shown for classifying six-channel EEG recorded from subjects performing five mental tasks. For this dataset, classification performance with other representations, including signal fraction analysis (SFA) (Kirby and Anderson (2003)), is shown to be considerably lower than in the short-term PCA analysis. This classification performance is better than the results we have achieved previously with the same data using more complex representations and classifiers (Garrett et al. (2003)), though recently we have achieved similar performance with a complex process that combines a clustering process with a decision tree classifier (Anderson et al. (2006)). The STPCA method is also applied to Data Set V from the BCI Competition III (BCI Competition III (2005)).

Section 15.3 defines the EEG representations studied here including the short-time PCA, the linear discriminant analysis (LDA) classifier, and the cross-validation procedure used for training and evaluating the representations and classifier. Section 15.4 describes the data used in our analysis, and section 15.5 presents the results of classification experiments that are discussed in section 15.6. Conclusions are stated in section 15.7.

15.3   Method

In this section, several EEG signal representations are defined including short-time PCA. Linear discriminant analysis and the cross-validation training procedures are also described.

15.3.1   EEG Signal Representations

Let $x_i(k)$ be the voltage sample at time index k from channel i. The $d+1$-dimensional time-embedded representation,

$$y_i(k) = (x_i(k), x_i(k+1), x_i(k+2), \ldots, x_i(k+d))$$

is created by combining samples at time k with d next samples for channel i (which we might say is a lag-d representation). These time-embedded samples for all n channels are concatenated into one column vector, $e(k) = (y_1(k), \ldots, y_n(k))^T$. So, for example, if we have a 6-channel recording and use a lag of 3, then $e(k)$ would have dimension 24 and would represent a space-time snapshot of the EEG dynamics. Combining these column vectors for all sample indices k results in a matrix X. For example, EEG in one trial for the five-task dataset was recorded for 10 s at 250 Hz resulting in $X = (e(1), \ldots, e(2500-d))$. The data for task t and trial r will be designated $X_d^{(t,r)}$.

In this chapter, we compare the following transformations of $X_d^{(t,r)}$ as feature representations with which data from different mental tasks are classified:

(1)   samples with no further transformations, $X_d^{(t,r)}$;
(2)   projections of time-embedded samples onto the PCA basis, $PV_d^{(t,r)}$;
(3)   projections onto the signal-to-noise maximizing SFA basis, $PS_d^{(t,r)}$;
(4)   the short-time PCA bases, $V_d^{(t,r)}$; and
(5)   the short-time SFA bases, $S_d^{(t,r)}$.

These transformations are performed by the following procedures.

Let the matrix L be formed by collecting all time-lagged samples,

$$L = \left[X_d^{(i,j)} \right]_{i=1:N_t, j=1:N_r}$$

where N_t is the number of tasks and N_r is the number of trials per task. If we have r channels, the columns of L will have dimension $r(d+1)$. Given lagged EEG data $X_d^{(t,r)}$, the features $PV_d^{(t,r)}$ are based on the projections of L onto the variance maximizing basis given by the eigenvectors of the covariance of the lagged EEG data. The eigenvectors V of the covariance of the lagged EEG data are found by the eigendecomposition $D = V^T LL^T V$, where V is an orthonormal basis for samples L and D is the diagonal matrix of eigenvalues. Before using V, the columns of V are ordered in decreasing order of their corresponding eigenvalues. L may be mean centered by subtracting from each sample (column) of L the mean of each component. The projections of lagged data for each trial are formed by $PV_d^{(t,r)} = V^T X_d^{(t,r)}$.

Similarly, given lagged EEG data $X_d^{(t,r)}$, the features $PS_d^{(t,r)}$ are based on the projections of L onto a signal-to-noise maximizing basis that is found by maximizing the ratio of projected signal to projected noise. To do so, a characterization of noise is required. Assumptions described by Hundley et al. (2002) lead to an estimation of noise covariance by the covariance of the difference between EEG samples at each electrode and the samples shifted in time by one interval (Knight (2003)). Let S be an operator that shifts all samples in a matrix by one time interval, so that the noise, N, of the signals in $X = (e(1), \ldots, e(2500-d))$ is given by $N = X - S(X)$ or $(e(2) - e(1), \ldots, e(2500-d) - e(2500 - d - 1))$. The desired basis is given by the solution to the generalized eigenvector problem $XX^T V = NN^T V D$. Before using V, the columns of V are ordered according to increasing order of their corresponding eigenvalues, and, as mentioned above, L may be mean centered by subtracting from each sample (column) of L the mean of each component. The projections of lagged data for each trial is formed by $PS_d^{(t,r)} = V^T X_d^{(t,r)}$. This representation is called signal fraction analysis, or SFA (Kirby and Anderson (2003)).

Representing signals from all trials by their projections onto the same basis may not capture variations that appear during short time intervals and that are not similar to other variations. One approach to capturing such short-term variations is to segment each trial into short, possibly overlapping, windows and to calculate new bases for each window. We construct windows of contiguous data from the time-lagged data so that $W_i = (e((i-1)h + 1), \ldots, e((i-1)h + s))$ are defined using s samples in time, each window shifted by h samples for $i = 1, \ldots, w$ where w is the number of windows. The samples in W_i may be mean centered by subtracting each sample from their mean. The variance-maximizing basis for each window is given by $D_i = V_i^T W_i W_i^T V_i$ and the sequence of these bases for one trial are collected into $\widetilde{V_d}^{(t,r)} = (V_1, \ldots, V_w)$. In addition, columns of V_i for which the first component is negative are multiplied by -1 to remove the variation in sign of basis vectors over multiple windows that results from the eigendecomposition algorithm. If we have r channels with lag d and we retain n basis vectors, then $V_d^{(t,r)}$ has dimension $r(d+1) \times n$, which we concatenate into a single "point" that has dimension $r(d+1)n$. This is the STPCA representation. We note for future reference that by construction, all STPCA points have the same norm, and so we are normalizing the data by putting them on the surface of a sphere of dimension $r(d+1)n$.

An example of a short-time PCA representation is shown in figure 15.1 for data from the first subject in the BCI Competition III, Data Set V (described in section 15.4), where we have a 32-channel signal preprocessed as described later in this section so that one window has 256 points, and three lags, and W_i has dimensions 96×256. PCA is performed on each window independently and the first four eigenvectors are concatenated into one column vector so that one STPCA "point" is a vector with $32 \cdot 3 \cdot 5 = 480$ dimensions. We note that a single data point is actually a summary of the variation in the space-time snapshots for a particular window.

In figure 15.1, the numerical values of each STPCA point are represented by greyscale patches. The data is sorted by task labels, which are plotted in the bottom graph. The greyscale display provides only a rough indication of patterns that might correlate with class; a reliable classification must take into account many of the components in each column. As described in section 15.5.2, approximately 62 percent of the windows from a second trial of test data are correctly classified using linear discriminant analysis.

Similarly, the signal-to-noise maximizing basis of a window, W_i, is given by $W_i W_i^T S_i = N_i N_i^T S_i D_i$ where $N_i = S(W_i)$. The sequence of these bases for one trial are collected into $\widetilde{S}_d^{(t,r)} = (S_1, \ldots, S_w)$, forming the short-time SFA representation.

As mentioned above, rather than using all basis vectors from each window for classification, a subset is selected from each. In the following experiments, all sequences of basis vectors are tested. A particular sequence is specified by the index of the first basis vector, f, and the number of basis vectors, m. Letting $C_{f,m}(V_i)$ be the selection operator that extracts the columns $f, \ldots, f+m-1$ from matrix V, the reduced data representations become $\tilde{V}_d^{(t,r)} = (C_{f,m}(V_1), \ldots, C_{f,m}(V_w))$ and $\tilde{S}_d^{(t,r)} = (C_{f,m}(S_1), \ldots, C_{f,m}(S_w))$. We first described these short-time representations and their use for mental-task EEG signals in Kirby and Anderson (2003) and Anderson and Kirby (2003).

15.3.2   Linear Discriminant Analysis

Linear discriminant analysis (LDA) is a simple probabilistic approach to classification in which the distribution of samples from each class are modeled by a normal distribution. The parameters for the distribution of each class are estimated, and are combined with Bayes' Rule to form discriminant functions that are linear in the features used to represent the data. LDA is summarized in this section; for a more detailed discussion, see Hastie et al. (2001).

The probability that the correct class is k given a data sample x can be defined using Bayes' Rule in terms of other probabilities by

$$P(C = k|x) = \frac{P(x|C = k)P(C = k)}{P(x)}.$$

The classification of a data sample x is given by $\mathrm{argmax}_k\, P(C = k|x)$ over all classes k. In this comparison, $P(x)$ may be removed and $P(C = k)$ may be removed as well if each class is equally likely a priori, which is assumed to be true for the experiments reported here. With these assumptions, $\mathrm{argmax}_k\, P(C = k|x) = \mathrm{argmax}_k\, P(x|C = k)$.

In LDA, the normal distributions, $P(x|C = k)$, for each class k are modeled using the same covariance matrix, Σ, and are defined as

$$P(x|C = k) = \frac{1}{(2\pi)^{\frac{p}{2}}|\Sigma|^{\frac{1}{2}}} e^{-\frac{1}{2}(x-\mu_k)^T \Sigma^{-1}(x-\mu_k)}.$$

Let C_k be the set of known samples from class k. The mean μ_k for each class and the common covariance matrix Σ is estimated by

$$\mu_k = \frac{1}{N_k} \sum_{x \in C_k} x$$

$$\Sigma = \frac{1}{N-K} \sum_{k=1}^{K} \sum_{x \in C_k} (x - \mu_k)^T (x - \mu_k)$$

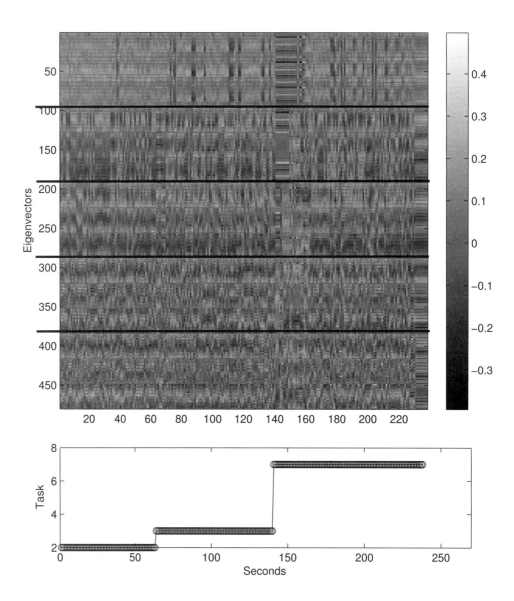

Figure 15.1   Example of STPCA representation. 32-channel EEG is augmented with three lagged samples, segmented into 256-point windows, and PCA performed on each window, where the first 5 eigenvectors are retained. Thus, each STPCA "point" is a vector with $32 \cdot 3 \cdot 5 = 480$ dimensions, and the values are displayed here as a column of greyscale patches. The bottom graph shows the corresponding class label indicating which mental task is being performed: 2 is imagined left hand movement, 3 is imagined right hand movement, and 7 is word generation.

where N_k is the number of samples in C_k, N is the total number of samples, and K is the number of classes.

To simplify the determination of the maximum $P(x|C=k)$, its logarithm is used. After removing common terms, the resulting comparison involves linear discriminant functions for each class of the form

$$\delta_k(x) = x^T \Sigma^{-1} \mu_k - \frac{1}{2} \mu_k^T \Sigma^{-1} \mu_k.$$

Defining weights $w_k = \Sigma^{-1} \mu_k$ and bias $b_k = -\frac{1}{2} \mu_k^T \Sigma^{-1} \mu_k$, each discriminant function simplifies to $\delta_k(x) = x^T w_k + b_k$.

Alternatively, with uniform priors, we can view LDA as using the Mahalanobis distance, where if we write the estimated covariance

$$\Sigma = R^T R,$$

then

$$(x - \mu_k)\Sigma^{-1}(x - \mu_k) = \|R^{-1}(x - \mu_k)\|^2,$$

so that if we transform the data by $\hat{x} = R^{-1}x$, then the class identification is made by finding the (transformed) class mean that is closest (for more details, see Duda et al. (2001), for example).

15.3.3   Cross-Validation Training Procedure

The five representations defined previously depend on the following parameters: the number of lags, d; the first basis vector, f; the number of basis vectors, m; and for the short-time representations, the window size s for fixed h of 32. The following cross-validation procedure was used to choose the best values of these parameters for each partitioning of the five trials into one test trial and four training trials.

For each set of parameter value to be tested, the training trials were randomly partitioned into 80 percent for constructing the classifier and 20 percent for evaluating it. This partitioning, construction, and evaluation process was repeated five times and the average performance in terms of percent of validation samples correctly classified was recorded. Once all parameter sets were tested, the parameter set resulting in the best validation performance was used to construct a new classifier using all the data in all training trials. This classifier was then applied to the data in the test trial.

15.4   Data

We are using two datasets for our analysis. The first dataset was provided by an earlier study (Keirn and Aunon (1990)), and we refer to this as the "five-task set." In this data, EEG signals were recorded from subjects performing the following five mental tasks: (1) resting task, in which subjects were asked to relax and think of nothing in particular; (2)

mental letter writing, in which subjects were instructed to mentally compose a letter to a friend without vocalizing; (3) mental multiplication of two multidigit numbers, such as 49 times 78; (4) visual counting, in which subjects were asked to imagine a blackboard and to visualize numbers being written on the board sequentially; and (5) visual rotation of a three-dimensional block of figures. For each task and trial, the recordings were from six electrodes $(C_3, C_4, P_3, P_4, O_1, O_2)$ for 10 s at 250 Hz, and each task was repeated five times (for a total of five trials per task). The order in which tasks were performed was randomized, and subjects did not practice the tasks beforehand.

The second dataset we use we refer to as the "three-task set." In June 2005, the Third International Brain-Computer Interface Meeting was held at Rensselaerville, New York. One of the events at this meeting was the culmination of the BCI Competition III (BCI Competition III (2005)) for which five datasets had been made publicly available and entries were collected from participants who provided implementations of classification schemes. The classifications schemes were then applied to test data that had not been publicly available.

The three-task dataset is Data Set V from the BCI Competition III, provided by J. del R. Millán of the IDIAP Research Institute, Martigny, Switzerland. It contains data from three subjects performing three tasks: imagined left hand movements, imagined right hand movements, and generation of words beginning with the same random letter. The subjects performed a given task for about 15 s and then switched randomly to another task at the operator's request.

EEG signals were recorded at 512 Hz using a Biosemi system from electrodes at 32 positions: Fp1, AF3, F7, F3, FC1, FC5, T7, C3, CP1, CP5, P7, P3, Pz, PO3, O1, Oz, O2, PO4, P4, P8, CP6, CP2, C4, T8, FC6, FC2, F4, F8, AF4, Fp2, Fz, and Cz. Approximately four minutes of data was recorded, followed by approximately four minutes of rest, and this was repeated to get three training sets and one test set of data.

15.5   Results

15.5.1   Five-Task Dataset

The resulting performance and chosen parameter values for the five-task dataset are shown in table 15.1 for each representation. Two parameters not shown in the table were also varied—the window size and whether data was mean centered. Sensitivity to these parameters is mentioned later in relation to figure 15.5.

Table 15.1 shows that the best results were obtained with the $V_d^{(t,r)}$ representation produced by the short-time PCA method with percentages of samples correctly classified ranging from 67.5 percent for the first trial to 87.7 percent for the fourth trial. The second best representation was short-time SFA with the highest percent correct being 64.8 percent.

The confusion matrix in table 15.2 shows the percent correct partitioned into actual and predicted classes, averaged over all five test trials. The task most often classified correctly is task 2, the mental letter writing task. Tasks 4 and 5, visual rotation and visual counting,

Representation	Test trial	Number of lags	First vector	Number of vectors	Mean CV percent correct	Mean test percent correct
X Untransformed X time-embedded	1	15			26.5	22.3
	2	0			23.5	18.3
	3	0			23.0	21.0
	4	0			23.6	17.1
	5	1			23.3	17.9
PV Projections onto single PCA basis	1	6	2	18 (of 42)	26.8	22.1
	2	2	4	7 (of 18)	24.2	18.9
	3	1	3	9 (of 12)	24.2	21.2
	4	2	1	11 (of 18)	23.6	17.4
	5	1	3	8 (of 12)	24.2	18.1
PS Projections onto single SFA basis	1	6	37	6 (of 42)	27.0	21.8
	2	4	19	12 (of 30)	23.8	17.7
	3	1	4	7 (of 12)	23.6	19.9
	4	2	4	15 (of 18)	23.6	17.2
	5	2	12	7 (of 18)	23.5	17.8
V Short-time PCA	1	2	1	18 (of 18)	**94.9**	**67.5**
	2	3	2	22 (of 24)	**93.7**	**72.3**
	3	3	1	23 (of 24)	**91.4**	**85.6**
	4	2	1	18 (of 18)	**91.1**	**87.7**
	5	3	1	23 (of 24)	**91.7**	**80.3**
S Short-time SFA	1	2	3	16 (of 18)	78.9	49.9
	2	2	2	17 (of 18)	77.8	49.3
	3	2	3	16 (of 18)	74.5	64.8
	4	2	3	16 (of 18)	73.8	64.8
	5	2	1	18 (of 18)	75.5	62.9

Table 15.1   The last two columns show the validation and test percent correct for each representation and for each test trial. The values in bold face designate the best validation and test data performance. Also shown are the numbers of lags, first basis vectors, and numbers of vectors (out of total number of vectors) that resulted in the best validation performance.

		Actual				
		Task 1	Task 2	Task 3	Task 4	Task 5
	Task 1	86.1	2.1	22.1	0.0	0.0
	Task 2	1.1	94.7	5.9	0.0	0.5
Predicted	Task 3	12.8	2.7	71.7	0.0	0.0
	Task 4	0.0	0.3	0.0	72.3	30.9
	Task 5	0.0	0.3	0.3	27.7	68.5

Table 15.2 Confusion matrix for short-time PCA representation, averaged over the five test trials. Tasks are (1) resting, (2) mental letter writing, (3) mental multiplication, (4) visual rotation, and (5) mental counting.

Subject	Number of Lags	First Vector	Number of Vectors
1	2	1	5
2	2	1	4
3	3	1	5

Table 15.3 Best parameters for the Three-Task data set, from BCI Competition Data Set V.

are often misclassified as the other. Task 3, mental multiplication, is often misclassified as task 1, the resting task.

To visualize the classification performed by the STPCA process, we can cluster the data in each class and look at a low-dimensional representation. To cluster the data, we used an Linde-Buzo-Gray (LBG) algorithm (Linde et al. (1980)) (or equivalently, a k-means clustering) to obtain fifty cluster points per class. We then performed a Sammon mapping (Sammon, Jr. (1969)) to get the low-dimensional visualization; the Sammon map is appropriate since it tries to maintain interpoint distances. Figure 15.2 shows the class separation for one particular trial.

15.5.2 Three-Task Dataset

We bandpass-filtered the data to 8–30 Hz and down-sampled to 128 Hz. The short-time PCA representation was calculated for the training data for a range of lags, first basis vectors, and numbers of vectors. One-second windows were used that overlap by one-sixteenth of a second. LDA was used to classify the transformed data. The cross-validation procedure described above was used to identify the best values for the number of lags, number of vectors, and first vector. The values producing the best validation classification accuracy were determined independently for the data from the three subjects. The resulting values are shown in the first row of table 15.3.

Once these parameters were determined by the validation procedure, they were used to obtain the short-time PCA representation of the test data. For each subject, an LDA

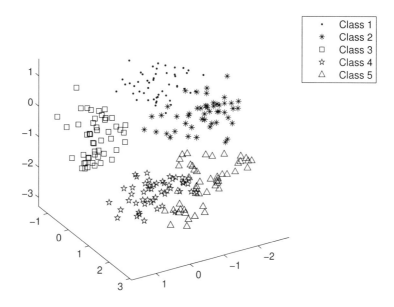

Figure 15.2   A low-dimensional visualization of the mental tasks for a single trial in the five-task set. Shown are the fifty cluster points per task, visualized using the Sammon map. Here we see that STPCA does indeed perform a good class separation.

	Subject 1	Subject 2	Subject 3	Average
Short-time PCA	62.3	57.6	47.5	55.8
S. Sun	74.3	62.3	52.0	62.8
A. Schlögl	69.0	57.1	32.3	52.7
E. Arbabi	55.4	51.8	43.6	50.2
A. Salehi	26.5	32.8	24.5	28.0

Table 15.4   Percent of test windows correctly classified. First row shows our result for short-time PCA. The other four rows are for the only entries to the BCI Competition III that classified the raw data from data set V.

classifier was calculated for all the training data and applied to the test data. As instructed by the requirements of the BCI Competition III for Data Set V, the classification result was smoothed by determining the most common predicted task label for eight consecutive windows, the equivalent of one half second of data. The percent of one-half-second spans of test data that were correctly classified is shown in table 15.4. This table also shows results from the BCI Competition III entries. The average performance of short-time PCA was within about 11 percent of the best approach submitted to the competition.

The submitted approaches are described at BCI Competition III (2005) and are summarized here. Sun et al. removed the data for seven electrodes judged to contain artifacts.

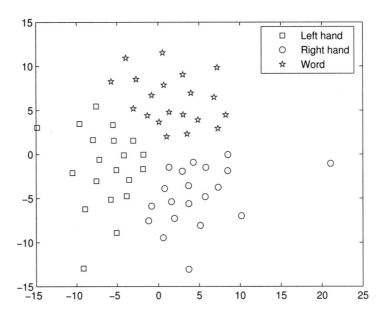

Figure 15.3 A low-dimensional visualization of the class separation for one training trial, subject 3, for the three-task dataset. Shown are twenty cluster points per task. The low-dimensional visualization was performed via the Sammon map. We see that the STPCA method does indeed give a good separation.

They were common-average referenced and bandpass filtered to 8–13 Hz for subjects 1 and 2 and to 11–15 Hz for subject 3. A multiclass approach to common spatial patterns is used to extract features and support vector machines are used to classify. Schlögl et al. down-sampled to 128 Hz, formed all bipolar channels and estimated autoregressive models for each channel, and also formed energy in α and β bands. The best single feature for which a statistical classifier best classified the data was then selected. Arbabi et al. down-sampled to 128 Hz and filtered to 0.5–45 Hz. Features based on statistical measures and on parametric models of one-second windows were extracted and classified using a Bayesian classifier. Best features were selected. Salehi used a combination of short-time Fourier transform energy values and time-domain features that were classified using a Bayesian classifier.

On average, the performance of the short-time PCA result surpasses all but one of the submitted entries. Perhaps the short-time PCA performance would be higher if the steps of electrode elimination and bandpass selection followed by the winning entry are similarly performed.

We again can visualize the class separation for a single training set by performing a clustering (20 clusters per task using the LBG algorithm discussed previously), and a low dimensional visualization using the Sammon map (referenced earlier). Recall that once the covariance matrix is estimated (section 15.3), we transform the data by $x \rightarrow R^{-1}x$. The result of the Sammon mapping is shown in figure 15.3.

	Without smoothing	With smoothing
Test trial 1	67.5	68.7
Test trial 2	72.3	74.9
Test trial 3	85.6	92.7
Test trial 4	87.7	92.7
Test trial 5	80.3	84.6
Mean	78.7	82.7

Table 15.5 Percent of test samples correctly classified without and with smoothing by binning classifier output into sequences of five samples and finding majority class.

15.6 Analysis and Discussion

For the five-task dataset, an analysis of the time course of the classifier output suggests that combining the output from successive samples might improve the performance. Figure 15.4 shows output of classifier versus sample index for each test trial for the short-time PCA representation. Sample index here refers to 125-sample windows of data, each shifted by 32 samples. Many of the incorrect classifications appear as single samples. One way to combine n successive classifications is to pick the class that appears most often. The percents of test samples correctly classified without and with this smoothing process for $n = 5$ are shown in table 15.5. Smoothing improves the mean percent correct from 78.7 percent to 82.7 percent. Since window size is 125 samples, or 1/2 second, and windows are shifted by 32 samples, or about 1/8 second, five successive classifier outputs cover $1/2 + 4(1/8) = 1$ second of time.

Indications of the sensitivity of the classification results for short-time PCA to each parameter are shown in figure 15.5. Each graph includes five curves showing the percent correct averaged over the validation samples taken from the four training trials remaining after choosing one of the five trials as the test trial. From the graphs we draw the following conclusions.

When the number of lags, d, is zero, only the current time sample enters into the representation. Including past samples improves performance. Results show that the best numbers of lags are 2 or 3. Two window sizes s were tested, 62 and 125, or 1/4 and 1/2 second. Windows of 1/2 second were always better. Only one value, 32, of window shift h was tested. The first basis vector used in the short-time PCA representation should appear early in their order. Performance drops quickly past about the twentieth vector. The performance versus the number of basis vectors climbs until about the twenty-second vector. The subtraction of the mean has minor effect on the results.

The interpretation of the resulting LDA classifiers is not obvious, due to the high-dimensional nature of the data resulting from the time-embedding. Here an initial analysis is performed by considering the weights of the linear discriminant functions. Figure 15.6 shows the variance of the weights over the five discriminant functions for the classifier trained on all but the first trial. The variance of weights corresponding to short-time PCA components from the first and last few basis vectors are highest, suggesting that it is these

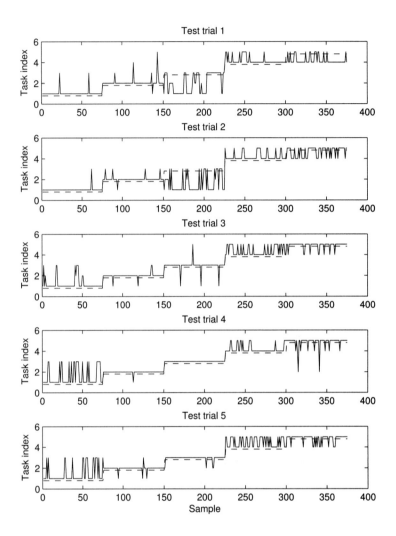

Figure 15.4   Output of classifier for sequences of data from the five mental tasks, using short-time PCA. The dashed line shows the true class index for each sample and the solid line shows the classifier's output. For each test trial, a classifier is trained on the remaining four trials and applied to the test trial, resulting in the five separate graphs.

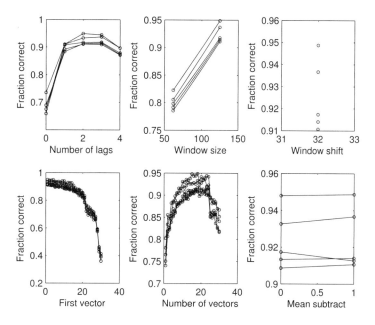

Figure 15.5   Sensitivity of fraction of average validation samples correctly classified to parameter values for short-time PCA representation.

components that most discriminate between the classes. The first few vectors indicate the directions in which the data varies the most and it is not surprising that they help discriminate, but the high variance of the last few vectors is intriguing—these low-variance directions may be capturing small variations in the data that relate strongly to the mental task being performed.

Another way to summarize the weights of the discriminant functions is to group them by their corresponding electrode. Figure 15.7 shows the variance of the weights grouped this way for a classifier trained on all but the first trial. For three of the trials, the P3 coefficients vary the most, while for the fourth trial, P4 coefficients vary the most. This simple analysis suggests that the parietal electrodes are most important for mental task discrimination.

15.7   Conclusion

Experiments showed that EEG representations based on short-time PCA can be classified by simple linear discriminant analysis (LDA) with an accuracy of about 80 percent correct classification of the correct mental task for the five-task dataset. This data was obtained from a single subject; tests on additional subjects are warranted to investigate the generality of this result. The three-task dataset—Data Set V from the BCI Competition III—includes data from three subjects performing three tasks. On this data, short-time PCA with LDA

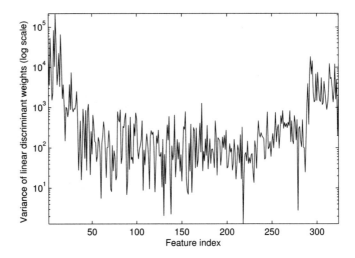

Figure 15.6   Variance (on logarithmic scale) of the weights over the five discriminant functions for the classifier trained on trials 2 through 4.

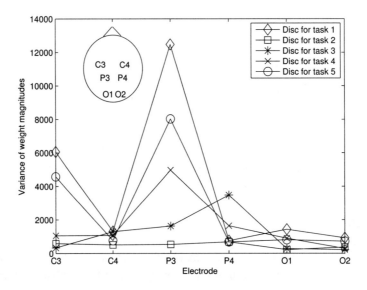

Figure 15.7   Variance of weights grouped by corresponding electrode. Each curve is formed by analyzing the weights for one discriminant function. There are five discriminant functions, one for each class, or mental task.

resulted in about 55 percent correct classification, placing it second among four entries to the competition. An analysis of the sensitivity of this result to the values of the representation parameters suggests that time-embedding is necessary for good performance and that the discriminatory information is not isolated to a small number of basis vectors.

Analysis of the classifiers' weights revealed that short-time PCA basis vectors late in the sequence play significant roles, suggesting that the low-variance activity represented by these vectors is strongly related to the mental task. This hypothesis warrants further study.

Information gleaned from analyses like those summarized in figures 15.6 and 15.7 can be used to select subsets of features to greatly reduce the dimensionality of the data and possibly improve the generalization performance of the classifiers. Extending this analysis to consider the time course of significant electrodes and basis vector directions could lead to hypotheses of the underlying cognitive activity.

Acknowledgments

This material is based upon work supported by the National Science Foundation under Grant No. 0208958. The authors would like to thank the organizers of BCI Competition III for providing access to the competition datasets. The authors also thank the reviewers for suggesting the application to the competition data.

Notes

E-mail for correspondence: anderson@cs.colostate.edu

16 Noninvasive Estimates of Local Field Potentials for Brain-Computer Interfaces

Rolando Grave de Peralta Menendez and Sara Gonzalez Andino
Electrical Neuroimaging Group
Department of Neurology
University Hospital Geneva (HUG)
1211 Geneva, Switzerland

Pierre W. Ferrez and José del R. Millán
IDIAP Research Institute   *Ecole Polytechnique Fédérale de*
1920 Martigny, Switzerland   *Lausanne (EPFL), Switzerland*

16.1   Abstract

Recent experiments have shown the possibility of using the brain electrical activity to directly control the movement of robots or prosthetic devices in real time. Such neuroprostheses can be invasive or noninvasive, depending on how the brain signals are recorded. In principle, invasive approaches will provide a more natural and flexible control of neuroprostheses, but their use in humans is debatable given the inherent medical risks. Noninvasive approaches mainly use scalp electroencephalogram (EEG) signals and their main disadvantage is that these signals represent the noisy spatiotemporal overlapping of activity arising from very diverse brain regions, that is, a single scalp electrode picks up and mixes the temporal activity of myriad neurons at very different brain areas. To combine the benefits of both approaches, we propose to rely on the noninvasive estimation of local field potentials (eLFP) in the whole human brain from the scalp-measured EEG data using a recently developed inverse solution (ELECTRA) to the EEG inverse problem. The goal of a linear inverse procedure is to deconvolve or unmix the scalp signals attributing to each brain area its own temporal activity. To illustrate the advantage of this approach, we compare, using identical sets of spectral features, classification of rapid voluntary finger self-tapping with left and right hands based on scalp EEG and eLFP on three subjects using different numbers of electrodes. It is shown that the eLFP-based Gaussian classifier outperforms the EEG-based Gaussian classifier for the three subjects.

16.2   Introduction

Recent experiments have shown the possibility of using the brain electrical activity to directly control the movement of robots or prosthetic devices in real time (Wessberg et al. (2000); Pfurtscheller and Neuper (2001); Taylor et al. (2002); Carmena et al. (2003); Mehring et al. (2003); Millán et al. (2004a); Musallam et al. (2004)). Such a kind of brain-controlled assistive system is a natural way to augment human capabilities by providing a new interaction link with the outside world. As such, it is particularly relevant as an aid for paralyzed humans, although it also opens up new possibilities in human-robot interaction for able-bodied people.

Initial demonstrations of the feasibility of controlling complex neuroprostheses have relied on intracranial electrodes implanted in the brains of monkeys (Wessberg et al. (2000); Taylor et al. (2002); Carmena et al. (2003); Mehring et al. (2003); Musallam et al. (2004)). In these experiments, one or more array of microelectrodes record the extracellular activity of single neurons (their spiking rate) in different areas of the cortex related to planning and execution of movements—motor, premotor, and posterior parietal cortex. Then, from the real-time analysis of the activity of the neuronal population, it has been possible to predict either the animal's movement intention (Mehring et al. (2003); Musallam et al. (2004)) or the monkey's hand trajectory (Wessberg et al. (2000); Taylor et al. (2002); Carmena et al. (2003)).

For humans, however, noninvasive methods based on electroencephalogram (EEG) signals are preferable because of ethical concerns and medical risks. The main source of the EEG—the brain electrical activity recorded from electrodes placed over the scalp—is the synchronous activity of thousands of cortical neurons. Thus, EEG signals suffer from a reduced spatial resolution and increased noise due to measurements on the scalp. As a consequence, current EEG-based brain-actuated devices are limited by a low channel capacity and are considered too slow for controlling rapid and complex sequences of movements. So far control tasks based on human EEG have been limited to exercises such as moving a computer cursor to the corners of the screen (Wolpaw and McFarland (1994)) or opening a hand orthosis (Pfurtscheller and Neuper (2001)). But recently, Millán et al. (2004a) have shown for the first time that asynchronous analysis of EEG signals is sufficient for humans to continuously control a mobile robot. Two human subjects learned to mentally drive the robot between rooms in a house-like environment using an EEG-based brain interface that recognized three mental states. Furthermore, mental control was only marginally worse than manual control on the same task. A key element of this brain-actuated robot is a suitable combination of intelligent robotics, asynchronous EEG analysis, and machine learning that requires only the user to deliver high-level commands, which the robot performs autonomously, at any time. This is possible because the operation of the brain interface is asynchronous and, unlike synchronous approaches (Wolpaw and McFarland (1994); Birbaumer et al. (1999); Donchin et al. (2000); Roberts and Penny (2000); Pfurtscheller and Neuper (2001)), does not require waiting for external cues that arrive at a fixed pace of 4–10 s.

Despite this latter demonstration of the feasibility of EEG-based neuroprostheses, it is widely assumed that only invasive approaches will provide natural and flexible control of robots (Nicolelis (2001); Donoghue (2002)). The rationale is that surgically implanted arrays of electrodes will be required to properly record the brain signals because the non-invasive scalp recordings with the EEG lack spatial resolution. However, recent advances in EEG analysis techniques have shown that the sources of the electric activity in the brain can be estimated from the surface signals with relatively high spatial accuracy. We believe that such EEG source analysis techniques overcome the lack of spatial resolution and may lead to EEG-based neuroprostheses that parallel invasive ones.

The basic question addressed in this chapter is the feasibility of noninvasive brain interfaces to reproduce the prediction properties of the invasive systems evaluated in animals while suppressing their risks. For doing that, we propose the noninvasive estimation of local field potentials (eLFP) in the whole human brain from the scalp-measured EEG data using a recently developed distributed linear inverse solution termed ELECTRA (Grave de Peralta Menendez et al. (2000, 2004))). The use of linear inversion procedures yields an online implementation of the method, a key aspect for real-time applications.

The development of a brain interface based on eLFP allows us to apply methods identical to those used for EEG-based brain interfaces but with the advantage of targeting the activity at specific brain areas. An additional advantage of our approach over scalp EEG is that the latter represents the noisy spatiotemporal overlapping of activity arising from very diverse brain regions, that is, a single scalp electrode picks up and mixes the temporal activity of myriad neurons at very different brain areas. Consequently, temporal and spectral features, which are probably specific to different parallel processes arising at different brain areas, are intermixed on the same recording. This certainly complicates the classification task by misleading even the most sophisticated analysis methods. For example, an electrode placed on the frontal midline picks up and mixes activity related to different motor areas known to have different functional roles such as the primary motor cortex, supplementary motor areas, anterior cingulate cortex, and motor cingulate areas. On the other hand, eLFP has the potential to unravel scalp signals, attributing to each brain area its own temporal (spectral) activity.

The feasibility of this noninvasive eLFP approach is shown here in the analysis of single trials recorded during self-paced finger tapping with right and left hands.[1] To illustrate the generalization of our approach and the influence of the number of electrodes, we report results obtained with three normal volunteers using either 111 or 32 electrodes. The capability to predict and differentiate the laterality of the movement using scalp EEG is compared with that of eLFP.

16.3 Methods

16.3.1 Data Recording

Three healthy young right-handed subjects completed a self-paced finger-tapping task. Subjects were instructed to press at their own pace the mouse button with the index finger of

a given hand while fixating on a white cross at the middle of the computer screen. Subjects'
arms rested on the table with their hands placed over the mouse. The intervals between
successive movements were rather stable for the three subjects, namely around 500 ms for
subject A and 2000 ms for subjects B and C. Subjects performed several sessions of the
task with breaks of around 5–10 minutes in between.

The EEG was recorded at 1000 Hz from 111 scalp electrodes (Electric Geodesic Inc.
system, subject A and B) and at 512 Hz from 32 scalp electrodes (Biosemi ActiveTwo
system, subject C). Head position was stabilized with a head and chin rest. In the first case
(i.e., 111 electrodes) offline processing of the scalp data consisted uniquely in the rejection
of bad channels[2] and their interpolation using a simple nearest-neighbor's algorithm.
This procedure was not necessary with the 32-electrode system. Since digitized electrode
positions were not available, we used standard spherical positions and the 10-10 system.
These positions were projected onto the scalp of the segmented Montreal Neurological
Institute (MNI) average brain, in preparation for the ELECTRA method that estimates
local field potentials.

The pace selected by the subjects allowed for the construction of trials aligned by the
response consisting of 400 ms before key press. In this way, the analyzed time window
contains mainly the movement preparation excluding the movement onset. For subject A
we recorded 680 trials of the left index tapping and 634 trials of the right index tapping, for
subject B we recorded 179 left trials and 167 right trials, while for subject C we recorded
140 left trials and 145 right trials. We did not apply any visual or automatic artifact rejection
and so kept all trials for analysis. After a visual a posteriori artifact check of the trials,
we found no evidence of muscular artifacts that could have contaminated one condition
differently from the other.

16.3.2   Local Field Potentials Estimates from Scalp EEG Recordings

The electroencephalogram (EEG) measures the extracranial electric fields produced by
neuronal activity within a living brain. When the positions and orientations of the active
neurons in the brain are known, it is possible to calculate the patterns of electric potentials
on the surface of the head produced by these sources. This process is called the forward
problem. If instead the only available information is the measured pattern of electric potential on the scalp surface, then one is interested in determining the intracranial distribution
of neural activity. This is called the inverse problem or the source localization problem, for
which there is no unique solution. The only hope is that additional information can be used
to constrain the infinite set of possible solutions to a single one. Depending on the additional information added, different inverse solutions—that is, different reconstructions of
neural activities with different properties—can be obtained (van Oosterom (1991); Scherg
(1994)).

Classical constraints used to solve the EEG inverse problem rely on considering the
neural generators as current dipoles (Ilmoniemi (1993)). In this case, the magnitude to
estimate is the dipole model supposed to represent a current density vector that can
be distributed over the whole grey matter mantle or confined to a single point. When
the dipole is assumed to be confined to a single or a few brain sites, the task is to

solve a nonlinear optimization problem aimed to find simultaneously the position and dipolar model of the dipoles (Scherg (1992); Mosher et al. (1999)). When the dipoles are distributed over a discrete set of solution points within the brain, the task is to find the magnitude of the dipolar model for each dipole leading to an under-determined inverse problem, which is usually solved by adding linear constraints such as minimum norm. (Hamalainen and Ilmoniemi (1994); Grave de Peralta Menendez and Gonzalez Andino (1998)). In both single-dipoles and distributed-dipole approaches the magnitude to be estimated is a vector field commonly termed the current density vector. However, in the approach with distributed models, the values of the current density vector are obtained for the whole grey matter akin to the tomographic images produced by other modalities of functional neuroimaging (fMRI, PET, or SPECT) but with temporal resolution in the order of milliseconds.

A change in the formulation of the EEG inverse problem takes place when the fact that neurophysiological currents are ohmic and can therefore be expressed as gradients of potential fields is included as a constraint in the formalism of the problem (Grave de Peralta Menendez et al. (2000)). With this neurophysiological constraint, we can reformulate the EEG inverse problem in more restrictive terms, providing the basis for the noninvasive estimation of intracranial local field potentials (a scalar field) instead of the current density vector (a 3D vector field) (Grave de Peralta Menendez et al. (2004)). This solution is termed ELECTRA.

ELECTRA can be described intuitively as the noninvasive estimation of local field potentials by means of virtual intracranial electrodes. The advantages of this method are

(1) mathematical simplicity and computational efficiency compared to models based on current density estimation, since the number of unknowns estimated by the inverse model is threefold fewer—that is, the unknowns decrease from a vector field to a scalar field;

(2) contrary to dipolar models, distributed linear solutions provide simultaneous temporal estimates for all brain areas not being confined to a few sites;

(3) the temporal reconstructions provided by linear distributed inverse solutions are better than those of discrete spatiotemporal models or L1-based reconstructions (Liu et al. (1998)). A few comparisons with intracranial data are also extremely appealing (Grave de Peralta Menendez et al. (2004)), systematically suggesting that temporal reconstructions of the generators are more reliable than their spatial counterparts; and

(4) since these are linear methods, computation of the intracranial estimates reduces to a simple inverse matrix by vector product, which warrants efficient online implementation.

The analysis that follows relies on the estimation for each single trial of the 3D distribution of the local field potentials (eLFP) using the ELECTRA source model. The eLFP were estimated at 4,024 voxels homogeneously distributed within the inner compartment of a realistic head model (Montreal Neurological Institute average brain). The voxels are restricted to the grey matter of this inner compartment and form an isotropic grid of 6 mm resolution.

16.3.3   Statistical Classifier

The different mental tasks are recognized by a Gaussian classifier trained to classify samples (single trials) as class "left" or "right" (Millán et al. (2002c, 2004a)). The output of this statistical classifier is an estimation of the posterior class probability distribution for a sample, that is, the probability that a given single trial belongs either to class "left" or class "right."

In our statistical classifier, we have for each mental task a mixture of several Gaussian units. We think of each unit as a prototype of one of the N_c mental tasks (or classes) to be recognized. The challenge is to find the appropriate position of the Gaussian prototype as well as an appropriate variance. We use several prototypes per mental task. We assume that the class-conditional probability density function of class C_k is a superposition of N_k Gaussians (or prototypes) and that classes have equal prior probabilities. In our case, all the classes have the same number of prototypes. In addition, we assume that all prototypes have an equal weight of $1/N_k$. Then, dropping constant terms, the activity a_k^i of the ith prototype of the class C_k for the input vector, or sample, x derived from a trial is

$$a_k^i(x) = \frac{\exp\left(-\frac{1}{2}(x - \mu_k^i)^T (\Sigma_k^i)^{-1}(x - \mu_k^i)\right)}{|\Sigma_k^i|^{1/2}} \tag{16.1}$$

where μ_k^i is the center of the ith prototype of the class C_k, Σ_k^i is the covariance matrix of the class C_k, and $|\Sigma_k|$ is the determinant of that matrix. Usually, each prototype has its own covariance matrix Σ_k^i. To reduce the number of parameters, we restrict our model to a diagonal covariance matrix Σ_k that is common to all the prototypes of the class C_k. Imposing diagonality equals an assumption of independence among the features. Even though we do not believe this assumption holds for our experiments in a strict sense, this has demonstrated to be a valid simplification of the model given the a posteriori good performance of the system. Now, the posterior probability y_k of the class C_k is

$$y_k(x) = p(x|C_k) = \frac{a_k(x)}{A(x)} = \frac{\sum_{i=1}^{N_p} a_k^i(x)}{\sum_{k=1}^{N_c} \sum_{i=1}^{N_p} a_k^i(x)} \tag{16.2}$$

where a_k is the activity of class C_k and A is the total activity of the network. The response of the network for the input vector x is the class C_k with the highest posterior probability provided that it is greater than a given probability threshold, otherwise the response is classified as "unknown" so as to avoid making risky decisions for uncertain samples. This rejection criterion keeps the number of errors (false positives) low, which is desired since recovering from erroneous actions has a high cost. In the experiments reported below, however, we do not use any rejection criterion because the probability threshold was put to 0.5, thus classifying all samples as belonging to one of the possible classes.

To initialize the center of the prototypes μ_k^i of the class C_k, we run a clustering algorithm—typically, self-organizing maps (Kohonen (1997)). We then initialize the diagonal covariance matrix Σ_k of the class C_k by setting

$$\Sigma_k = \frac{1}{|S_k|} \sum_{x \in S_k} (x - \mu_k^{i^*})(x - \mu_k^{i^*})^T \tag{16.3}$$

where S_k is the set of the training samples belonging to the class C_k, $|S_k|$ is the cardinality of this set, and i^* is the nearest prototype of this class to the sample x. During learning we improve these initial estimations iteratively by stochastic gradient descent so as to minimize the mean square error[3]

$$E = \frac{1}{2} \sum_{k=1}^{N_c} (y_k - t_k)^2 \tag{16.4}$$

where t_k is the kth component of the target vector in the form 1-of-c, for example, the target vector for class 2 is coded as $(0,1)$ if the number of classes N_c is 2. Taking the gradients of the error function yields

$$\Delta \mu_k^i(x) = \alpha \frac{\partial E}{\partial \mu_k^i}(x) = \alpha \frac{a_k^i(x)}{A(x)} \frac{x - \mu_k^i}{\Sigma_k^i}$$
$$\times \left((y_k(x) - t_k(x)) - \sum_j^{N_c} y_j(x)(y_j(x) - t_j(x)) \right) \tag{16.5}$$

$$\Delta \Sigma_k^i(x) = \beta \frac{\partial E}{\partial \Sigma_k^i}(x) = \beta \frac{1}{2} \frac{a_k^i(x)}{A(x)} \frac{(x - \mu_k^i)^2 - \Sigma_k^i}{(\Sigma_k^i)^2}$$
$$\times \left((y_k(x) - t_k(x)) - \sum_j^{N_c} y_j(x)(y_j(x) - t_j(x)) \right) \tag{16.6}$$

where α and β are the learning rates. After updating μ_k^i and Σ_k^i for each training sample, the covariance matrices of all prototypes of the same class are averaged to obtain the common class covariance matrix Σ_k. This simple operation leads to better performance than if separate covariance matrices are kept for each individual prototype. The interpretation of this rule is that, during training, the centers of the Gaussians are pulled toward the EEG samples of the mental task they represent and are pushed away from EEG samples of other tasks.

16.3.4   Feature Extraction

To test the capability of our eLFP approach to discriminate between left and right finger movements, we have done a tenfold cross-validation study and also have compared the performance of the eLFP-based classifier to an EEG-based classifier. This means that all the available single trials of each class are split in ten different subsets, and then we take nine of them to train the classifier and select the hyperparameters of the classifier (learning rates and number of prototypes), whereas the remaining subset is used for testing the generalization capabilities. This process is repeated ten times to get an average of the performance of the classifier based on PSD features computed either on scalp EEG or eLFP.

In the case of using scalp EEG signals, each single trial of 400 ms of raw EEG potentials is first transformed to the common average reference (CAR)[4] (removal of the average activity over all the electrodes). The superiority of spatial filters and CAR over raw potentials for the operation of a brain interface has been demonstrated in different studies (e.g., Babiloni et al. (2000)). Then the power spectral density (PSD) in the band 7.5–30 Hz with a resolution of 2.5 Hz, thus yielding ten values per channel, was estimated for the 10 channels CPz, Pz, FC3, FC4, C3, C4, CP3, CP4, P3, and P4, which cover the motor cortex bilaterally. We have successfully used these PSD features in previous experiments (Millán et al. (2002c, 2004a)). In particular, we have computed the PSD using modern multitaper methods (Thomson (1982)). These methods have shown to be particularly well suited for spectral analysis of short segments of noisy data, and have been successfully applied to the analysis of neuronal recordings in behaving animals (e.g., Pesaran et al. (2002)). Specifically, the PSD was estimated using seven Slepian data tapers.

In the case of the classifier based on eLFP, we also have computed the PSD in the band 7.5–30 Hz using multitaper methods with seven Slepian data tapers. In this case, we used three values per channel to limit the dimensionality of the input space for the statistical classifier. The PSD was estimated for each single trial of 400 ms on the 50 most relevant voxels (out of 4,024) as selected by a feature selection algorithm that is a variant of the so-called Relief method (Kira and Rendell (1992)). Relief has been successfully applied to the selection of relevant spectral features for the classification of EEG signals (Millán et al. (2002b)).

Feature selection was applied only to the eLFP because of the large number of potential voxels that can be fed to the classifier. Feature selection was done on the training set of each cross-validation step. In the case of scalp EEG, it has been widely shown that only channels over the motor cortex suffice for good recognition of bimanual movements. Indeed, feature selection on subject C yielded the before-mentioned channels as the most relevant ones, and using more than ten channels did not improve performance. On the other hand, the choice of fifty voxels as input to the eLFP classifier was motivated by the desire of keeping the dimensionality similar to that of the scalp EEG classifier. A small comparative study on subject B showed that the optimal number of voxels was around fifty, although differences in performance were not highly statistically significant (especially when compared to larger numbers of voxels).

16.4   Results

Table 16.1 shows the results of this comparative study based, as explained, in a tenfold cross-validation using the Gaussian classifier to get an average of the performance of the classifier based on PSD features computed either on scalp EEG or eLFP.

Classification based on scalp EEG achieves error rates similar to previous studies (10.8% on average for the three subjects), and that despite the short time windows used to estimate the PSD, namely 400 ms. In particular, performance is worse for subject A than for subjects B and C (11.6% vs. 10.4% and 10.5%), which illustrates the difficulty of recognizing rapid motor decisions (500 ms tapping pace vs. 2000 ms) based on short segments of brain electrical activity.

On the contrary, the performance of the Gaussian classifier based on eLFP is extremely good as it only makes 3.7 percent, 0.6 percent, and 4.9 percent errors for subjects A, B,

Method	Subject		
	A, 111 elect	B, 111 elect	C, 32 elect
EEG	11.6% ± 2.7	10.4% ± 4.1	10.5% ± 3.7
LFP	3.7% ± 1.2	0.6% ± 1.2	4.9% ± 2.5

Table 16.1   Error rates (mean ± standard deviation) in the recognition of "left" versus "right" finger movements for three subjects made by a Gaussian classifier based on PSD features computed either on scalp EEG or noninvasive eLFP using the multitaper method. Results are the average of a tenfold cross-validation.

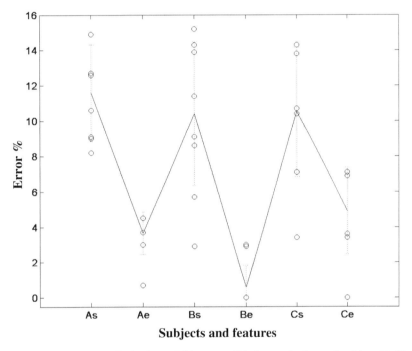

Figure 16.1   Plot of all results in the tenfold cross-validation study, for each subject (A, B, C) and type of features (s, scalp EEG, or e, eLFP). Circles indicate individual values, dotted lines show error bars with unit standard deviation, and the solid line connects mean values.

and C, respectively. These performances are 3, 17, and 2 times better than when using scalp EEG features, respectively, and are statistically significant ($p = 0$ for subjects A and B; $p < 0.001$ for subject C). This is particularly the case for subject B for whom we recorded from 111 electrodes. It is also worth noting that performance is still very good for subject C even though eLFP were estimated from only 32 scalp electrodes.

Figure 16.1 shows a plot of all results in the tenfold cross-validation study, for each subject and type of features, illustrating the amount of variation in the values.

Regarding the spatial distribution of the voxels selected by the feature selection algorithm, the voxels form clusters located on the frontal cortex with the tendency to have the most relevant ones at the dorsolateral premotor cortex.

16.5   Discussion

The goal of a linear inverse procedure is to deconvolve or unmix the scalp signals attributing to each brain area its own temporal activity. By targeting the particular temporal/spectral features at specific brain areas, we can select a low number of features that capture information related to the state of the individual in a way that is relatively invariant to time. Eventually, this may avoid long training periods and increase the reliability and efficiency of the classifiers. For the case of paralyzed patients, the classification stage can be improved by focusing on the specific brain areas known to participate and code the different steps of voluntary or imagined motor action through temporal and spectral features.

Distributed inverse solutions, as any other inverse method, suffer from limitations inherent to the ill-posed nature of the problem. The limitations of these methods have been described already (Grave de Peralta Menendez and Gonzalez Andino (1998)) and basically concern: (1) errors on the estimation of the source amplitudes for the instantaneous maps and (2) inherent blurring, that is, the spatial extent of the actual source is usually overestimated. However, several theoretical and experimental studies showed that spectral and temporal features are quite well preserved by these methods (Grave de Peralta Menendez et al. (2000)) that surpass nonlinear and dipolar methods (Liu et al. (1998)). Consequently, our approach relies on temporal and spectral features disregarding estimated amplitudes so as to alleviate these limitations.

It is also worth noting that, since the head model is stable for the same subject over time, the inverse matrix requires that it be computed only once for each subject and is invariant over recording sessions. Online estimation of intracranial field potentials is reduced to a simple matrix-by-vector product, a key aspect for real-time applications. However, despite a careful positioning of the electrodes and the regularization[5] used to deal with the noise associated with electrode misplacement, the estimated activity might still be displaced to a neighbor location out of the strict boundaries defined in the anatomical atlas. This could happen because of the differences between the subject's head and the average MNI head model, or because of the differences in electrode locations from one session to another. Based on the results of the extensive studies of presurgical evaluations of epileptic patients, we should expect low errors using realistic head models based on a subject's MRI. However, since presurgical studies barely use more than one EEG recording session, the second source of error requires further study.

Regarding the possibility of using biophysically constrained inverse solutions for brain-computer interfaces, the results reported here are highly encouraging. They suggest that recognition of motor intents is possible from nonaveraged inverse solutions and are superior to systems based on scalp EEG. While prediction of the upcoming movements' direction is possible from invasive recordings from neuronal populations in the motor cortex of monkeys (Carmena et al. (2003)) as well as from local field potentials recorded from the motor cortex of monkeys (Mehring et al. (2003); Musallam et al. (2004)), the possibility of doing the same noninvasively is appealing for its much higher potential with humans. Finally, the use of noninvasive estimations of local field potentials at specific brain areas allows us to rely on features with a priori established neurophysiological information.

16.6   Conclusion

In conclusion, this study shows the advantage of using noninvasive eLFP over scalp EEG as input for a brain-computer interface, as it considerably increases the accuracy of classification. It also suggests that the prediction capabilities of brain interfaces based on noninvasive eLFP might parallel those of invasive approaches. Moreover, it indicates that eLFP can be reliably estimated even with a reduced number of scalp electrodes.

These conclusions are supported by other studies on tasks not related to brain-computer interfaces, such as visuomotor coordination, with more than twenty-five subjects and several experimental paradigms (Grave de Peralta Menendez et al. (2005a)). These studies showed that the discriminative power of eLFP is higher than that of scalp EEG. Also, for a couple of patients where it was possible to record intracranial potentials directly, eLFP and intracranial potentials had similar predicting power, indicating that ELECTRA correctly retrieves the main attributes of the temporal activity of different brain regions.

Acknowledgments

This work is supported by the Swiss National Science Foundation through the National Centre of Competence in Research on "Interactive Multimodal Information Management (IM2)" and grant 3152A0-100745, and also by the European IST Programme FET Project FP6-003758. This chapter reflects only the authors' views and funding agencies are not liable for any use that may be made of the information contained herein.

Notes

E-mail for correspondence: jose.millan@idiap.ch, rolando.grave@hcuge.ch

(1)   As described in section 16.3.1, the experimental setup in this chapter does not allow us to implement an asynchronous BCI as used previously in our group because the time window of EEG is time-locked to the response. However, subjects can still work asynchronously since they decide the response time.

(2)   Bad channels were detected by visual inspection combined with an automatic rejection criterion based on their amplitudes.

(3)   An alternative to gradient descent for training the Gaussian classifier is expectation-maximization (Hastie et al. (2001)). The former, however, is better suited for online adaptation (see chapter 18).

(4)   Studies comparing CAR and spatial filters like the Laplacian did not show any statistical difference in classification performance between them.

(5)   The regularization parameters were tuned during a previous study with epileptic data where we dealt with the challenging problem of computing inverse solutions for spontaneous EEG (in contrast to averaged EEG that is the standard and well known problem).

17   Error-Related EEG Potentials in Brain-Computer Interfaces

Pierre W. Ferrez and José del R. Millán
IDIAP Research Institute
1920 Martigny, Switzerland

Ecole Polytechnique Fédérale de
Lausanne (EPFL), Switzerland

17.1   Abstract

Brain-computer interfaces (BCI), as any other interaction modality based on physiological signals and body channels (e.g., muscular activity, speech, and gestures), are prone to errors in the recognition of subject's intent. An elegant approach to improve the accuracy of BCIs consists in a verification procedure directly based on the presence of error-related potentials (ErrP) in the EEG recorded right after the occurrence of an error. Most of these studies show the presence of ErrP in typical choice reaction tasks where subjects respond to a stimulus and ErrP arise following errors due to the subject's incorrect motor action. However, in the context of a BCI, the central question is: Are ErrP also elicited when the error is made by the interface during the recognition of the subject's intent? We have thus explored whether ErrP also follow a feedback indicating incorrect responses of the interface and no longer errors of the subjects themselves. Four healthy volunteer subjects participated in a simple human-robot interaction experiment (i.e., bringing the robot to either the left or right side of a room), which seemed to reveal a new kind of ErrP. These "interaction ErrP" exhibit a first sharp negative peak followed by a broader positive peak and a second negative peak ($\sim$270, $\sim$400, and $\sim$ 550 ms after the feedback, respectively). But to exploit these ErrP, we need to detect them in each single trial using a short window following the feedback that shows the response of the classifier embedded in the BCI. We have achieved an average recognition rate of correct and erroneous single trials of 83.7 percent and 80.2 percent, respectively. We also show that the integration of these ErrP in a BCI, where the subject's intent is not executed if an ErrP is detected, significantly improves the performance of the BCI.

17.2   Introduction

BCIs, as any other interaction modality based on physiological signals and body channels (e.g., muscular activity, speech, and gestures), are prone to errors in the recognition of subject's intent, and those errors can be frequent. Indeed, even well-trained subjects rarely reach 100 percent success. A possible way to reduce errors consists in a verification procedure whereby each output consists of two opposite trials, and success is required on both to validate the outcome (Wolpaw et al. (1998)). Even if this method greatly reduces the errors, it requires much more mental effort from the subject and reduces the communication rate.

In contrast to other interaction modalities, a unique feature of the "brain channel" is that it conveys both information from which we can derive mental control commands to operate a brain-actuated device as well as information about cognitive states that are crucial for a purposeful interaction—all this on the millisecond range. One of these states is the awareness of erroneous responses, which a number of groups have recently started to explore as a way to improve the performance of BCIs (Schalk et al. (2000); Blankertz et al. (2003); Parra et al. (2003)). Since the late 1980s, different physiological studies have shown the presence of error-related potentials (ErrP) in the EEG recorded right after people become aware that they have made an error (Gehring et al. (1990); Carter et al. (1998); Falkenstein et al. (2000); Holroyd and Coles (2002)). Apart from Schalk et al. (2000) who investigated ErrP in real BCI feedback, most of these studies show the presence of ErrP in typical choice reaction tasks (Carter et al. (1998); Falkenstein et al. (2000); Blankertz et al. (2003); Parra et al. (2003)). In this kind of task, the subject is asked to respond as quickly as possible to a stimulus, and ErrP (sometimes referred to as "response ErrP") arise following errors due to the subject's incorrect motor action (e.g., subjects press a key with the left hand when they should have responded with the right hand). The main components here are a negative potential showing up 80 ms after the incorrect response followed by a larger positive peak showing up between 200 and 500 ms after the incorrect response. More recently, other studies have shown the presence of ErrP in typical reinforcement learning tasks where the subject is asked to make a choice and ErrP (sometimes referred to as "feedback ErrP") arise following the presentation of a stimulus that indicates incorrect performance (Holroyd and Coles (2002)). The main component here is a negative deflection observed 250 ms after presentation of the feedback indicating incorrect performance. Finally, other studies reported the presence of ErrP (that we will refer to as "observation ErrP) following observation of errors made by an operator during choice reaction tasks (van Schie et al. (2004)) where the operator needs to respond to stimuli. As in the feedback ErrP, the main component here is a negative potential showing up 250 ms after the incorrect response of the subject performing the task. ErrP most probably are generated in a brain area called anterior cingulate cortex (ACC), which is crucial for regulating emotional responses (Holroyd and Coles (2002)).

An important aspect of the first two described ErrP is that they always follow an error made by the subjects themselves. First the subjects make a selection, and then ErrP arise either simply after the occurrence of an error (choice reaction task) or after a feedback

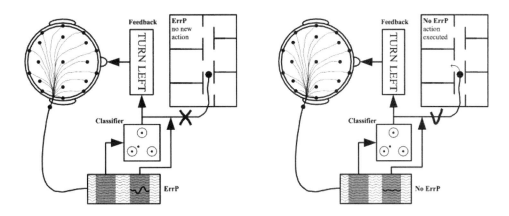

Figure 17.1 Exploiting error-related potentials (ErrP) in a brain-controlled mobile robot. The subject receives feedback indicating the output of the classifier before the actual execution of the associated command (e.g., "TURN LEFT"). If the feedback generates an ErrP (left), this command is simply ignored and the robot will keep executing the previous command. Otherwise (right), the command is sent to the robot.

indicating the error (reinforcement learning task). However, in the context of a BCI or human-computer interaction in general, the central question is: Are ErrP also elicited when the error is made by the interface during the recognition of the subject's intent?

To consider the full implications of this question, let's imagine that the subject's intent is to make a robot reach a target to the left. What would happen if the interface fails to recognize the intended command and the robot starts turning in the wrong direction? Are ErrP still present even though the subject did not make any error but only perceives that the interface is performing incorrectly?

The objective of this study is to investigate how ErrP could be used to improve the performance of a BCI. Thus, we will first explore whether or not ErrP also follow a feedback indicating incorrect responses of the interface and no longer errors of the subjects themselves. If ErrP are also elicited in this case, then we could integrate them in a BCI in the following way as shown in figure 17.1: After translating the subject's intention into a control command, the BCI provides a feedback of that command, which actually will be executed only if no ErrP follows the feedback. This should greatly increase the reliability of the BCI, as we see in section 17.4. Of course, this new interaction protocol depends on the ability to detect ErrP no longer in averages of a large number of trials, but in each single trial using a short window following the feedback that shows the response of the classifier embedded in the BCI.

In this chapter, we report recently published results with volunteer subjects during a simple human-robot interaction (i.e., bringing the robot to either the left or right side of a room) that seem to reveal a new kind of ErrP, which is satisfactorily recognized in single trials in Ferrez and Millán (2005). These recognition rates significantly improve the performance of the brain interface.

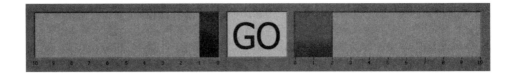

Figure 17.2   Left and right horizontal progress bars. The goal of an interaction experiment is to fill one of the bars, which simulates a real interaction with a robot that needs to reach one side of a room (left or right). The system fills the bars with an error rate of 20 percent; that is, at each step, there was a 20 percent probability that the incorrect progress bar was filled.

17.3   Experimental Setup

To test the presence of ErrP after a feedback indicating errors made by the interface in the recognition of the subject's intent, we have simulated a real interaction with a robot where the subject wishes to bring the robot to one side of a room (left or right) by delivering repetitive commands until the robot reaches the target. This virtual interaction is implemented by means of two horizontal progress bars made of ten steps each. One of the bars goes from the center of the screen to the left side (left bar), and the other bar progresses to the right side (right bar). Figure 17.2 shows the left and right horizontal progress bars used as feedback.

To isolate the issue of the recognition of ErrP from the more difficult and general problem of a whole BCI where erroneous feedback can be due to nonoptimal performance of both the interface (i.e., the classifier embedded into the interface) and the users themselves, in the following experiments the subjects deliver commands manually and not mentally. That is, they simply press a left or right key with the left or right hand. In this way, any error feedback is due only to a wrong recognition of the interface of the subject's intention.

Four healthy volunteer subjects participated in these experiments. The subjects press a key after a stimulus delivered by the system (the word "GO" appears on the screen). The system filled the bars with an error rate of 20 percent; that is, at each step, there was a 20 percent probability that the incorrect progress bar was filled. Subjects performed ten series of five progress bars, the delay between two consecutive steps (two consecutive GOs from the system) was 3–4 s (random delay to prevent habituation). Duration of each interaction experiment (i.e., filling a progress bar) was about 40 s, with breaks of 5–10 minutes between two series but no break between interaction experiments of the same series.

EEG potentials were acquired with a portable system (Biosemi ActiveTwo) by means of a cap with 32 integrated electrodes covering the whole scalp and located according to the standard 10-20 international system. The sampling rate was 512 Hz and signals were measured at full DC. Raw EEG potentials were first spatially filtered by subtracting from each electrode the average potential (over the 32 channels) at each time step. The aim of this re-referencing procedure is to suppress the average brain activity, which can be seen as underlying background activity, so as to keep the information coming from local sources below each electrode. Then, we applied a 1–10 Hz bandpass filter, as ErrP are known to be a relatively slow cortical potential. Finally, EEG signals were subsampled from 512 Hz to 128 Hz (i.e., we took 1 point out of 4) before classification, which was entirely based on temporal features. Indeed, the actual input vector for the statistical classifier described below is a 0.5-s window starting 150 ms after the feedback and ending 650 ms after the feedback for channels Cz and Fz. The choice of these channels follows the fact that ErrP are characterized by a fronto-central distribution along the midline. Thus, the dimensionality of the input vector is 128, that is, concatenation of two windows of 64 points (EEG potentials) each.

The two different classes are recognized by a Gaussian classifier trained to classify single trials as "correct" or "error" (Millán et al. (2004a)). The output of the statistical classifier is an estimation of the posterior class probability distribution for a single trial, that is, the probability that a given single trial belongs to class "correct" or class "error." In this statistical classifier, every Gaussian unit represents a prototype of one of the classes to be recognized, and we use several prototypes per class. During learning, the centers of the classes of the Gaussian units are pulled toward the trials of the class they represent and pushed away from the trials of the other class. For more details about this Gaussian classifier, see chapter 16.

No artifact rejection algorithm (for removing or filtering out eye or muscular movements) was applied and all trials were kept for analysis. It is worth noting, however, that after a visual a posteriori check of the trials, we found no evidence of muscular artifacts that could have contaminated one condition differently from the other.

17.4 Experimental Results

With this protocol, it is first necessary to investigate whether or not ErrP are present no more in reaction to errors made by the subjects themselves, but in reaction to erroneous responses made by the interface as indicated by the feedback visualizing the recognized subjects' intentions. Figure 17.3 shows the difference error-minus-correct for channel Cz for the four subjects plus the grand average of the four subjects. A first sharp negative peak (Ne) can be seen 270 ms after the feedback (except for subject 2). A later positive peak (Pe) appears between 350 and 450 ms after the feedback. Finally, an additional negative peak occurs ~550 ms after the feedback. Figure 17.3 also shows the scalp potentials topographies, for the grand average EEG of the four subjects, at the occurrence of the maximum of the Ne, the Pe, and the additional negative peak: a first frontal negativity appears after 270 ms, followed by a fronto-central positivity at 375 ms, followed by a fronto-central negativity at 550 ms. All four subjects show very similar ErrP time courses whose amplitudes slightly differ from one subject to the other. Indeed, subject 2 shows no initial negative peak whereas subject 4 shows an important one. Subjects 3 and 4 show a larger positive potential, but all four subjects show similar amplitudes for the second negative peak.

These experiments seem to reveal a new kind of error-related potentials that, for convenience, we call "interaction ErrP." The general shape of this ErrP is quite similar to the shape of the response ErrP in a choice reaction task, whereas the timing is similar to the

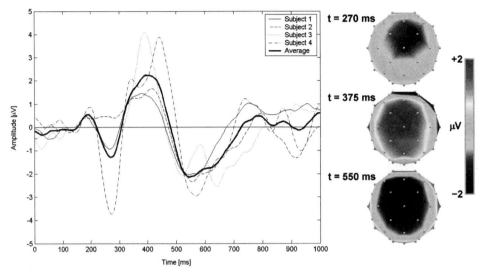

Figure 17.3 Left: Average EEG for the difference error-minus-correct at channel Cz for the four subjects plus the grand average of them. Feedback is delivered at time 0 seconds. The negative (Ne) and positive (Pe) peaks show up about 270 ms and between 350 and 450 ms after the feedback, respectively. An additional negative peak occurs ∼550 ms after the feedback. Right: Scalp potentials topographies, for the grand average EEG of the four subjects, at the occurrence of the peaks. Small filled circles indicate positions of the electrodes (frontal on top), Cz being in the middle of the scalp.

feedback ErrP of reinforcement learning tasks and to observation ErrP. As in the case of response ErrP, interaction ErrP exhibit a first sharp negative peak followed by a broader positive peak. However, interaction ErrP are also characterized by a second negative peak that does not appear in response ErrP. This is quite different from the shape of feedback ErrP and observation ErrP that are only characterized by a small negative deflection. On the other hand, the time course of the interaction ErrP bears some similarities to that of the feedback ErrP and observation ErrP: In both cases, the first distinctive feature (negative peak and negative deflection, respectively) appears ∼250 ms after feedback. This delay represents the time required by the subject to "see" the feedback. The time course of response ErrP is definitely different. The peaks show up much faster because the subjects are aware of their errors before they perform the wrong actions. In this case, the real initial time ($t = 0$) is internal and unknown to the experimenter.

17.5   Single-Trial Classification

To explore the feasibility of detecting single-trial erroneous responses, we have done a tenfold cross-validation study where the testing set consists of one of the recorded sessions. In this way, testing is always done on a different recording session to those used for training the model.

Table 17.1 reports the recognition rates (mean and standard deviations) for the four subjects plus the average of them. The different hyperparameters—that is, the learning rates

Subject	Error %	Correct %
#1	87.3 ± 11.3	82.8 ± 7.2
#2	74.4 ± 12.4	75.3 ± 10.0
#3	78.1 ± 14.8	89.2 ± 4.9
#4	80.9 ± 11.3	87.3 ± 5.2
Average	80.2 ± 5.4	83.7 ± 6.2

Table 17.1   Percentages of correctly recognized error trials and correct trials for the four subjects and the average of them.

of the centers and diagonal covariance matrices, number of prototypes, and common/single covariance matrices for each class—were chosen by model selection in the training sets. Regarding the learning rates, usual values were 10^{-4} to 10^{-6} for the centers and 10^{-6} to 10^{-8} for the variances, while the usual number of prototypes was rather small (from 2 to 4). These results show that single-trial recognition of erroneous responses is 80 percent on average, while the recognition rate of correct responses is slightly better (83.7 percent). Quite importantly, even for the subject with the worse detection rates, they are around 75 percent. Beside the crucial importance to integrate ErrP in the BCI in a way that the subject still feels comfortable, for example, by reducing as much as possible the rejection of actually correct commands, a key point for the exploitation of the automatic recognition of interaction errors is that they translate into an actual improvement of the performance of the BCI, which we can measure in terms of the bit rate.

17.6   Bit Rate Improvement

A traditional measure of the performance of a system is the bit rate, the amount of information communicated per unit time. The bit rate usually is expressed in bits per trial (bits per selection). If a single trial has N_c possible outcomes, if the probability p that this outcome is correct (accuracy of the BCI), and if finally each of the other outcomes has the same probability of selection (i.e., $(1 - p)/(N_c - 1)$), then the information transfer rate in bits per trial BpT is

$$BpT = \log_2(N_c) + p \log_2(p) + (1 - p) \log_2 \left(\frac{1 - p}{N_c - 1} \right). \qquad (17.1)$$

This formula makes the assumption that BCI errors and ErrP detection errors are independent, which might not always be the case in particular situations like lack of concentration, longer lasting artifacts, or fatigue. Let's consider now how the performance of the BCI changes after introducing ErrP, and that the system detects a proportion e of erroneous trials and a proportion c of correct trials. In the general case, after detecting an erroneous trial the outcome of the interface is simply stopped and not sent to the brain-actuated device. The new accuracy p' of the BCI becomes $p' = pc/p_t$ where $p_t = pc + (1 - p)(1 - e)$ is the proportion of the commands that are effectively sent to the device. Now the new

Subject	$N_c = 3$			$N_c = 2$				
	Initial	**Stop**		**Initial**	**Stop**		**Replace**	
	BpT	*BpT*	**Gain**	*BpT*	*BpT*	**Gain**	*BpT*	**Gain**
1	0.66	0.91	37%	0.28	0.53	91%	0.36	29%
2	0.66	0.73	10%	0.28	0.40	42%	0.19	-32%
3	0.66	0.92	38%	0.28	0.52	86%	0.44	59%
4	0.66	0.91	37%	0.28	0.52	86%	0.42	50%
Average	**0.66**	**0.86**	**30%**	**0.28**	**0.49**	**76%**	**0.34**	**23%**

Table 17.2   Performances of the BCI integrating ErrP for the four subjects and the average of them.

information transfer rate in bits per trial, which takes into account the fact that there are now fewer outcomes, becomes

$$BpT = p_t \left(\log_2(N_c) + p' \log_2(p') + (1 - p') \log_2 \left(\frac{1 - p'}{N_c - 1} \right) \right). \tag{17.2}$$

In the case of a two-class BCI ($N_c = 2$), after detecting an erroneous trial, it could be possible to replace the "wrong" outcome by the opposite one, what yields an accuracy $p'' = pc + (1 - p)e$. The information transfer rate in this case is calculated by replacing p by p'' in (17.1), because now there is no stopped outcome.

   Table 17.2 reports the theoretical performances of a BCI that integrates ErrP for the four subjects and the average of them, where we have assumed an accuracy of 80 percent the recognition of the subject's intent. These figures are to be compared to the performance of a standard BCI (i.e., without integrating ErrP). We have also reported the performances in the case $N_c = 3$, as the mind-controlled robot described by Millán et al. (2004a). In the case of standard two-class and three-class BCI, their performances are 0.28 and 0.66 bits per trial, respectively. Results indicate there is a significant improvement in performance in the case of stopping outcomes, which is above 70 percent on average and higher than 90 percent for one of the subjects. Surprisingly, replacing the wrong outcome leads to smaller improvements and, in the case of subject 2, even to a significant degradation.

17.7   Error-Related Potentials and Oddball N200 and P300

Since our protocol is quite similar to an oddball paradigm, the question arises of whether the potentials we describe are simply oddball N200 and P300. An oddball paradigm is characterized by an infrequent or especially significant stimulus interspersed with frequent stimuli. The subject is accustomed to a certain stimulus and the occurrence of an infrequent stimulus generates a negative deflection (N200) about 200 ms after the stimulus, followed by a positive peak (P300) about 300 ms after the stimulus. Our protocol is very close to an oddball paradigm in the sense that the subject is accustomed to seeing the increase in stages of the "correct" progress bars, and the increase in stages of the "wrong" progress bar is the infrequent stimulus. To clarify this issue, we have run new series of experiments for the ErrP study.

In the new series of experiments, the interface executed the subject's command with an error rate of 50 percent and, so, error trials are no longer less frequent than correct trials. Analysis of the ErrP for different subjects using error rates of 20 and 50 percent show no difference between them except that the amplitude of the potentials are smaller in the case of an error rate of 50 percent, but the time course remains the same. This is in agreement with all previous findings on ErrP that show that the amplitude is directly proportional to the error rate. It is worthwhile to note that the average classification rate with an error rate of 50 percent was 75. We can conclude then that, while we cannot exclude the possibility that N200 and P300 contribute to the potentials in the case of an error rate of 20 percent, the oddball N200 and P300 are not sufficient to explain the reported potentials.

17.8   Ocular Artifacts

In the reported experiments, subjects look in the middle of the two progress bars, awaiting the central *GO* to press the key corresponding to the desired bar. After the feedback, the subjects become aware of the correct or erroneous response and they will shift their gaze to the side of the progress bar that has just been filled, so that there is a gaze shift in every single trial. Nevertheless, it is possible that the subjects concentrate upon the side of the progress bar they want to complete. After an erroneous trial, they will shift their gaze to the other side, so that the gaze shift could be present in erroneous trials only. The statistical classifier could therefore pick those gaze shifts since several prototypes per class were used.

To demonstrate that there is no systematical influence of gaze shifts on the presented ErrP as well as on classification results, we have calculated the different averages of the single trials with respect to the side of the progress bar that was intended to be completed: left error, right error, left correct, right correct. Figure 17.4 shows these four averages at channel Cz. The top left graph shows the average of erroneous single trials when the left progress bar was selected for the four subjects and the average of them. The top right graph shows the average of erroneous single trials with respect to the right bar. The bottom left and right graph show the average of correct trials with respect to the left and right progress bar, respectively.

The left and right erroneous averages as well as the left and right correct averages are very similar whereas the left erroneous and correct as well as the right erroneous and correct are very different. So it appears that there is no systematical influence of gaze shifts on the reported potentials.

Eye blinks are another potential source of artifacts. Indeed, it is conceivable that subjects may blink more frequently after one of the two conditions, and so the classifier could partly rely on eye blinks to discriminate error and correct trials. However, the scalp topographies of figure 17.3 show that the three ErrP components do not have a front focus, which would be expected in blink-related potentials. So, as for the gaze shifts, it appears that there is no systematical influence of eye blinks on the reported results.

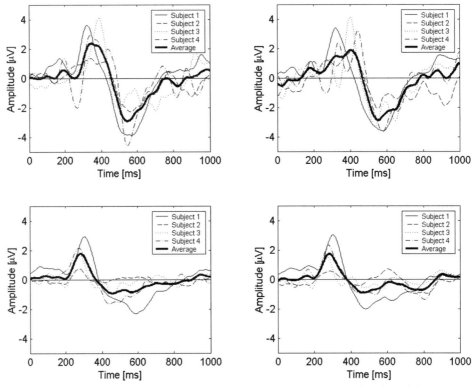

Figure 17.4 Averages of the single trials at channel Cz with respect to the side of the progress bar that was intended to be completed for the four subjects and the average of them. There are four cases: erroneous trials when the left bar was selected (top left), erroneous trials with the right bar (top right), correct trials with the left bar (bottom left), and correct trials with the right bar (bottom right). The left and right erroneous averages as well as the left and right correct averages are very similar, whereas the left erroneous and correct as well as the right erroneous and correct are very different. This probably excludes any artifacts due to gaze shifts.

17.9   Discussion

In this study we have reported first results on the detection of the neural correlate of error awareness for improving the performance and reliability of BCI. In particular, we have found what seems to be a new kind of error-related potential elicited in reaction to an erroneous recognition of the subject's intention. An important difference between response ErrP, feedback ErrP, and observation ErrP on one side and the reported interaction ErrP on the other side is that the former involve a stimulus from the system for every single trial whereas the latter involve a choice of a long-term goal made by the subjects themselves (choice of the progress bar). More importantly, we have shown the feasibility of detecting single-trial erroneous responses of the interface that lead to significant improvements of the information transfer rate of a BCI even though these improvements are theoretical. Indeed, the introduction of an automatic response rejection strongly interferes with the BCI. The user needs to process additional information that induces higher workload and may considerably slow down the interaction. These issues will be investigated when running online BCI experiments integrating automatic error detection.

Given the promising results obtained in a simulated human-robot interaction, we are working on the actual integration of ErrP detection into our BCI system. In parallel, we are exploring how to increase the recognition rate of single-trial erroneous and correct responses. A basic issue here is to find what kind of feedback elicits the strongest "interaction ErrP." The feedback can be of very different nature—visual, auditory, somatosensory, or even a mix of these different types. More importantly, we will need to focus on alternative methods to exploit at best the current "interaction ErrP." In this respect, Grave de Peralta Menendez et al. (2004) have recently developed a technique that estimates the so-called local field potentials (i.e., the synchronous activity of a small neuronal population) in the whole human brain from scalp EEG. Furthermore, recent results show significant improvements in the classification of bimanual motor tasks using estimated local field potentials (LFP) with respect to scalp EEG (Grave de Peralta Menendez et al. (2005b)). Consequently, we plan to use this method to best discriminate erroneous and correct responses of the interface. As a matter of fact, a key issue for the success in the above-mentioned study was the selection of those relevant voxels inside the brain whose estimated LFP were most discriminant. It turns out that the sources of the ErrP seem to be very well localized into the anterior cingulate cortex and thus we may well expect a significant improvement in recognition rates by focusing on the LFP estimated in this specific brain area.

More generally, the work described here suggests that it could be possible to recognize in real time high-level cognitive and emotional states from EEG (as opposed, and in addition, to motor commands) such as alarm, fatigue, frustration, confusion, or attention that are crucial for an effective and purposeful interaction. Indeed, the rapid recognition of these states will lead to truly adaptive interfaces that customize dynamically in response to changes of the cognitive and emotional/affective states of the user.

Acknowledgments

This work is supported by the Swiss National Science Foundation NCCR "IM2" and by the European IST Programme FET Project FP6-003758. This chapter reflects only the authors' views and funding agencies are not liable for any use that may be made of the information contained herein.

Notes

E-mail for correspondence: jose.millan@idiap.ch

18   Adaptation in Brain-Computer Interfaces

José del R. Millán and Anna Buttfield
IDIAP Research Institute
1920 Martigny, Switzerland

*Ecole Polytechnique Fédérale de
Lausanne (EPFL), Switzerland*

Carmen Vidaurre and Rafael Cabeza
Department of Electrical and Electronic Engineering
Public University of Navarre
Pamplona, Spain

Matthias Krauledat, Benjamin Blankertz, and Klaus-Robert Müller
Fraunhofer–Institute FIRST
Intelligent Data Analysis Group (IDA)
Kekuléstr. 7, 12489 Berlin, Germany

*Technical University Berlin
Str. des 17. Juni 135
10 623 Berlin, Germany*

Alois Schlögl and Gert Pfurtscheller
Graz University of Technology
Graz, Austria

Pradeep Shenoy and Rajesh P. N. Rao
Computer Science Department
University of Washington
Seattle, USA

18.1   Abstract

One major challenge in brain-computer interface (BCI) research is to cope with the inherent nonstationarity of the recorded brain signals caused by changes in the subject's brain processes during an experiment. Online adaptation of the classifier embedded in the BCI is a possible way of tackling this issue. In this chapter, we investigate the effect of adaptation on the performance of the classifier embedded in three different BCI systems, all of them based on noninvasive electroencephalogram (EEG) signals. Through this adaptation we aim to keep the classifier constantly tuned to the EEG signals it receives in the current session. Although the experimental results reported here show the benefits of online adaptation, some questions still need to be addressed. The chapter ends discussing some of these open issues.

18.2   Introduction

One major challenge in brain-computer interface (BCI) research is coping with the inherent nonstationarity of the recorded brain signals caused by changes in the subject's brain processes during an experiment. The distribution of electrical brain signals varies between BCI sessions and within individual sessions due to a number of factors including changes in background brain activity, fatigue and concentration levels, and intentional change of mental strategy by the subject. This means that a classifier trained on past EEG data probably will not be optimal for following sessions. Even with a subject who has developed a high degree of control of the EEG, there are variations in the EEG signals over a session. In a subject who is first learning to use the BCI, these variations are going to be more pronounced as the subject has not yet learned to generate stable EEG signals.

The need for adaptation in BCI has been recognized for some time (Millán (2002); Wolpaw et al. (2002)); however, little research has been published in this area (Buttfield et al. (2006); Millán (2004); Shenoy et al. (2006); Vidaurre et al. (2006)). In this chapter, we investigate the effect of adaptation on the performance of the classifier embedded in three different BCI systems, all of them based on noninvasive electroencephalogram (EEG) signals. Through this adaptation we aim to keep the classifier constantly tuned to the EEG signals it receives in the current session. In performing online adaptation (i.e., while the subject is interacting with the BCI and receiving feedback), we are limited in both time and computing resources. The BCI system classifies the incoming signals in real time, and we do not want to reduce the rate at which we can sample data and make decisions by using an adaptation strategy that takes too much time. So in most cases with online learning, we will use each data sample only once and in chronological order, since we adapt the classifier based on each new sample as it is presented and then discard the sample. This is in contrast to techniques such as stochastic gradient descent, which also takes samples individually but is not limited to taking samples in order and can reuse samples as many times as necessary for convergence. A range of techniques has been developed to address the problem of online learning (Saad (1998)).

During initial training, we know what class the subject is trying to generate at all times, so we can use supervised methods to adapt the classifier at this stage. The same techniques could be applied during ongoing use (where we don't know the exact intention of the subject) as a periodic recalibration step. In either case, the goal is to adapt the classifier to compensate for the changes in the signal between sessions, and then track the signals as they vary throughout the session.

In this chapter, we first examine data recorded during a text spelling experiment. For this offline study, we propose several adaptive classification schemes and compare their performances. An interesting result of this study is that most sources of nonstationarity seem to be eliminated by the feature extraction method such that only slight, or even no, adaptivity is needed. Second, we suggest an approach to adapt online the classifier embedded into a cue-based BCI. In this online study, we explore different methods to tune a classifier based on discriminant analysis. A large comparative study shows that subjects using an online adaptive classifier outperform those who do not. Finally, the third study investigates online adaptation for asynchronous BCI based on stochastic gradient descent. We discuss online experiments where the subject performed three mental tasks to mentally control a simulated wheelchair. Experimental results show the feasibility and benefits of the approach. A significant result is that online adaptation makes it possible to complete the task from the very first trial.

18.3   Adaptation in CSP-Based BCI Systems

Matthias Krauledat, Pradeep Shenoy, Benjamin Blankertz, Rajesh P. N. Rao, Klaus-Robert Müller.

18.3.1   Experimental Setup

We investigate data from a study of three subjects using the BBCI system with visual feedback. The BBCI system was developed by Fraunhofer FIRST in cooperation with the Department of Neurology of the Charité University Medicine Berlin (see also chapter 5). For the translation of brain activity into device commands, we use features reflecting changes of ongoing bandpower in subject-specific topographical patterns and subject-specific frequency bands. These event-related (de)synchronization (ERD/ERS) phenomena of sensorimotor rhythms (cf. Pfurtscheller and Lopes da Silva (1999)) are well-studied and consistently reproducible features in EEG recordings, and are used in a number of BCI systems (e.g., Guger et al. (2000); Dornhege et al. (2004a)).

We recorded data from three subjects, of which one subject was a naive BCI user and the other two subjects had some previous experience. The experiments consisted of two parts: a calibration measurement and a feedback period. In the calibration measurement, visual stimuli L, R (for imagined left and right hand movement), and F (for imagined foot movement) were presented to the subject. Based on recorded data from this measurement, the parameters of a subject-specific translation algorithm were estimated (semiautomatically): selection of two of the three imagery classes and frequency bands showing best discriminability, common spatial pattern (CSP) analysis (Guger et al. (2000)) and selection of CSP filters, and calculation of a linear separation between bandpower values in the surrogate CSP channels of the two selected classes by linear discriminant analysis (LDA). Details can be found in chapter 5 and Blankertz et al. (2005).

The translation of ongoing EEG during the feedback period into a real-valued control signal then proceeded as follows: EEG signals were acquired from 64 channels on the scalp surface, at a sampling frequency of 100 Hz and bandpass-filtered to a specifically selected frequency band. The common spatial filters, calculated individually from the calibration data, were then applied. A measure of instantaneous bandpower in each of the surrogate

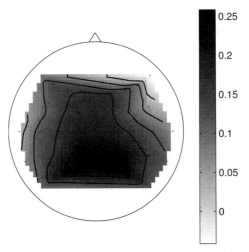

Figure 18.1   This figure shows the shift in the power of the selected frequency band in terms of r-values in one subject. Positive values indicate increased bandpower in the selected frequency band in the calibration measurement compared to the feedback session.

CSP channels was estimated by calculating the log-variance in sliding windows of 750-ms length. Finally, these values were linearly weighted by the LDA classifier generated from the initial calibration session. The resulting real number was used to move a cursor horizontally on the screen.

18.3.2   Lessons Learned from an Earlier Study

In our earlier BBCI feedback experiments (Blankertz et al. (2005)), we encountered in many cases a strong shift in the features from training to feedback sessions as the major detrimental influence on the performance of the classifier. Accordingly, we introduced an adaptation of the classifier's bias as a standard tool in our system. To investigate the cause of this shift in data distributions, we compared the brain activity during calibration measurement versus feedback situation using the biserial correlation coefficient r, which was calculated between bandpower values of each channel. The topography of one representative subject shown in figure 18.1 suggests that in the former case a strong parietal α rhythm (idle rhythm of the visual cortex) is present due to the decreased visual input during the calibration measurement, while that rhythm activity is decreased in online operation due to the increased demand for visual processing (Shenoy et al. (2006)).

18.3.3   Mental Typewriter Feedback

Since the mental engagement with an application is one additional possible source of non-stationarity, we believe that the investigation of nonstationarity issues is most interesting during the control of real applications. Therefore, we chose a mental typewriter application that the subjects used for free spelling. Furthermore, this application has the benefit that even in a free-operation mode it is possible to assign labels (i.e., subject had intended to

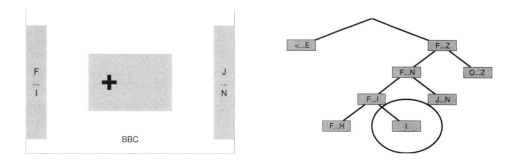

Figure 18.2 The figure on the left is a screenshot of the feedback that was given to the subjects. The position of the cross was controlled by the classification output of the current EEG signal. By moving the cross into the right or left box, the respective set of letters was selected. To complete the acronym *BBCI*, the subject would try to select the left box, since the letter *I* is associated with it. A unique series of decisions (right–left–left–right) leads to the selection of this letter; this corresponds to the binary decision tree shown in the right figure.

move the cursor left or right) to ongoing EEG in an a posteriori fashion: After the correct completion of a word, one can decide for preceding trials the direction in which the subject was trying to move the cursor. This also applies if the intended word is not known to the experimenter beforehand.

There are various ways in which a one-dimensional continuous output of a BCI can be used to enter text (e.g., Birbaumer et al. (1999); Wolpaw et al. (2000b); Obermaier et al. (2003); Millán et al. (2004b)). The basis for our mental typewriter is a continuous movement of the cursor in the horizontal direction. We use a "rate-controlled" scenario, that is, at the beginning of each trial, the cursor is placed in a deactivated mode in the middle of the screen. Every 40 ms, the current classifier output is added to the position of the cursor, thus moving it left or right. The feedback enables the subjects to type letter by letter on the basis of binary choices. The alphabet is divided into two contiguous sets of letters with approximately equal probability of occurrence in the German language. The first and last letter of each division appear in a rectangle on the left and right end of the computer screen; see figure 18.2. By moving the cursor into one of the targets, the subjects can choose the set of letters containing the one they wish to type. The chosen set is then divided into smaller sets, until a single letter is selected. For correction purposes, one further symbol ($<$) for deleting one letter is added to the alphabet. In the case of failing to hit the correct letter, the subject can then try to select this deletion symbol to erase the erroneous letter. Note that after an error of only one binary choice, it is impossible for the subject to get back to the node of the decision tree containing the correct letter. Thus, a wrong letter will be selected regardless of the next decisions. In our experiments, subjects often used this period to relax or stretch. This period of the experiment, however, does not contribute to the relearning schemes, since it does not contain useful information about the intended task.

18.3.3.1   *Labeling Data from Online Feedback*

The subjects were instructed to use the mental typewriter interface to write error-free sentences over a period of 30 minutes. We recorded the data and assigned labels a posteriori to the binary choices (trials), depending on the desired outcome of the letter.

Since we presented feedback in asynchronous mode (i.e., starting and end point of each trial were not given at a fixed rate by the application, but were based solely on the output of the classifier), the lengths of the trials range from less than one second up to tens of seconds. For this analysis, we take into account only the last 750 ms before the completion of the trial.

18.3.4   Adaptation Algorithms

The adaptive classification methods investigated are

ORIG: This is the unmodified classifier trained on data from the calibration session, and serves as a baseline.

REBIAS: We use the continuous output of the unmodified classifier and *shift* the output by an amount that would minimize the error on the labeled feedback data.

RETRAIN: We use the features as chosen from the offline scenario, but retrain the LDA classifier to choose the hyperplane that minimizes the error on labeled feedback data.

RECSP: We completely ignore the offline training data, and perform CSP feature selection and classification training solely on the feedback data.

These schemes are listed in increasing order of change to the classifier. Note that RETRAIN also includes the choice of a bias as in REBIAS, and RECSP requires the retraining of the hyperplanes as in RETRAIN. In all adaptive methods, we need to make a trade-off: Taking more training samples for retraining gives more stable estimates, but on the other hand it makes the method less adaptive, that is, the policy should be to take as little training samples for retraining as possible but enough to allow estimations with reasonable stability. Here we estimate the number of training samples necessary for retraining separately for each method and each subject.

18.3.5   Results

For validation of the proposed classification schemes, we select for each trial from the feedback experiment a preceding window of specified size for retraining. Using the CSP filters and the classifier from the calibration measurement and these new training trials, we update the classifier and apply it to the current test trial. Then we compare the predicted laterality with the actual labels. Figure 18.3 shows the influence of the number of training trials on the accuracy of each adaptation method. In all methods under investigation, the error rate decreases with the used amount of training data. The method RECSP, however, does not produce satisfactory results when used with less than twenty training samples per class. With more samples, the curve stabilizes at a low error rate for one subject, while

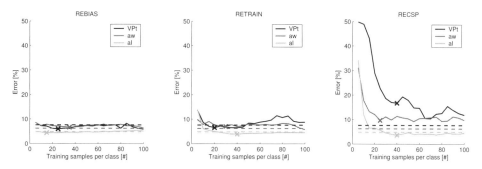

Figure 18.3 The solid lines show the dependency of each algorithm on the number of training samples. For each subject, a sliding window containing the indicated amount of training samples per class (x-axis) was used for adaptation in the recording of the feedback session, and the resulting classifier was applied to the current sample. The average classification error on the test samples is shown on the y-axis in %, and the position of the optimal adaptation window is marked with a cross. The dashed horizontal lines indicate the respective errors of the ORIG classifier, applied to all samples of the feedback session.

Table 18.1 Validation errors for different adaptation methods, evaluated with a sliding window with an individually chosen number of training trials. The error rates are given in percent. The number in brackets denotes the optimal window size (trials per class) for each subject under each method. Only the two numbers printed in bold differ significantly from the ORIG classifier.

Subject	ORIG	REBIAS		RETRAIN		RECSP	
al	4.9	4.4	(15)	3.9	(40)	3.6	(40)
aw	6.2	6.6	(35)	7.0	(30)	**9.7**	(25)
VPt	7.6	6.0	(25)	6.6	(20)	**16.7**	(40)
mean	6.2	5.7		5.8		10.0	

remaining far above the baseline of ORIG for the other two subjects. Methods REBIAS and RETRAIN perform more stably, producing a reliable estimation with only a few adaptation trials.

Table 18.1 shows the classification errors of all presented adaptation methods, evaluated for a window size that is optimal in the sense that increasing the window sizes by up to ten trials per class will not decrease the classification error. This window size is also denoted in the table. For subject "al," all suggested adaptation methods show an improvement over the performance of the original classifier, where the gain is increasing with the complexity of the adaptation. However none of these improvements reaches the level of significance (using McNemar's test, with a confidence level of $\alpha = 5\%$; see Fleiss (1981) for details). For subject "aw," the opposite effect can be observed. For the last subject, REBIAS and RETRAIN again show some improvement while RECSP performs poorly. Taking into account that in this analysis the window size for adaptation was chosen a posteriori to fit optimally to the test (i.e., the evaluation is biased in favor of the adaptive methods), one must conclude that *in this data* the original classifier can hardly be outperformed by any relearning method.

18.4   Adaptive Online Discriminant Analysis for Cue-Based BCI

Carmen Vidaurre, Alois Schlögl, Rafael Cabeza, Gert Pfurtscheller.

The top panel of figure 18.4 depicts a block diagram where the adaptation of the classifier embedded into a cue-based BCI can be accomplished in a variety of ways. The adaptation trigger is divided into two parameters: trigger start, or "initial time" ($Tini$ in bottom panel of figure 18.4), and trigger stop. The number of samples acquired between trigger start and trigger stop is called "adaptation window" (N in bottom panel of figure 18.4). In this diagram, the current samples are used to update the classifier. Adaptation starts at initial time and stops after the adaptation window. As shown in figure 18.4, a delay of the updated classifier is introduced to avoid overfitting in the classification of dependent samples. After the delay, the old classifier is replaced by the updated one.

The initial time for the adaptation window $Tini$ is estimated for each trial using an online estimate of the maximum class-separability. This estimate is motivated by and closely related to the mutual information (MI) (Schlögl et al. (2003)) because, unlike the error rate, it also takes into account the magnitude of the output. The online estimation of maximum class-separability, $\widehat{\mathbf{MI}}_t$, is obtained using a moving average algorithm:

$$\widehat{\mathbf{MI}}_t = \mathbf{mi} \cdot UC_{tini} + \widehat{\mathbf{MI}}_{t-1} \cdot (1 - UC_{tini}) \tag{18.1}$$

$$Tini = t|_{max(\widehat{\mathbf{MI}}_t)} \tag{18.2}$$

where $\mathbf{mi}$ is the output of the classifier multiplied by the class label of the current trial, and UC_{tini} is an update coefficient, the speed of adaptation of mutual information. The time when the maximum of $\widehat{\mathbf{MI}}_t$ appears is selected as $Tini$ for the next trial.

The classifier is based on linear discriminant analysis (LDA). In such a classifier, the decision rule for a new sample x is $[w^T \cdot (x - b)]$ and its weight vector $[b, w^T]$ can be estimated online with Kalman filtering. The update equations for Kalman filtering can be summarized as follows:

$$e_k = y_k - H_k \cdot \widehat{w}_{k-1} \tag{18.3}$$

$$H_k = [1,\ x_k^T] \tag{18.4}$$

$$Q_k = H_k \cdot A_{k-1} \cdot H_k^T + v_k \tag{18.5}$$

$$k_k = \frac{A_{k-1} \cdot H_k^T}{Q_k} \tag{18.6}$$

$$\widehat{w}_k = \widehat{w}_{k-1} + k_k \cdot e_k \tag{18.7}$$

$$\tilde{A}_k = A_{k-1} - k_k \cdot H_k \cdot A_{k-1} \tag{18.8}$$

$$A_k = \frac{trace(\tilde{A}_k) \cdot UC}{p} + \tilde{A}_k \tag{18.9}$$

$$v_k = 1 - UC \tag{18.10}$$

where e_k is the one-step prediction error, y_k is the current class label, H_k is the measurement matrix, $\widehat{w}_k$ is the state vector (the estimated weights for LDA), x_k is the current

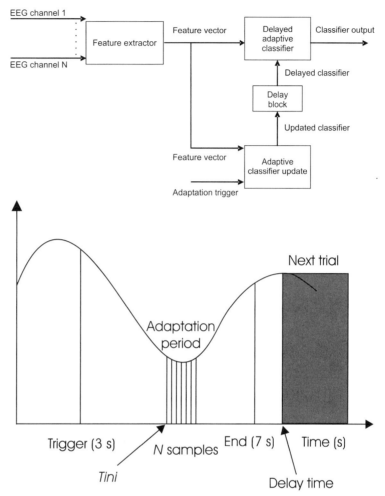

Figure 18.4   Adaptation diagram for a cue-based BCI.

sample vector, Q_k is the estimated prediction variance, $\tilde{A}_k$ is an intermediate value needed to compute A_k (a priori state error correlation matrix), v_k is the variance of the innovation process, k_k is the Kalman gain, p is the number of elements of $\widehat{w}_k$, and UC is the update coefficient (given in samples as it represents the "memory" of the process).

More details about this adaptive online LDA scheme, as well as comparison to other adaptive and nonadaptive approaches based on discriminant analysis, can be found in Vidaurre (2006).

18.4.1   Parameter Initialization and Features

The starting values for A_0 and $\widehat{w}_0$ were computed from data previously recorded from seven subjects in different sessions. As for the parameters UC, N, and UC_{tini}, their values were obtained by optimization with prerecorded data from six naive subjects (different from the previous seven). All these subjects performed feedback experiments of left- versus right-hand motor imagery (Pfurtscheller and Neuper (2001)).

During the optimization procedure, the range of the parameters were 8 to 440,000 for UC, changing in logarithmic scale in 25 steps, 1 to 128 for N, changing in logarithmic scale in 7 steps, and $1/20$ to $1/1024$ for UC_{tini}, changing in logarithmic scale in 9 steps. Each parameter set was analyzed and the set of values that provided the maximum MI was selected for running the online experiments.

The input to the adaptive classifier was a vector containing two types of features, namely adaptive autoregressive parameters (AAR) and logarithmic bandpower estimates (BP). The AAR model had order 3, found by optimization over the group of 6 subjects. To compute the BP features, the EEG signals were bandpass-filtered in the bands 10–12 Hz and 16–24 Hz. The filtered signal was squared and averaged over one second, then the logarithm was taken.

18.4.2 Experimental Results

Experiments were carried out with six able-bodied naive subjects without previous BCI experience, but started with seven subjects. One subject was rejected because he could not avoid producing artifacts during the feedback period. They performed motor imagery experiments using the "basket paradigm" (Krausz et al. (2003)). Each subject conducted three different sessions, with 9 runs per session and 40 trials per run. For each of them, 1,080 trials were available (540 trials for each class). The system was a two-class cue-based and EEG-based BCI and the subjects had to perform motor imagery of the left or right hand depending on the cue. They were asked to maintain their strategy for at least one run.

The recording was made using a g.tec amplifier (Guger Technologies OEG Austria) and Ag/AgCl electrodes. Two bipolar EEG channels were measured 2.5 cm above and below the positions C3 and C4. EEG signals were filtered between 0.5 and 30 Hz and sampled at 125 Hz.

In the basket paradigm, subjects sat on a relaxing chair with armrests. In each trial the subject saw a black screen for a fixed period (3 s). Then two different colored baskets (green and red) appeared at the bottom of the screen as did a little green ball at the top of the screen. At second 4, the ball began to fall downward with constant speed for 3 s. The horizontal position of the ball was directly controlled by the output of the classifier. The duration of each trial was 7 s, with a random interval between trials from 1 to 2 s. The order of the left and right cues was random.

The results were obtained by single trial analysis of the online classification output of each experimental session. As performance measurements, the minimum error rate (ERR) and maximum MI of such analysis were used. The learning process of the subjects was analyzed by comparing sessions. To discover whether the differences between sessions were statistically significant, the difference between the ERR and MI of each pair of sessions was calculated for each subject and compared to 0. One sample parametric and permutation tests were performed on these results. The α-level was corrected for multicomparison with α_e where α_e is the overall type I error fixed to 10 percent, resulting in 3.45 percent. Each population for the statistical analyses had six observations (one from each subject).

Table 18.2 reports the results of the experiments for the six subjects over the three sessions. The last rows give the average and standard error of the mean of each session. Subjects achieved stable results and improved from session 1 to session 3 a 12.04±3.32 [%] in ERR and a 0.290±0.091 [bits] in MI.

Looking at table 18.2, we see that all subjects improved in performance from session 1 to session 2 and from session 2 to session 3. This steady increase is expected when the subject is able to learn, although, as reported in Guger et al. (2001) this does not always occur. We also see that the time point when minimum ERR and maximum MI take place varies from subject to subject and from session to session. This phenomenon could suggest that an updating of the adaptation initial time is a good approach.

The last rows of table 18.2, illustrate the clear improvement of the subjects from session 1 to session 3, demonstrating the success of the feedback. Parametric tests found significant differences among sessions with this system, particularly between sessions 1 and 3, and 2 and 3. The values for the comparison between sessions 1 and 2 are on the limit of the significance level. Permutation tests found significant differences in all the possible combinations. The result is an increase of the maximum MI and a decrease of the minimum ERR, meaning that the data separability improves over time. It is therefore possible to run successful experiments using this combined feature technique and online adaptive LDA cue-based BCI system.

With regard to the time points between sessions, no significant difference was found between them. It is interesting to see that the latest time for ERR was found in the first session; nevertheless, the time difference between sessions is so small (7 ms) that the subjects could not notice it. In the case of time points for MI, they slightly increased over sessions (8 ms), but again the difference was too small to be noticed.

An important issue that arises when studying the topic of adaptive classifiers is whether continuously adaptive classifiers are better than discontinuously adaptive ones. Discontinuously adaptive classifiers have always been used in BCI research, but the decision of when to update them was mainly based on the researcher's experience and the subject's control; therefore, it is not easy to simulate such a system, and online experiments are preferable.

Taking this into account, we performed online experiments with a discontinuously adaptive LDA classifier, using again the basket paradigm. Six new subjects participated in these experiments, all being naive. For these experiments, the general scheme for when to update the discontinuously adaptive classifier was as follows: The first classifier used with every subject was the general classifier. After three runs, the LDA classifier was updated (using these three runs) and used for the next three runs. Then a classifier using the six runs already recorded was calculated for the next three runs. For the next session, the classifier of the session carried out the day before was calculated and used (nine runs). The day after again three, six, and nine runs were used for the calculation of the classifier and so on. However, this scheme could vary depending on the feedback received with the updated classifier. When the feedback was worse and/or the subject felt less control with the new than with the old classifier, the run was stopped and started again with the classifier

Table 18.2 Experimental results, minimum ERR and maximum MI from single trial analysis of each session of subjects S1 to S6.

Subject	Session	ERR[%]	Time[s]	MI[bits]	Time[s]
S1	1	38.06	4.29	0.033	4.23
	2	35.83	4.14	0.046	4.23
	3	22.22	4.00	0.281	4.14
S2	1	32.22	6.40	0.103	6.45
	2	14.72	5.87	0.536	6.64
	3	08.06	6.33	0.786	6.50
S3	1	33.33	5.24	0.094	5.06
	2	31.39	4.66	0.114	4.65
	3	23.33	4.60	0.242	4.33
S4	1	18.61	5.18	0.327	5.25
	2	18.33	5.28	0.433	5.26
	3	15.83	5.39	0.472	5.50
S5	1	31.67	4.73	0.074	4.81
	2	16.94	5.86	0.390	5.90
	3	16.11	5.79	0.491	5.68
S6	1	14.17	6.54	0.519	6.54
	2	11.39	6.15	0.599	5.96
	3	10.28	5.90	0.616	6.74

Mean±SEM					
Session 1		28.01±3.83	5.40±0.37	0.192±0.078	5.39±0.38
Session 2		21.43±4.01	5.33±0.32	0.353±0.092	5.44±0.37
Session 3		15.97±2.50	5.34±0.36	0.481±0.083	5.48±0.44

Session comparison, α-level=3.45%

		Sess.1–2	Sess.1–3	Sess.2–3
Parametric test p-values	ERR	4.20%	**0.75%**	**2.17%**
	MI	3.55%	**1.24%**	**1.16%**
Permutation test p-values	ERR	**1.56%**	**1.56%**	**1.56%**
	MI	**1.56%**	**1.56%**	**1.56%**

Time points in session comparison, α-level=3.45%

		Sess.1–2	Sess.1–3	Sess.2–3
Parametric test p-values	ERR	39.98%	41.15%	46.91%
	MI	42.13%	34.20%	40.63%
Permutation test p-values	ERR	43.75%	42.19%	54.69%
	MI	40.63%	29.69%	42.19%

Table 18.3   Minimum ERR and maximum MI of online and discontinuously adaptive LDA classifiers.

Subject	Session	ERR[%]	MI[bit]	Subject	Session	ERR[%]	MI[bit]
	1	40.00	0.011		1	38.06	0.033
D1	2	21.94	0.315	S13	2	35.83	0.046
	3	18.06	0.349		3	22.22	0.281
	1	21.67	0.321		1	32.22	0.103
D2	2	17.22	0.507	S14	2	14.72	0.536
	3	20.28	0.351		3	08.06	0.786
	1	25.28	0.234		1	33.33	0.094
D3	2	17.22	0.399	S15	2	31.39	0.114
	3	21.11	0.351		3	23.33	0.242
	1	40.56	0.022		1	18.61	0.327
D4	2	37.78	0.046	S16	2	18.33	0.433
	3	35.56	0.041		3	15.83	0.472
	1	41.39	0.021		1	31.67	0.074
D5	2	24.17	0.255	S17	2	16.94	0.390
	3	17.78	0.391		3	16.11	0.491
	1	38.61	0.020		1	14.17	0.519
D6	2	34.44	0.090	S18	2	11.39	0.599
	3	38.61	0.041		3	10.28	0.616
Session		ERR±SEM	MI±SEM	Session		ERR±SEM	MI±SEM
1		34.58±3.56	0.105±0.056	1		28.01±3.83	0.192±0.078
2		25.46±3.57	0.269±0.072	2		23.09±1.96	0.301±0.050
3		25.23±3.80	0.254±0.068	3		15.97±2.50	0.481±0.083

that seemed to provide better feedback. In any case, the minimum number of runs for the calculation of the classifier was three.

The performance of these new six subjects (D1–D6) was then compared to that of the subjects who used the online adaptive LDA classifier (S1–S6). Table 18.3 reports these results.

In table 18.3, we see that subjects D1 and D5 could improve from session to session, D4 improved a bit but with a poor performance. D2 performed similarly in sessions 1 and 3 but best was session 2; the same goes for D6 but this subject had a poor performance. Finally, D3 performed best in session 2, although session 3 was better than session 1. ERR and MI mean values of session 1 for the online adaptive system were better than the ones obtained with the discontinuously adaptive system, but the difference was not significant (see table 18.5); session 2 of both systems were very similar and finally session 3 of the online adaptive system showed better results than the manually adaptive system (see table 18.5). Looking at the mean values of sessions 2 and 3 of the discontinuously adaptive system, both performed similarly (see table 18.4). Contrarily to this trend, sessions 2 and 3 of the online adaptive system were significantly different (see table 18.2).

Table 18.4   P-values from session comparison of discontinuously adaptive LDA classifiers.

P-values, α-level=3.45%

Session comparison		Sess.1–2	Sess.1–3	Sess.2–3
Parametric test	ERR	**1.11%**	4.12%	45.32%
	MI	**0.58%**	3.76%	36.37%
Permutation test	ERR	**1.56%**	**3.13%**	48.44%
	MI	**1.56%**	**1.56%**	32.81%

Table 18.5   P-values from the comparison of discontinuously and online adaptive classifiers in each session.

P-values, α-level=5%

		Sess.1	Sess.2	Sess.3
Parametric test	ERR	11.87%	23.51%	**3.47%**
	MI	19.30%	24.38%	**3.02%**
Permutation test	ERR	11.69%	23.27%	**3.90%**
	MI	19.70%	23.81%	**3.14%**

Table 18.5 shows the difference between discontinuous and online updating of the classifier over three sessions. Independent samples permutation and parametric tests were performed in each session.

Table 18.5 shows that during the first and second sessions subjects performed similarly with the two systems, whereas the last session (which also contains most of the information about the learning process of the subjects) was significantly better with the online adaptive system.

18.5   Online Classifier Adaptation in an Asynchronous BCI

Anna Buttfield, José del R. Millán.

As an initial experiment to test feasibility of supervised online adaptation in the IDIAP BCI (see chapter 6), we have implemented basic gradient descent to adapt the classifier during initial subject training. Previous preliminary work (Millán (2004)) evaluated the advantages of using continued online learning with the basic gradient descent algorithm on a Gaussian classifier. Since then we have been investigating extensions of the basic gradient descent algorithm such as stochastic meta descent (Schraudolph (1999)), which accelerates training by adapting individual learning rates for each parameter of the classifier. BCI experiments at IDIAP generally are performed in an asynchronous or self-paced paradigm—that is, the subjects are not tied to a cue from the system but perform the tasks at their own pace, and the command signals are extracted from spontaneous brain activity.

18.5.1   Statistical Gaussian Classifier

We use a Gaussian classifier to separate the signal into the different classes of mental task. Each class is represented by a number of Gaussian prototypes, typically fewer than four. That is, we assume that the class-conditional probability function of class C_i is a superposition of N_j Gaussian prototypes. We also assume that all classes have equal prior probability. All classes have the same number of prototypes N_p, and for each class each prototype has equal weight $1/N_p$.

Dropping the constant terms, we can define the posterior probability y_c of the class c in terms of the total activation of the classifier (A) and the activation of class c (a_c):

$$A = \sum_{i=1}^{N_c} \sum_{j=1}^{N_p} a_{ij} \tag{18.11}$$

$$a_c = \sum_{j=1}^{N_p} a_{cj} \tag{18.12}$$

$$y_c = \frac{a_c}{A} \tag{18.13}$$

where N_c is the number of classes and a_{ij} is the activation level of the jth prototype of class C_i, with center μ_{ij} and diagonal covariance matrix Σ_i, for a given sample $\mathbf{x}$

$$a_{ij} = \frac{1}{\prod_k \Sigma_{ik}} \exp\left(-\frac{1}{2} \sum_k \frac{(\mathbf{x}_k - \mu_{ijk})^2}{\Sigma_{ik}} \right). \tag{18.14}$$

In this equation, μ_{ijk} is the kth element of the vector μ_{ij}, and Σ_{ik} is the element (k,k) of the diagonal matrix Σ_i. Usually each prototype of each class would have an individual covariance matrix Σ_{ij}, but to reduce the number of parameters, the model uses a single diagonal covariance matrix common to all the prototypes of the same class.

The decision of the classifier for input vector $\mathbf{x}$ is now the class with the highest probability, provided that the probability is above a given threshold; otherwise the result is "unknown."

Training of the classifier starts from an initial model that can be either a previously trained classifier or a new classifier created by estimating the prototype centers with a clustering algorithm. This initial estimate is then improved by stochastic gradient descent to minimize the mean square error given by

$$E = \frac{1}{2} \sum_{i=1}^{N_c} (y_i - t_i)^2 \tag{18.15}$$

where $\mathbf{t}$ is the target vector in the form 1-of-C, that is, if the second of three classes was the desired output, the target vector is (0,1,0).

This optimization is performed on the mean and covariance of each prototype. We calculate the derivative of the error with respect to element l of the mean and the covariances respectively, for prototype p of class c:

$$\frac{\partial E(x)}{\partial \mu_{cpl}} = \frac{a_{cp}}{A} \frac{[x_l - \mu_{cpl}]}{\Sigma_{cl}} \left[(y_c - t_c) - \sum_{i=1}^{N_c} (y_i (y_i - t_i)) \right] \qquad (18.16)$$

$$\frac{\partial E(x)}{\partial \Sigma_{cpl}} = \frac{1}{2} \frac{a_{cp}}{A} \frac{[x_l - \mu_{cpl}]^2 - \Sigma_{cpl}}{(\Sigma_{cl})^2} \left[(y_c - t_c) - \sum_{i=1}^{N_c} (y_i (y_i - t_i)) \right]. \qquad (18.17)$$

The gradient descent update equations are now defined as follows, with learning rates for the centers and covariances α and β, respectively:

$$(\mu_{cpl})_{t+1} = (\mu_{cpl})_t - \alpha \cdot \frac{\partial E(\mathbf{x}_t)}{\partial \mu_{cpl}} \qquad (18.18)$$

$$(\Sigma_{cpl})_{t+1} = (\Sigma_{cpl})_t - \beta \cdot \frac{\partial E(\mathbf{x}_t)}{\partial \Sigma_{cpl}}. \qquad (18.19)$$

At each step, the updates to the covariance matrices are computed individually and then averaged over the prototypes of each class to give Σ_c.

When updating the covariance matrices, it is important to ensure that they never become negative. One way to do this is simply to impose a small positive lower limit on $(\Sigma_{cpl})_{t+1}$. An alternative method is to use exponentiated gradient descent to update the covariances (Kivinen and Warmuth (1995)), which ensures that the covariances are always positive:

$$(\Sigma_{cpl})_{t+1} = (\Sigma_{cpl})_t \cdot \exp\left(-\beta \cdot \frac{\partial E(\mathbf{x}_t)}{\partial \Sigma_{cpl}} \right). \qquad (18.20)$$

18.5.2   Stochastic Meta Descent

Stochastic meta descent (SMD) (Schraudolph (1999)) is an extension of gradient descent that uses adaptive learning rates to accelerate learning. The SMD algorithm is a nonlinear extension of earlier work (Sutton (1992)).

The SMD algorithm is applied to each parameter in the classifier separately (the center and covariance of each Gaussian prototype), and each parameter maintains and adapts an individual learning rate. This is in contrast to basic gradient descent, which uses a single learning rate for all parameters. Thus, the parameters $\boldsymbol{\mu}_{ij}$ and $\boldsymbol{\Sigma}_{ij}$ of prototype j of class i have learning rates $\mathbf{p}_{ij}$ and $\mathbf{q}_{ij}$, respectively; gradient traces $\mathbf{v}_{ij}$ and $\mathbf{w}_{ij}$, respectively; and gradients $(\boldsymbol{\delta\mu}_{ij})_t$ and $(\boldsymbol{\delta\Sigma}_{ij})_t$, respectively. For simplicity, the indices i and j have been dropped from the following equations.

The equation for adapting the Gaussian prototype center $\boldsymbol{\mu}$ with respect to the error function E and input $\mathbf{x}_t$ is

$$\boldsymbol{\mu}_{t+1} = \boldsymbol{\mu}_t + \mathbf{p}_t \cdot (\boldsymbol{\delta\mu})_t, \text{ where } (\boldsymbol{\delta\mu})_t \equiv -\frac{\partial E(\mathbf{x}_t)}{\partial \boldsymbol{\mu}}. \qquad (18.21)$$

This equation is an extension of the gradient descent update rule, since if we replaced the vector of learning rates $\mathbf{p}_t$ with a scalar we have the basic gradient descent update rule. We update the learning rates by exponentiated gradient descent, which allows the learning rates to cover a large range of positive values:

$$\mathbf{p}_t = \mathbf{p}_{t-1} \cdot \exp(\alpha \, (\boldsymbol{\delta}_{\boldsymbol{\mu}})_t \, \mathbf{v}_t). \tag{18.22}$$

In this equation, the term α is the meta-learning rate for the centers. The term $\mathbf{v}_t$ is the gradient trace, which projects forward into time the effect of a change in learning parameter on the variables, and is defined as $\mathbf{v}_t \equiv -\frac{\partial \boldsymbol{\mu}_t}{\partial \ln(\mathbf{p})}$. From this we can derive an iterative update rule:

$$\mathbf{v}_{t+1} = \mathbf{v}_t + \mathbf{p}_t \left((\boldsymbol{\delta}_{\boldsymbol{\mu}})_t - (\mathbf{H}_{\boldsymbol{\mu}})_t \mathbf{v}_t \right) \tag{18.23}$$

where $(\mathbf{H}_{\boldsymbol{\mu}})_t$ is the Hessian matrix of E with respect to $\boldsymbol{\mu}$.

A similar system of equations is derived for the covariance updates. Using linear gradient descent would give us a parallel system of equations to those for the centers. If we choose to use exponentiated gradient descent, we need to derive a new set of equations:

$$\boldsymbol{\Sigma}_{t+1} = \boldsymbol{\Sigma}_t \cdot \exp(\mathbf{q}_t(\boldsymbol{\delta}_{\boldsymbol{\Sigma}})_t), \text{ where } (\boldsymbol{\delta}_{\boldsymbol{\Sigma}})_t \equiv -\frac{\partial E(\mathbf{x_t})}{\partial \boldsymbol{\Sigma}}. \tag{18.24}$$

The learning rate update for the covariance is then

$$\mathbf{q}_t = \mathbf{q}_{t-1} \cdot \exp(\beta \, (\boldsymbol{\delta}_{\boldsymbol{\Sigma}})_t \, \mathbf{w}_t) \tag{18.25}$$

with β being the meta-learning rate for the covariances. The gradient trace $\mathbf{w}$ for the covariance is derived as

$$\mathbf{w_{t+1}} = \exp(\mathbf{q_t}(\boldsymbol{\delta}_{\boldsymbol{\Sigma}})_t) \cdot [\mathbf{w_t} + \boldsymbol{\Sigma}_t \mathbf{q}_t \left((\boldsymbol{\delta}_{\boldsymbol{\Sigma}})_t - (\mathbf{H}_{\boldsymbol{\Sigma}})_t \mathbf{w_t} \right)] \tag{18.26}$$

where $(\mathbf{H}_{\boldsymbol{\Sigma}})_t$ is the Hessian matrix of E with respect to $\boldsymbol{\Sigma}$.

The complicating factor when implementing SMD is the calculation of the Hessians in (18.23) and (18.26). While there is a method of efficiently calculating the product of a Hessian and a vector, this method is extremely cumbersome for a Gaussian classifier. An alternative to using the exact Hessian is to use an approximation such as the Levenberg-Marquardt or outer product approximation. This approximation is based on the properties of the error function, (18.15). The elements of the Hessian with respect to the vector $\boldsymbol{\mu}$, where μ_m and μ_n are the mth and n^{th} elements of $\boldsymbol{\mu}$, can be approximated by

$$\mathbf{H}_{\mu(m,n)} = \frac{\partial^2 E}{\partial \mu_m \partial \mu_n} \approx \sum_k \frac{\partial y_k}{\partial \mu_m} \frac{\partial y_k}{\partial \mu_n}. \tag{18.27}$$

This approximation is valid only for a well trained network, since the elements that it ignores are negligible only on a trained network but not on an untrained network. We further simplify this approximation by neglecting the off-diagonal elements. A similar approximation is obtained for $\mathbf{H}_{\boldsymbol{\Sigma}}$.

18.5.3   Experimental Results

The IDIAP BCI is based on a portable BioSemi acquisition system. The electrode caps contain either 32 or 64 electrodes covering the whole scalp.

The IDIAP BCI uses EEG rhythm modulation as a control signal and operates asynchronously. The subjects are trained to perform three mental tasks while being given feedback on their performance. The system analyzes the EEG signals to distinguish between the tasks, which may include imagination of left and right hand movement, arithmetic operations, rotation of geometrical objects, and language tasks. The most common combination is imagination of left and right hand movement and a language task, specifically a vocabulary search. Classification is performed by calculating the frequency components on sliding half-second windows of a selection of electrodes (in between 8 and 12) over a relevant feature band (typically between 8Hz and 30Hz, with a resolution of 2 Hz), and passing these frequency features to the statistical Gaussian classifier. This system has been used in the past to operate simple computer games, use a virtual keyboard, and navigate a robot through a model house–like environment (Millán et al. (2004b,a)).

The experimental setup that we tested the system on was a computer simulation of driving a wheelchair through a corridor while avoiding obstacles. A key aspect is the combination of the subject's high-level commands with advanced robotics that implement those commands efficiently (Millán et al. (2004a)). The subject was guided by an operator who told the subject which task to attempt to produce as the wheelchair moved through the corridor. In this way the data was labeled with the target classes and the subject was learning to generate the BCI tasks while becoming accustomed to the simulator interface. In this task, samples are not necessarily balanced between classes, and the length of time each class is generated for varies. The more complicated, "real-world" setup also makes it more difficult for the subjects to concentrate on the mental tasks, as they can be distracted by watching the wheelchair and anticipating its movements.

One performance measure used in this task was the time the subject took to steer the wheelchair to the end of the corridor and back again. Times over a number of days are shown in figure 18.5.

We want to compare the online classification results against the offline performance of static classifiers. For these experiments we take an initial classifier, adapt it online throughout the session, and produce the final classifier (which then becomes the initial classifier for the next session). We measure the classification rates of the initial classifier and the final classifier on this session, and compare with the online classification rate. Tables 18.6 and 18.7 show the online classification rates of the classifier, compared to the static initial and final adapted classifiers, in terms of bit rate[1] and correct-error-rejection rates, respectively. The online classification rates are much higher than the static classifiers. Also, in each session the online adaptation produces a final classifier that outperforms the initial classifier. A t-test on the bit rates shows that differences are statistically significant.

Figures 18.6 and 18.7 show the probabilities of each sample for session 4; figure 18.6 is the online classification rate and figure 18.7 is the offline performance of the final classifier. The online classification rates track the EEG signals well, with no clear bias between classes. The final classifier can be seen to perform well on the last part of the session

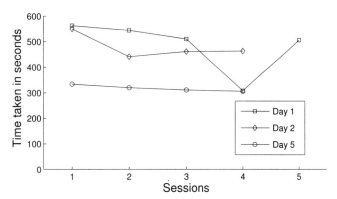

Figure 18.5   Times, in seconds, to navigate the wheelchair to the end of the corridor and back. The wheelchair needs to avoid obstacles along the corridor.

Table 18.6   Classification of four sessions from Day 5—bit rate.

Session	Initial classifier	Online classification	Final classifier
1	0.29	1.44	0.65
2	0.20	1.41	0.67
3	0.14	1.34	0.71
4	0.18	1.34	0.67
Average	0.20 ± 0.06	1.38 ± 0.05	0.67 ± 0.02

Table 18.7   Four sessions from Day 5—percentage of correct, error, and rejected trials.

Session	Initial classifier Cor - Err - Rej	Online classification Cor - Err - Rej	Final classifier Cor - Err - Rej
1	20.1 - 37.5 - 42.3	64.3 - 11.7 - 24.0	40.3 - 26.4 - 33.3
2	26.9 - 45.0 - 28.1	63.9 - 12.2 - 23.8	43.3 - 26.9 - 29.8
3	23.6 - 48.7 - 27.7	62.2 - 13.4 - 24.4	41.0 - 24.2 - 34.8
4	23.9 - 46.3 - 29.8	61.1 - 12.8 - 26.1	41.3 - 26.1 - 32.6
Av. Cor	23.6 ± 3.0	62.9 ± 1.5	41.4 ± 1.3
Av. Err	44.4 ± 5.3	12.5 ± 0.7	25.9 ± 1.2
Av. Rej	32.0 ± 8.0	24.6 ± 1.0	32.6 ± 2.1

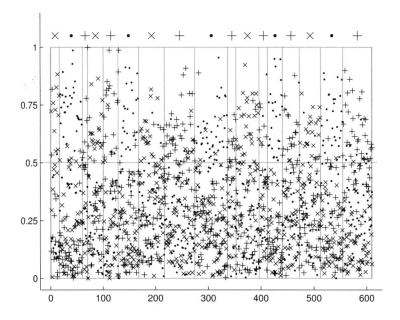

Figure 18.6   Probability of each of the classes ($\times$, $\bullet$, $+$) for each data sample when using online adaptation (session 4 in tables 18.6 and 18.7). The target class is the symbol above the line at probability 1, and points above the threshold (0.5) are decisions by the classifier. This shows the classifier tracking the EEG signals throughout the session.

but less well on the early part of the session. This is consistent with drift in the signal, which means that the final classifier is tuned to the later part of the session but does not classify well on the different signals from the early part of the session.

In all the experiments, the online adaptation seems to be providing consistent feedback to the subject, allowing for predictable responses from the classifier. This can be observed in the consistent online classification rates and the stable time taken to complete the task. Finally, it is worth noting that online adaptation makes it possible to complete the task from the very first trial.

18.6   Discussion

Although the experimental results reported here show the benefits of online adaptation, some questions still need to be addressed. The first of them is how to combine the strengths of each of the approaches explored here for different scenarios. In this respect, a second issue is a better understanding of EEG variation. We believe online classifier adaptation would improve the performance of a BCI because of the high variability in EEG signals, but no systematic study has been done to formally analyze the extent of signal variation

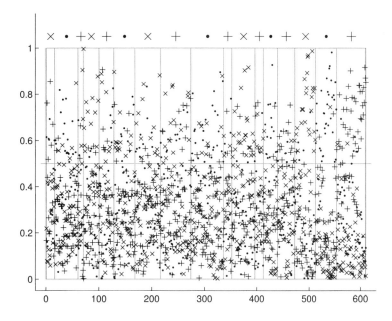

Figure 18.7 Probability of each of the classes ($\times$, $\bullet$, $+$) for each data sample when using the final classifier generated by online adaptation, measured without adaptation (session 4 in tables 18.6 and 18.7). Again, the target class is the symbol above the line at probability 1, and points above the threshold (0.5) are decisions by the classifier. Inspection shows that the classification rate of this static classifier is high toward the end of the session but lower toward the start. This supports the hypothesis that adapting the classifier online tracks drifts in the signal, so the final classifier is tuned to the data of the later part of the session but is not valid for the beginning.

through different stages in a subject's usage of a BCI. Such a study would be helpful in justifying the use of online adaptation and determining whether it is necessary in all cases.

In fact, as shown in section 18.3, adaptive methods such as readjusting bias and angle of the LDA classifier using feedback data improve the classifier, but do not necessarily result in a significant increase of the performance. Note that this by no means indicates nonstationarities were absent in the EEG signals, but it indicates that the BBCI classifier successfully extracted relevant information from sensorimotor areas while filtering out contributions from sources of nonstationary characteristics like the visual cortex. Figure 18.1, which shows an enormous difference between the brain activity during calibration measurement and feedback operation, was calculated from one of the experiments of this study.

Based on the results presented here, one could conjecture that in the ideal case, feature extraction and classification can be successful in extracting a control signal that is not affected by the nonstationarities in the EEG. Nevertheless, experience with other data has shown that change of mental state when turning from the calibration measurement to online operation sometimes needs to be compensated by a robust adaptive method like bias correction or covariate shift compensation (Shenoy et al. (2006); Sugiyama and Müller (2005)).

Finally, the main research issue is adaptation throughout ongoing use, where we don't have explicit information about which is the user's intent. In this situation, we need to develop other methods for online classifier adaptation that are not supervised. Reinforcement learning (Sutton and Barto (1998)) is a framework that could be useful for this situation. The problem that reinforcement learning attempts to address is that of learning when we receive only occasional feedback on how well or poorly we are performing, rather than explicitly being told what the correct response should have been for each sample. That is, we could use whatever partial information we can glean about BCI performance during ongoing use to improve the classifier. In particular, we can gain some partial information by examining the EEG signals or examining how the BCI task is being performed. One approach that might be able to give us some information about the performance of the classifier is the recognition of cognitive error potentials (see chapter 17). Error potentials are the reaction in the subject's brain to a mistake made by the interface. Thus, if an error potential is detected when the classifier makes a wrong classification, we know which class the subject was not attempting to produce, even though we don't know what the actual target was. If we can reliably recognize these error potentials, we know when the classifier has made a mistake in the recognition of the subject's intent, and we can update the classifier based on this information. In this case, we have rapid feedback on whether a classification was erroneous, and we can use this negative feedback to update the classifier. An alternative source of information is contextual information about how well the brain-controlled device is operating, for example, evaluating the quality of the robot's path in a robot navigation problem or noting when the subject deletes letters in a keyboard application. An example of this approach to determining the subject's intent is the mental typewriter application presented in section 18.3, where the labels are currently assigned through an a posteriori analysis of the sequence of decisions. In these situations, we can only make occasional guesses at the true intention of the subject, so we have only occasional feedback on how well or poorly the classifier is performing, which is the type of situation addressed by reinforcement learning.

Acknowledgments

Matthias Krauledat, Pradeep Shenoy, Benjamin Blankertz, Rajesh P. N. Rao and Klaus-Robert Müller thank G. Dornhege, A. Schwaighofer, and G. Curio for helpful discussions.

José del R. Millán and Anna Buttfield[1,2]'s work is supported by the Swiss National Science Foundation NCCR "IM2," by the European IST Programme FET Project FP6-003758, and by the European Network of Excellence "PASCAL," Author Carmen Vidaurre was supported by the Spanish Ministry of Education and Culture (Grant AP-2000-4673). Authors Alois Schlögl and Gerd Pfurtscheller were supported by the Austrian Fonds zur Förderung der Wissenschaftlichen Forschung project 16326-BO2. The work of Matthias Krauledat, Benjamin Blankertz, and Klaus-Robert Müller was supported in part by grants of the Bundesministerium für Bildung und Forschung (BMBF), FKZ 01 IBE 01A/B, by the Deutsche Forschungsgemeinschaft (DFG), FOR 375/B1, and MU 987/1-1, and by the IST Programme of the European Community, under the PASCAL Network of Excellence, IST-2002-506778. Rajesh P. N. Rao was supported by NSF grant 130705 and the Packard Foundation. This publication reflects only the authors' views.

Notes

E-mail for correspondence: jose.millan@idiap.ch

(1)   The expression that estimates the bit rate takes into account the rejection rates of the classifier as described in Millán et al. (2004a).

19   Evaluation Criteria for BCI Research

Alois Schlögl
Institute for Human-Computer Interfaces
University of Technology Graz
Krenngasse 37, A-8010 Graz

Julien Kronegg
Computer Vision and Multimedia Laboratory
Computer Science Department
University of Geneva, Switzerland

Jane E. Huggins
Department of Physical Medicine and Rehabilitation and Biomedical Engineering
University of Michigan
Ann Arbor, USA

Steve G. Mason
Neil Squire Society
220 2250 Boundary Rd.
Burnaby, BC Canada

19.1   Abstract

To analyze the performance of BCI systems, some evaluation criteria must be applied. The most popular is accuracy or error rate. Because of some strict prerequisites, accuracy is not always a suitable criterion, and other evaluation criteria have been proposed. This chapter provides an overview of evaluation criteria used in BCI research. An example from the BCI Competition 2005 is used to display results using different criteria.

Within this chapter, evaluation criteria for BCI systems with more than two classes are presented, criteria for evaluating discrete and continuous output are included, and the problem of evaluating self-paced BCI operation is addressed. Special emphasis is put on discussing different methods for calculating the information transfer rate. Finally, a criterion for taking into account the response time is suggested.

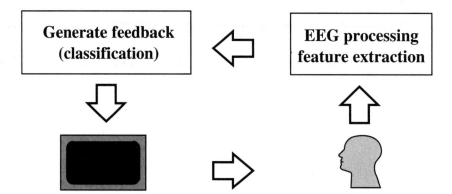

Figure 19.1   Scheme of a BCI. A typical BCI consists of the data acquisition, the feature extraction, a classification system for combining the feature and generating the feedback, the actual presentation of the feedback, and a (ideally motivated and cooperating) subject. The subjects receive real-time feedback to train their own strategy for generating repeatable patterns.

19.2   Introduction

At present, the communication capacity (i.e., information tranfer rate) of current BCI systems is not sufficient for many real-world applications. To increase the information transfer rate, possible improvements in signal processing and classification must be investigated and compared. It is reasonable to assume that the quest for the best methods requires efficient evaluation criteria.

The performance of BCI systems can be influenced by a large variety of methodological factors: experimental paradigms and setups that include trial-based (system-paced) or asynchronous (self-paced) modes of interaction; the type and number of EEG features (e.g., spectral parameters, slow cortical potentials, spatiotemporal parameters, nonlinear features); and the type of classifier (e.g., linear and quadratic discriminant analysis, support vector machines, neural networks, or a simple threshold detection) and the target application as well as the feedback presentation. BCI systems can consist of almost any arbitrary combination of these methods. To compare different BCI systems and approaches, consistent evaluation criteria are necessary.

Which criterion to use depends on what is being evaluated. The highest-level evaluation studies the operation of useful BCI applications, like the evaluation of a spelling device or a controlled wheelchair. Here, application-specific tests must be applied. For example, the operation of a spelling device could be assessed by "letters per minute." However, a criterion of "letters per minute" has a different meaning depending on whether the speller includes word prediction.

The evaluation of BCI systems is also complicated by the fact that most systems include a feedback loop (see figure 19.1). Each component within this feedback loop can fail. If one component fails (e.g., bad EEG features, bad classifier, low subject motivation, or poor feedback presentation), the whole BCI system may not work. If this happens, it can be very difficult to determine which component caused the problem. To address these

Class	Y	N
Y	Hits (TP)	Misses (FN)
N	FA (FP)	CR (TN)

Table 19.1 Example of a confusion matrix with two states. If a two-class problem consists of one active and one passive state, the terms *true positives* (TP), *false negatives* (FN), *false positives* (FP), and *true negative* (TN) are used for *hits*, *misses*, *false activation* (FA), and *correct rejection* (CR), respectively.

Class	1	2	3	4	Total
1	73	17	7	8	105
2	10	87	3	5	105
3	6	13	74	12	105
4	2	4	7	92	105
Total	91	121	91	117	420

Table 19.2 Example of a Confusion matrix for $M = 4$ classes. The result is one submission in the BCI Competition 2005 for Data Set IIIa. More results are available in table 19.3.

difficulties, online and offline analysis must be performed. All of these analyses use criteria for measuring the performance.

In this chapter, an overview of evaluation criteria used in BCI research is presented and discussed. Three methods of estimating the information transfer are presented. Cue-paced BCI data from the last BCI competition is used as an example. The shortcomings of the most frequently used evaluation criterion—the error rate or accuracy—is discussed and alternative criteria presented. Evaluation criteria of the response speed of BCIs and the evaluation of asynchronous BCI data are presented, too. Note, the BioSig project at http://biosig.sf.net provides a software library that contains the software implementation of the evaluation criteria presented below.

19.3 The Confusion Matrix

For a M-class classification problem, the results are best described by a confusion matrix. The confusion matrix shows the relationship between the output classes the user intended (the true classes) and the actual output of the classifier (i.e., the predicted class). Two examples of confusion matrices are shown in tables 19.1 and 19.2. If a two-class problem consists of one active and one passive (no control) state, the terms *true positives* (TP), *false negatives* (FN), *false positives* (FP), and *true negative* (TN) are used for *hits*, *misses*, *false activation* (FA), and *correct rejection* (CR), respectively (see table 19.1). If the classes all represent intentional control states, for example, *1* and *2*, *left* and *right*, or more than two classes, no special denotation is used for the fields of the confusion matrix (see table 19.2).

The elements n_{ij} in the confusion matrix indicate how many samples of class i have been predicted as class j. Accordingly, the diagonal elements n_{ii} represent the number of correctly classified samples. The off-diagonal n_{ij} represent how many samples of class i have been incorrectly classified as class j. The total number of samples is $N = \sum_{i=1}^{M} \sum_{j=1}^{M} n_{ij}$. Asymmetrical confusion matrices can be used to reveal a biased classifier. Despite its advantages, the confusion matrices are rarely presented; usually some summary statistic (see section 19.4) is calculated and presented. Partly, this can be explained by the difficulty of comparing two confusion matrices.

19.4   Classification Accuracy and Error Rate

The classification accuracy (ACC) or the error rate (ERR = 1-ACC) are the most widely used evaluation criteria in BCI research. Nine out of fourteen datasets in the BCI competitions 2003 and 2005 used the accuracy or the error rate as the evaluation criterion. One possible reason for its popularity is that it can be very easily calculated and interpreted.

However, it is important to note that the accuracy of a trivial (random) classifier is already $100\%/M$, (e.g., for $M = 2$ classes 50% are correct just by chance). If the ACC is smaller than this limit, an error occurred and further exploration is required. On the other hand, the maximum accuracy can never exceed 100%. Sometimes, this could be a disadvantage, especially when two classification systems should be compared and both provide a result close to 100%.

$$ACC = p_0 = \frac{\sum_{i=1}^{M} n_{ii}}{N} \tag{19.1}$$

The ACC also can be derived from the confusion matrix and has been called the overall accuracy. Some limitations of accuracy as evaluation criterion are based on the facts that (1) the off-diagonal values of the confusion matrix are not considered and (2) classification accuracy of less frequent classes have smaller weight.

19.5   Cohen's Kappa Coefficient

Cohen's kappa coefficient κ addresses several of the critiques on the accuracy measure. The calculation of κ uses the *overall agreement* $p_0 = ACC$, which is equal to the classification accuracy, and the *chance agreement* p_e

$$p_e = \frac{\sum_{i=1}^{M} n_{:i} n_{i:}}{N^2} \tag{19.2}$$

with $n_{\cdot i}$ and $n_{i\cdot}$ are the sum of the ith column and the ith row, respectively. Note, $n_{\cdot i}/N$ and $n_{i\cdot}/N$ are the a posteriori and a priori probability. Then, the estimate of the kappa coefficient κ is

$$\kappa = \frac{p_0 - p_e}{1 - p_e} \tag{19.3}$$

and its standard error $\sigma_e(\kappa)$ is obtained by

$$\sigma_e(\kappa) = \frac{\sqrt{(p_0 + p_e^2 - \sum_{i=1}^{M} [n_{\cdot i} n_{i\cdot}(n_{\cdot i} + n_{i\cdot})]/N^3)}}{(1 - p_e)\sqrt{N}}. \tag{19.4}$$

The kappa coefficient is zero if the predicted classes show no correlation with the actual classes. A kappa coefficient of 1 indicates perfect classification. Kappa values smaller than zero indicate that the classifier suggests a different assignment between output and the true classes.

Sometimes, the specific accuracy $specACC$ for each class i is calculated, too.

$$specACC_i = \frac{2n_{ii}}{n_{i\cdot} + n_{\cdot i}} \tag{19.5}$$

For more details on Cohen's kappa coefficient, see also Cohen (1960); Bortz and Lienert (1998); Kraemer (1982). Cohen's kappa coefficient addresses several of the criticisms of the accuracy measure: (1) it considers the distribution of the wrong classifications (i.e., the off-diagonal elements of the confusion matrix); (2) the frequency of occurrence is normalized for each class—classes with less samples get the same weight as classes with many samples; and (3) the standard error of the kappa coefficient easily can be used for comparing whether the results of distinct classification systems have statistically significant differences.

If the actual (or the predicated) number of samples are equally distributed across classes, the chance expected agreement is $p_e = 1/M$, and the Kappa coefficient and the accuracy are related by the following equalities:

$$\kappa = \frac{p_0 - p_e}{1 - p_e} = \frac{Mp_0 - 1}{M - 1} \tag{19.6}$$

$$ACC = p_0 = \frac{M\kappa - \kappa + 1}{M}. \tag{19.7}$$

The kappa coefficient has been used in Schlögl et al. (2005) and was also the evaluation criterion for dataset IIIa of the BCI competition 2005 (BCI Competition III (2005a)). The result of one submission is shown in figure 19.3; the kappa coefficient was calculated for every point in time across all trials of the test set.

19.6   Mutual Information of a Discrete Output

One of the ultimate goals of a BCI system is to provide an additional communication channel from the subjects' brains to their environment. Therefore, the communication theory of Shannon and Weaver (1949) can be applied directly to quantify the information transfer. Based on this idea, several attempts have been suggested.

Farwell and Donchin (1988) calculated the information transfer for M classes as

$$I = \log_2 (M). \tag{19.8}$$

For example, a two-class system can provide one bit, a four-class system can provide two bits. This information rate assumes an error-free system; it provides an upper limit for a discrete M-class system. Therefore, this suggestion is not useful for comparing different BCI systems.

Based on Pierce (1980), Wolpaw et al. (2000a) suggested the following formula for calculating the information transfer rate for M classes and $ACC = p_0$:

$$B[bits] = \log_2 (M) + p_0 \cdot \log_2 (p_0) + (1 - p_0) \log_2 (1 - p_0)/(M - 1). \tag{19.9}$$

The formula holds under the following conditions:

(1) M selections (classes) are possible,
(2)   each class has the same probability,
(3)   the specific accuracy (see section 19.4) is the same for each class, and
(4)   each undesired selection must have the same probability of selection.

Often these assumptions are not fulfilled. In the example in table 19.2, the conditions (3) and (4) are not fulfilled.

The information transfer rate can also be derived from the confusion matrix, which provides a transition matrix of a communication channel between the input X and the output Y. The random variable X models the user intention and can take M possible values according to the selected tasks. The random variable Y models the classifier output and can take M possible values, or $M+1$ if the clasifier supports trial rejection. The entropy $H(X)$ of a discrete random variable is defined as

$$H(X) = - \sum_{j=1}^{M} p(x_j) \cdot log_2(p(x_j)). \tag{19.10}$$

Nykopp (2001) derived the information transfer for a general confusion matrix:

$$I(X;Y) = H(Y) - H(Y \mid X) \tag{19.11}$$

$$H(Y) = - \sum_{j=1}^{M} p(y_j) \cdot log_2(p(y_j)) \tag{19.12}$$

with

$$p(y_j) = \sum_{1=1}^{M} p(x_i) \cdot p(y_j \mid x_i) \tag{19.13}$$

$$H(Y \mid X) = -\sum_{i=1}^{M} \sum_{j=1}^{M} p(x_i) \cdot p(y_j \mid x_i) \cdot log_2(p(y_j \mid x_i)) \tag{19.14}$$

$$I(X;Y) = \sum_{i=1}^{M} \sum_{j=1}^{M} p(x_i) \cdot p(y_j \mid x_i) \cdot log_2(p(y_j \mid x_i)) - \sum_{j=1}^{M} p(y_j) \cdot log_2(p(y_j)) \tag{19.15}$$

where $I(X;Y)$ is the mutual information, $p(x_i)$ is the a priori probability for class x_i, and $p(y_j \mid x_i)$ is the probability to classify x_i as y_j.

While the definition in (19.15) is more precise than (19.9), it is not frequently used in practice because it requires the confusion matrix and the a priori class probabilities. The prerequisites for (19.9) say $p(x_i) = 1/M$ (classes have the same a priori probability), $p(y_i \mid x_i) = p_0$ (accuracy for each class is equal), and for $j \neq i$ is $p(y_j \mid x_i) = (1 - p_0)/(M - 1)$ (each undesired selection is equally distributed); accordingly, the entropies are $H(Y) = log_2(M)$ and

$$H(Y \mid X) = -\sum_{i=1}^{M} 1/M [p_0 \cdot log_2(p_0) + \sum_{j \neq i} (1 - p_0)/(M - 1) \cdot log_2((1 - p_0)/(M - 1))].$$

It follows that $I(X;Y) = log_2(M) + p_0 \cdot log_2(p_0) + (1 - p_0) \cdot log_2((1 - p_0)/(M - 1))$, which is equivalent to (19.9). Thus, equation (19.15) is a general version of equation (19.9) (Kronegg and Pun (2005); Kronegg et al. (2005)).

These criteria have been applied mostly to BCI systems operating on a trial-by-trial basis. In figure 19.3, these criteria were applied to each sample within the trial, providing a time course of these criteria.

19.7   Mutual Information of a Continuous Output

The criteria in section 19.6 are based on discrete magnitudes of the BCI output. Evaluation criteria are also needed for continuous magnitudes such as those to move a cursor in the horizontal or vertical direction. The information content of such continuous output will affect the subject's training. BCI experiments with continuous (in time and magnitude) feedback have been described in Neuper et al. (1999), BCI Competition III (2005b), and Schlögl (2000a). Thus, quantifying this information content is of crucial interest.

Shannon's communication theory (Shannon and Weaver (1949)) also is applicable to these continuous signals. It is reasonable to assume that the BCI output Y is a stochastic process. Moreover, the output can be decomposed into a *signal* component X and a *noise* component Z. The signal component X is due to the *will* or *deliberate action* of the

Criterion	Measure	Class 1	Class 2	Class 3	Class 4
Error	22.4 %				
Accuracy	77.6 %				
Specific Accuracy		74.5	77.0	75.5	82.9
Kappa	0.70 ± 0.05				
I(Wolpaw)	0.88 bit				
I(Nykopp)	0.92 bit				
I(Continous)	1.24 bit	0.30	0.28	0.31	0.35
max. STMI	0.64 bit/s	0.21	0.18	0.14	0.14
SNR		0.51	0.48	0.53	0.63
Parametric correlation		0.67	0.69	0.68	0.77
Rank correlation		0.67	0.69	0.68	0.77
AUC		0.85	0.87	0.87	0.88

Table 19.3 Summary results. The results are derived from the time point with the largest κ at $t = 6.80s$. The one-versus-rest results for each class are presented for the two-class criteria. The time courses are shown in figure 19.3.

user, as it contains the user's intention; the second component contains all uncorrelated (noise) terms Z including the background brain activity, amplifier noise, etc. Implicitly, it is assumed that the subject was motivated and deliberately performed the mental task. If the subject was not cooperative, the subject's activity would be counted as background noise. The signal component can be obtained from the correlation between the output and the actual class labels (intentional state); the noise is the component of the output that does not contain any class-related information. Note, the signal and the noise are uncorrelated and provide an additive noise model (see also Schlögl et al. (2002, 2003)).

According to communication theory, the entropy of the output $H(Y)$ is the sum of the entropy of the input $H(X)$ and the entropy of the (additive) noise $H(Z)$. In other words, the difference between the entropies of the output and the noise is the entropy of the input. This entropy difference is also the mutual information between the input and the output, also called the information transfer $I(X;Y)$. That is, the mutual information is the amount of information that can be interfered with from the output.

The mutual information is

$$I(X;Y) = H(X) - H(X|Y) \qquad (19.16)$$

and can be alternatively written as

$$I(X;Y) = H(Y) - H(Y|X). \qquad (19.17)$$

The next step consists of estimating the entropy $H(X)$ of a stochastic process X. The entropy of a stochastic process with the probability distribution $p(x)$ is

$$H(x) = \int_x p(x)log(p(x)). \qquad (19.18)$$

Accordingly, the probability density of X must be known. The probability density can be obtained empirically from the histogram of X. However, if the number of samples is too small, it is reasonable to use second order statistics only; in this case, only the mean and variance have to be estimated, assuming all higher order moments are zero. This corresponds to the assumption of a Gaussian distribution.

The entropy of a Gaussian process with variance σ_x^2 is (Rieke et al. (1999) Appendix 9, pp. 316–317)

$$H(X) = \frac{1}{2} \log_2 (2\pi e \sigma_x^2). \tag{19.19}$$

The entropy of the noise component $H(Y \mid X)$ is based on within-class variance $\sigma_{withinclass}^2$ (the variance when the input X, i.e., the class c, is fixed) of the system output. The entropy of the total process $H(Y)$ is based on the total variance σ_{total}^2 of the output. The difference in entropy indicates the information of the *input* X transferred to the output Y.

$$I(X, Y) = H(Y) - H(Y \mid X) \tag{19.20}$$

$$= \frac{1}{2} \log_2 (2\pi e \sigma_{total}^2) - \frac{1}{2} \log_2 (2\pi e \sigma_{withinclass}^2) \tag{19.21}$$

$$= \frac{1}{2} \log_2 \left(\frac{\sigma_{total}^2}{\sigma_{withinclass}^2} \right) \tag{19.22}$$

The mutual information indicates the input information that passes through a noisy communication channel and can be obtained at the output.

The above formula can be rewritten such that the total variance is the sum of the noise (i.e., within-class) variance and the signal variance, assuming that noise and signal are uncorrelated. Accordingly, we get

$$I = H(Y) - H(Y \mid X) = \frac{1}{2} \log_2 \left(\frac{\sigma_{signal}^2 + \sigma_{noise}^2}{\sigma_{noise}^2} \right) = \frac{1}{2} \log_2 (1 + SNR) \tag{19.23}$$

whereas

$$SNR = \frac{\sigma_{signal}^2}{\sigma_{noise}^2} = \frac{\sigma_{total}^2}{\sigma_{noise}^2} - 1 \tag{19.24}$$

indicates the signal-to-noise ratio.

Intuitively, the SNR also can be obtained visually, comparing the means and the variances of the output for each class. This approach has been proposed for evaluating cue-based BCI with two classes (i.e., intentional control states) with a continuous output (Schlögl (2000a); Schlögl et al. (2002, 2003)). For the interpretation of M-states, M discriminant functions are obtained (using a one-versus-rest scheme), and each provides a continuous output for which the mutual information can be obtained. The total amount of information can be obtained by summing up the mutual information of the M one-versus-rest outputs. This approach has been used in figure 19.3 for four-class data. Accordingly, it is also possible to extend this approach toward M classes.

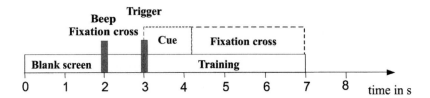

Figure 19.2   Paradigm used for the experiment in BCI Competition III (2005a). Results are shown in figure 19.3.

19.8   Criteria for Evaluating Self-Paced BCI Data

The previous criteria usually are applied to system outputs obtained in individual trials sychronized to an external "go-now" cue. As such trial-based analysis has been referred to as *synchronous*, *cue-paced*, or *intermittent* analysis. The results in figure 19.3 and tables 19.2 and 19.3 were obtained in this way.

For certain applications, we want subjects to operate the BCI in a self-paced (or asynchronous) mode. To support this, the BCI system is specially designed to produce outputs in response to intentional control as well as periods of no control (Mason and Birch (2000)). For investigations of self-paced control, we need to identify the subject's intention to control at arbitrary times and distinguish it from periods of no control. Thus, we need to evaluate the continuous (nonstop) data stream produced by the BCI. The terms *asynchronous*, *self-paced*, and *continuous* analysis have been used for this kind of evaluation. (Remark: In this context the term *continuous* is used differently than in section 19.7, where we used the terms *continuous in magnitude* and *continuous in time within a trial*).

Unlike intermittent analysis, where the timing of intended control is tied to experimental cues, the identification of the intended output in continuous (nonstop) analysis is more problematic. The intended output is often estimated from observations of the subject's behavior in relation to the experimental protocol or through subject self-report. This can result in fuzzy time estimates, which impact the analysis. There is no strict algorithm for defining the intended output sequence, and it remains up to the experimenter how to do this. In any case, the method used to define the intended output sequence is essential information and should be accurately reported in research papers.

19.8.1   HF-Difference

The University of Michigan group has developed a validation criterion for continuous analysis called the *HF-difference* (Huggins et al. (1999)). The HF-difference is a cost function that combines the likelihood of event detection and the accuracy of detected events. The HF-difference has been used only in a single-event state-versus-idle/no-control state discrimination task. The HF-difference is created by subtracting a false detection percentage (F) from a hit percentage (H). H is the percentage of events that are detected within specified timing constraints. F is the percentage of detections that are not correct and therefore is a measure describing the trustworthiness of the detections produced by

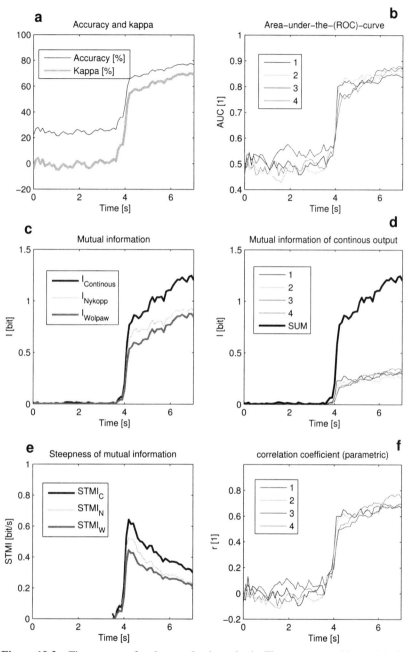

Figure 19.3   Time course of various evaluation criteria. The accuracy and kappa (a), the area-under-the-curve for each of the four one-versus-rest evaluation (b), Wolpaw's and Nykopp's discrete mutual information together with the sum of the continuous mutual information (c), and the continuous mutual information for each of the one-versus-rest evaluation together with its sum (d), the "steepness of mutual information" $I(t)/(t - t_0,$ for the continuous "C," Nykopp's "N" and Wolpaw's "W" formula (e), and finally the parametric correlation coefficient (f) are shown. Before cue-onset (at $t_0 = 3s$), no separability is observed, the accuracy is 1/4=25%, kappa is 0, AUC is 0.5, I=0 bit, and the correlation is 0. After the cue onset, the separability increases.

the method. The H and F percentages are subtracted to produce the HF-difference, which varies between 100 percent for perfect detection and -100 percent. Equal weighting of the H and F metrics are used typically.

The hit rate H (also called Sensitivity Se or Recall) is defined as

$$H = Se = \frac{TP}{TP + FN}. \tag{19.25}$$

The false detection rate F is defined as

$$F = \frac{FP}{TP + FP}. \tag{19.26}$$

Note, $1 - F$ (also called the positive predictive value or Precision Pr) is not the same as the specificity ($Sc = \frac{TN}{TN+FP}$). In asynchronous mode, the specificity Sc cannot be obtained because the number of true negatives TN is not defined. In the field of information retrieval (Rijsbergen (1979)), the harmonic mean of *Precision* and *Recall* is called the F_1-measure

$$F_1 = 2\frac{Se \cdot Pr}{Se + Pr} = \frac{2 \cdot TP}{2 \cdot TP + FN + FP}. \tag{19.27}$$

In the field of BCI research, the Hit/False–difference has been more used widely and is defined as

$$HFdiff = H - F = \frac{TP}{TP + FN} - \frac{FP}{TP + FP} = Se + Pr - 1. \tag{19.28}$$

Computing false detections in this way emphasizes the operational cost of false positives (to the user of the interface) more than sample-based metrics. For example, suppose a 100-second segment of data sampled at 200 Hz and containing 20 event triggers was used as the test data and a detection method produced 20 detections, of which 10 were wrong. With a sample-by-sample classification, 10 false detections in 100 s would yield a false positive rate of 10/(100 * 200) = 0.05%, giving a false sense of confidence in a method that was wrong half the time. However, the HF-difference calculation would produce an H of 50% (half of the events detected), an F of 50% (half of the detections incorrect) and an HF-difference of 0.

On the other hand, the HF-difference ignores important timing characteristics such as the time over which the measurement was made and the time between events. So, while the same HF-difference may describe the performance for 5 events over a 10 second period and over a 10 minute period, this level of performance over the longer period means a much larger number of correctly classified nonevent samples. Further, the HF-difference formula does not specify the criteria by which a detection is classified as a hit or a false detection, allowing the adjustment of these criteria for the particular application under consideration.

As a cost function, the HF-difference provides a user-centered evaluation criteria. However, HF-difference values can be directly compared only when the criteria used to define a hit are the same and over data with similar event spacing.

19.8.2 Confusion Matrix for Self-Paced Data

Because of the limitations of the HF-difference and the lack of an alternative, there is currently no commonly accepted criterion available for evaluating self-paced BCI data. An important step toward such a standard is the paper of Mason et al. (submitted) defining the relevant terms and providing some cornerstones for such criterion. Currently, there are two approaches under consideration—both are confusion matrices (Mason et al. (2005a)). In the first approach, the confusion matrix is obtained on a sample-per-sample basis. Each sample of the BCI output is compared with the label of the intended output for that sample. The second approach is a transition-based confusion matrix. Each transition of the BCI output is compared to the intended output to determine whether it is a desired or undesired transition. Currently, there is no consensus on how to create the confusion matrix and the issue is an ongoing research topic.

19.9 Other Criteria

19.9.1 Receiver-Operator Characteristics (ROC)

There are several other criteria that can be used; one is the receiver-operator characteristics (ROC) curve. The ROC curve obtained by varying the detection threshold and plotting the *Sensitivity* (fraction of true positives) versus $1 - Specificity$ (fraction of false positives). Several summary statistics can be derived from ROC curves. A-prime (A') and d-prime (d') describe the separability of the data and are based on a detection threshold (Pal (2002)), whereas no detection threshold is needed for the area under the (ROC) curve AUC. ROC curves also have other interesting properties (for more details, see Stanislaw and Todorow (1999)). ROC-based criteria have been used for evaluating different artifact detection methods (Schlögl et al. (1999a,b)), in the BCI competition 2005 for feature selection (Lal et al. (2005b)), and by Rohde et al. (2002) for *self-paced* evaluation using AUC for comparing different detectors and for selecting detection thresholds.

19.9.2 Correlation Coefficient

The correlation coefficient is used sometimes for feature extraction or for validation. The Pearson correlation (i.e., the parametric correlation) is defined as

$$r = \frac{\sum_i (y_i - \bar{y})(x_i - \bar{x})}{\sqrt{(\sum_i (y_i - \bar{y})^2)(\sum_i (x_i - \bar{x})^2)}} \tag{19.29}$$

where x_i is the class label, y_i is the output value, and $\bar{x}_i$ and $\bar{y}_i$ denote the mean values of x_i and y_i, respectively. Alternatively, the rank correlation is computed by replacing the sample values x_i and y_i by its ranks $rank(x_i)$ and $rank(y_i)$ (19.29). The rank correlation should be used for non-Gaussian data, while for Gaussian data the parametric correlation is recommended. The correlation coefficient r can range from -1 to 1 with an $r = 0$ indicating no correlation between the output and the class label. The time courses of the parametric and the rank correlation are presented in figure 19.3. The squared correlation coefficient r^2 has been used by Wolpaw's group (Wolpaw et al. (2000b)) for selecting the electrode position and the frequency band. The correlation coefficient can be computed for two classes, and also for more classes if the classes are ordered (e.g., if more than two target classes are available on a one-dimensional scale). The dataset used in table 19.2 and figure 19.3 does not provide such an ordering; therefore, the results of the two-class correlation coefficient are presented only for each of the individual one-versus-rest comparisons.

19.9.3   Evaluation of Continuous-Input and Continuous-Output Systems

So far, all the presented evaluation criteria require a discrete target class for reference. However, BCI systems with continuous output information have been developed recently by groups such as Donoghue et al. at Brown University (Gao et al. (2003a); Wu et al. (2004a, 2005)). Within the evelution of these systems, the task of the subject is to track a target in a two-dimensionsional space. The reference information (the 2D position of the target) as well as the BCI output are continuous variables. For the evaluation of this type of BCI system, the mean squared prediction error (MSE)

$$MSE = 1/N \cdot \sum_{t=1}^{N} \left((x_t - \hat{x}_t)^2 + (y_t - \hat{y}_t)^2 \right) \qquad (19.30)$$

and the correlation coefficient in the x and y direction have been used

$$CC_x = \frac{\sum_i (x_i - \bar{x})(\hat{x}_i - \bar{\hat{x}})}{\sqrt{(\sum_i (x_i - \bar{x})^2)(\sum_i (\hat{x}_i - \bar{\hat{x}})^2)}} \qquad (19.31)$$

$$CC_y = \frac{\sum_i (y_i - \bar{y})(\hat{y}_i - \bar{\hat{y}})}{\sqrt{(\sum_i (y_i - \bar{y})^2)(\sum_i (\hat{y}_i - \bar{\hat{y}})^2)}} \qquad (19.32)$$

in several works (Gao et al. (2003a); Wu et al. (2004a, 2005)) for comparing different decoding algorithms. Here, (x, y) and $(\hat{x}, \hat{y})$ indicate the position target and the output, respectively. Note, the correlation coefficient here is the same in (19.29), only the symbols are used differently. Here, the two-dimensional input and output are denoted by (x, y) and $(\hat{x}, \hat{y})$, respectivly; in (19.29), the one-dimensional input and ouput are denoted by x and y, respectively.

However, they recommend the MSE over the correlation coefficients, because "MSE is more meaningful for prosthetic applications, where the subjects need precise control of cursor positions; [they] observed decoding results with relatively high correlation coefficients that were sometimes far from 2D hand trajectory" (Wu et al. (2005)(pp. 93–94)).

19.9.4   Response Time

The previous paragraphs were dedicated to evaluation criteria that measure the separability of the data (through accuracy, mutual information, etc.). However, what happens if the perfect data processing method has been developed, but the result is obtained one hour after the subject actually performed the action? Even if we could speed up the method to a one-minute delay, the BCI will not be accepted by users. In other words, the response time is also a crucial parameter in assessing the performance of a BCI.

To take into account not only the separability but also the response time, the maximum *steepness of the mutual information* has been used as the evaluation criterion in BCI Competition III (2005b).

$$STMI(t) = \frac{I(t)}{t - t_0} \tag{19.33}$$

whereas t_0 is the time for the cue onset and $I(t)$ is the continuous mutual information. The maximum mutual information is the slope of that tangent on the curve $I(t)$ that goes through point $(t, I) = [t_0, 0]$.

The results in figure 19.3 provide some information about time course of the detection accuracy. The data were recorded according to a cue-based paradigm (figure 19.2) with the cue presented at time $t_0 = 3s$; afterward the separability (figure 19.3) increases up to a maximum time $t = 7.0s$ giving a response time of $4.0s$ for optimum accuracy. However, the maximum steepness of $0.64bit/s$ is obtained at $t = 4.2s$.

The steepness can also be calculated for any other criterion; for the BCI competition, the steepness of the mutual information was chosen because the mutual information provides a smooth curve and is, therefore, most suitable.

The BCI system with the largest maximum steepness provides the fastest and most accurate feedback at the output. The steepness will be especially useful for investigating signal processing and feature extraction methods. For example, it can be used to identify the optimum window length (trade-off between estimation accuracy and delay time). Furthermore, the steepness of the mutual information also provides an upper limit of the theoretical information transfer rate (amount of information per time unit) of a specific BCI design.

19.10   Discussion

Three approaches (19.9), (19.15), and (19.23) for estimating the mutual information have been described. The first approach uses the (overall) accuracy, the second approach uses the confusion matrix to estimate the mutual information, and the third approach evaluates the information content of the continuous output. All approaches were derived from the communication theory of Shannon and Weaver (1949). The differences in the results (see figure 19.3 and table 19.3) are due to different a priori assumptions, which are not always fulfilled. Especially (19.9) has some strong preconditions (e.g., equal distribution of wrong classifications), which are rarely fulfilled. Consequently, methods taking into account the whole confusion matrix should be preferred in case of a discrete output. For the evaluation of continuous BCI output, the mutual information for continuous output is recommended; it does not require thresholding, and the magnitude information is taken into account. The derivation of the equations also points out the possibility of a more refined analysis, for

Criterion	Units	# classes	min/chance/max	Threshold required
ERR	%	M	$0/\frac{M-1}{M}100\%/100\%$	YES
ACC	%	M	$0/\frac{100\%}{M}/100\%$	YES
Kappa	[1]	M	-1/0/1	YES
I_{Wolpaw}	[bit]	M	$0/0/\log_2(M)$	YES
I_{Nykopp}	[bit]	M	$0/0/\log_2(M)$	YES
$I_{Continuous}$	[bit]	$2, M^1$	$0/0/\inf$	NO
$STMI$	[bit/s]	2	$0/0/\inf$	NO
SNR	1	2	$0/0/\inf$	NO
Correlation r	[1]	$2, M^2, cont.^4$	$-1/0/1$	NO
AUC	[1]	2	0/0.5/1	NO
A'	[1]	2	0/0.5/1	YES
d'	[1]	2	$-\inf/0/\inf$	YES
F_1	[1]	2	0/0.5/1	YES
HF-diff	%	1^3	-100%/-/100%	YES
MSE	$[cm^2]$	$cont.^4$		NO

Table 19.4 Overview of evaluation criteria. The # classes column indicates whether the criterion is suitable for a two-class or for an M-class problem. Nevertheless, the two-class criteria also can be applied to each class of an M-class problem if each class is evaluated against the rest (one-vs.-rest scheme). The column min/chance/max indicates the range (min/max) and the result of a chance classification. The threshold column indicates whether a known threshold value is necessary (YES) or if the performance can be computed without determining a certain threshold (NO).
[1]The mutual information for continuous output is defined by two classes, and can be extended to M classes by summing up the information of each 1-vs.-rest output. [2]The correlation coefficient r can be applied to $M > 2$ classes only if the classes can be ordered such that $c_1 < c_2 < \cdots < c_M$. [3]The $HF - diff$ is used for evaluating one active state versus a resting state. [4]The reference information is not discrete but continuous, no class information but, e.g., target trajectory is provided.

example, the assumption of Gaussianity can be replaced by more accurate estimates of the actual output distribution.

Although evaluation criteria have not received much attention in BCI research, complete definitions, further discussion, and sound application of these criteria will improve the overall evaluations of BCI systems. To simplify the usage of various criteria, the software implementation of the evaluation criteria is available through the BioSig project http://biosig.sf.net/.

Notes

E-mail for correspondence: alois.schloegl@tugraz.at

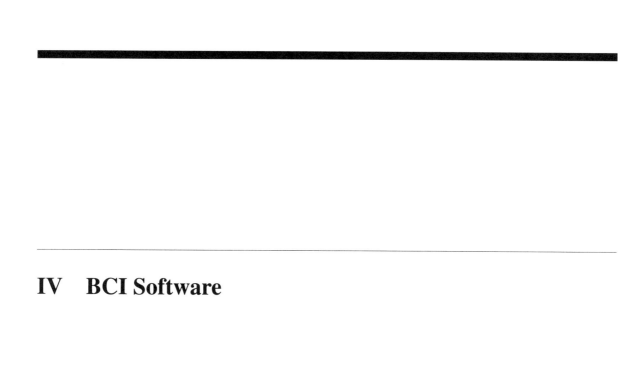

IV BCI Software

Introduction

In this part, we introduce two software packages for BCI that are freely available for research and include a set of useful tools to process EEG signals for real-time BCI. Note that the subsequent chapters are intended as practical references for a quick start to the new BCI researcher.

In chapter 20, Schlögl et al. introduce the Graz BioSig toolbox. Besides an interface to many different data formats of EEG recordings, the toolbox supports several-signal processing and artifact reduction, feature extraction, and classification methods. The software package is freely available licensed with the GNU General Public License. It allows for the use of several programming languages and computer platforms.

In chapter 21, Mellinger and Schalk introduce the EEG software toolbox BCI 2000 developed in cooperation of the Wadsworth Center in Albany and the University of Tübingen. The system has been developed mainly for real-time BCI applications and provides the user with general data acquisition techniques and a general framework where a research group is able to use their own signal processing, user application, and operator modules. The software is freely available for research and education. However, it is restricted to Windows platforms and C++ programming.

Note that a number of further software packages are available in the field of EEG processing (see section 20.2 for an overview) and BCI. The licensing schemes and the technical scope of these packages vary strongly. Mostly they are software libraries that are assembled by the respective local BCI group with varying degrees of documenting the package functionalities. For example, in the case of Berlin, the BBCI toolbox is part of a larger software library of general machine learning and signal processing, parts of which contain patented technology; therefore, the software is only commercially available.

Guido Dornhege and Klaus-Robert Müller

20   BioSig: An Open-Source Software Library for BCI Research

Alois Schlögl, Clemens Brunner, Reinhold Scherer, and Andreas Glatz
Institute for Human-Computer Interfaces
University of Technology Graz
Krenngasse 37, A-8010 Graz

20.1   Abstract

BioSig is an open-source software library for biomedical signal processing. Besides several other application areas, BioSig also has been developed for BCI research. It provides a common interface to many different dataformats, it supports artifact processing and quality control, it provides adaptive signal processing and feature extraction methods that are very suitable for online and real-time processing, it supports handling of missing values, and it includes several classification methods for single-trial classification of EEG.

This chapter provides an overview of the current status and an outline of future possibilities. BioSig is licensed with the GNU General Public License; it provides an open development platform unencumbered from legal restrictions. Therefore, it is also an ideal tool for research and development.

20.2   Overview

Besides several proprietary software packages, several open-source software tools are available in the field of EEG processing. Currently, we know of the following packages: EEGLAB by Makeig and Delourme, BioSig (http://biosig.sf.net), OpenEEG, Bioelectromagnetism toolbox (http://eeg.sf.net), EMEGS, FieldTrip, LORETA by Pascual-Marqui, and BCI2000 (http://www.bci2000.org) (see also table 20.1). The first five are licensed with the GNU General Public License (GPL); thus, the user has the freedom to *run, copy, distribute study, change, and improve* the software. EEGLAB, Bioelectromagnetism toolbox, EMEGS, FieldTrip, and LORETA are designed for classical offline EEG analysis.

Table 20.1 Software packages for EEG analysis.

Package	License	Language	Requirements
BCI2000	?	C++	Windows
Bioelectromagnetism	GPL	Matlab	Matlab
BioSig	GPL	Octave, Matlab, Simulink, C/C++, Qt, Java, Python	various
EEGLAB	GPL	Matlab	Matlab (5+)
EMEGS	GPL	Matlab	Matlab (6+)
FieldTrip	GPL	Matlab	Matlab
LORETA	?	unknown	Windows
OpenEEG	GPL	various	various

Table 20.2 The library of m-functions is organized along the following subtasks or topics.

(i)	Data acquisition
(ii)	Data formats and storage
(iii)	Preprocessing
(iv)	Signal processing and feature extraction
(v)	Classification and statistics
(vi)	Evaluation criteria
(vii)	Visualization
(viii)	Interactive viewer and scoring

The packages BioSig and BCI2000 are dedicated to BCI research. BCI2000 is described in detail in chapter 21, while the BioSig project is discussed here.

A major aim of BioSig is to provide an open-source software library for BCI research; it is available from http://biosig.sf.net. In the following chapter, we outline the general structure of BioSig and highlight some important components.

20.3   BioSig for Octave and MATLAB

The BioSig project was started as a library for MATLAB with an attempt to be compatible with Octave (http://www.octave.org). The first toolbox already contained several subtasks (see table 20.2). With the advent of other subprojects (rtsBCI, C/C++, SigViewer, etc.) this part was renamed "Biosig for Octave and MATLAB."

20.3.1   Data Formats and Storage

The "data format module" implements a common interface to various data formats; currently, more than fourty different data formats are supported. This is more than any other project in the field of biomedical signal processing.

Automated detection of the file format is supported. The range of supported formats includes data formats of equipment providers (e.g., ACQ from BIOPAC or CNT from NeuroScan), specific research projects (e.g., Physiobank format from MIT, or the BCI2000 format), and standards and quasi-standards (e.,g., EDF, SCP, or MFER formats), and also supports several audio and sound formats.

The various data formats contain many encoding schemes using different bit depths, allowing single or multiple sampling rates, and they contain different header information. With the common interface implemented in BioSig, the users do not need to care which data format is actually used or how the proper scaling of the amplitude values is obtained or from where to obtain the sampling rate. The interface also supports simple preprocessing like the selection of specific data channels and overflow detection (if supported by the underlying data format). If an overflow is detected, the corresponding sample value is replaced by *not-a-number* (NaN) (IEEE754). This feature of automated overflow detection can be turned off, but by default it is on.

However, none of these data formats contains all the features needed for BCI research. Therefore, the advantages of various data formats were used to construct the general data format (GDF) for biomedical signal processing (by Schlögl). Besides several other improvements, an encoding scheme for events and annotations is part of the GDF definition (see table 20.3). The codes are grouped according to different application areas, for example, EEG artifacts have the code range 0x0100–0x010f, while the range of 0x0300–0x3ff is reserved for BCI experiments.

The GDF format has been used already in several BCI studies, for example, the datasets IIIa and IIIb of the BCI competition 2005 have been exchanged in the GDF format. Also, the "rtsBCI" and the "biofeedpro" (see sections 20.4 and 20.6) are using GDF as the standard data format for data recording.

20.3.2 Preprocessing

Methods for preproccessing are applied at an intermediate state between data access and feature extraction. Accordingly, this module contains several useful preprocessing routines. One of the most often used functions is probably the function for triggering the data, that is, to extract data segments relative to a given trigger. Also available is a function for extracting the trigger time points from a continuous trigger channel, as well as some simple resampling methods. Some advanced algorithms for artifact processing are also included: a method for quality control using histogram analysis (Schlögl et al. (1999c)), an algorithm for reducing EOG artifacts based on regression analysis, and a method for detecting muscle artifacts based on inverse filtering.

20.3.3 Signal Processing and Feature Extraction

Naturally, signal processing is one of the core components of a biomedical signal processing toolbox. Many signal processing methods are already available elsewhere. Unfortunately, it is rare that any signal processing toolbox supports the handling of missing data.

Table 20.3 Predefined event codes for BCI experiments. The complete list is available from http://biosig.cvs.sourceforge.net/biosig/biosig/doc/eventcodes.txt

###	Table of event codes.
#	
###	table of event codes: lines starting with # are omitted
###	add 0x8000 to indicate end of event
###	0x010_ EEG artifacts
0x0101	artifact:EOG (blinks, fast, large amplitude)
...	
###	0x011_ EEG patterns
0x0111	eeg:Sleep spindles
...	
###	0x012_ Evoked potentials
0x0121	VEP: visual EP
...	
###	0x013_ Steady State Evoked potentials
0x0131	SSVEP
...	
###	0x03__ BCI: Trigger, cues, classlabels,
0x0300	Start of Trial, Trigger at t=0s
0x0301	Left - cue onset (BCI experiment)
0x0302	Right - cue onset (BCI experiment)
0x0303	Foot - cue onset (BCI experiment)
0x0304	Tongue - cue onset (BCI experiment)
0x0306	Down - cue onset (BCI experiment)
0x030C	Up - cue onset (BCI experiment)
0x030D	Feedback (continuous) - onset (BCI experiment)
0x030E	Feedback (discrete) - onset (BCI experiment)
0x030F	cue unknown/undefined (used for BCI competition)
0x0311	Beep (accustic stimulus, BCI experiment)
0x0312	Cross on screen (BCI experiment)
0x0313	Flashing light
0x031B	- 0x037f reserved for ASCII characters #27-#127
0x0381	target hit, task successful, correct classification
0x0382	target missed, task not reached, incorrect classification
0x03ff	Rejection of whole trial
###	0x00__ user specific events
0x0001	condition 1
0x0002	condition 2
...	

Exceptions are the "time series analysis (TSA) toolbox" and the NaN toolbox. Both are part of OctaveForge and are distributed with BioSig.

The NaN toolbox contains methods for statistical analysis that support data with missing values encoded as not-a-number (NaN) according to the IEEE754 standard. The basic functionality of the NaN toolbox is a function called `sumskipnan.m`, which skips all NaNs, and sums and counts all numerical values. The two return values SUM and COUNT are sufficient to calculate the mean of the data. This principle also can be used to calculate the expectation value of any statistic including covariance matrices and more advanced statistics. Whether or not this principle can be applied to more advanced signal processing methods is being investigated.

The TSA toolbox contains many functions for parametric modeling, that is, autoregressive estimators. It contains the well-known Burg and Levinson-Durbin algorithms for estimating autoregressive (AR) parameters of single-channel stationary processes. Adaptive autoregressive (AAR) estimators (Schlögl (2000a)) like Kalman filtering, and RLS and LMS algorithms are available. Multivariate autoregresssive (MVAR) estimators like the Nuttall-Strand method (multichannel Burg) or the multichannel Levinson algorithm have been included. Furthermore, the adaptive estimation of some standard EEG parameters (e. g., bandpower, Hjorth (1970) and Wackermann (1999) parameters) are also supported. The adaptive estimation does not require downsampling and is still computationally efficient. Accordingly, the features are obtained with the same sampling rate as the input data. All these functions can deal also with missing data encoded as NaN. This represents an efficient way of handling missing data values and can be used easily in combination with artifact detection methods, for example, saturation or muscle artifacts.

20.3.4   Classification

This module has been developed according to the needs of the Graz BCI system (see chapter 4) using the advantage of statistical classifiers (e.g., robustness) like linear and quadratic discriminant analysis. This use allowed the possibility of a continuous feedback (in time as well as magnitude). A classifier combines various features into a single output, and the time lag of classification should be as small as possible. Often, one wants to know how well the classifier is able to separate the training data. To prevent overfitting, cross-validation is required. Finally, the optimal time point for applying the classifier must be identified in BCI research.

To fulfill the various needs, a wrapper function (`findclassifier.m`) has been developed that includes the required functionality. In the first version, a linear discriminant analysis (LDA) for two classes was implemented. Later, quadratic classifiers and an interface to support vector machines (SVM) were added; multiple classes $N > 2$ are supported (using a one-versus-rest scheme). Another important issue was the selection of the proper time segment for estimating a classifier. For this purpose, the data were triggered and separability was calculated for each time segment. The length of each segment can be varied from 1 to N samples; typically, a fixed segment length of a fraction of a second (e.g., 0.2 s or 0.125 s; 8 to 25 samples depending on the sampling rate) is used. For the search step, the relative separability is sufficient; the cross-validation is omitted in this step. In the next step, a trial-based leave-one-out method (LOOM) is used for cross-validation.

The samples from the chosen segment of all but one trial are used to train the classifier, and this classifier is applied to all samples of the testing trial; this provides a time course of the output for the specific trial. This procedure is repeated until each trial has been used once as test trial. When all permutations are finished, a time course of the output is obtained from each trial. This outcome is then evaluated for different evaluation criteria like error rate, SNR, mutual information, and kappa. An example is shown in section 19.6.

Results have been used in several works (e.g., Blankertz et al. (2004); Schlögl et al. (2002, 2003, 2005). This classifier was also used in the BCI competition 2005 on dataset I (rank 7) and IVa (rank 8). Moreover, the general classifier was obtained from the data of the selected segment. This classifier has been used together with "rtsBCI" in several BCI experiments (Scherer et al. (2004b); Vidaurre et al. (2004a,b)).

20.3.5   Evaluation Criteria

Several different evaluation criteria are used in BCI research (for details, see also chapter 19): Implemented are accuracy (error rate), information transfer (Schlögl et al. (2002, 2003)), Cohen's kappa coefficient (Schlögl et al. (2005)), and several others. Moreover, functions for analyzing the time courses of the different criteria are provided. The implementation of these functions were also used for analyzing results of the BCI competition 2003 (dataset III) (Blankertz et al. (2004)) and BCI competition 2005 (dataset IIIa and IIIb).

20.3.6   Visualization

Visualization is always an important issue. Currently, the function `plota.m` is a wrapper function for displaying various results. The presented result depends on the input data and which function has generated a certain result. For example, the outcome of `findclassifier.m` for two classes is presented as time courses of the error rate, SNR, and the mutual information. If the result stems from $N > 2$ classes, the time course of the accuracy and the kappa coefficient are displayed.

Another useful function is `sview`, which is able to present the raw EEG data in a compressed form on a single screen. It also includes any event information (if available). Within MATLAB it is possible to zoom into specific segments. The `sview` function is useful to get an overview of the available data. Another important functionality is the scoring of EEG data. Two packages—SViewer and SigViewer—support the viewing and the scoring of EEG data and are described in more detail in section 20.5.

20.3.7   SViewer – a viewing and scoring software

`SViewer` is written in MATLAB, and it uses the MATLAB GUI functions and the functions for reading the data and for writing event information. Because it is based on the common interface, it can read any data format supported by *Biosig for Octave and*

Figure 20.1   SViewer: a viewing and scoring software based on the graphical user interface of MATLAB.

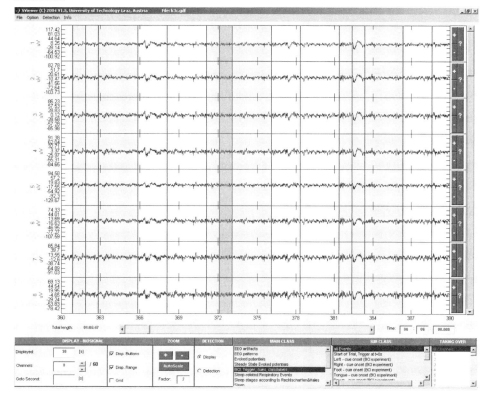

MATLAB. The annotations, markers, and events can be edited and stored in a separate event file. A screenshot of SViewer is shown in figure 20.1. SViewer must not be confused with SigViewer, which is a stand-alone program and does not require MATLAB; SigViewer is described in section 20.5.

20.4   Real-time BCI System Based on MATLAB/Simulink—rtsBCI

The Graz BCI (see chapter 4) open-source software package rtsBCI provides a framework for the development and rapid prototyping of real-time BCI systems. The software is licensed under the GNU GPL and based on MATLAB/Simulink (The Mathworks, Inc., Natick, MA, USA) running on Microsoft Windows (Microsoft Corporation, Redmond, WA, USA). To enable hard real-time computing on Windows platforms, the Real-Time Windows Target (RTWT) and, for the generation of stand-alone C code, the Real-Time Workshop (RTW) are required. Both toolboxes are extensions of Simulink. Furthermore, BioSig for Octave and MATLAB is required for data format handling, and the TCP/UDP/IP toolbox of P. Rydesäter (http://www.mathworks.com/matlabcentral/fileexchange/) is required for network communication support. In addition, to the software requirements, a data acquisition card is needed to sample the biosignals.

After installation, all rtsBCI modules are listed in the Simulink Library Browser and can be used to design (model) the BCI system (figure 20.2). Several MATLAB functions and Simulink blocks are available for (1) data acquisition and conversion; (2) storage (using the open data format GDF (Schlögl (2006))); (3) digital signal processing (e.g. bandpower feature estimation, adaptive autoregressive parameters (AAR) estimated with Kalman filtering (by Schlögl (2000a)), or linear discriminant analysis (LDA)); (4) visualization (e.g. signal scope, presentation of cue information, or feedback of a moving bar); (5) paradigm control (synchronous and asynchronous operation mode); and (6) network support (e.g., remote monitoring).

Tunable parameters as well as other information relevant for the experiment (e.g., subject information, amplifier settings, electrode setup, and paradigm timing) are stored in an individual configuration file (INI file). Before a model is executed, the configuration is transferred to the model and stored altogether with the biosignals for further analysis. The division of model and parameters makes it very easy to deal with changes: For example, a new classifier requires only the replacement of the classification block. A new subject requires only the modification of the related data in the configuration file.

Most of the online BCI feedback experiments reported from the Graz research group (see chapter 4) in the past few years are based on rtsBCI and come along with the package: the standard Graz BCI training without feedback (Pfurtscheller and Neuper (2001)), the standard two-class Graz BCI training with feedback (Pfurtscheller and Neuper (2001)), and the two-class basket paradigm (Krausz et al. (2003)). Generally, the first paradigm is used to collect data for analysis and setup of the classifier. The second provides a simple feedback in the form of a bar moving either toward the left or right side of the screen. The third paradigm provides feedback in the form of a ball falling from the top to the bottom of the screen at a constant speed with the task of hitting the correct target at the bottom of the screen by moving the ball either to the left or right side (figure 20.2).

20.5   SigViewer

SigViewer is a viewing and scoring program for biosignals, originally designed to process electroencephalogram (EEG) signals. SigViewer can load multichannel signals, such as EEG, ECG, EMG, and EOG recordings, and display these in various scales. For example, figure 20.3 shows the viewer displaying five EEG channels simultaneously. Besides the viewing functions of SigViewer, the other major application is the scoring of biosignals, which permits the user to make annotations to the signals (e.g., mark segments as artifact or mark specific events) and save this information to a file (either in the original data file, a copy of the data file, or in a file that contains only these annotations). In the example in figure 20.3, an EOG artifact is marked inside the left light grey area. The right light and dark grey rectangles label two overlapping events; for instance, the light grey area might denote an EEG trial and the dark one might indicate the period where an arrow (a cue) is displayed to the subject.

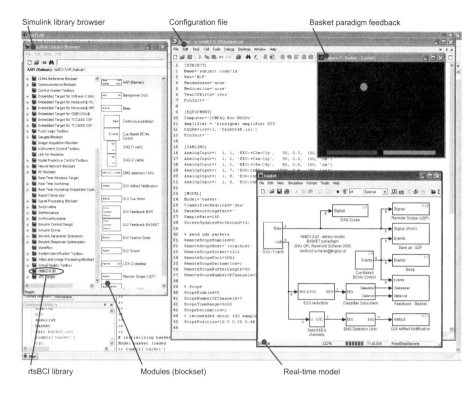

Figure 20.2   The screenshot shows the development environment: the basic platform MATLAB, Simulink with rtsBCI, an editor with configuration file, and a real-time model of the Basket paradigm with feedback window.

It is also possible to view basic information about a specific file (e.g., number of channels, sampling frequency, number of events, time of recording). In addition to graphically scoring the data, a list-based widget is available for viewing and deleting all events (annotations) manually. In the future, adding new events that way will also be possible.

Currently, the software supports only GDF files as input and output signals, but thanks to its modular structure it can be extended to support other file formats. In principle, any kind of signal data (including audio files) is a candidate to be displayed. The availability of new import and export filters is planned for in the separate subproject called "BioSig for C++" (or biosig4c++ for short), which can be used not only by SigViewer but also by other programs.

SigViewer is written in C++ using the platform-independent graphical user interface (GUI) toolkit QT4. One major design specification was that SigViewer be able to run under many different operating systems such as Linux, Windows, and MacOS and thus be designed as platform-independent. Moreover, SigViewer does not depend on any proprietary software, making it a truly free program.

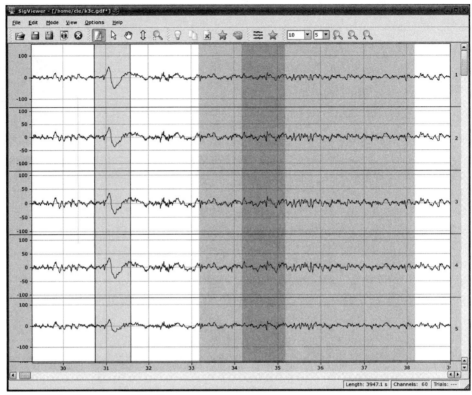

Figure 20.3   Screenshot of SigViewer.

20.6   BioProFeed

BioProFeed is a data acquisition module based on the real-time application interface (RTAI http://www.rtai.org/). Currently, BioProFeed can be used with the following data acquisition hardware:

(1)   g.mobilab from g.tec
(2)   NI-6024e PCMCIA from National Instruments
(3)   ModularEEG from OpenEEG

Support for further hardware modules is in preparation.

The name *BioProFeed* stands for Portable **Bio**signal acquisition, real-time **Pro**cessing and **Feed**back generation framework. The biosignal acquisition chain consists of one or more transducers, a biosignal amplifier, an analog-digital converter (ADC) and a processing and storage unit. BioProFeed is a software framework for the processing and storage unit that is often a standard personal computer. It is licensed under the GPL and is a part of the Biosig project.

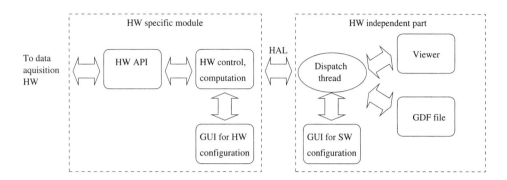

Figure 20.4   Software structure of BioProFeed.

BioProFeed was written with the following specifications in mind:

(1)   it should be platform independent
(2)   it should be modular to support different data aquisition hardware
(3)   real-time data processing should be possible
(4)   storage of the data in GDF format (Schlögl (2006)) should be possible

Currently, BioProFeed runs on Linux (i386, ppc, arm), MacOS, and Windows XP with Cygwin. Autotools (by Vaughan et al.), like autoheader, autoconf, and automake, are used to build software framework. These help to build the software by ensuring correct byte ordering for the different hardware platforms. The byte ordering is important when storing the data in GDF format (by Schlögl).

Gimp-Toolkit (GTK) has been used to write the user interface of the software. It can be integrated into any C/C++ program and is also highly portable. In fact, many GLib (glib) functions have been used to make BioProFeed more portable. In addition to the gLib functions, standard POSIX functions have been used.

The main structure of BioProFeed can be seen in figure 20.4. BioProFeed consists of two parts: the main part where data can be processed, displayed and stored, and the module part that controls and gets samples from the data acquisition hardware. The interface between the main part and the module part is called HAL (hardware abstraction layer). The modules supporting the data aquisition hardware are present in the CVS Tree of BioProFeed.

BioProFeed is a tool for data acquisition, processing, storage, and feedback generation. It is not restricted to specific data acquisition hardware or to specific data processing and storage hardware, and can store the data in GDF format (by Schlögl) for further offline data processing.

20.7   Summary

There are plans to improve almost every part of BioSig. The common interface to access different file formats will be translated into the languages C/C++, Java, and Python. Improvements in artifact processing and quality control should be evaluated offline, and, if successful, implemented online. Support for additional signal processing and feature extraction methods needs to be developed including the ability to handle missing values. Further data formats should be supported in SigViewer. Although each component of BioSig can be improved, it provides a working environment that has been used already in several BCI projects. BioSig contains modules for data acquistion, for BCI experiments with online feedback, viewing and scoring software for reviewing the raw data, functions for offline analysis of BCI data, and for obtaining a classifier that can be applied in online experiments, and many more. It contains everything for running BCI experiments, analyzing the data, and obtaining classifiers.

Almost all components can be used with free software; the M-code is also compatible with Octave (http://www.octave.org). Exceptions are the SViewer (which requires the graphical user interface of MATLAB) and rtsBCI (which requires the MATLAB, Simulink, and the Real-Time Workshop from Mathworks). SigViewer is a viewing and scoring software that can be used to replace SViewer as it requires only open-source software. Despite this deviations, the overall commitment to the open source philosophy is substantiated through the GNU General Public License (GPL).

Notes

E-mail for correspondence: alois.schloegl@tugraz.at

21   BCI2000: A General-Purpose Software Platform for BCI

Jürgen Mellinger
Institute of Medical Psychology and Behavioural Neurobiology
Eberhard-Karls-University Tübingen
MEG Center, Otfried-Müller-Str. 47
72076 Tübingen, Germany

Gerwin Schalk
Wadsworth Center
New York State Department of Health
E1001 Empire State Plaza
Albany, New York 12201

21.1   Abstract

BCI2000 is a flexible general-purpose platform for brain-computer interface (BCI) research and development that is aimed mainly at reducing the complexity and cost of implementing BCI systems. Since 2000, we have been developing this system in a collaboration between the Wadsworth Center of the New York State Department of Health in Albany, New York, and the Institute of Medical Psychology and Behavioral Neurobiology at the University of Tübingen, Germany. This system currently is used for a variety of studies in more than 110 laboratories around the world. BCI2000 currently supports a variety of data acquisition systems, brain signals, and feedback modalities and can thus be configured to implement many commonly used BCI systems without any programming. We provide the source code and corresponding documentation with the system to facilitate the implementation of BCI methods that are not supported by the current system. This process, and thus the evaluation of different BCI methods, is further encouraged by the modular design of BCI2000, which is designed such that a change in a module or a component requires little or no change in other modules or components. In summary, by substantially reducing labor and cost, BCI2000 facilitates the implementation of different BCI systems and other psychophysiological experiments. It is available with full documentation and free of charge for research or educational purposes and is currently being used in a variety of studies by many research groups (http://www.bci2000.org).

21.2 Overview

BCI2000 is a flexible general-purpose platform for brain-computer interface (BCI) research and development. It also can be used for simple data acquisition and auditory or visual stimulus presentation using a variety of data acquisition devices. BCI2000 has been in development since 2000 in a joint project between the Wadsworth Center of the New York State Department of Health in Albany, New York, USA, and the Institute of Medical Psychology and Behavioral Neurobiology at the University of Tübingen, Germany. Many other laboratories, most notably the BrainLab at Georgia State University and Fondazione Santa Lucia in Rome, Italy, have contributed to the project also.

The goals of the BCI2000 project are (1) to create a system that can facilitate the implementation of any BCI system, (2) to incorporate into this system support for the most commonly used BCI methods, and (3) to disseminate the system and associated documentation to other laboratories. BCI2000 should thus facilitate progress in laboratory and clinical BCI research by reducing the time, effort, and expense of testing new BCI methods, by providing a standardized data format for offline analyses, and by allowing groups lacking high-level software expertise to engage in BCI research. As of February 2007, BCI2000 has been adopted by more than 110 laboratories around the world that use the system for a variety of studies.

To achieve these three goals, BCI2000 decomposes a BCI into four independent and interchangeable modules that represent the four essential functions of any BCI system: signal acquisition, signal processing, user feedback, and operating protocol. These four modules and their components, and the interfaces between them, are designed such that a change in a module or a component requires little or no change in other modules or components. This feature facilitates evaluation of different BCI methods.

To date, BCI2000 has been used to implement BCI methods that can use a variety of data acquisition devices, that can make use of sensorimotor rhythms, cortical surface rhythms, slow cortical potentials, and the P300 potential, and that can provide the different outputs needed for several kinds of cursor and robotic arm control, sequential menu selection, and selection from a matrix. The growing number of contributions from laboratories using BCI2000 ensures that new methods are being developed continually.

To facilitate integration in other environments, the BCI2000 system can run on standard PC hardware, and supports a variety of data acquisition devices. Because it is written in C++, it makes efficient use of computational resources and can satisfy the real-time requirements of BCI operation.

21.3   Dissemination of BCI2000

BCI2000 is an open system that is available free of charge for research and educational purposes (http://www.bci2000.org). As of January 2006, seventy laboratories have acquired
BCI2000 and are using it for a variety of studies. Most of these laboratories follow one of
the three following patterns:

(1)   they use the existing BCI2000 system without changing the software,
(2)   they implement new methods or system capabilities into BCI2000, and/or
(3)   they use BCI2000 as a real-time signal acquisition platform to develop systems for
      research not related to brain-computer interfaces.

Investigators planning to use the existing system are provided with example configurations, descriptive documentation, and tutorial introductions. Extensions to the existing
BCI2000 system are encouraged and supported by a simple and robust programming interface, tutorials, and sample code illustrating its use. An online bulletin board system allows
for efficiently asking support questions and sharing answers.

21.4   BCI Model and Modules

BCI2000 is based on a model that can describe any BCI system. This model, shown in
figure 21.1, consists of four modules that communicate with each other: Source (data
acquisition and storage), Signal Processing, User Application, and Operator Interface. The
modules communicate through a network-capable protocol based on TCP/IP. Each may
be written in any programming language and can be run on any machine on a network.
Communication between modules uses a generic protocol that can transmit all information
(e.g., signals or variables) needed for operation. Thus, the protocol does not need to be
changed when changes are made in a module. Brain signals are processed synchronously,
in blocks containing a fixed number of samples that are acquired by the Source module.
Each time a new block of data is acquired, the Source module sends it to Signal Processing,
which extracts signal features, translates those features into control signals, and sends them
on to the User Application module. Finally, the Application module sends the resulting
event markers back to the Source module where they and the raw signals are stored to disc.
The contents of the data file thus allow for full reconstruction of an experimental session
during offline analyses.

The choice of block size is determined by processing resources as well as timing precision considerations. In the BCI2000 online system, the duration of a block corresponds
to the temporal resolution of stimulus presentation and to the cursor update rate during
feedback, suggesting small block sizes. On the other hand, real-time operation implies that
the average time required for processing a block and communicating it between modules
(roundtrip time) is less than a block's duration. Thus, processing resources (and network
latencies in a distributed system) impose a lower limit on the block size. A typical configuration, for example, sampling 16 channels at 160 Hz and processing blocks of 10 samples

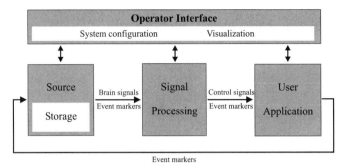

Figure 21.1 The four modules in BCI2000: Operator Interface, Source, Signal Processing, and User Application. The operator module acts as a central relay for system configuration and online presentation of results to the investigator. It also defines onset and offset of operation. During operation, information (i.e., signals, parameters, or event markers) is communicated from Source to Signal Processing to User Application and back to Source.

each, will result in a cursor update rate of 16 Hz with small output latency (table 21.2). When using data sources that can acquire data only at specific block sizes (e.g., the TCP-based data acquisition schemes in figure 21.1), BCI2000 block size will be further constrained to multiples of the source's block size.

21.4.1 Source Module and File Format

The Source module digitizes and stores brain signals, and passes them on without any further preprocessing to Signal Processing. It consists of a data acquisition component (table 21.1 lists data acquisition hardware currently supported by BCI2000), and a data storage component that implements the BCI2000 file format. This file format consists of an ASCII header that defines all parameters used for this particular experimental session, followed by binary signal sample and event marker values. The file format can accommodate any number of signal channels, system parameters, or event markers. It supports 16- and 32-bit integer formats as well as the IEEE 754 single precision (32-bit) floating point format.

21.4.2 Signal Processing Module

The Signal Processing module converts signals from the brain into signals that control an output device. This conversion is done in two stages, feature extraction and translation, and realized using a chain of signal filters, each of which transforms an input signal into an output signal. The individual signal filters are designed to be independent of each other and can thus be combined or interchanged without affecting others.

The first stage, feature extraction, is currently comprised of three filters. The first filter realizes a linear calibration routine that converts signals from A/D units into μV. The second filter can implement any linear spatial filtering operation by calculating a matrix multiplication of the input signals with a spatial filtering matrix. The third filter is called "temporal filter." To date, we have created six variations of this temporal filter: a slow wave

Vendor	Product	Type
National Instruments DAQ	ADC boards	Driver library
Data Translation	ADC boards	Driver library
Measurement Computing/Computer Boards	ADC boards	Driver library
g.tec	g.USBamp	Driver library
g.tec	g.MOBIlab	Driver library
Cleveland Medical Devices	BioRadio 150	Driver library
OpenEEG	ModularEEG	Serial port protocol
BrainProducts	BrainAmp	TCP based protocol
Neuroscan	SynAmps2	TCP based protocol
BioSemi		Driver library
TuckerDavis	Pentusa	Driver library
Refa Sytem (TMSI, Inc.)		TCP based protocol
Micromed EEG Systems		TCP based protocol

Table 21.1   Support for data acquisition systems in BCI2000. An up-to-date list is maintained at http://www.bci2000.org.

filter that can process slow cortical potentials, autoregressive spectral estimation, spectral estimation based on the fast fourier transform (FFT), a general finite impulse response filter (FIR) that can process sensorimotor rhythms, a peak detection routine that extracts firing rates from neuronal action potentials, and a filter that averages evoked responses (e.g., P300s).

The second stage, feature translation, translates the extracted signal features into device-independent control signals. This is done by two filters. The first applies a linear classifier, and the second filter normalizes the output signals such that they have zero mean and a specific value range. The output of this procedure is the output of the signal processing module.

An additional statistics component can be enabled to update in real time certain parameters of the signal processing components such as the slope and intercept (i.e., baseline) of the linear equation the normalization filter applies to each output channel; this allows to compensate for spontaneous or adaptive changes in the distribution of the control signal values.

21.4.3   User Application Module

The User Application module receives control signals from Signal Processing and uses them to drive an application. In most present-day BCIs, the user application is presented visually on a computer screen and consists of the selection of targets, letters, or icons.

Existing user application modules in BCI2000 implement one- to three-dimensional cursor movement paradigms for feedback of sensorimotor rhythm amplitude or slow cortical potential amplitude, two-dimensional robotic arm control, presentation of auditory and visual stimuli with optional feedback of evoked potential classification result, and a

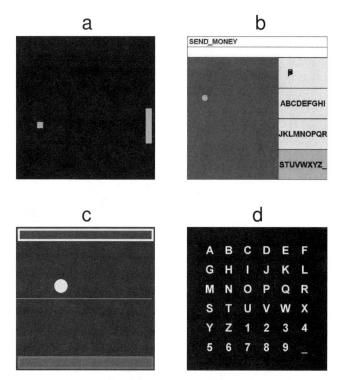

Figure 21.2   Output screens for four BCI2000 implementations tested to date. **(a)** Sensorimotor rhythm control of cursor movement to a variable number of targets. **(b)** A simple spelling application using sensorimotor rhythm control. **(c)** Slow cortical potential (SCP) control of cursor movement to two possible selections. **(d)** A spelling application based on P300 evoked potentials. In (a)–(c), the cursor moves from left to right at a constant rate with its vertical movement controlled by the user's brain signals. In (d), rows and columns of the matrix flash in a block-randomized fashion.

matrix spelling application based on P300 evoked potentials. Figure 21.2 shows the user screens for four of these applications.

21.4.4   Operator Interface Module

The Operator Interface module provides the investigator with a graphical interface that displays current system parameters and real-time analysis results (e.g., frequency spectra) communicated to it from other modules. It allows the investigator to start, stop, suspend, resume, or reconfigure system operation. In a typical BCI2000 configuration, user feedback is displayed on one monitor, and the Operator module's graphical interface (i.e., the interface to the investigator) is displayed on a second monitor.

21.4.5   System Variables

BCI2000 incorporates three types of system variables: parameters, event markers, and signals. System parameters are those variables that do not change throughout a data file (i.e., during a specified period of online operation). In contrast, event markers record events that occur during operation and that can change from one data sample to the next. The inclusion of all event markers in the data file allows full offline reconstruction and analysis of the experimental session. Each module has access to these event markers, and can modify and/or simply monitor them. Finally, system signals are functions of the user's brain signals that are received and modified by the modules.

Each module can request that the Operator module create any number of system parameters (of different data types such as numbers, vectors, matrices, or strings) or event markers (each 1–16 bits long). For example, the Source module might request a parameter that defines the signal's sampling rate. This parameter is constant during some defined period of online operation, is available to all other modules, and is recorded automatically in the data file. Similarly, a Signal Processing filter designed to detect artifacts (such as ones created by muscle movements) might request an event marker with which to mark artifacts in the signal, and an Application module might request an event marker to record stimulus conditions.

21.4.6   System Requirements and Real-Time Processing

As a run-time environment, the current implementation of BCI2000 requires Microsoft Windows 2000 or a more recent Windows-based operating system, any recent desktop or laptop computer, and one of the data acquisition devices that BCI2000 supports (see table 21.1).

A BCI system must acquire and process brain signals (potentially from many channels at high sampling rates) and respond with appropriate output within a short time period (i.e., latency) with minimal variation (i.e., latency jitter). To give an impression of the timing performance of BCI2000 in actual online operation, table 21.2 illustrates system performance for different configurations. While Windows is not a real-time operating system and thus does not guarantee specific timing of events, in each test case, system latency and latency jitter easily satisfied the real-time requirements of BCI operation (e.g., latencies are well below 20 ms). Furthermore, processor load was sufficiently low to guarantee reliable operation. This indicates that even on the modest hardware tested, BCI2000 could have handled even higher sampling rates, larger numbers of channels, or more complex signal processing methods.

21.4.7   Offline Analysis Tools

We currently provide tools to visualize signals in the time domain, to get information on the configuration stored in a data file, and to convert data files to ASCII and MATLAB.

The standard installation of BCI2000 also comes with an easy-to-use analysis tool developed by Febo Cincotti at Fondazione Santa Lucia in Rome, Italy. This software, called "Mario," supports data recorded from sensorimotor rhythm experiments and from P300 evoked potential experiments conducted using BCI2000. For analysis of sensorimotor rhythms, it produces statistical analyses of frequency components for the different experimental conditions. For analysis of P300-evoked potentials, it produces statistical analyses

PC Cfg	Processing configuration	Output latency (ms)	Latency jitter (ms)	System clock jitter (ms)	Processor load (%)
1	A	4.26	0.57	4.31	15
1	B	15.11	0.57	2.65	36
2	A	3.22	0.67	0.57	23
2	C	11.02	0.75	0.69	59

Table 21.2 Performance measures for two different hardware configurations and three different data acquisition/signal processing implementations. PC configuration 1 was a machine with a 1.4 GHz Athlon processor, 256 Mb RAM, IDE I/O sub-system, and Data Translation DT3003 data acquisition board, running Windows 2000. PC configuration 2 was a machine with a 2.53 GHz Pentium 4 processor, 1 Gb RAM, SCSI I/O sub-system, and National Instruments NI 6024E data acquisition board, running Windows XP. Both configurations provided real-time display of the raw signals; and for both the User Application was one of the two cursor movement applications (section 21.4.3). In configuration A, the Source module sampled and stored 16 channels at 160 Hz each and 16 times/s sent the results (i.e., all 16 channels at 10 values per channel) to the Signal Processing module. The Signal Processing module extracted signal features from all channels by using an autoregressive method to calculate voltage spectra. (All voltage spectra were displayed in real time.) Configuration B was the same as configuration A, except that 64 channels were acquired and processed. In configuration C, the Source module sampled 16 channels at 25 kHz each and 25 times/s sent the results (i.e., all 16 channels at 1000 values per channel) to the Signal Processing module. The Signal Processing module used a simple spike detection method to extract spike firings from all 16 channels. For each configuration, Output Latency was the average time between acquisition of a block of data and feedback output reflecting that block, and Latency Jitter was its standard deviation. System Clock Jitter was the standard deviation of the intervals between successive completions of acquisitions of blocks of data.

of the signal time course for different conditions. In both cases, the results can be mapped topographically to standard EEG electrode locations.

Additionally, we created a framework to compile and link BCI2000 signal processing components (filters) as command-line programs that read BCI2000 parameter, state, and signal data from standard input, apply the filter they represent, and write the result to standard output. This allows for offline processing of recorded data using the same code that is used in the online system. For high sampling rates and/or large numbers of channels, the memory efficiency of stream-based command line processing may make it the preferred choice for data preprocessing and data reduction prior to statistical analysis.

Similar to the command line programs, BCI2000 filters may also be compiled into dynamically loaded libraries (DLLs), and thus be called from any program, for example, from MATLAB. In BCI development, signal processing routines that exist as a MATLAB prototype may be implemented in C++ as a BCI2000 filter, and then called from MATLAB, allowing comparison of the C++ and the MATLAB versions of this filter. A detailed example script is provided with the DLL framework, demonstrating how to call a filter DLL through MATLAB's *loadlibrary* generic DLL interface.

21.4.8 Rapid Prototyping with MATLAB

For rapid prototyping of signal processing algorithms, BCI2000 comes with a Signal Processing module that exports most of the BCI2000 filter interface to the MATLAB side. There, a filter implementation consists of a set of scripts called from BCI2000 to perform various aspects of initialization and processing of data blocks. From within these scripts, MATLAB code can

(1) act on blocks of brain signal data in real-time,
(2) request its own parameters and event markers,
(3) read and modify parameter and marker values, and
(4) report configuration and run-time errors.

21.5 Future Development

Hardware support: Data acquisition systems tend to be the most expensive components in BCI systems, and laboratories often already own such equipment. Thus, the utility of the BCI2000 system could be increased if it supported all commonly used data acquisition systems. Table 21.1 provides a list of data acquisition systems that are currently supported. We plan to add support for additional devices if there is sufficient demand.

Platform independence: In its current implementation, BCI2000 depends on the Borland C++ compiler and the Borland VCL application framework. By moving toward platform-independent libraries, and by replacing nonportable portions from the code base, we plan to make future versions of BCI2000 compatible with multiple compilers and operating systems, in particular gcc and Linux but also WindowsCE and Mac OS X.

Clinical implementations: In clinical settings, it is critical to make BCI setup, operation, and analyses available to users who are not experts on BCI technology. Thus, it is necessary to create versions of BCI2000 that might be less complex and flexible, but also easier to use. We plan to create initial versions of such clinical versions of BCI2000, which will support simple menu selection using sensorimotor rhythms and P300-evoked potentials.

Integration with other software: Real-world applications of a BCI could often benefit from the plethora of existing software that specialize in stimulus presentation, augmentative control (such as the University of Rome's ASPICE project), or efficient low-bandwidth communication (such as the Dasher project developed at Cambridge University). Interfacing BCI2000 with such external software is an important goal of its future development.

21.6 Availability

BCI2000 is available at http://www.bci2000.org. This Web site provides additional information for and from the growing number of BCI2000 users.

While access to BCI2000 source code and executables is free of charge for research and educational purposes, Wadsworth requires execution of a Material Transfer Agreement between a user's institution and Wadsworth. At present, this agreement is paper-based. This process will soon be simplified and made available through a Web-based interface. This agreement mainly prohibits commercial use and limits liability. Wadsworth is prepared for potential commercial licensing.

Compilation of the full BCI2000 source code requires version 5.4 of the Borland C++ compiler and version 6.0 of the Borland VCL application framework (both of which are part of the Borland C++ Builder 6 Development Studio 2006 development environment), but otherwise does not rely on third-party components. The Borland C++ compiler (without IDE and VCL, available free of charge from the vendor's Web site) is sufficient to build the offline signal processing environment (command line programs and DLLs).

Acknowledgments

Initial development of BCI2000 has been sponsored by a NIH Bioengineering Research Partnership grant (EB00856) to Jonathan Wolpaw. Current development is sponsored by a NIH R01 grant (EB006356) to Gerwin Schalk.

Many individuals contributed to the development of BCI2000. These include, in alphabetical order, Erik Aarnoutse, Brendan Allison, Simona Bufalari, Bob Cardillo, Febo Cincotti, Emanuele Fiorilla, g.tec, Thilo Hinterberger, Jenny Hizver, Sam Inverso, Vaishali Kamat, Dean Krusienski, Marco Mattioco, Dennis McFarland, Melody M. Moore-Jackson, Yvan Pearson-Lecours, Chintan Shah, Mark Span, Chris Veigl, Janki Vora, Adam Wilson, Shi Dong Zheng.

Notes

E-mail for correspondence: juergen.mellinger@uni-tuebingen.de

V Applications

Introduction

The promise of BCI technology is to augment human capabilities by enabling people to interact with a computer through a conscious and spontaneous modulation of their brainwaves after a short training period. Indeed, by analyzing brain electrical activity online, several groups have designed brain-actuated systems that provide alternative channels for communication, entertainment, and control. Thus, a person can write messages using a virtual keyboard on a computer screen and also browse the internet. Alternatively, subjects can operate simple computer games, or brain games, and interact with educational software. Researchers have also been able to train monkeys to move a computer cursor to desired targets and also to control a robot arm. Work with humans has shown that it is possible for them to move a cursor, open and close a hand orthosis, and even to drive a mobile robot through rooms in a house model. It is worth noticing that for brain-actuated robots, contrarily to augmented communication through BCI, fast decision-making is critical. In this sense, real-time control of brain-actuated devices, especially robots and neuroprostheses, is the most challenging application for BCI.

Some of these BCI prototypes have been described in previous chapters, especially in parts I and II. The chapters in this part illustrate other possible applications of BCI technology. Kübler et al. (see chapter 22) give a review of clinical applications of BCI, highlighting the low number of paralyzed patients using BCI technology and experiments carried out by patients without the expert assistance. In particular, the authors report their experience with patients in the complete locked-in state. Leeb et al. (see chapter 23) describe a virtual reality system controlled through a BCI. They report experiments on navigation in virtual environments with a cue-based (synchronous) and an uncued (asynchronous) BCI. The authors conclude with a discussion on the possible uses and advantages of virtual reality for improving BCI performance and speeding up BCI training.

The last two chapters in this part deal with a different way of brain-computer interaction, namely, recognition of brain phenomena for monitoring purposes. The basic idea is to recognize neural correlates of some cognitive states such as mental workload (see chapter 24) and visual recognition events (see chapter 25) and use them for improving the performance of the system in which they are embedded. Kohlmorgen et al. (see chapter 24) present an EEG-based system able to detect high mental workload in drivers operating under real traffic conditions. After detection of this high workload, the system automatically reduces workload, thus leading to an increase of the driver's overall performance. Sajda et al. (see chapter 25) describe an EEG-based system for single-trial detection of visual recognition events. They exploit basic neuroscience findings for the development of a system that achieves high-throughput image triage. Experimental results show that their brain technology improves image search over a strictly behavioral paradigm.

Altogether these applications show that the field of BCI, although still in its infancy, is no longer in the realm of science fiction. It will not be long before it is possible to operate mentally complex systems that will restore mobility and communication capabilities to disabled people, thus helping them increase their independence and facilitate their participation in society. This is the main driving force behind the development of BCI technology. But to achieve the promise of augmenting the mental capabilities, it is first necessary to improve the performance and robustness of BCI technology so that it can be taken out of the laboratory and used in real-world situations. The previous chapters provide a rather large, but not exhaustive, set of approaches that currently are being explored in this rapidly developing field.

Of course, BCI is also relevant for healthy people. However, its development is more pressing for disabled people since the former will start using BCI systems only when new sensor technology is developed and performance and robustness will become sufficiently high, as it is the case today with speech recognition technology. In the meantime, though, applications such as those illustrated by Ferrez and Millán, Kohlmorgen et al., and Sajda et al. in chapters 17, 24, and 25, respectively, may well lead to new paradigms of human-computer interaction based on BCI technology. In this case, classical interaction, control, or supervision tasks are extended with real-time recognition of particular brain phenomena, thus yielding substantial improvements in performance and, more importantly, achieving the development of truly adaptive systems that customize dynamically in response to changes of the cognitive and emotional/affective states of the user.

José del R. Millán

22   Brain-Computer Interfaces for Communication and Motor Control— Perspectives on Clinical Applications

Andrea Kübler and Femke Nijboer
Institute of Medical Psychology and Behavioural Neurobiology
Eberhard-Karls-University Tübingen, Gartenstr. 29
72074 Tübingen, Germany

Niels Birbaumer

Institute of Medical Psychology and　　　　*National Institute of Health (NIH)*
Behavioural Neurobiology　　　　　　　　　*NINDS*
Eberhard-Karls-University Tübingen　　　　*Human Cortical Physiology Unit*
Gartenstr. 29　　　　　　　　　　　　　　　　*Bethesda, USA*
72074 Tübingen, Germany

22.1   Abstract

In this overview of the state-of-the-art of clinical applications of BCIs and outlook for the future, we focus on interfaces aiming at maintaining or restoring lost communication and motor function using the electric and magnetic activity of the human cortex.

22.2   Introduction

In 2001 we presented our first review on BCIs and we identified five groups that worked with disabled patients, three of which had more or less experience with patients in the field (Kübler et al. (2001a)). Only one patient from our group in Tübingen has been using the BCI system without experts from the lab being present for private communication with his friends, such that he wrote and printed letters with the BCI.[1] A caregiver was needed only to put the letter into an envelope and to bring it to the post office. None of the patients used the BCI for communication or environmental control in daily life. In the past ten years, the number of laboratories involved in BCI research and development augmented from about 5 in 1994 (Vaughan et al. (1996)),[2] about twenty-two in 1999 (Wolpaw et al. (2000a)),

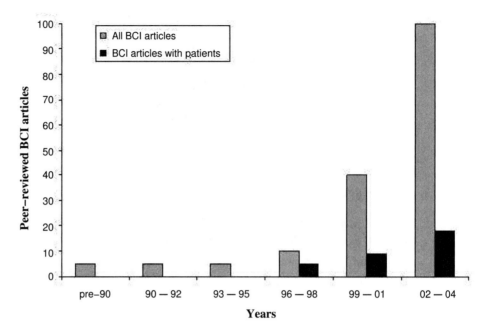

Figure 22.1 Number of peer-reviewed BCI publications as a function of time. Grey columns represent all BCI articles (from J. R. Wolpaw with kind permission). Black columns represent BCI publications that include patients regardless of their disease, whether data of the same patients were published under different aspects, and whether the same patients took part in different studies. Only publications in which patients received feedback (closed-loop) are included. Publication output in 2002–2004 is tenfold that of the prenineties and doubles that of the turn of the twentieth century. In 1997 the first publications with patients appear and are also constantly increasing, but are by far outnumbered by technical papers based on data from healthy participants.

twenty-eight in 2002 (Vaughan et al. (2003b)), to more than fifty in 2005[3] (Vaughan and Wolpaw (2006)). Currently, seventy groups are using the BCI2000 as a general purpose brain-computer interface (Schalk et al. (2004)) (http://www.bciresearch.org). Figure 22.1 illustrates the increase of people working in the BCI field on the basis of the publication output.

Tremendous improvements have been achieved in brain signal classification and patient training resulting in as many as ten brain-controlled selections per minute (see section on P300 in 22.4). More studies (mainly from the same laboratories as reviewed in 2001) have been published on results with patients (Kübler et al. (2004, 2005a); Wolpaw and McFarland (2004); Neuper et al. (2003); Pfurtscheller et al. (2003b); Sellers and Donchin (2006)) (figures 22.1 and 22.2). Despite these positive and encouraging results and developments, the number of patients in the field using the system without experts from the BCI group being present has not increased and still—to our knowledge—none of the patients is using a BCI for communication and control in daily life. Additionally, and of utmost importance, we have not yet successfully restored even basic communication (yes/no) in patients who

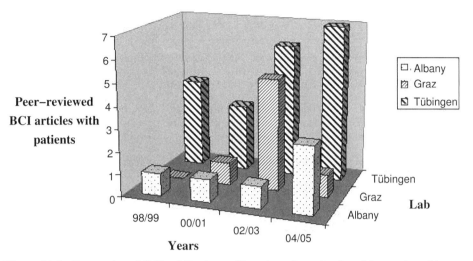

Figure 22.2 Peer-reviewed BCI publications with patients from the three laboratories with most patient experience (in terms of patient numbers and BCI training in the lab and at the patients' home).

are in the complete locked-in state (CLIS; see next section). These patients, however, need most urgently a BCI to restore communication and interaction with the environment.

22.3 The Locked-In Syndrome

Several neurological diseases with different neuropathology may lead to the so-called locked-in state (LIS) in which only residual voluntary muscular control is possible. Such a state in which sensory, emotional, and cognitive processing remains largely intact (depending on the disease) may be the result of a traumatic brain injury, hypoxia (e.g., due to heart attack), stroke, encephalitis, tumor, chronic Guillain Barré syndrome, or neurodegenerative diseases such as amyotrophic lateral sclerosis (ALS). Despite different disease etiology, the affected patients are very similar such that they can hardly communicate, have no control over limb movement, depend on intensive care, are artificially fed and often also ventilated, and lack immediate reinforcement of thoughts and intentions (see section 22.5). In almost all cases, residual muscular control like blinking and eye movement remains available. However, patients may also be in or enter—with disease progression—the complete locked-in state in which no muscular control, and thus no communication, is possible.

The specifics with regard to ALS are that the disease progresses over, on average, three years (sometimes only months, sometimes many years) from the first symptoms of muscular or respiratory weakness to respiratory failure. Thus, these patients are in a unique manner confronted with the end-of-life decision. They have the possibility to continue their life beyond respiratory failure if they consent to invasive ventilation. Issues on quality of life and ethical considerations with regard to the LIS and in relation to assisted suicide go beyond the scope of this chapter. The interested reader is referred to Kübler et al. (2006, 2005b); Birbaumer (2005).

22.4   State-of-the-Art in Clinical Application of BCIs

In the following paragraphs, we refer only to results achieved with patients. We do so because many impressive classification results have been achieved with healthy participants (e.g., Dornhege et al. (2004a); Blankertz et al. (2003)). However, as the neurophysiology and topography of the brains of all patients who are in need of a BCI, are altered—due to lesions, degeneration, reorganization, and possibly nonuse—results from healthy controls have to prove their validity in patient groups before we may consider the used brain signal and its classification method as a potential means of communication or neuroprosthesis control. Moreover, several reviews without restriction to patient groups are available (Kübler et al. (2001a); Donoghue (2002); Kübler and Neumann (2005); Nicolelis (2003); Curran and Stokes (2003); Wolpaw et al. (2002); Schwartz (2004b)). We also refrain from going into the details of signal analysis and classification for the different BCI approaches (see part III) and rather focus on the control and command outcome within the patient population.

22.4.1   Non-Invasive BCIs—Electrical and Magnetic Brain Activity (EEG, MEG)

Noninvasive BCIs use the electrical activity of the brain (electroencephalogram, EEG) recorded with single or multiple electrodes from the scalp surface as input signal for BCI control. Such BCIs we refer to as EEG-BCIs. We summarize results of EEG-BCIs used to restore communication and motor control. Noninvasive BCIs on the basis of the magnetic activity of the brain (magnetoencephalogram, MEG) are introduced and discussed in the last section of this chapter.

22.4.1.1   EEG-BCIs

The brain signals that have been used as input signals for BCI to maintain or reinstall motor control are slow cortical potentials (SCP) (Kübler et al. (1999); Birbaumer et al. (1999); Hinterberger et al. (2004b)), sensorimotor rhythms (SMR) (Wolpaw and McFarland (2004); Pfurtscheller et al. (2000b); Neuper et al. (2005); McFarland et al. (1993)), or a combination of both (Dornhege et al. (2004a)), and the P300 response of the visually and auditorily evoked potential (Sellers and Donchin (2006); Farwell and Donchin (1988)). Both the SCP-BCI and the SMR-BCI require regulation of the brain response whereas the P300-BCI requires the specific evoked potential to be present in the EEG. Patients learn to regulate the SCP amplitude or to modulate SMR when presented with continuous feedback of the EEG signal of interest. Over the past ten years, we have confronted thirty-five patients with one or each of the EEG-BCIs; such a huge patient sample is unique in the BCI community. Thirty patients were diagnosed with ALS, five of which were in the LIS and five in the CLIS, one patient was in the LIS after brain stem stroke, two as a consequence of

Degree of success*	Degree of physical impairment				
	Limb movement restricted, but possible; speech	Limb movement intact, no speech	Limb movement very restricted, speech impaired	Locked-in state (LIS) residual muscular control (eye movement, lip twitch, etc.)	Complete locked-in state (CLIS)
None			2**	1	7
Significant control over a brain or other physiological response	7	1	9	7	1 (pH)
Copy spelling	1	1	6	4	
Free spelling		1	2	3	
Internet			1	1	
Number of patients	7	1	12	8	7

Table 22.1 Overview of the degree of success achieved by patients from our group who have been confronted with a BCI on the basis of SCPs, SMR, or P300. All patients were severely disabled ranging from being able to control limb movement and speech (although almost always restricted) to being left with only residual muscular control (LIS) or even with no motor control (CLIS).
* Multiple entries of patients possible. For example, the one patient with intact limb movement but no speech achieved significant control over a brain response and succeeded in copy and free spelling.
** We were unable to analyze data of one patient due to trainer failure.

muscular dystrophy, one CLIS patient suffered from hypoxia after a heart attack, and one had chronic Guillan Barré syndrome. The table 22.1 provides an overview of the degree of physical impairment and the degree of successful BCI control (significant control over the brain signal) and communication (significant spelling results). With the exception of two patients, who were still able to walk or use a wheelchair without a caregiver and came to our institute for the training sessions, all patients were trained in their home environment. In the following three paragraphs, we review the results of our and other patient groups using these BCIs for communication and motor control.

SCP-BCI

Slow cortical potentials depend on sustained afferent intracortical or thalamocortical input to cortical layers I and II and on simultaneous depolarization of large pools of pyramidal neurons. The depolarization of cortical cell assemblies reduces their excitation threshold, and firing of neurons in regions responsible for specified motor or cognitive tasks is facilitated (Birbaumer et al. (1990)). The anterior brain systems are particularly important for regulation of SCPs (Lutzenberger et al. (1980)). Over the past ten years we trained thirty-two disabled patients with our SCP-BCI. We record the EEG with single electrodes and feedback is provided from Cz (Jasper (1958)). To learn regulation of the SCP amplitude, patients are presented with two targets: one at the top and one at the bottom of the screen. We provide continuous feedback in discrete trials via cursor movement on a computer screen. A negative SCP amplitude—compared to a baseline recorded at the beginning of each trial—leads to cursor movement toward the top, and a positive SCP amplitude toward the bottom of the screen. For details of patient training and signal processing, the reader is referred to our other publications (Kübler et al. (1999); Hinterberger et al. (2004b); Kübler et al. (2001b, 2003); Hinterberger et al. (2003a)). Twenty patients have been participating in SCP-BCI training for the purpose of communication. Eight patients were trained with the SCP-BCI for the purpose of being examined with functional magnetic resonance imaging during SCP amplitude regulation. These patients were trained only until they achieved significant control, but were not further trained to use this ability for communication. Many of the patients achieved significant cursor control within a few training sessions (Kübler et al. (2004, 1999, 1998)). However, to use this ability for communication, patients need to be able to regulate their SCP amplitude with at least 70 percent accuracy (Kübler et al. (2004, 1999, 1998); Perelmouter and Birbaumer (2000)). Five patients were trained long enough to achieve such a high accuracy and used this ability to select letters in a language support program (Perelmouter et al. (1999)). Over weeks and months, patients learn in small steps the dual task of regulating their SCP amplitude and selecting letters or items on the screen. To achieve this goal, we present patients with words to copy. If they master this task with 75 percent accuracy, we confront them with the multiple task of SCP amplitude regulation, and letter selection, as well as thinking of what to communicate and how to spell these words (Kübler et al. (2001b)). Figure 22.3 shows selection of the letter "O" in the free spelling mode of our language support program. At the uppermost level of the LSP, the patient is presented with the entire alphabet subdivided in halves for presentation. After selection of one half by producing a positive SCP amplitude shift, this half is again split in two and this goes on until a single letter is presented for selection. Although the SCP-BCI takes quite a while until patients are able to communicate, it is—to our knowledge—still the only BCI with which severely disabled and LIS patients have communicated messages of considerable length (Neumann et al. (2003); Birbaumer et al. (1999); Kübler et al. (2001b); Kübler (2000)). Two of our patients are surfing the Net with Nessi, a BCI-adapted Internet browser, which allows the patients a selection of links by presenting them in a binary mode; all the links of one Web site are assigned to either the top or bottom half of the screen. As in the language support program, the number of links per target is divided after selection until a single link is presented for selection (Karim et al. (2006); Mellinger et al. (2003)).

SMR-BCI

Sensorimotor or μ rhythm refers to 8–12 Hz EEG activity that can be recorded in awake people over primary sensory or motor cortical areas (Niedermeyer (2005a)). It is usually accompanied by 18–25Hz β rhythms. It decreases or desynchronizes with movement or preparation for movement (event-related desynchronization—ERD) and increases or synchronizes (event-related synchronization—ERS) in the postmovement period or during

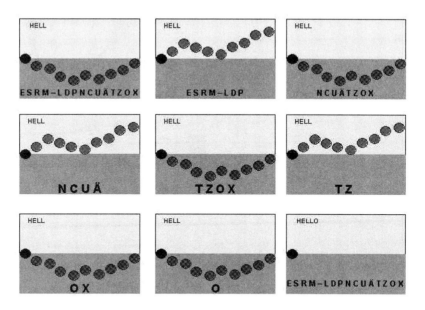

Figure 22.3 Spelling with the language support program in the free spelling mode (Kübler et al. (2001b)). Letters are presented in the bottom half of the screen for selection. If the target letter is in the presented string of letters, the patient has to produce cortical positivity to select the bottom half. If not the patient must reject the letter string by producing a cortical negativity which moves the cursor into the upper half of the screen. In the case of selecting of the letter "O," 8 consecutive steps are needed corresponding to a minimum of 32 seconds if no error occurs.

relaxation (Pfurtscheller (2005); Pfurtscheller and Aranibar (1979)). Operant learning of SMR regulation is achieved through activation and deactivation of the central motor loops. To learn to modulate the power of SMR, patients are also presented with feedback, for example, cursor movement on a computer screen in one or two dimensions (Wolpaw et al. (1991); Wolpaw and McFarland (1994)). During each trial of one-dimensional control, users are presented with a target consisting of a red vertical bar that occupies the top or bottom half of the right edge of the screen and a cursor on the left edge. The cursor moves steadily across the screen, with its vertical movement controlled by the SMR amplitude. The patients' task is to move the cursor to the level of the target so that it hits the target when it reaches the right edge. Low SMR amplitude following movement imagery moves the cursor to the bottom bar, high SMR amplitude following thinking of nothing in particular ("relaxation") moves the cursor toward the top bar. Cursor movement to different targets can also be achieved by different movement imagery (e.g., left vs. right hand or feet vs. hand movement). Using this SMR-BCI, we have shown that ALS patients are able to achieve SMR regulation of more than 75 percent accuracy within less than twenty training

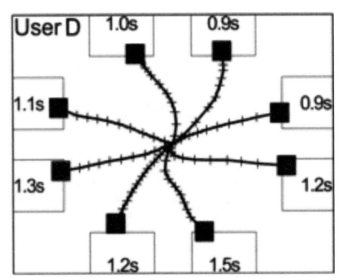

Figure 22.4   Feedback screen of the two-dimensional SMR-BCI with eight targets. Participant's task is to move the cursor to one of the targets. Cursor movement starts in the center of the screen (Wolpaw and McFarland (2004)). The trajectories of the best of four users are depicted. Within 0.9–1.5 s he was able to move the cursor to the targets without hitting one of the neighbor targets erroneously (from PNAS, Vol. 101, No. 51, 2004, p. 17852, with permission).

sessions (Kübler et al. (2005a)). With such control over SMR amplitude, a binary "yes/no" answer is possible. On the basis of their tremendous expertise with SMR regulation, classification, and feedback, Wolpaw, McFarland, and their colleagues recently realized two-dimensional control with cursor movement to eight targets (figure 22.4) (Wolpaw and McFarland (2004)). To date, Wolpaw et al. have trained two patients with spinal cord injury (C6, T7) (Wolpaw and McFarland (2004); McFarland et al. (2005)), two patients with cerebral palsy (McFarland et al. (2003)), two patients with ALS (Wolpaw et al. (1997); Miner et al. (1998)), and one patient with abnormal gait (Schalk et al. (2000)) to control cursor movement in one or two dimensions toward two to eight targets via regulation of the SMR amplitude. In one study, participants used SMR regulation to answer yes or no questions such that the two targets were replaced by the words YES and NO (Miner et al. (1998)).

Event-related desynchronization (ERD) of SMR as a function of motor imagery is also used by the Graz group (Pfurtscheller et al. (2003c)). BCI training with the Graz system typically involves moving a cursor to one of two possible targets for the purpose of communication or controlling a neuroprosthesis.

In 2003, Neuper et al. (in cooperation with the Tübingen group) reported results of a patient with infantile cerebral paresis, who was trained over a period of several months with the SMR-BCI (Neuper et al. (2003)). The patient was trained with a two-target task and was provided with feedback of ERD in the alpha band (8–12 Hz). Eventually, the targets were replaced by letters and the patient could spell with the system, using a so-called virtual keyboard (Obermaier et al. (2001)). The virtual keyboard has the same function

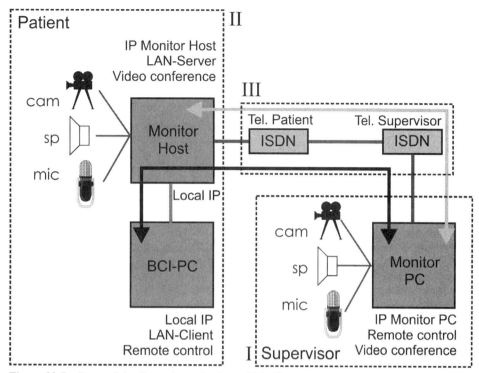

Figure 22.5 Setup of the Graz telemonitoring, which allows experts to supervise patient training, to analyze data immediately, and to correct parameters if necessary in the laboratory (Müller et al. (2003b)) (from IEEE Trans Neural Syst Rehabil Eng, Vol. 11, No. 1, 2003, p. 55, with permission).

as the language support program from our group (Perelmouter et al. (1999)): It allows patients to select letters in successive binary steps. A different set of letters is presented at the top and the bottom of the screen and the patient has to move the cursor into that half of the screen that contains the desired letter. The spelling rate varied between 0.2 and 2.5 letters per minute. Although this rate may seem slow, Neuper et al. showed for the first time that SMR-BCIs could provide communication for patients in the LIS. Müller et al. (2003) implemented a telemonitoring system during SMR-BCI training with the same patient diagnosed with cerebral palsy (figure 22.5). Since this patient lived in Germany 850 kilometers (approximately 530 miles) away from the Graz lab, the training was conducted by a local caregiver and supervised by the Graz group by means of a Web camera and online control of the EEG and BCI settings (Müller et al. (2003b)). Via telemonitoring, the authors conducted thirty-nine BCI training sessions over twenty-two weeks occasionally supervised directly by a BCI trainer from the Tübingen group.

Besides communication, the Graz group implemented SMR-BCI mediated neuroprosthesis control in two exemplary patients. First, a tetraplegic patient, whose residual muscle activity of the upper limbs was restricted to the left biceps after spinal cord injury, learned to open and close his hand with the aids of an orthosis that reacted upon changes in the SMR ERD (Pfurtscheller et al. (2000a)). The authors report an accuracy rate of almost

100 percent. In a second study with the same patient, grasping movement was realized via SMR-BCI-controlled functional electrical stimulation (FES). To execute a grasping movement first, the finger and thumb extensors were stimulated for hand opening. Closing of fingers was achieved by deactivation of the finger extensors and moderate activation of finger and thumb flexors. To close the thumb, the thumb extensor was deactivated and finger and thumb flexors fully activated. Reopening of the hand followed deactivation of finger and thumb flexors and reactivation of finger and thumb extensors. An idling state of hand muscles was achieved by deactivating finger and thumb extensors (Pfurtscheller et al. (2003b)). The patient could induce FES sequentially by foot movement imagery that was accompanied by increased power in the β band (15–19 Hz). In an interview, the patient stated that with only minimal help from his family he can perform simple grasp functions, for example, he can now grasp a glass of milk and drink it instead of having to ask one of his family members to hold the cup for him (http://www.bci-info.tugraz.at/).

Another patient with spinal cord injury (C5) was available for only three training days. Müller-Putz et al. demonstrated that the patient gained control over the SMR-BCI system for the control of a neuroprosthesis within a very short training period (Müller-Putz et al. (2005b)). The patient was trained with the so-called Basket paradigm. A trial consisted of a ball descending from the top to the bottom of a black screen. Baskets (serving as cues) positioned either on the left or the right half of the screen indicated by their color (red: target; green: nontarget) which type of imagery the patient should perform to move the ball into the basket. Imagery of left hand movement was the strategy that worked best for the patient. Then the BCI was coupled with the neuroprosthesis. Each detection of a left hand motor imagery task subsequently switched the neuroprosthesis to grasping movement (see FES). Krausz et al. trained four wheelchair-bound paraplegic patients with the Basket paradigm. After a few sessions over some weeks, all patients learned to control the BCI with the best session between 77 and 95 percent accuracy (Krausz et al. (2003)).

In summary, SMR-BCIs have been successfully tested in ALS, cerebral palsy, and spinal cord injury patients and may provide communication or restoration of lost motor function.

P300-BCI

The P300 is a positive deflection in the electroencephalogram (EEG) time-locked to auditory or visual stimuli. It is seen typically when participants are required to attend to rare target stimuli presented within a stream of frequent standard stimuli (Squires et al. (1977)), an experimental design referred to as an oddball paradigm (Fabiani et al. (1987)). In the P300-BCI, participants are presented with a 6×6 matrix where each of the 36 cells contains a character or a symbol (Farwell and Donchin (1988)) (figure 22.6). This design becomes an oddball paradigm by first intensifying each row and column for 100 ms in random order and second by instructing participants to attend to only one of the 36 cells. Thus, in one trial of 12 flashes (6 rows and 6 columns), the target cell will flash only twice, constituting a rare event compared to the 10 flashes of all other rows and columns, and will therefore elicit a P300. For details of design and signal classification, the reader is referred to Sellers and Donchin (2006), Sellers et al. (2006b), and Xu et al. (2004).

Using data from 10 able-bodied participants and 4 paraplegic patients, Donchin et al. predicted from offline analysis a spelling rate of 7.8 characters per minute for able-bodied

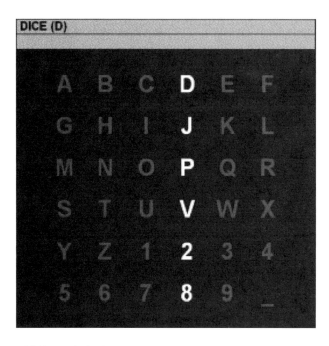

Figure 22.6   The P300 matrix in the copy-spelling mode. The patients' task is to copy the word given by the trainer. Rows and columns are intensified in random order. In each trial, the target letter is shown in parentheses following the word to copy. Selected letters appear in the second line. The patients must count how often the target letter flashes.

participants and a spelling rate of 5.9 characters per minute for patients with an accuracy of 80 percent (Donchin et al. (2000)). In 2003, Sellers et al. published the first results of an ALS patient using the P300 Speller (Sellers et al. (2003)). In recent studies, Sellers et al. and Nijboer et al. presented preliminary results of the P300 Speller used by ALS patients indicating that ALS patients are able to use the P300-BCI with accuracies up to 100 percent (Sellers et al. (2006b)). To date, we have presented 8 ALS patients in different stages of the disease with the P300 spelling matrix. In all but one we were able to detect a P300 in response to the target letters, and all patients spelled above chance level (Kübler et al. (in preparation)). Two of the patients spelled with 100 percent accuracy and four were transferred to free spelling. By further adapting the classification to the patients' P300 response, we succeeded in reducing the number of flashes per letter to four in one patient. This presentation rate resulted in a character selection time of 5.25 s with an accuracy of 80 percent using a 7 × 7 matrix (67.23 bits/min not including time between characters or 22.96 bits/min including the time between characters) (Nijboer et al. (submitted)). This is the highest communication speed ever achieved with a BCI. This result is very promising because it was achieved with ALS patients. Both patients were severely disabled (patient A had limb movement but no speech and patient G was wheelchair bound, almost quadriplegic, and had largely impaired speech) but not in the LIS or CLIS. Thus, it remains to be shown that the P300-BCI is also useful for LIS and CLIS patients. The main problem with using P300-BCI for these patients is that eye movement becomes weaker so that they may no longer be able to fixate on all cells of the matrix; the matrix then has to be reduced in size according to the individual patients' capacity to control gaze. CLIS patients, in fact, are no longer able to use a BCI based on vision. For CLIS patients, all BCIs must work with auditory stimulation completely independent of vision. First results with a four-choice auditory oddball in four patients who were in the CLIS for several years have not been promising.

22.4.1.2 MEG-BCI

Magnetoencephalography (MEG) measures magnetic fields generated by the electrical currents in the brain. MEG sensors are induction coils statically arranged in a helmet, and the position of a participant's head relative to the helmet is controlled using three localization coils attached to the head. In contrast to EEG-BCIs, the MEG-BCI is confined to the laboratory and only patients who manage to get to the lab can participate. We used a whole-head MEG system comprising 151 first-order gradiometers (CTF Inc., Vancouver, Canada) placed in a magnetically shielded room. The MEG-BCI provides visual real-time feedback of μ (8–12 Hz) or β (18–25 Hz) amplitudes. MEG yields a more localized SMR of higher amplitude compared to EEG, even allowing discrimination of fingers (Braun et al. (2000)), because brain magnetic fields are not attenuated and distorted on their way from the cortical generators to the MEG dewar containing the recording SQUIDs. Feedback consisted of the speed of a cursor projected onto a screen. The cursor moved from left to right and the participants' task was to move it up or down by regulating the amplitude of their SMR. All five (healthy) participants learned to control their SMR amplitude. In all cases, accuracy reached a high level toward the end of the first session. Maximum accuracy exceeded 90 percent for four participants, and one participant achieved 80 percent accuracy. Performance stabilized above the level achieved in session one (Mellinger et al. (2005)). Recently, we were able to detect SMR modulation related to left- and right-hand movement imagery in one of our ALS patients in whom EEG recording provided no classifiable results. In the MEG, however, a right hemispheric dipole field related to imagery of left-hand versus right-hand movement was identified and SMR amplitude varied as a function of imagery (figure 22.7). With this patient, we will now continue EEG-SMR-BCI training with electrode position, frequency range, and feedback design as suggested by the MEG results.

On the basis of these results, Birbaumer et al. at the National Institute of Neurological Diseases and Stroke (NINDS) together with the Tübingen group (Mellinger et al. (2005)) further developed the MEG-BCI for motor restoration (Birbaumer and Cohen (2005)). They train patients with no residual hand movement one or more years after stroke with an MEG-controlled hand orthosis for ten to twenty sessions. The head of the patient is fixated in the dewar and the fingers are attached to the orthosis that opens and closes the hand contingent on SMR increase or decrease, respectively. The patients receive proprioceptive feedback from their own movement simultaneously with visual feedback by means of cursor movement on a screen in relation to the SMR amplitude. After successful hand-

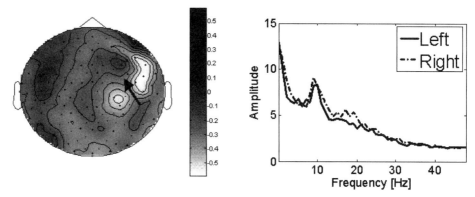

Figure 22.7   Results of an SMR screening session with an ALS patient in the MEG. Left: Topographical plot of signal amplitude differences (in arbitrary units) in the frequency range from 18 to 21 Hz, taken between left-hand and right-hand imagined movement. On the right hemisphere, negative difference values (white) form the field of a dipolar source located roughly at the position indicated by the arrow. Right: Amplitude spectra for the two conditions of imagined hand movements (in arbitrary units). SMR activity appears in the form of amplitude peaks at around 9 Hz (basis frequency) and 18 Hz (first harmonic), with modulation being larger for the first harmonic.

opening, closing, and grasping by means of SMR regulation, the patients are transferred to a mobile EEG-BCI controlled by SMR wearing the same orthosis (Birbaumer (2006a)). As a positive side effect, the patient experienced complete relief of the hand spasticity after several training sessions with the MEG-BCI (Birbaumer (2006a)).

22.4.2   Invasive BCIs—Epidural, Subdural, and Intracortical Recordings

Most of the data on invasive recordings for motor control stem from animal experiments (Schwartz (2004b); Nicolelis et al. (2003); Serruya et al. (2002)) that will not be reviewed here due to the focus on clinical application of BCIs. Few studies were conducted with patients. In the first part of this section we report first results of BCIs on the basis of the electrocorticogram (ECoG), and in the second part we review studies with intracortical recordings. These BCI approaches require brain surgery and long-term stability of the implanted electrode grids (ECoG) or microelectrode arrays (intracortical recordings).

22.4.2.1   ECoG-BCI

The ECoG is measured with strips or arrays epidurally or subdurally from the cortical surface. Its advantages compared to scalp-recorded EEG lay in the broader bandwidth that allows recording of γ band activity (> 30Hz), the higher spatial resolution, and the reduced vulnerability to artifacts such as muscular activity (Leuthardt et al. (2004)). All published data on ECoG-BCIs have been acquired with epilepsy patients in whom electrode grids were implanted for the purpose of later brain surgery to treat epilepsy. In all studies, modulation of the ECoG as a function of actual or imagined movement or both has been recorded (Leuthardt et al. (2004); Lal et al. (2005a); Brunner et al. (2005); Graimann et al. (2004)) and classification accuracies of up to 100 percent have been reported. Leuthardt et al. and Lal et al. closed the loop and provided participants with feedback. Presented with a one-dimensional binary task, patients achieved 74–100 percent accuracy by imagery of speech, hand, and tongue movement. Hinterberger et al. presented their participants with a spelling program and also achieved accuracies up to 100 percent within one training session (Hinterberger et al., unpublished data). Encouraged by these results, we were quite optimistic about being able to reinstall communication in an ALS patient who recently entered the CLIS. She gave informed consent to subdural implantation of a 64-electrode grid to record ECoG. Wilhelm et al. established communication in the otherwise completely locked-in patient by changes in the saliva pH as a function of food imagery (Wilhelm et al. (2006)). When asked to imagine lemon, the saliva pH increased, and after imagery of milk decreased. The authors measured the pH in the mouth cavity mucosa and assigned counterbalanced "yes" and "no" to "milk" and "lemon." Responding with pH manipulation, however, was lost after implantation. Slowing of the ECoG and complete absence of gamma-band activity characterizes her recordings. She responded to sensory stimulation (finger and mouth) and the corresponding areas in S1 were perfectly localizable (figure 22.8), but when regulation of this activity was required by imagery of finger and tongue movement, no classification of the signal was possible. This underlines convincingly and dramatically that results of healthy BCI users or patients diagnosed with other diseases than those that lead to paralysis of the motor system are not sufficient to claim that a BCI is suitable to maintain communication and control in LIS and CLIS patients.

22.4.2.2 *Intracortical Recording*

Intracortical signal acquisition can be realized with single, few, or multiple electrodes that capture spike or field potentials or both simultaneously. Kennedy and Bakay have shown in a few ALS patients that humans are able to modulate the action potential firing rate when provided with feedback (Kennedy and Bakay (1998); Kennedy et al. (2000)). The authors implanted into the motor cortex a single electrode with a glass tip containing neurotrophic factors. Adjacent neurons grew into the tip and, after a few weeks, action potentials were recorded. One patient was able to move a cursor on a computer screen to select presented items, but the time needed for a selection is unclear. The patient had residual muscular control that was also used for system control (Kennedy et al. (2000)).

Several groups use multielectrode recording to detect activation patterns related to movement execution in animals (Carmena et al. (2003); Paninski et al. (2004); Taylor et al. (2002); Musallam et al. (2004)). The action potential firing rate in motor areas contains sensory, motor, perceptual, and cognitive information, which allows us to estimate a subject's intention to execute a movement; it was shown that hand trajectories can be derived from the activity pattern of neuronal cell assemblies in the motor cortex (Serruya et al. (2002)). After training, even complex motor patterns can be reconstructed from a small number of cells located in the motor or parietal areas (Carmena et al. (2003); Taylor et al. (2002); Musallam et al. (2004)). Taylor et al. trained rhesus macaques to move a brain-

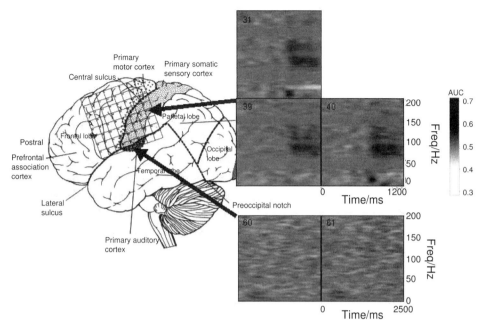

Figure 22.8   Separability of time-frequency features that characterize sensory-evoked responses in the ECoG of one of our patients. A 64-electrode grid has been implanted subdurally as shown on the left-hand side. Panels on the right-hand side show AUC scores as a function of frequency and time after stimulation: midgrey indicates no separability (AUC=0.5; see chapter 19) as exemplified by the horizontal stripes at 50 Hz (mains electricity) and its second harmonic at 150 Hz. Lighter and darker tones indicate better separability. Support-vector classification of the spectrograms of electrodes 31, 39, and 40 following tactile stimulation of the lip resulted in a mean estimated accuracy of 77% (varying from 68 to 86% across 8 sessions). The classifier consistently made use of the frequency range 80–120 Hz about 850 ms after stimulation (see upper right panels). With auditory stimulation, a weakly discriminating feature was visible in several of the sessions in the 5–10 Hz region, also about 850 ms after stimulation (see the bottom right panels—note the different time scale), although classification of spectrograms and of a time-domain representation of the signal was never possible above 55%. Arrows indicate electrode positions from which spectrograms are shown.

controlled robot arm in virtual reality while neural activity was recorded from 18 cells only (Taylor et al. (2003)), and then to feed themselves with a real robot arm (Schwartz (2004a)). Donoghue et al. implanted for the first time such an electrode array in the hand motor area of a patient with quadriplegia following spinal cord injury (Hochberg et al. (2006)). Neural activity from field potentials was translated into movement of a robotic arm and continuous mouse movement on a computer monitor, which was comparable to the multidirectional SMR-controlled cursor movement reported by Wolpaw and McFarland (2004). None of the invasive procedures allowed restoration of skillful movement in animals or humans in daily life situations. All the animals participating in BCI research (Donoghue (2002); Nicolelis (2003)) were healthy, performed real arm movement first, and then learned through food reward to move a robotic arm while movement of the intact arm was restricted in highly artificial laboratory situations. Any generalization from these results with animals to paralyzed, LIS, and CLIS patients seems somewhat premature (Birbaumer (2006a)).

22.5   Some Thoughts about Learning, Thinking, and Communication in the Complete Locked-in State

Despite the view of some neurologists that the CLIS does not exist, we have encountered five patients in the CLIS as a result of degenerative neurological disease. All but one responded to auditory stimulation with oddball (P300) and semantic (N400) paradigms, indicating at least some cognitive processing (Kotchoubey et al. (2002, 2005); Kotchoubey (2005)). Of the two patients we met before they were completely locked-in, both still had control of eye movement. Both responded to auditory stimulation with oddball and semantic paradigms when they entered the CLIS, but lost this ability after months and years in the CLIS.[4]

22.5.1   Operant Conditioning of Autonomic Functions

During the late sixties and early seventies, Miller and colleagues showed that autonomous functions such as heart rate or blood pressure can be brought under voluntary control by means of operant conditioning (Miller (1969)). Curarized rats even after weeks of artificial nutrition and ventilation learned to increase and decrease heart rate, renal blood flow, dilation, and constriction of peripheral arteries in an operant conditioning paradigm rewarding (brain stimulation) the animals for changes in their physiological parameters. These were landmark results because it was believed that the autonomous system is autonomous and independent of the central nervous system. However, in the eighties Miller and his students failed to replicate these results (Dworkin and Miller (1986)). Dworkin, the most productive of Miller's students, attributed this failure to the missing homeostatic effect of the reward: The reward acquires its positive outcome through the homoeostasis-restoring effects, that is, ingestion of food restores glucostatic and fluid balance. In the curarized rat, where all bodily functions are kept artificially constant, the homeostatic function of the reward is no longer present because imbalances of the equilibrium do not occur.

Chronically curarized rats and patients in the CLIS who are artificially fed and ventilated share many similarities. The up-to-date unsuccessful efforts to restore communication in these patients by means of BCI and the failure of the curarized rat to achieve voluntary control of autonomous parameters may have a common reason.

22.5.2   Event-Related Potentials and Regulation of Brain Responses in CLIS

Most often, the lack of communication in the CLIS as a result of ALS or Guillan Barré syndrome is assumed to be due to deterioration of cognitive functions preventing learning and communication. It is difficult to reject this argument empirically because neuropsychological testing for cognitive function is impossible in a completely paralyzed person.

The only possible channel to get information about cognitive processing is the brain itself. Consequently, we developed an event-related brain-potential test battery with a series of cognitive paradigms ranging from simple oddball P300 evoking tasks to highly complex semantic mismatch N400 and personalized memory tasks eliciting late cortical positivities (Kotchoubey et al. (2002, 2005); Kotchoubey (2005); Hinterberger et al. (2005c)).

None of five patients—three of which had ALS—starting BCI-training *after* entering the CLIS acquired stable regulation of a brain response, neither SCP nor SMR. Furthermore, we confronted two patients with an auditory oddball in which a high tone was assigned to "yes" and a low tone to "no." We detected an N100 in both patients showing that the patients heard the tones, but found no P300 response indicating that the lower probability of the target tones was not processed. One of these five patients was implanted with subdural electrodes over the left frontal cortex (figure 22.8). Despite clean ECoG recordings and extensive learning attempts over weeks neither regulation of a brain response nor communication was achieved.

More than one hundred patients in responsive and nonresponsive vegetative states and seventeen ALS patients at different stages of the disease were tested. The relationships between the complexity of a cognitive task and the presence or absence of a particular component in the EEG were rather inconsistent (Kotchoubey et al. (2005)), meaning a patient may show absent early cortical components like the N100 but normal P300, or absent P300 to simple tones but intact P600 to highly complex verbal material. With one exception, all CLIS patients had ERP-responses to one or more of the complex cognitive tasks, indicating at least partially intact processing stages in CLIS (Hinterberger et al. (2005c)). Patients in CLIS and patients in advanced stages of ALS show slowing of the waking EEG with increased θ band activity. This slowing may at least in part be caused by episodes of anoxia due to inadequate artificial respiration (e.g., every time patients are transferred from their beds into a wheelchair they are disconnected from the ventilator). It is often difficult to decide whether the patient is awake or asleep in stage 1 or 2.

These ERP data do not prove or disprove normal information processing in CLIS but suggest some intact "processing modules" in most ALS patients with CLIS (ALS-CLIS) despite a reduced general arousal. Assuming partially intact processing in ALS-CLIS, the question remains of why the patients who entered the CLIS *before* learning BCI use have not acquired control of their brain signals. We confronted them with the SCP-BCI, SMR-BCI, and auditory P300 oddball paradigm, but found no classifiable response.

22.5.3   Why Do We Fail in Patients with CLIS?

The failure to replicate operant (voluntary) learning of visceral functions (Dworkin and Miller (1986)) may provide an answer to this question: Chronically curarized rats and people with longer time periods in CLIS may lose the contingency between the required physiological behavior (SMR decrease, SCP amplitude changes, or heart rate increase) and its consequences (brain stimulation reward in the curarized rat, and letter selection in the patient). From the viewpoint of learning psychology, extinction sets in between the few reinforced learning trials in the rat. In the patient with CLIS, no contingency remains: Thoughts and intentions are never followed by their anticipated consequences in one's own behavior, and thoughts, imagery, and goal-directed feelings extinguish. Theories of consciousness come to a similar conclusion as the just-mentioned learning theory accounts of extinction of thinking (the interested reader is referred to Birbaumer (2006a,b)). The resulting cognitive state and remaining information processing capacities remain unclear until the first CLIS patient communicates. From the failure to control autonomic functions with operant learning in the curarized rat, the studies on contingency perception and will, and the—at least—intact sensory event-related cognitive potentials, we may conclude that passive sensory information processing seems to be intact even at the most complex semantic processing levels. It may be the motor control element that is responsible for the cessation of voluntary cognitive activity, goal-directed thinking, and imagery supporting a "motor theory of thinking" already discussed by James (1983).

22.6   Summary and Outlook for the Future

Compared to the number of studies published under the scope of BCI for communication and control for paralyzed patients, only few exist that include the target patient population. It has been shown that the SCP-BCI enables severely paralyzed and LIS patients to communicate, albeit slowly, and several messages of considerable length were formulated. The P300-BCI provides a tremendous increase of the spelling-per-minute rate and has proved its feasibility for severely disabled patients but not yet for patients in the LIS[5] or CLIS. After extensive training, the SMR-BCI allows patients multidirectional cursor control comparable to that achieved with intracortical recording, which seems, however, to require less training time. The ECoG-BCI allowed epilepsy patients to acquire SMR regulation and spelling with high accuracy within one training session, but failed to do so for an ALS-CLIS patient despite weeks and months of training. The MEG-BCI may constitute a unique approach to restore motor function after stroke. Neuroprosthesis control on the basis of intracortical signals and noninvasive SMR regulation has been established in three exemplary patients. Irrespective of the purpose—communication or neuroprosthesis control—none of the BCIs has been used by patients in their daily life, with the one exception described in the introduction. However, encouraged by recent success with the P300- and SMR-BCI, we are setting up BCIs at three patients' homes and will teach caregivers to handle the system. We will supervise the "laymen training" by means of telemonitoring introduced by the Graz group. The major drawback of BCI use in daily life expressed by our patients is the still complicated and time-consuming setup of the system including an electrode cap with which patients are uncomfortable. For the caregivers who have to supervise the system at least to checking if EEG signals are too bad to start the BCI and if the BCI is not running properly, the many degrees of freedom of the BCI2000 may constitute a constant source of errors if not completely automatized. With the P300- and SMR-BCI we have now achieved a considerable selection-per-minute rate so that we are quite optimistic that BCIs will become attractive for daily use in paralyzed patients, provided we can reduce the complexity of the system and the number of electrodes needed for signal analysis and classification. The invasive BCIs have to prove their superiority to the EEG-BCIs, and for which patients they might be specifically suitable to justify brain surgery needs to be defined. We doubt that patients will consent to implantation of an electrode grid for ECoG or a microelectrode array for intracortical recordings unless the results of invasive BCIs exceeds that of EEG-BCIs. Whether we will be able to restore communication in CLIS patients remains an open question.

Acknowledgments

We thank all our patients and our colleagues from the Institute of Medical Psychology and Behavioral Neurobiology in Tübingen and the Wadsworth Center in Albany who contributed to this work: Michael Bensch, Christoph Braun, Jeremy Hill, Thilo Hinterberger, Navin Lal, Miguel Jordan, Ahmed el Karim, Boris Kleber, Tamara Matuz, Jürgen Mellinger, Dennis McFarland, Ursula Mochty, Nicola Neumann, Hubert Preissl, Gerwin Schalk, Michael Schröder, Eric Sellers, Theresa Vaughan, Slavica von Hartlieb, Cornelia Weber, and Jonathan Wolpaw. This work is funded by the Deutsche Forschungsgemeinschaft (DFG) and the National Institutes of Health (NIH).

Notes

E-mail for correspondence: andrea.kuebler@uni-tuebingen.de

(1)   These data have not been published due to the private nature of the communicated messages. After the patient had written several letters we asked him whether he would be ready to write a letter for us and, thus, for the scientific community. This resulted in the longest BCI message ever communicated, in which the patient described his strategy to control cursor movement (Neumann et al. (2003)).

(2)   BCI workshop at the 13th Annual Carmel Workshop.

(3)   Numbers derived from participating groups at the International Meetings on BCI research and development. In 1999. 40 scientists participated, in 2002 roughly 100, in 2005 150.

(4)   Some of the considerations in this section are from Birbaumer (2006a,b).

(5)   By the time of proof-reading we have confronted an ALS patient in the US with the 6×6 matrix. She had a text book P300 and had copy and free spelling runs with 100 percent accuracy. She has participated in three training sessions and will be provided with a P300-BCI for daily use.

23 Combining BCI and Virtual Reality: Scouting Virtual Worlds

Robert Leeb, Reinhold Scherer, Claudia Keinrath, and Gert Pfurtscheller
Laboratory of Brain-Computer Interfaces
Institute for Knowledge Discovery
Graz University of Technology
Krenngasse 37, A-8010 Graz, Austria

Doron Friedman
Department of Computer Science
University College London
Gower Street
WC1E 6BT London, United Kingdom

Felix Y. Lee and Horst Bischof
Institute for Computer Graphics and Vision
Graz University of Technology
Inffeldgasse 16, A-8010 Graz, Austria

Mel Slater
Department of Computer Science   *Department Llenguatges i Sistemes*
University College London   *Informàtics*
Gower Street   *Universitat Politècnica de Catalunya*
WC1E 6BT London, United Kingdom   *E-08028 Barcelona, Spain*

23.1   Abstract

A brain-computer interface (BCI) is a closed-loop system with feedback as one important component. Dependent on the BCI application either to establish communication in patients with severe motor paralysis, to control neuroprosthesis, or to perform neurofeedback, information is visually fed back to the user about success or failure of the intended act. One way to realize feedback is the use of virtual reality (VR). In this chapter, an overview is given of BCI-based control of VR. In addition, four examples are reported in more detail about navigating in virtual environments with a cue-based (synchronous) and an uncued (asynchronous) BCI. Similar results in different virtual worlds with different types of motor imageries could be achieved, but no significant differences in the BCI classification accuracy were observed between VR and non-VR feedback. Nevertheless, the use of VR stimulated the subject's task performances and provided motivation.

23.2   Introduction

Brain-computer interface (BCI) technology deals with the development of a direct communication channel between the human brain and machines that does not require any motor activity (Wolpaw et al. (2002)). This is possible through the real-time analysis of electrophysiological brain signals recorded by electroencephalogram (EEG) or electrocorticogram (ECoG). Voluntary mental activity (e.g., a sequence of thoughts) modifies bioelectrical brain activity and consequently the EEG and ECoG. A BCI is able to detect such changes and generate operative control signals. Particularly for people suffering from severe physical disabilities or who are in a "locked-in" state, a BCI offers a possible communication channel.

Before a BCI can be used for control purposes, several training sessions are necessary. Two sorts of learning can occur in BCI: (1) the users learn to control their own brain activity (operant conditioning) and (2) the machine learns to recognize mentally modified brain patterns (machine learning). Operant conditioning is exploited by feeding back raw signals, or extracted parameters, as real-time changes to the user. Machine learning employs adaptive algorithms to detect brain patterns. For this purpose, signals first need to be recorded and analyzed, and a classifier must be setup, before feedback can be provided. The duration of the training varies strongly from subject to subject and can last from several hours to many months; therefore, a fundamental goal of BCI research is to reduce this period.

The presentation of visual feedback plays a major role during the training (Neuper and Pfurtscheller (1999)). Visual input has a strong impact on motor cortex activity (Rizzolatti et al. (2001)). Not only the primary and higher order visual areas are activated, but also the activities in motor and premotor areas are affected. This raises the question of which type of visualization best facilitates online learning and therefore improves the performance of a BCI system. Virtual reality (VR) might be a useful tool in providing visual feedback since it provides a class of user interfaces able to create "realistic" artificial (virtual) environments by means of three-dimensional, usually stereoscopic, computer graphics. The immersion into the virtual environment (VE) should allow users to be shielded from the outside world (Slater et al. (2002)) and therefore be able to focus on the required mental task. The use of VR as feedback medium may be more motivating and entertaining than standard feedback representations and therefore represents a crucial component during learning processes. The field of presence research (Slater and Usoh (1993)) aims to create VR where people feel and respond similarly to an equivalent real-world situation. If a VR keeps this promise, then feedback would be as natural as a real-world feedback could be. For example, users would control a locomotion device and actually feel themselves moving.

The technological progress in the past decade has made VR systems attractive for various research fields and applications ranging from aviation and military applications to simulation and training programs (where real-life training is too expensive or difficult to monitor and control), and from psychotherapy (Huber (2005)) to medical surgery. In particular, the area of medical rehabilitation exploits the possibilities and advances available from VR systems. Precisely, it encourages the rehabilitation of motor functions (Holden (2005)) including stroke rehabilitation (upper and lower extremity training) (Jack et al. (2001)), spatial and perceptual motor training, Parkinson's disease, orthopedic rehabilitation (Girone et al. (2000)), balance training, and wheelchair mobility (Webster et al. (2001)). A major finding in this field is that people with disabilities can perform motor learning in VR that can then be transferred to reality. In some cases it is even possible to generalize to other untrained tasks including improved efficiency of virtual training and learning (Holden (2005); Todorov et al. (1997)). It is important to note that VR is not a treatment by itself, and therefore it is impossible to study whether it is effective or not for rehabilitation. Although VR rehabilitation was undertaken for patients with acquired brain injury or damage with some success (Rose et al. (2005)), it is rather a new technological tool, which may be exploited to enhance motor retraining. Finally, virtual reality technology has positively influenced many other fields in neuroscience (Sanchez-Vives and Slater (2005); Tarr and Warren (2002)).

This chapter focuses on the benefits and impacts of such a technology on brain-computer interface (BCI) research, starting with a description of the background and related work and followed by a discussion of several results from various applications of BCI-based control of VR.

23.3   Background and Related Work

This section introduces two kinds of research in the context of virtual environments (VEs). Previous research has been established suggesting that a BCI may be used to control events within immersive VEs. Additionally, a second line of research is presented that did not use VEs but related technologies such as video games.

23.3.1   BCI and Immersive Systems

Nelson et al. (1997) were interested in BCI as a potential application for increasing the effectiveness of future tactical airborne crew stations. CyberLink is an interface that uses a combination of EEG and electromyographic (EMG) biopotentials as input signals in a single-axis continuous control task. The participants used the interface to navigate along a predetermined flight course that was projected onto a 40-foot diameter dome display. Continuous feedback was provided by a graphical head-up display. Participants were not given any BCI instructions. Scores of effective task performance gradually increased with training.

Bayliss and Ballard (2000) used the P300-evoked potential (EP) component, a positive waveform occurring approximately 300–550 ms after an infrequent task-relevant stimulus.

They used a head mounted display – (HMD) based VR system. Subjects were instructed to drive a modified go-cart within a virtual town and stop at red lights while ignoring both green and yellow lights. The red lights were made to be rare enough to receive full attention, which usually causes a clear P300 component. Results showed that a P300 EP indeed occurs at red lights and was absent at yellow lights, with recognition rates high enough to serve as a suitable BCI communication medium. In further research, Bayliss (2003) continued exploring the usage of the P300 component in VR. Subjects were asked to control several objects or commands in a virtual apartment: a lamp, a stereo system, a television set, a "Hi" command, and a "Bye" command, in several nonimmersive conditions, and with an HMD. Using BCI, subjects could switch the objects on and off or cause the animated character to appear or disappear. The BCI worked as follows: Approximately once per second a semitransparent sphere appeared for 250 ms on a randomly selected object. Subjects were asked to count the flashes on a specific object (to focus their attention) and to make the stimulus task-related, which is necessary to obtain a P300 component. During every run a written text instruction on the bottom of the screen indicated the goal object. The subject had to count the flashes for that object only and a visual feedback was given when the goal was achieved, that is, when a P300 event was recorded. Subjects were able to achieve approximately three goals per minute. Bayliss found no significant difference in BCI performance between VR and the standard computer paradigm, but individually most subjects preferred the VR environment.

Ron Angevin et al. (2004) proposed a training paradigm using VR techniques to avoid early fatigue from the learning process. In this work they used a virtual driving simulator inside an HMD, whereby the subjects had to control the car's left/right position to avoid an obstacle placed on the street by the imagination of hand movements. Five out of eight subjects were able to achieve suitable results. They noted that the control group (standard BCI feedback) reacted faster than the VR group; however, the VR group achieved less error than the control group.

Finally, the Graz-BCI also was used to control VR applications. Leeb et al. (2003, 2005) described the possibility of exploring a virtual conference room by the imagination of left and right hand movements using an HMD setup with success rates up to 100 percent. In further research, Leeb and Pfurtscheller (2004) and Pfurtscheller et al. (2006b) reported on an experiment concerned with subjects moving through a virtual environment by thought ("walking from thought") based on the imagination of foot movements, whereby after an HMD training, the subjects were able to move through a virtual street displayed on a highly immersive projection environment (Leeb et al. (2006)).

23.3.2   BCI-Based Control of Game-Like Environments

Middendorf et al. (2000) harnessed the steady-state visually evoked potential (SSVEP), a periodic response elicited by the repetitive presentation of a visual stimulus, as a communication medium for the BCI. One of the presented experiments involved controlling a flight simulator, where the roll position of the flight simulator was controlled with BCI. The "airplane" rolled right or left depending on the SSVEP amplitude over a half-second period. Most operators were able to successfully control the airplane after thirty minutes of training.

Lalor et al. (2005) used the SSVEP as a control mechanism for a 3D game. By looking on the checkerboard (either left or right of the character) the player good countersteer when the character was going to lost its balance on the robe. They reported robust BCI control and attributed relative success to motivation. Both approaches are based on visually evoked responses, which typically force the subject to focus visual attention and therefore may be unnatural.

Pineda et al. (2003) used the similarity or the difference in the μ activity (8–12 Hz) over the two hemispheres to control movements in a video game environment. After ten hours of training the subject played a high-resolution 3D first-person shooter game on a desktop monitor, whereby the forward and backward movements were controlled by the keyboard but the left and right movements were controlled by high and low μ, respectively.

Mason et al. (2004) applied their low-frequency asynchronous switch design (LF-ASD) to control a video game-like environment. The LF-ASD has been derived from signal characteristics observed in the 1–4 Hz frequency band of a feature vector based on nine electrodes over the primary and supplementary motor cortex. After a training session (six trials), a test with a simple video game was performed. A white circle (user's avatar) was moving with continuous speed over the monitor and was bouncing off obstacles (walls or pillars). An activation of the brain-switch would cause the avatar to turn left. Subjects self-reported an error (the avatar either failed to turn when intended or turned unintentionally) with a pneumatic sip-n-puff switch. They report that the performances of four able-bodied subjects and four subjects with high-level spinal cord injuries (level of injury between C3-4 and C5-6) were similar.

23.4   Combination of BCI and VR

23.4.1   Graz-BCI

The basic principle of the Graz-BCI is the detection and classification of motor-imagery-related EEG patterns, whereby the dynamics of sensorimotor rhythms are analyzed (as described in chapter 4; Pfurtscheller and Neuper (2001); Pfurtscheller et al. (2003c)). In particular, hand and foot motor imagery makes it possible to realize a BCI (Pfurtscheller et al. (2005a)).

Over the sensorimotor hand and foot representation areas two (C3 and C4) or three (C3, Cz and C4) EEG-electrode pairs are placed according to the international 10-20 system (2.5 cm anterior and posterior to the named electrode positions). The ground electrode is positioned on the forehead. The EEG is bipolarly recorded at a bandwidth of 0.5–30 Hz from sintered Ag/AgCl electrodes and sampled with 250 Hz. For online classification, two frequency bands (logarithmic bandpower, BP) of the specific EEG channels are used. These features are classified with Fisher's linear discriminant analysis (LDA, Bishop (1995)) and transformed into a control signal (for details, see Pfurtscheller et al. (2005a)). For offline processing, all trials are visually controlled for artifacts and affected trials are excluded from further analyses.

To calculate the classifier setup, motor imagery data must be acquired for each subject. In general, one run consists of fourty trials in a randomized order, twenty trials for each type of imagery. The task is to perform a cue-dependent (synchronous) mental activity following a predefined, repetitive time-scheme. The visual cue, for example, an arrow pointing either to the left or right side, indicates the imagination of a left or right hand movement, respectively. The imagination has to be performed for a predefined period (usually 4 s, see figure 23.1b), followed by a random-length pause usually between 4 and 5 s. Afterward the classifier, trained with these trials, is subsequently used for the online feedback training. The task is to move the feedback cursor toward the direction indicated by the arrow by performing the same mental activity previously trained to do. By updating the classifier with this new data, the human brain and the classifier are mutually adapting (Pfurtscheller and Neuper (2001)). In the presented experiments, the classifiers were updated only after the first two feedback sessions, and afterward used for all further sessions.

The Graz-BCI consists of an EEG amplifier (g.tec, Graz, Austria), a data acquisition card (National Instruments, Austin, Texas, USA) and a commercial desktop PC running WindowsXP (Guger et al. (2001)). The BCI algorithms are implemented in MATLAB 6.5 and Simulink 5.0 (The MathWorks, Natick, Mass., USA) using rtsBCI and the open source package BIOSIG (http://biosig.sf.net).

23.4.2   Virtual Environments

Virtual reality generates three-dimensional stereoscopic representations of computer-animated worlds. Present VR systems need either a large-scale display with shutter or polarization glasses, or an HMD to separate the two stereoscopic images generated for each eye of the observer. The basic idea is to let a user become immersed in a 3D scene. The highest immersion can be achieved in a multiprojection stereo-based and head-tracked VE system commonly known as a "Cave" (Cruz-Neira et al. (1993)). A special feature of any multiwall system is that the images on the adjacent walls are joined together seamlessly, so that participants do not see the physical corners but the continuous virtual world that is projected with active stereo (Slater et al. (2002)).

The creation of the 3D virtual environment consisted of two consecutive steps: first the creation of a 3D model of the scene and second the generation of a VR-application that controls and animates the modeled scene. In our studies, the 3D modeling software packages Performer (Silicon Graphics, Mountain View, Calif., USA) and Maya (Alias, Toronto, Canada) were used. The experiments reported are performed with a Virtual Research V8 HMD (Virtual Research Systems, Aptos, Calif., USA) with a resolution of 640 x 480 pixels at a refresh rate of 60 Hz driven by VRjuggler (http://www.vrjuggler.org), with a single back-projected wall and shutter glasses driven by Coin3D (http://www.coin3d.org) or the Studierstube Augmented Reality framework (http://www.studierstube.org), or with a ReaCTor, a Cave-like system using the DIVE software (Frecon et al. (2001)) with CrystalEye (StereoGraphics, Beverly Hills, Calif., USA) stereo glasses. All VR systems have also the possibility to include tracking information, but because BCI experiments require a subject in a sitting position, no positional information had to be considered. Additionally, rotational information from the tracking system was ignored because rotation should be controlled by the BCI in the following Graz-BCI-specific VR applications.

23.5   Graz-BCI-Specific VR Applications

23.5.1   Study 1: Rotation in a Virtual Environment by Left- and Right-Hand Motor Imagery

In the first application, the imagination of left and right hand movement was applied to control VR feedback. For evaluation purposes three different conditions were compared: (1) a standard horizontal bar graph on a desktop monitor (Pfurtscheller et al. (2003c)), (2) a virtual conference room presented with an HMD (Leeb et al. (2005)), and finally (3) a virtual pub populated with animated avatars, including background music and chatter of the avatars (see figure 23.1a) in a Cave. The subject was either sitting in front of an LCD monitor, wearing an HMD, or sitting in the middle of this virtual pub.

Three subjects, two male and one female (23, 26, and 28 years old), participated repeatedly in this study over a period of seven months. The order of feedback conditions was standard bar graph, HMD, Cave, HMD, standard bar graph (see figure 23.1d–f). The participants were instructed to imagine left or right hand movements, depending on an acoustic cue (single or double beep). During the feedback time, the output of the classifier controlled either the length and the orientation of the horizontal bar graph in case of the standard BCI feedback, or the rotation angle and direction within VR. During the BCI experiments the cue was given at second 3 and the feedback was presented continuously for 4 s (see figure 23.1b) (Pfurtscheller and Neuper (2001)). The feedback on the screen was updated 25 times per second and either the length of the bar graph was changed or the rotation angle was modified. Thereby, the subject perceived the feeling of rotating with constant speed (24 degrees/s) to the right and left depending on the imagined movement. In this way, the rotation information was integrated over one trial (cumulative feedback). The maximum achievable gyration was ± 90 degrees within one trial, increasing linearly to this maximum over the feedback time. A random classification would result in an expected rotation of 0 degrees.

The mean rotation achieved by one exemplary subject (S1, HMD condition, session 4, run 6), is plotted in figure 23.1c by averaging all 20 trials for right hand imagination and all 20 trials for left hand imagination. In this run, the subject had problems with the right class during second 4.25 and 5; therefore, the rotation angle moved first to the left and afterward from a negative angle straight to the right side. The mean of the achieved rotation over all trials of this run is 70 degrees for right-hand and -79 degrees for left-hand motor imagery. The reason for the larger standard deviation (SD) at second 8 compared to second 5, for example, is due to the cumulative presentation of the results. The subjects obtained promising results with the three feedback systems. For comparison reasons, the rotational information of the runs recorded with standard BCI feedback were simulated offline and

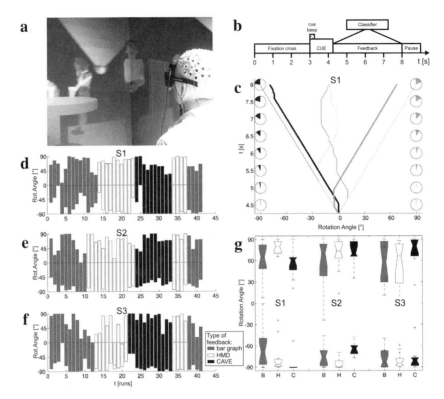

Figure 23.1   (a) Picture of a subject in the virtual pub room. The pub is populated with animated avatars (guests and barman). The subject wears shutter glasses and an electrode cap. (b) Timing of the used paradigm. Between seconds 3 and 4.25 the cue information is presented by an arrow pointing to the left, the right, or downward, depending on the motor imagery used. The cue information of the synchronous two-class BCI is also given acoustically as a single or double beep. In the case of feedback sessions, the classifier output is not presented until second 8. (c) Plot of the achieved rotation angle of one exemplary run of 40 trials of subject S1. Mean angles are plotted in thick and mean ± one SD in thin lines. Right-hand imagery is plotted in light and left-hand in dark colors. The maximum achievable angle is ±90° at second 8, whereby the two outer lines reach these points. The small circles on the left and right side are a more convenient illustration of the mean rotation angle at that specific time point, whereby the pie slices are the actually reached gyrations. (d)–(f) Achieved rotation angle over all runs for subjects S1, S2, and S3. Each vertical bar corresponds to the rotation angle of one run (final value of panel c), whereby the upper bar indicates the rotation to the right and the lower bar the rotation to the left. Runs with bar graph feedback are plotted in grey, with HMD feedback in white and Cave feedback in black. (g) Boxplot of all rotation angles of all subjects and feedback types, whereby the upper boxplot indicates the rotation to the right and the lower boxplot the rotation to the left. The diagram consists of 3 groups each corresponding to one subject. Within these groups the left plots correspond to standard BCI feedback B, the middle to HMD feedback H and the right one to Cave feedback C. Each boxplot has lines at the lower quartile, median, and upper quartile values.

therefore these runs can be compared to the VR experiments. Subject S1 achieved the best performance with HMD feedback and worst with standard bar graph feedback (see figure 23.1d and g). Subject S3 was best in Cave condition followed by HMD and bar graph (see figure 23.1f and g). Interestingly, no differences between HMD and Cave feedback could be found because some subjects performed better with HMD and some better with Cave feedback, but all subjects performed at least as well with VR feedback compared to standard bar graph feedback (see figure 23.1g). The number of trials contaminated with movement, muscle, or eye-movement artifacts were always between 0 and 5 out of 40 trials, but no differences between the various feedback conditions could be found.

Subjects noted that the virtual pub in the Cave feedback had two areas: The virtual characters concentrated in one area, whereas the other side of the room was empty. It did not even contain furniture (only a disco-style chandelier). Subjects reported that BCI control was more difficult in the empty space because no clear spatial information was obtained. Some subjects found the audio chatter in the Cave condition a bit distracting, but none of them reported problems in identifying the auditory cues.

23.5.2   Study 2: Moving Forward in a Virtual Street by Foot Motor Imagery

In this experiment, the imagination of foot movement was used to walk through a VE based on the previously applied BCI paradigm (see figure 23.1b). The subject was instructed to imagine a right hand movement (arrow to the right and single beep) or a foot movement (arrow pointing downward and double beep). Three healthy male volunteers aged 23, 28, and 30 years participated several times in this study (Leeb et al. (2006)). The task given to each participant was to walk to the end of a virtual street (see figure 23.2a) and in the case of successful foot motor imagery only, a motion would occur. Correct classification of foot motor imagery was accompanied by forward movement at constant speed (1.3 length units/s) in the virtual street, whereas a correct classification of hand motor imagery stopped the motion. Incorrect classification of foot motor imagery also resulted in halting, and incorrect classification of hand motor imagery resulted in backward motion (same speed). The walking distance was scored as a "cumulative achieved mileage" (CAM; Leeb and Pfurtscheller (2004)), which was the integrated forward/backward distance covered during foot movement imagination, and was used as performance measurement.

The output of the online classification was used either to control the length and orientation of the bar graph feedback or to move through a virtual street (HMD or Cave condition). The order of feedback conditions was as follows: standard bar graph, HMD, Cave, HMD, standard bar graph (see figure 23.2d–f). For comparison reasons, the CAM performances of the bar graph feedback experiments were simulated offline.

In figure 23.2b and c, the performed CAM of exemplary results of subject S1 (session 2, run 4) and subject S3 (session 2, run 5) are plotted. Both the theoretically possible CAM (dashed line) and the real-achieved CAM (full line) are plotted. Due to the different sequences of the twenty foot (F) and twenty right-hand (R) motor imageries, which were randomly distributed to avoid adaptation, the theoretical pathways are different in all pictures. Nevertheless, the number of trials for both classes is the same and therefore the maximum possible CAM also. A CAM of 100 percent corresponds to a correct classifi-

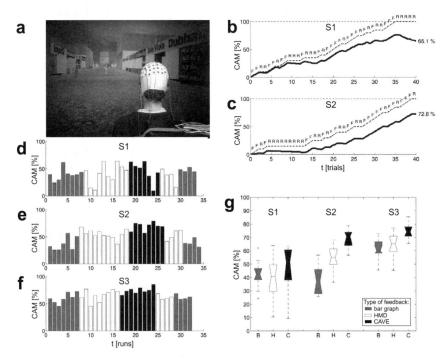

Figure 23.2 (a) Participant in the virtual main street with shops and animated avatars. The subject wears an electrode cap and shutter glasses. (b) and (c) Exemplary task performances displayed in the theoretical possible CAM (dashed line) and the real CAM (full line) of one run of two subjects. The cue class indicated is written above the line. Due to the random cue sequence, each participant had a different theoretical pathway (dashed line). (d)–(f) Achieved walking distances over all runs for subjects S1, S2, and S3. Each vertical bar corresponds to the CAM of each run (end value of picture b or c). Runs with bar graph feedback are plotted in grey, with HMD feedback in white and Cave feedback in black. (g) Boxplot of all achieved CAMs of all subjects and feedback types. The diagram consists of 3 groups, each corresponding to a subject. Within these groups, the left plots corresponds to standard BCI feedback B, the middle to HMD feedback H and the right one to Cave feedback C.

cation of all fourty imagery tasks over the entire feedback time. A random classification would result in an expected CAM of 0 percent. It is almost impossible to achieve the maximum attainable CAM of 100 percent, because every small procrastination or hesitation of the participant results in reduced mileage. In the example presented in figure 23.2b, a close-to-perfect performance at least up to trial 35 is shown, followed by a small breakdown. A possible explanation for the problems in the performance results of subject S3 (in figure 23.2c) could be that between trial 4 and 14 the same class performance was required, which is the "standing class" (right hand movement), but the participant was not able to remain stationary for such a long period. A similar effect can be observed at the end of the run plotted in the bottom row of figure 23.2b. A faster alternation between the two classes might achieve better results, but the sequence of cues was randomized automatically through each run.

All subjects were able to walk through the virtual city. The use of VR as feedback stimulated the participant's performances. All subjects achieved their best results within the Cave and the worst in the standard BCI conditions (see figure 23.2g). In particular, subjects S2 and S3 improved by using VR feedback (see figure 23.2e and f). Only subject S1 showed a different behavior, due to a high variability over the runs in the VR feedback (see figure 23.2d). One possible interpretation is that VR feedback amplifies both positive and negative feedback effects on the performance. The wrong-behaving rich visual feedback can modify the EEG activity and thereby result in a further deterioration of performance. It must be noted that during the Cave experiments, a competition arose between subjects S2 and S3, which might have influenced the performances positively.

The number of trials contaminated with electrode movement, muscle, or eye-movement artifacts were always less than six out of fourty trials, but trials with VR feedback had no more artifacts than the trials with standard feedback.

These data indicate that foot motor imagery is a suitable mental strategy to control events within the VEs. Imagination of feet movement is a mental task that comes very close to that of natural walking. Especially in the Cave condition (highest immersion), the performance of two participants was excellent (up to 100 percent BCI classification accuracy of single trials), although variability in the classification results among individual runs occurred.

23.5.3   Study 3: Scouting through a Virtual Apartment

The next important step was to incorporate free will decisions (intentional control, IC) in a synchronous (cue-based) BCI. Although a predefined time window (with variable length) was used for feature extraction and classification, the user could choose which imagined movement to perform after each cue. In a pilot study, a virtual apartment (see figure 23.3a) was used as feedback presented on a single back-projected stereoscopic wall. In this apartment the subject could freely decide where to go, but walking was only possible along predefined pathways through the corridors or rooms (Leeb et al. (in revision)). At every junction the subject could decide to go in one of two directions that were indicated by a "neutral" cue consisting of arrows (see figure 23.3b). The size of the arrow was modulated depending on the BCI classification output, so the subject received feedback. The analysis was performed until a threshold was exceeded (huge arrow), and the subject was turned to the right, left, or straight. Afterward, the system automatically guided the subject to the next junction. Additionally, a small map of the apartment was inserted in the bottom right corner of the display. In this study a cue-based BCI was still used, but the cues were completely embedded in the given task or experiment and the duration of the trials was variable, depending on the performance of the subject only. Four naive subjects (three male and one female, between 21 and 27 years) without any prior BCI experience participated in this study. Before placing the subjects into the VE, two training sessions (each with four runs) without feedback and two sessions with feedback were performed. The resulting classification errors are presented in table 23.1.

Each subject performed eleven runs with variable duration in the virtual apartment, but all runs started at the same point (entrance door). During the first run, no instructions were given to the subjects, so they could walk freely through the apartment for five minutes

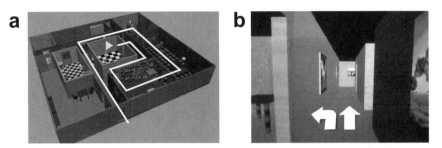

Figure 23.3   (a) View into a virtual apartment with one possible pathway. The target room is marked with a small flag pole (e.g., the room in the middle of the apartment). (b) First-person view of the virtual apartment with two arrows indicating the possible directions to go. The size of the arrow indicates the BCI classification output.

to become familiar with the VE. In all other runs the subjects were instructed to go to a predefined target room. A small flag pole on the map indicated the destination, which should be reached by using the shortest way through the maze-like apartment. In the first four runs only one target was given, but in further runs the number of targets was increased and only one target was visible each time. If this target was reached, either the follow-up target was inserted or the run was finished. Dividing the number of wrong decisions by the total number of turnarounds results into the classification performance of the VE task (see table 23.1). Different from the previous examples, the number of trials/decisions in a run varied depending on the chosen path. Furthermore, the analysis was more demanding since one wrong decision required several correct decisions to reach the same goal.

The time necessary for a decision at the junctions varied for all subjects between 2.2 and 5.9 s, with a mean $\pm$ SD of 2.9 ± 0.5 s. The naive subjects achieved a BCI classification error of less than 20 percent after two feedback sessions. Interestingly, two subjects revealed worse results within the first feedback session than they achieved in the training period without FB. However, the second feedback session resulted in reduced error. The subjects obtained comparable performances with the standard feedback (error rates between 1 and 33 percent) and the virtual apartment feedback (error rates between 7 and 23 percent). The subjects noted that the task in the virtual apartment was much harder compared to the prior feedback training because not only the "correct" imagination must have been performed, but also the shortest way had to be found. Despite the undefined trial length (the duration of the trial depended on how fast or slow the subject could perform a decision) and variable interdecision time, no dramatic change in the performance could be found.

23.5.4   Study 4: Asynchronous freeSpace Experiments

Our first paradigm designed to train and evaluate asynchronous control was called the "freeSpace virtual park" (see figure 23.4a). The VE consisted of hedges, a tree, and three coins to collect. The subject was sitting in front of a stereoscopic projection wall and wearing shutter glasses.

Table 23.1 Classification performance for each subject and each feedback type. The classification error in percent is given for training and standard feedback sessions, and the percentage of wrong turnarounds is given for sessions in the virtual apartment. The number of trials/junctions of these sessions are in brackets.

Subject	Training with no feedback		Standard feedback				Virtual apartment	
			Session 1		Session 2			
S1	7.9%	(240)	1.9%	(160)	1.0%	(160)	8.8%	(96)
S2	18.2%	(240)	28.4%	(160)	17.0%	(160)	28.6%	(136)
S3	29.7%	(240)	32.8%	(160)	19.1%	(160)	25.2%	(206)
S4	26.4%	(240)	20.2%	(160)	15.9%	(160)	20.8%	(133)

The aim of the paradigm was to explore the VE and collect the scattered items. Turn left and right and move forward were the navigation commands used to move through the freeSpace (IC). Whenever an IC command was detected by the BCI, the corresponding command was sent to the VE. When no IC pattern was detected (noncontrol state, NC) accordingly no navigation was performed. By using this simple navigation strategy, each corner of the VE was accessible. To realize this navigation, however, it was necessary to detect three different motor imagery–modulated brain patterns in the ongoing EEG. For more details on the setup of recordings and signal processing, see chapter 4.4.3 and Scherer et al. (in revision).

Figure 23.4a shows a picture taken during a feedback experiment. In the lower part of the screen feedback arrows were displayed, indicating the actual navigation command. Figure 23.4b shows the bird's view map of the freeSpace park. The dark line illustrates the selected pathway of the subject. The starting point is marked with an "x" and the light grey circles indicate the items to collect. The collection starts each time the path intersects with an item, marked with a small dark circle. Additionally, the map shows that an infinite number of ways to collect the three items exist. The selected path, however, is dependent on the will of the subject only. For comparison, the corresponding BCI classification output (navigation) sequence is shown in figure 23.4c. The items were collected at time points (t), 40, 72, and 182 s (vertical line). By using this command sequence it is possible to reconstruct the pathway. With 36 percent, as required by the paradigm, the moving forward command had the highest frequencies of occurrence (f_{OCC}). With 26 and 24 percent, left and right turn were balanced. NC was detected in 13 percent of the cases (see figure 23.4d).

Although the NC at the actual stage was not explicitly tested and evaluated, high classification accuracy was very important for the motivation of the subjects. Since each run lasted several minutes, it was difficult to keep the concentration and therefore periods of NC were required. If NC was not properly detected, navigation commands were sent to the freeSpace and this was extremely frustrating for subjects.

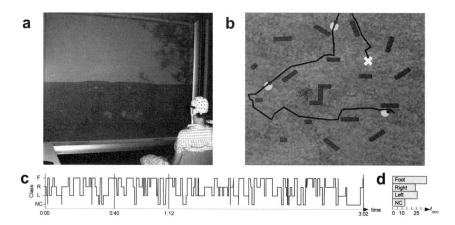

Figure 23.4 (a) Picture of the freeSpace VR experiments. (b) Bird's view of the park with the selected pathway (dark line), items to collect (light grey circle), pick-up position (small dark circle), and starting point (x). (c) BCI navigation command sequence. To operate the BCI, left hand (L), right hand (R), and foot (F) motor imagery were used. Also the noncontrol state (NC) was detected. The marked time (vertical lines) indicates the pick-up time. (d) The histogram on the right shows the frequency of occurrence for each class.

23.6 Discussion and Conclusion

The presented studies describe the possibility and feasibility of using a motor imagery–based BCI with VR as feedback medium. Similar results in different virtual worlds with different types of motor imageries (left-hand, right-hand, and foot movement imagination) could be achieved but no significant differences in the BCI performance were observed between VR and non-VR feedback.

At this time it is unknown whether the feedback in form of a realistic VE can improve the BCI performance or not. However, there is strong evidence that observation of moving body parts can modify the sensorimotor activity (Pfurtscheller et al. (2007); Rizzolatti et al. (2001)), whereas observations of non-body parts have less influence on the brain activity (Altschuller et al. (2000)). With the coupling of BCI and VR a new research tool is available for investigating different research questions, for example, the impact of VR feedback to shorten the training time. Nevertheless, VR provides an excellent training and testing environment for procedures that may apply later in reality. One important application might be the use of VE for people with severe motor disabilities. If it can be shown that within VE people can learn to control their movements through space, the much greater expense of building physical devices (e.g., neuroprosthesis or a robotic arm) controlled by a BCI will be justified. One goal could be to move with a wheelchair through a virtual environment and afterward through the real world solely by the imagination of movements.

It must be noted, however, that in some experiments with VR feedback the task of the subjects was more challenging than in the experiments with the standard BCI feedback.

In the presented experiments, all subjects achieved their best results within the VEs (either HMD or Cave) and the worst results in the standard BCI conditions. One possible interpretation is that VR feedback amplifies both positive and negative feedback effects on the performance: Generally, good performance is enhanced, but if the performance is not satisfactory, the VR feedback distracts and leads to higher frustration compared to the standard BCI feedback. Nevertheless, the use of VR stimulated the subject's performances and provided motivation.

High classification accuracy (low error rate) can be achieved only when the subjects correctly perform the indicated mental task. This not only requires focused attention to the corresponding body part, but also a withdrawal of attention from other body parts. Because one run lasts several minutes, the subject must be vigilant the whole time, that is, concentrate on the task, anticipate and process the cue stimuli, and perform the indicated imagery task. This high mental load during each run and the performance of three to four consecutive runs within one recording (approximately 1 hour including electrode montage) can lead to a temporary drop in attention and an increased rate of misclassifications and errors. Presenting such an erroneous feedback to the subject can modify the EEG activity and result in a further deterioration of performance. Therefore, it is not surprising that in nearly all sessions and different conditions individual runs with inferior and superior performance were found (see figure 23.1d–f and 23.2d–f).

Concerning the difference between Cave, HMD and desktop PC experiments, the following observations are of interest:

(1) Subjects felt more natural in VE compared with BCI experiments with standard feedback.
(2) Each subject preferred the Cave experiments to the HMD and both were favored over BCI session on a desktop PC.
(3) Motivation (e.g., to "walk from thought" in a virtual street) seems to improve the BCI performance, but too much excitement might also distract the subject.
(4) Despite distraction from auditory and moving visual stimuli in VE, motor imagery and its classification in the ongoing EEG is still possible.

The research reported in this work is a further step to the long-range vision for interaction in multisensory environments exploiting mental-only activity.

Acknowlegments

This work was supported by the European FET Program, PRESENCIA IST-2001-37927 and PRESENCCIA IST-2006-27731, and in part by the Austrian Science Fund ("Fonds zur Förderung der wissenschaftlichen Forschung") project P16326-B02 and Hewlett-Packard. Thanks to Angus Antley, Maia Garau, Marco Gillies, Christoph Guger, Gernot R. Müller, Christa Neuper, Anthony Steed, David Swapp, Vinoba Vinayagamoorthy, and Selina Wriessnegger.

Notes

E-mail for correspondence: robert.leeb@tugraz.at

24   Improving Human Performance in a Real Operating Environment through Real-Time Mental Workload Detection

Jens Kohlmorgen, Guido Dornhege, and Mikio L. Braun
Fraunhofer–Institute FIRST
Intelligent Data Analysis Group (IDA)
Kekuléstr. 7, 12489 Berlin, Germany

Benjamin Blankertz and Klaus-Robert Müller
Fraunhofer–Institute FIRST   *Technical University Berlin*
Intelligent Data Analysis Group (IDA)   *Str. des 17. Juni 135*
Kekuléstr. 7, 12489 Berlin, Germany   *10 623 Berlin, Germany*

Gabriel Curio
Department of Neurology, Neurophysics Group
Campus Benjamin Franklin, Charité University Medicine Berlin
Hindenburgdamm 30, 12200 Berlin, Germany

Konrad Hagemann, Andreas Bruns, Michael Schrauf, and Wilhelm E. Kincses
DaimlerChrysler AG
Group Research, HPC 50-G024
71059 Sindelfingen, Germany

24.1   Abstract

The ability to directly detect mental over- and under-load in human operators is an essential feature of complex monitoring and control processes. Such processes can be found, for example, in industrial production lines, in aviation, as well as in common everyday tasks such as driving. In this chapter, we present an EEG-based system that is able to detect high mental workload in drivers operating under real traffic conditions. This information is used immediately to mitigate the workload typically induced by the influx of information that is generated by the car's electronic systems. Two experimental paradigms were tested: an auditory workload scheme and a mental calculation task. The result is twofold. The system's performance is strongly subject-dependent; however, the results are good to excellent for the majority of subjects. We show that in these cases an induced mitigation of a reaction time experiment leads to an increase of the driver's overall task performance.

24.2   Introduction

The detection of mental workload is considered an important issue in fields where operational alertness and elevated concentration is crucial, as it is, for example, for pilots, flight controllers, or operators of industrial plants. The output of such a workload detector could be integrated with existing systems to control the information flow to the operator in order to maximize the performance. One approach consists of creating a closed-loop system in which the system's interaction with the operator is adjusted according to the operator's mental workload measured by the workload detector. Another possibility consists of using the workload detector as an objective measure of mental workload to develop improved modes and organizations of human-machine interaction.

In this chapter, we follow the first approach and use a workload detector to reduce the imposed workload, thereby improving the operator's overall performance. We study the problem of workload detection and performance improvement in the context of driving a car while performing additional tasks that model interaction with the car's systems. The motivation for the present work was to obtain a system that is able to measure *and* mitigate mental workload (1) in real time and (2) in a real operational environment, ultimately to detect, or even to avoid, stressful and cognitively demanding situations for human operators in critical monitoring or control tasks.

Approaches to mental workload detection are largely based on the electroencephalogram (EEG) and have so far been investigated mainly under controlled laboratory conditions, for example, by using tasks that involve the subject's short-term memory (Gevins et al. (1997, 1998); Low et al. (1999); Schack et al. (2002); Stipacek et al. (2003); Howard et al. (2003)), by mimicking in-flight tasks of a pilot (Pope et al. (1995); Prinzel et al. (2000); Smith et al. (2001)), or by simulating air traffic control (Brookings et al. (1996)). Attempts to measure mental workload in real operational environments have so far been limited to an offline analysis after the recording (Sterman and Mann (1995); Hankins and Wilson (1998)), lacking the possibility of online feedback to actually control the workload as discussed above (see Scerbo et al. (2003) for a more comprehensive review of the field).

The utility of these studies for our current application is rather limited. While the studies have identified some neurophysiological effects of mental workload, the results do not provide clear evidence due to the heterogeneity of the studied tasks. In the works cited above, the workload is induced either visually or by memory tasks, and it is unclear if these observations carry over to the setting of car driving, a task that is rather visually demanding by itself.

Also, most of the results were obtained using laboratory experiments conducted under relatively controlled conditions, and it is unclear how the observations of these experiments translate to the more complex real-world setting. It is important to note that the analysis of EEG data under real operating conditions is significantly more challenging than under controlled laboratory conditions. Besides uncontrollable sources of distraction and consequently a larger degree of uncertainty about the subject's true mental state, the EEG signals can be heavily contaminated by artifacts, primarily due to facial muscle activity.

Finally, previous work in the field of single-trial EEG analysis has shown large intra- as well as interindividual differences. Consequently, it does not seem realistic at this point to build a universally applicable detector with fixed parameters. It is our belief that any realistic workload detector currently must have some means of adaption to the individual under consideration.

Based on these considerations as well as on the results reported in the literature, we follow a flexible approach that takes into account the observed neurophysiological effects while at the same time addressing the uncertainty and variability of the experimental and physiological conditions. This is realized by designing a highly parameterized workload detector that can detect the reported neurophysiological effects, but is not restricted to a particular feature. The high dimensionality of the parameter set and the noisy nature of the EEG signals then pose the challenge of robustly estimating the parameters. This task is addressed by using methods from machine learning.

24.3   The Experimental Setup

The goal of the current study was to develop a system that is able to measure and mitigate mental workload in real time and in real operational environments. Operating a vehicle under real conditions, including the execution of secondary tasks not related to driving such as interacting with other vehicle occupants or with the electronic equipment of the vehicle, represents a complex operational task. We exemplarily used this task to develop our approach and prove its success.

Twelve male and five female subjects age 20 to 32 years old performed the experiment. The subjects were instructed to drive at approximately 100 km/h on the highway in moderate traffic conditions. Note, however, that the traffic intensity was not controllable. The experiments took place on the public German highway B10 (between Esslingen am Neckar and Wendlingen) during the usual daytime traffic (figure 24.1). The subjects were instructed not to speak during the experiment in order to avoid additional workload as well as a systematic activation due to muscle artifacts.

The subjects were instructed to perform three types of tasks: a *primary task* (driving the vehicle), a *secondary task*, and a *tertiary task*.

The secondary task was an auditory reaction time task mimicking the interaction with the vehicle's electronic warning and information system. It was important to choose a simple task that would most likely *not* impose any significant amount of additional cognitive workload on the driver. The task was used to measure the driver's performance in terms of reaction time: voice recordings of the German words *links* (left) and *rechts* (right) were randomly presented every 7.5 s via the car's audio system and had to be acknowledged as quickly as possible by pressing corresponding buttons mounted on both index fingers.

The tertiary task was designed to induce high mental workload. We studied two different types of workload. The first type was a *mental calculation task* (mimicking "thinking

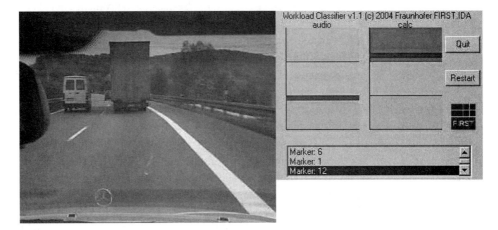

Figure 24.1   The mental workload detector in operation, during a mental calculation task performed by the driver (a scene from one of the experiments). Two gauges (right) separately indicate auditory and mental calculation workload. Each indicator bar can move over a green (lower), yellow (middle), and red (top) background, indicating the amount of detected workload. In the snapshot, the bars correctly indicate low auditory and high calculation workload.

processes") that stressed the driver's working memory. In this condition, the drivers are asked to silently count down in steps of twenty-seven, starting from an initially given three-digit random number (between 800 and 999). After two minutes, the subjects were stopped by the beep of a timer and verbally asked for the final result. The second type of workload-inducing task was an *auditory task* in which the drivers had to direct their attention to one of two simultaneously presented voice recordings, replicating a situation in which several vehicle occupants are talking at the same time: A female news reader and a male voice reciting from a book. The subjects were instructed to follow the latter. To verify whether the subjects were engaged or not, they had to answer related questions. To avoid artifact contamination of the EEG, the questions were presented during the turning points of the course, where EEG was not analyzed.

The entire experiment is organized in a block structure with a block length of two minutes each (see figure 24.2). A *high-workload block* of two minutes' length, comprising all three tasks, was alternated with a *low-workload block*, in which the subjects performed the primary task (driving) and the secondary task (reaction time task), but not the tertiary task. Experience from pilot testings shows that it is possible to perform the tertiary tasks for two minutes at the same attention level without getting tired.

One full pass of the experiment consisted of three pairs of high and low blocks in a row, with different initial three-digit numbers and with different parts of the story. Each pass is performed two times by each subject to get sufficiently many changes in workload level for the subsequent performance analysis of the detector.

A crucial purpose of the experiment is to investigate whether the output of the workload detector can be used to control the secondary task such that the performance of the subject is improved. This is accomplished by making the secondary task a controllable task interrupted by the workload detector each time the system identifies a high workload

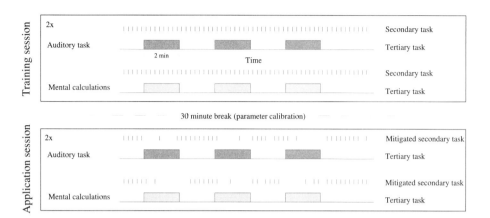

Figure 24.2   Illustration of the experimental procedure. The experiment consists of two consecutive sessions, *training* and *application*, joined by a short break in which the parameters of the workload detector are computed from the training session data. Each session consists of two runs for each tertiary task, and a run consists of three high workload blocks of two minutes length, followed by a low workload block of the same length. In the training session, the secondary task (reaction time experiment) is performed throughout the session, whereas in the application session it is controlled by the workload detector. If a high workload condition is detected, the secondary task is suppressed in order to improve the performance for this task as measured by the average reaction time.

condition. This serves to mitigate the workload imposed on the driver. The performance is measured by the average reaction time over the course of the experiment.

This experiment provides two measures for our method: the accuracy of the prediction of a high workload condition, and the performance increase as measured by the reaction times.

As stated, our workload detection method is highly parameterized to be able to adapt to the environmental conditions, the task, and the driver. To estimate these parameters, one experiment consists of two sessions: a training and an application session. The training session is performed without running the detector. Immediately after the training session, the recorded EEG data is used to train the detector, that is, its parameters are computed from the data. In the subsequent application session, the trained workload detector is applied to continuously analyze the ongoing EEG measurement in real time and to output a high or low workload indication. In case of a high workload indication, the secondary task automatically gets suppressed without external intervention until the detector indicates low workload again (mitigation strategy). Both sessions are performed on the same day with an intermediate break of roughly thirty minutes in which the detector is trained.

24.4   Online Detection of Mental Workload

In this section, we describe the workload detector and the procedure for parameter calibration. To test whether it is possible to distinguish types of workload, we use two independent

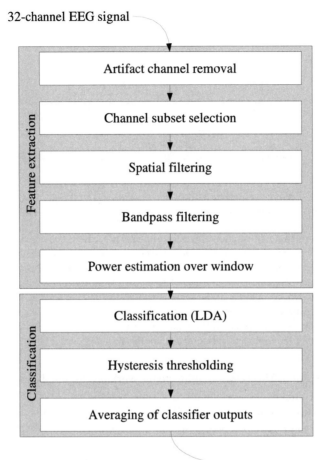

Figure 24.3 The workload detector predicts two different workload conditions in real time from an ongoing 32-channel EEG measurement. The detector consists of two stages: Feature extraction and classification.

workload detectors per subject, one for each paradigm. As mentioned, we observed a large inter- and intrasubject variability of the EEG in precursory investigations. We therefore adopted a rather general approach and designed a workload detector with subject- and task-specific parameters.

24.4.1   The Workload Detector

Each detector consists of two parts: feature extraction and classification. The feature extraction component extracts neurophysiologically interesting features, which are then used by the classifier to predict the workload (see figure 24.3).

The feature extraction consists of the following four steps: (1) removal of artifact contaminated EEG channels, (2) selection of a subset of the remaining channels, (3) spatial filtering, and (4) computing the power in a selected frequency band. The possible

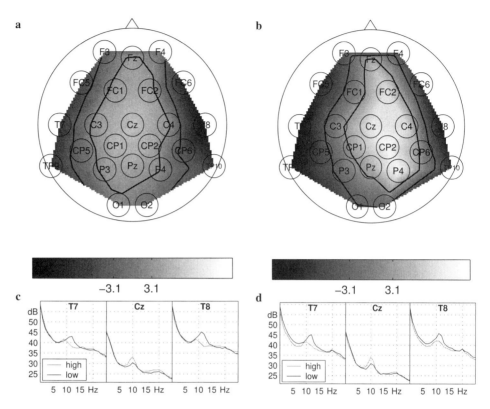

Figure 24.4   Spectral differences in EEG between low and high workload condition (on the average). Left: for auditory workload. Right: for mental calculation workload. (a), (b): t-statistics of 8–12 Hz and power, interpolated between the electrode positions of subject *ps*. The contour lines denote $P = 0.001$, i.e., bandpower differences in central and temporal areas are significant ($P < 0.001$). The central locations exhibit *more* bandpower under the high workload condition, the temporal locations *less*. (c), (d): power spectra of three discriminative EEG channels of subject *ps*. Clear differences are found at the 10 Hz α peaks.

parameters for each of these steps (and also for the classification stage) are listed below. The sets of candidate parameters were designed on the basis of neurophysiological findings that have been reported in the literature. A specific parameterization is chosen after the initial training session and kept constant for the entire application.

EEG channels:[1] (F# denotes the whole F-row, see figure 24.4a and b)
{FC#, C#, P#, CP#};
{F#, FC#, C#, P#, CP#, O#};
{F#, FC#, C#, P#, CP#, O#, T7, T8};
{FC#, C#, P#, CP#, T7, T8}.

Spatial filter: common median reference or none.

Frequency band: 3–15, 7–15, 10–15, 3–10 Hz.

Window lengths and integrate values: 10 s and 10; 15 s and 5; 30 s and 1.

Classifier parameters: real number weight for each remaining channel.

Hysteresis thresholds: two real numbers m_l and m_h.

Starting with 32 recorded EEG channels, the first step of data processing is the exclusion of channels that are contaminated with artifacts during the training session. More precisely, channels containing muscle or eye-movement artifacts that are correlated with a particular workload condition are identified based on their frequency spectra and excluded. This is a crucial step and prevents the classifier from being driven by artifacts rather than neurophysiological effects. Therefore, frequencies above 20 Hz and below 6 Hz are scanned for significant broadband differences between the two workload conditions. Such broad-band differences are characteristic for muscle artifacts (> 20 Hz) or eye artifacts (< 6 Hz). The channels that exhibit those differences are excluded.

Next, a subset of the remaining EEG channels is selected for further processing. This subset is one of four candidate sets that potentially include frontal, occipital, and temporal scalp positions. By using these sets, a rough preselection of EEG channels is achieved. Each of the selected channels is then optionally normalized by the common median reference signal (the median of all channels is subtracted from each channel), which is a variation of the commonly employed common average reference filter. We choose the median because it is more robust than the mean with respect to measurement outliers, which we expect to occur more often in the given real-world setting.

The signal is then processed through a subject- and task-specific bandpass filter using one of the bands listed above. The actual input to the workload classifier is the power of each bandpass-filtered channel in a time window of specific length (within 10–30 s), sampled every 200 ms. The use of time windows shorter than 10 s typically leads to a clear degradation of the classifier performance, which reflects the difficulty of distinguishing between the high and low workload class. Indeed, for the shorter window lengths we use an average of the classifier output for a predefined number of successive predictions to get a more robust result (i.e., 10 successive predictions for 10 s. window length, 5 for 15 s). Interestingly, in 82 percent of the cases, a 10 s window was finally chosen by our method. From this feature extraction stage, every 200 ms, we obtain a feature vector which is then fed into the classifier.

For classification, we use a linear model whose parameters are computed by standard linear discriminant analysis (LDA) of the feature vectors obtained from the high and low workload conditions of the training session (Fisher (1936)). Nonlinear methods, such as regularized kernel ridge regression (Poggio and Girosi (1990)) or support vector machines (Vapnik (1998)), produced comparable results but no improvements in offline analyses.

The output of the classifier is a scalar value representing the estimated degree of low workload (values below zero) or high workload (values above zero). We then map this real-valued output to a binary quantity that indicates the two states, high and low workload, by means of a threshold scheme that employs a hysteresis, which makes the classification substantially more robust. It consists of two thresholds, $m_l < m_h$, such that switching to a *high workload* indication takes place once the output exceeds m_h, while switching to a *low workload* requires that the output falls below the lower value m_l. The values m_l and m_h are subject- and task-specific, and therefore are calibrated on the training data also.

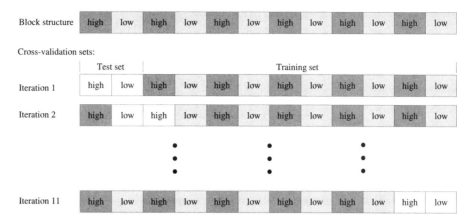

Figure 24.5   Recorded EEG signals typically are highly correlated locally. Therefore, the cross-validation scheme has to be set up properly to obtain a realistic estimate of the true generalization error. This can be accomplished by splitting the datasets based on the block structure of the experiment. For each of the eleven iterations, the workload detector is trained on ten blocks (dark and light grey). The detector is then applied to the two remaining blocks (white) to obtain an estimate of the performance on new, unseen data. The eleven individual performance estimates finally are averaged to obtain a robust estimate of the generalization error.

24.4.2   Parameter Calibration

The set of possible parameters, as specified in the last section, results in a controlled flexibility of the workload detector. The detector can adjust itself to the most discriminative features, individually for each subject and each task (and it thereby accounts for the known inter- and intrasubject variability). On the other hand, this adaptation is limited to a scope that is neurophysiologically reasonable.

This flexible approach poses the problem of robustly identifying the most suitable parameter set in each experiment. Therefore, to find suitable values for all the previously mentioned subject- and task-specific parameters, we use the well known cross-validation technique (Cover (1969)), taking into account the particular block structure of our experiment. The rationale of this technique is to find parameters that *generalize well*, that is, lead to good performance on new, unseen data, given just a fixed training dataset. For the training data, the class labels are known, in this case *high* or *low workload*, whereas for new data they must be inferred by the model (i.e., the workload detector). To avoid *overfitting* the training data, resulting in inferior performance on new data, new data is simulated in this approach by splitting the training dataset into two sets: One is used to fit the model to the data, and the other one, the *validation set*, is used to assess the quality of the model.

It is important to note that for time series data like EEG signals, some care has to be taken to perform the split such that the estimated generalization error is realistic. Since data points that are close in time are likely to be highly correlated, the split cannot be performed by selecting a random subset. This would result in many almost identical data points in both sets, such that the training and validation sets would be very similar and thus useless for testing the generalization performance. Instead, the validation set should be a single block of consecutive data points (see figure 24.5). For the same reason, if there is a block structure of the class labels, the two split points should be at the class label boundaries. Finally, to make the estimate of the generalization error more robust, it is useful to perform the split in two subsets several times in different ways and then average over all individual generalization errors. We therefore perform the splits by leaving out two consecutive high- and low-workload blocks for validation and repeat the estimation of the generalization error for all subsequent pairs of blocks, which thus results in an *elevenfold cross-validation*. This procedure is performed for each possible combination of parameter candidates in the feature extraction part (EEG channel subset, spatial filter, frequency band, window length): the corresponding features are extracted and a classifier is trained on the extracted features by using LDA.

For each classifier obtained in this way, the hysteresis thresholds are then determined using the workload predictions of the classifier for the data in the training set. Recall that these are real numbers below or above zero, representing the estimated degree of low or high workload, respectively. The idea behind using a threshold scheme is to identify an uncertainty interval by a lower and upper threshold, m_l and m_h, in which outputs are generated almost equally likely from data of both classes. In this region of uncertain predictions, the system should stick to its previous class decision, exploiting the fact that changes in workload are slow in comparison to the frequency at which predictions are made.

The thresholds lie in the interval spanned by the smallest and largest classifier output. In this range, there exists a decision threshold m_0 that attains maximum classification accuracy on the training set (without hysteresis). A candidate pair for m_l and m_h is then given as the smallest and largest threshold such that the classification accuracy is still larger than $\eta\, m_0$, with η being a value between 0.9 and 1.0. Such candidate pairs are generated for a number of η-values. The pair that maximizes the training set accuracy resulting from classification *with* hysteresis is ultimately selected.

The workload detector fully specified in this way then predicts the workload on the two left-out blocks, resulting in a cross-validation error. Each complete set of parameters is evaluated in this fashion, and the winning configuration is finally chosen among the candidates with the smallest cross-validation error.

24.5   Results

We discuss the results of our experiment with respect to three different criteria: neurophysiological interpretation of the results, the accuracy of the workload detector, and the performance increase obtained by using the workload detector to mitigate the workload in high workload conditions.

24.5.1 Neurophysiological Interpretation

A comparison of the relevant discriminating quantities, the channel-wise power spectra, reveals a strong intersubject variability. Only some subjects exhibit clear α peaks (8–12 Hz). There also is no clear unique neurophysiological effect that can be observed.

The best performing subject *ps* not only has very pronounced α peaks, but also displays clear differences in the amount of α power for the two workload conditions (at least in the overall average), which explains the good performance (figure 24.4). Remarkably, there is an *increase* in α power under the high workload condition (at and around Cz in figure 24.4), which also can be observed in eleven other subjects (mainly parietal). This is somewhat in contrast to the work of others, where α generally decreases (Scerbo et al. (2003))—an effect that we find in only about half of the subjects (and also in figure 24.4, e.g., at T7 and T8). A reason for this difference could be the complexity and real-world nature of our experiment, but most likely it is because our workload-inducing tasks are not visual, as opposed to a large number of experiments reported in the literature.

In summary, the large intersubject variability justifies our highly adaptable approach, which automatically adjusts the workload detector to these neurophysiological variations.

24.5.2 Accuracy of the Workload Detector

The quality of the workload detector is assessed by comparing the indicated workload with the high/low block structure of the experiment. The presented results reflect the performance of the subject- and task-specific workload detectors after training, that is, in the (real-time) application session.

As an example, the exact time course of the workload detector output for the best performing subject, *ps*, is depicted in figure 24.6. For this subject, the *continuous* classifier output (lower line) already exhibits a remarkable correlation with the block structure of the experiment. For the other subjects, this correlation was less prominent and there the hysteresis mechanism, which finally yields the binary high/low workload indication, significantly improved the classification performance.

The results for all subjects are shown in figure 24.7 as the percentage of correctly classified time points. The first few seconds of each task block that amount to the window length (i.e., typically 10 s) were excluded from the assessment, since this is the potential response time of the system. One can see that the intersubject variability is very large, but nevertheless a classification accuracy of more than 70 percent for eight out of seventeen subjects for the auditory task and for eleven out of seventeen subjects for the mental calculation task was achieved. The best performing subject, *ps*, achieved classification accuracies greater than 90 percent for both the auditory and the classification task.

24.5.3 Performance Improvement

The binary detector output was used to mitigate the workload of the subject by suppressing the auditory reaction task when the workload indication is *high*. By comparing the (unmitigated) training session with the (mitigated) application session, we see that the mitigation

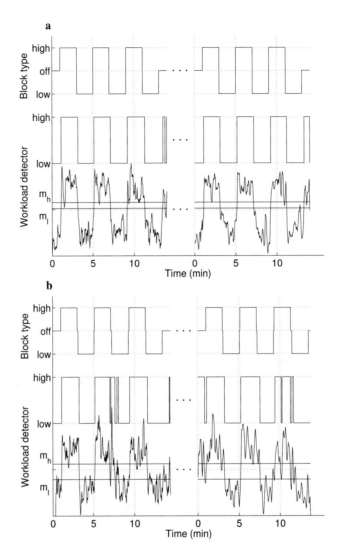

Figure 24.6   The exact time course of the classifier output for the best performing subject, *ps*, and the corresponding binary high/low workload indication used to control the mitigation, in comparison with the true high and low workload conditions. (A) For auditory workload (95.6% correct); (B) For mental calculation workload (91.8% correct).

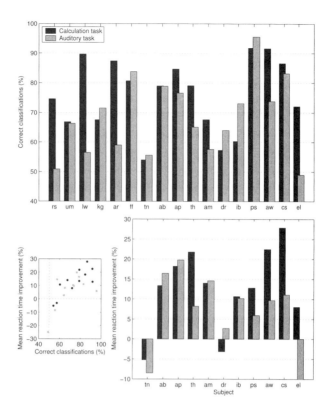

Figure 24.7   Experimental results. Top: Percentage of correctly classified workload for each subject (in chronological order). In some cases the classifier could not find sufficiently discriminating features in the EEG since even a random classification would already yield a rate of 50%. Bottom right: The average improvement of the reaction time of each subject due to the workload mitigation strategy (10% typically corresponds to an improvement of about 100 ms). Mitigation was introduced after the first six subjects and consists in the temporary suppression of the reaction task. Degradation of average reaction times happens only in cases where the classifier does not perform well. Bottom left: The correlation between classification performance and mean reaction time improvement.

strategy leads to significantly better reaction times on average (figure 24.7, bottom right). This is due mainly to the circumstance that reaction times are typically longer in the high workload phase. That clearly degrades the average performance in the training session, but it almost does not affect the performance in the application session, where the subject is largely exempted from reacting during the high workload condition because of the successfully activated suppression of the reaction task. Thus, the mitigation strategy effectively improves the performance of the subject by circumventing the periods of potentially long reaction times.

24.6   Discussion

In conclusion, we showed that mental workload detection in real-time and in real operating environments is possible and can lead to an improved performance of a subject by mitigating the workload in high workload conditions. In the context of driving, the mitigation of high mental workload can be of vital importance since a reaction time improvement of 100 ms, as achieved in the experiments, reduces the braking distance by 2.8 meters when driving at 100 km/h. This could be enough to prevent a collision.

We also have seen that the strong intersubject variability of the EEG makes the use of a highly adaptable system necessary. The performance of the workload detector is nevertheless strongly subject-dependent and depends on the existence of differences in the EEG power spectra for different workload conditions. These differences can be localized in different frequency bands and channels. Therefore, it seems unlikely that one can obtain good results by using a fixed neurophysiological feature. Instead, a system is required that can select from a number of neurophysiologically sensible features in a robust fashion. The presented feedback system is based on a *parameterized* EEG analysis, in which the parameters are adapted to the subject and the task in an initial training session. For future research, one major challenge is to reduce the amount of data necessary for the adaptation of the workload detector.

Acknowledgments

We gratefully acknowledge S. Willmann and S. Rothe for helpful support. The authors Konrad Hagemann, Andreas Bruns, Michael Schrauf, and Wilhelm E. Kincses were partly supported by DARPA grant NBCH 3030001.

Notes

* The first three authors contributed equally to this work.
E-mail for correspondence: jek@first.fhg.de

(1)   The EEG signals are recorded from Ag/AgCl electrodes at positions according to the international 10-20 system. The actual sampling frequency of 500 Hz was down-sampled to 100 Hz.

25 Single-Trial Analysis of EEG during Rapid Visual Discrimination: Enabling Cortically Coupled Computer Vision

Paul Sajda, Adam D. Gerson, and Marios G. Philiastides
Department of Biomedical Engineering
Columbia University
New York, NY 10027, USA

Lucas C. Parra
Department of Biomedical Engineering
City College of New York
New York, NY 10031, USA

25.1 Abstract

We describe our work using linear discrimination of multichannel electroencephalography for single-trial detection of neural signatures of visual recognition events. We demonstrate the approach as a methodology for relating neural variability to response variability, describing studies for response accuracy and response latency during visual target detection. We then show how the approach can be used to construct a novel type of brain-computer interface, which we term "cortically coupled computer vision." In this application, a large database of images is triaged using the detected neural signatures. We show how "cortical triaging" improves image search over a strictly behavioral response.

25.2 Introduction

Running in the park with your head phones on, listening to your favorite tune, and concentrating on your stride, you look up and see a face that you immediately recognize as a high school friend. She is wearing a hat, glasses, and has aged fifteen years since you last saw her. You and she are running in opposite directions so you only see her for a fleeting moment, yet you are sure it was her. Your visual system has just effortlessly accomplished a feat that has thus far baffled the best computer vision systems. Such ability for rapid processing of visual information is even more impressive in light of the fact that neurons are relatively slow processing elements compared to digital computers, where individual transistors can switch a million times faster than a neuron can spike.

Noninvasive neuroimaging has provided a means to peer into the brain during rapid visual object recognition. In particular, analysis of trial-averaged event-related potentials (ERPs) in electroencephalography (EEG) has enabled us to assess the speed of visual recognition and discrimination in terms of the timing of the underlying neural processes (Thorpe et al. (1996)). More recent work has used single-trial analysis of EEG to characterize the neural activity directly correlated with behavioral variability during tasks involving rapid visual discrimination (Gerson et al. (2005); Philiastides and Sajda (2006)). These results suggest that components extracted from the EEG can capture the neural correlates of the visual recognition and decision-making processing on a trial-by-trial basis.

In this chapter, we consider how such EEG components might be used for constructing a brain-computer interface (BCI) system for rapidly assessing streams of natural images. Traditionally, noninvasive BCI systems have been based on one of the following paradigms: (1) having a subject consciously modulate brain rhythms (e.g., Pfurtscheller (1989); Wolpaw et al. (1991); Delorme and Makeig (2003)), (2) having a subject consciously generate a motor plan and/or visual imagery (Pfurtscheller and Neuper (2001); Wolpaw and McFarland (2004)), (3) directly modulating the subject's cortical activity by the stimulus frequency (e.g., steady-state visually evoked potentials (SSVEP)) (Kelly et al. (2005); Cheng et al. (2002)), or (4) exploiting specific ERPs such as the novelty/oddball P300 (Kaper et al. (2004)). The approach and system we describe is most similar to the latter, though our focus is on single-trial detection of ERPs and their relationship to visual discrimination and recognition.

We begin this chapter by providing a brief review of the linear discrimination methods we employ to extract task-specific components in the EEG. We then show how such components are in fact directly coupled with the visual discrimination and decision-making processes for stimuli involving rapid sequences of natural images. For example, we show that we can construct neurometric functions from the EEG components that are indistinguishable from the corresponding psychometric functions for a rapid serial visual presentation (RSVP) task. We also investigate the neural correlates of response time variability responsible for such perceptual decision-making processes. We then describe how we use this approach to develop a BCI system for high-throughput imagery triage. We term our system *cortically coupled computer vision* since we leverage the robust recognition capabilities of the human visual system (e.g., invariance to pose, lighting, scale), and use a noninvasive cortical interface to intercept signatures of recognition events—that is, the visual processor performs perception and recognition and the EEG interface detects the result (decision) of that processing.

25.3   Linear Methods for Single-Trial Analysis

The goal of a BCI system is to detect neuronal activity associated with perceptual and/or cognitive events. Detecting such events implies detecting when an event occurred and identifying its significance. The task is greatly simplified if the timing information is provided by an external observable event. Thus, the conventional paradigm of the evoked response considers the neuronal activity following the presentation of a stimulus. In our work, we have adopted this paradigm by analyzing the EEG activity of multiple electrodes following presentation of an image. For simplicity, we aim to identify only one type of event, visual target recognition, and differentiate this from other visual processing. The task is therefore a binary classification based on the temporal and spatial profile of the potentials evoked following stimulus presentation. In every trial, an image is presented and in some trials the image contains a target object, which we assume is recognized by the subject. The EEG activity following each stimulus is recorded as $D \times T$ values, where D is the number of channels and T is the number of samples. Typically, we record data at 1000 Hz in up to 64 channels. With a time window of half a second following the presentation of the stimulus, one would acquire 32,000 samples. This is a rather large feature vector considering that typically there are fewer than $N = 100$ exemplars (trials) to train a classifier. In addition, EEG signals have a very low signal-to-noise ratio (SNR) and brute-force classification of this 32,000-dimensional feature vector will typically fail.

To obtain reasonable classification performance, we exploit prior information on the temporal characteristics of the signal and noise with the following steps: (1) Reduce the trial-to-trial variability by filtering the signal to remove 60 Hz interference and slow drifts (slower than 0.5 Hz). This assumes that slow constant currents below 0.5 Hz carry no information, (2) reduce the dimensionality of the problem by grouping the signal into blocks of L samples assuming that the signal of interest does not change much within this window in time, and (3) increase the number of exemplars by using the L redundant samples in each classification window. This implies that the variation within L samples is considered noise, that is, for $L = 50$ the signal of interest is at 10 Hz while faster signal variation are considered noise. Steps (2) and (3) taken together will transform the original data for each trial with TD dimensions into L exemplars of only DT/L dimensions. As an example, with $L = 50$ and $N = 100$ one will acquire 5,000 training examples, which can be used to train a classifier with a 640-dimensional feature vector. Admittedly these samples are not independent, but they are useful as they capture the noise in the data at least for frequencies above 10 Hz.

We have obtained good classification results with a simple linear classifier of these DT/L-dimensional feature vectors. The classification method is demonstrated in figure 25.1 for the simple case of a single training window ($L = T$ and D-dimensional feature vector). Linear classification means that the feature vector $\mathbf{x}$ is projected onto an orientation defined by vector $\mathbf{w}$ such that the projection, $y = \mathbf{w}^T\mathbf{x}$, optimally differentiates between the two classes. This is a traditional problem in pattern recognition with various solutions depending on the exact optimality criteria. In an offline processing mode, we use penalized logistic regression as it gives us the best generalization performance on this data (Parra et al. (2005)). For well-separated classes, this linear classification method is equivalent to linear support vectors. In a real-time processing mode, we use Fisher linear discriminants as the required means and covariances can easily be updated online as more trials become available for training. For a discussion on the relative benefits of various linear classification methods with EEG data, see Müller et al. (2003a) and Parra et al. (2005). Classification performance is measured with the conventional receiver operating characteristic (ROC) curve (Green and Swets (1966)), specifically the area under the ROC curve (A_z). We report in all cases the cross-validated test-set performance using a leave-one-out procedure where we leave out all samples belonging to one trial.

One can conceive of many other ways of classifying the spatiotemporal evoked responses including nonlinear methods. In fact, many different algorithms have been proposed, which exploit different prior assumptions on the signals (Parra et al. (2005); Lemm et al. (2005); Luo and Sajda (2006); Bronstein et al. (2005)). We are partial toward linear methods for two reasons: (1) The linear combination of voltages has an immediate interpretation as a current (tissue is primarily resistive with coupling coefficients representing conductivity). The coefficients that couple this current with the observed voltages are given for the linear model by $\mathbf{a} = \langle \mathbf{x}^T y \rangle / \langle y^2 \rangle$ where the angular brackets indicate the average over trials and samples. Specifically, coefficients $\mathbf{a}$ describe the coupling (and correlation) of the discriminating component y with the sensor activity $\mathbf{x}$. Both $\mathbf{a}$ and $\mathbf{x}$ are D-dimensional vectors (row and column, respectively). Strong coupling indicates low attenuation of the component and can be visualized as intensity maps that we call the "sensor projections" (Parra et al. (2005)). (2) Linear methods are easy to implement and are fast, permitting real-time operation. The disadvantage of our method is that it does not capture synchronized activity above 10 Hz, and neither does it capture activity that is not at a fixed distance in time from the stimulus; instead only phase-locked activity is detected.

In the remaining sections, we give several examples of how this linear discrimination method is used to identify the neural correlates of decision-making and response time variability, as well as how it can be integrated into a BCI system for image triage.

25.4   EEG Correlates of Perceptual Decision Making

Identifying neural activity directly responsible for perceptual decision-making is a major challenge for noninvasive BCI systems. A number of investigators have studied the neural correlates of decision-making in awake behaving animals, in particular primates, where single and multiunit recordings have been analyzed using signal detection theory (Green and Swets (1966)) and subsequently correlated with the animal's observed behavior (Britten et al. (1992, 1996); Newsome et al. (1989)). These approaches consist mainly of direct comparisons between psychometric and neurometric functions since this enables researchers to relate the variability of the neural activity to the variability observed in the behavioral response. The technique has been applied in a variety of perceptual decision-making paradigms including discrimination of visual objects such as faces (Keysers et al. (2001)). The approach, though powerful, has been limited to animal studies that use inva-

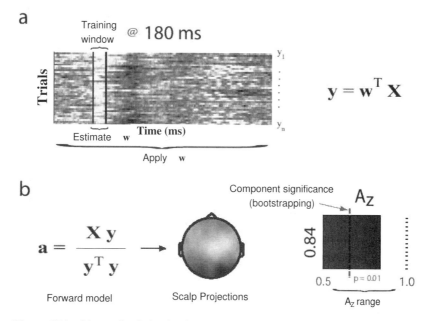

Figure 25.1   Linear discrimination in EEG: (a) The D-dimensional EEG activity, $\mathbf{X}$, is projected onto a single dimension $\mathbf{y}$. ($\mathbf{X}$ is a matrix of channels by samples, and $\mathbf{y}$ is a row vector containing multiple samples). The row vectors, $\mathbf{y}$, containing the samples that follow each target stimulus presentation, can be arranged for multiple trials as a matrix. This matrix ($\mathbf{y_{target}}$ - mean($\mathbf{y_{non-target}}$)) is displayed here as an image with white and black representing the largest and smallest values, respectively. The projection vector $\mathbf{w}$ is chosen so that the values $\mathbf{y}$ within the training window differ maximally between target and non-target trials. (b) The sensor projections $\mathbf{a}$ are computed for the samples within the training window. (In this equation, the inner product computes the average over trials and samples. Therefore, matrix $\mathbf{X}$ and vector $\mathbf{y}$ extend here over the training samples from all trials.) The resulting values of $\mathbf{a}$ are displayed at the corresponding scalp locations as a color-map with white and black representing the largest and smallest values respectively. When the intensity $\mathbf{y}$ averaged within the specified time window is used as classification criteria, we achieve on this data an A_z-value of 0.84. The probability of obtaining an A_z of this magnitude by chance is less than 1% ($p < 0.01$).

sive recordings of single-trial neural activities. Yet to be demonstrated, however, is whether decision-making could be studied in a similar fashion, noninvasively, in humans.

  We use single-trial linear discrimination analysis, as outlined in the previous section, to identify the cortical correlates of decision-making during rapid discrimination of images. Psychophysical performance is measured for several subjects during an RSVP task, where a series of target (faces) and non-target (cars) trials are presented in rapid succession (figure 25.2a) while simultaneously recording neuronal activity from a 64-channel EEG electrode array. Stimulus evidence is varied by manipulating the phase coherence (Dakin et al. (2002)) of the images (figure 25.2b). Within a block of trials, face and car images over a range of phase coherences are presented in random order. We use a set of 12 face (Max Planck Institute face database) and 12 car greyscale images (image size 512 x 512 pixels, 8-bits/pixel). Both image types contained equal numbers of frontal and side views (up to ±45 degrees). All images are equated for spatial frequency, luminance, and contrast. Subjects are required to discriminate the type of image (face or car) and report their decision by pressing a button.

EEG data is acquired simultaneously in an electrostatically shielded room (ETS-Lindgren, Glendale Heights, Ill.) using a Sensorium EPA-6 Electrophysiological Amplifier (Charlotte, Vt.) from 60 Ag/AgCl scalp electrodes and from 3 periocular electrodes placed below the left eye and at the left and right outer canthi. All channels are referenced to the left mastoid with input impedance $< 15k\Omega$ and chin ground. Data are sampled at 1000 Hz with an analog pass band of 0.01–300 Hz using 12 dB/octave high-pass and eighth-order elliptic low-pass filters. Subsequently, a software-based 0.5-Hz high-pass filter is used to remove DC drifts, and 60 and 120 Hz (harmonic) notch filters are applied to minimize line noise artifacts. These filters are designed to be linear-phase to minimize delay distortions. In all our experiments, we also record EOG signals and remove motion and blink artifacts using linear methods as described in Parra et al. (2005). Motor response and stimulus events recorded on separate channels are delayed to match latencies introduced by digitally filtering the EEG.

Using a linear discriminator, we identify EEG components that maximally discriminate between the two experimental conditions. At each phase coherence level, and between the stimulus onset and the earliest reaction time, we identify two time windows that give the most discriminating components. For this paradigm, an early ($\approx$ 170 ms following stimulus) and a late component ($>$ 300 ms following stimulus) can be identified. To be able to compare directly the neuronal performance at these two times, to the psychophysical sensitivity as captured by the psychometric functions (Green and Swets (1966)), we construct neurometric functions by plotting the area under the ROC curves (A_z values) against the corresponding phase coherence levels. A linear discriminator is trained by integrating data across both time windows ($2D$-dimensional feature vector). With this approach, we generally observe for the discriminator improved performance (and hence higher A_z values) compared to when training is performed on the individual components in isolation. Figure 25.3 shows a comparison of the psychometric and neurometric functions for one subject in the dataset. To demonstrate that the EEG-derived neurometric functions can account for psychophysical performance, a likelihood-ratio test is used (Hoel et al. (1971)), which shows that for all the subjects a single function can fit the behavioral and neuronal datasets as well as the two separate functions.

For both the early (the well-known N170 (Rossion et al. (2003); Puce et al. (1996); Jeffreys (1996))) and late face selective components, at each phase coherence level, we construct discriminant component maps to help us visualize the temporal evolution of the discriminating activity across trials. Data is analyzed for both stimulus and response-locked conditions, showing that both face selective components appear to be more correlated with the onset of visual stimulation than the response, as shown in figure 25.4 for one subject. In addition, we construct scalp maps of these discriminating components. The spatial distribution of activity seems to indicate signaling between occipito-parietal and centro-frontal networks, consistent with several ERP/MEG and functional neuroimaging studies (Hasson et al. (2002); Heekeren et al. (2004); Liu et al. (2002); Rossion et al. (2003); VanRullen and Thorpe (2001)). The A_z values that describe the discriminator's performance at each phase coherence level are also shown. For the subject shown in figure 25.4, the discriminant activity is statistically significant down to a 30 percent phase coherence for both the early and late components as assessed by a bootstrapping technique. Specifically, we compute a significance level for A_z by performing the leave-one-out test after randomizing the truth labels of our face and car trials. We repeat this randomization process one hundred times to produce an A_z randomization distribution and compute the A_z leading to a significance level of $p < 0.01$. Additional results and details can be found in Philiastides and Sajda (2006) and Philiastides et al. (2006).

Our results demonstrate that neural correlates of perceptual decision-making can be identified using high-spatial density EEG and that the corresponding component activities are temporally distributed. Important to the identification of these neural correlates is the spatial and, to a lesser extent, the temporal integration of the EEG component activities. This approach is complementary to those using single and multiunit recordings since it sacrifices spatial and some temporal resolution (local field potentials versus spike-trains) for a more spatially distributed view of the neural activity during decision-making. The fact that we are able to identify neural correlates of perceptual decision-making using relatively poor spatial resolution of EEG suggests that these neural correlates represent strong activities of neural populations and not the activity of a small number of neurons. As such, this approach can be especially useful in designing noninvasive BCI systems that reliably predict behavioral responses.

25.5   Identifying Cortical Processes Leading to Response Time Variability

Significant variability in response time is observed across trials in many visual discrimination and recognition tasks. A variety of factors may account for response time variability ranging from the difficulty in discriminating an object on any given trial, to trial-by-trial variability of the subject's engagement in the task, to intrinsic variability of neural processing. Identifying neural activity correlated with response time variability may shed light on the underlying cortical networks responsible for perceptual decision-making processes and the processing latencies that these networks may introduce for a given task.

We study visual target detection using an RSVP paradigm and use single-trial spatial integration of high-density electroencephalography to identify the time course and cortical origins leading to response time variability. The RSVP task emulates natural saccadic scene acquisition and requires high vigilance. The RSVP paradigm is illustrated in figure 25.5. Activity associated with recognition has been identified with the RSVP paradigm as early as 150 ms after stimulus presentation (Thorpe et al. (1996)). More recent work argues that this activity is associated with differences in low-level features of the imagery rather than target recognition (Johnson and Olshausen (2003)). The varied scale, pose, and position of target objects (people) requires subjects to recognize objects rather than low-level features. During this task, participants are presented with a continuous sequence of natural scenes. Participants completed four blocks of fifty sequences each with a rest period lasting no more than five minutes between blocks. Each sequence consists of fifty images and has a 50 percent chance of containing one target image with one or more people in a natural

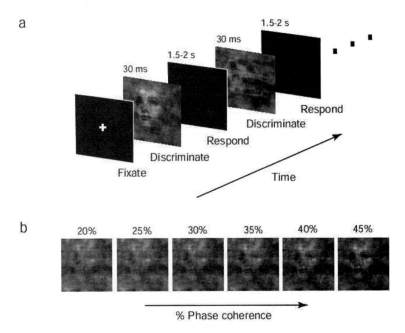

Figure 25.2 Schematic representation of the behavioral paradigm. (a) Within a block of trials, subjects are instructed to fixate on the center of the screen and are subsequently presented, in random order, with a series of different face and car images at one of the six phase coherence levels shown in (b). Each image is presented for 30 ms followed by an interstimulus-interval lasting between 1500–2000 ms during which subjects are required to discriminate among the two types of images and respond by pressing a button. A block of trials is completed once all face and car images at all six phase coherence levels are presented. (b) A sample face image at six different phase coherence levels (20, 25, 30, 35, 40, and 45%).

scene. These target images can appear only within the middle thirty images of each fifty-image sequence. The remaining natural scenes without a person are referred to as distractor images. Each image was presented for 100 ms. A fixation cross is displayed for 2 s between sequences. Participants are instructed to press the left button of a generic three-button mouse with their right index finger while the fixation cross is present, and release the button as soon as they recognize a target image.

Linear discrimination is used to determine spatial weighting coefficients that optimally discriminate between EEG resulting from different RSVP task conditions (e.g., target versus distractor images) over specific temporal windows between stimulus and response. Integration across sensors enhances signal quality without loss of temporal precision common to trial averaging in ERP studies. The resulting discriminating components describe activity specific to target recognition and subsequent response for individual trials.

Intertrial variability is estimated by extracting features from discriminating components. While robust extraction of component onset from individual trials is extremely difficult due to the stochastic nature of EEG, there is evidence of strong correlation between ERP peak and onset times (Scheffers et al. (1991)). The peaks of spatially integrated discriminating

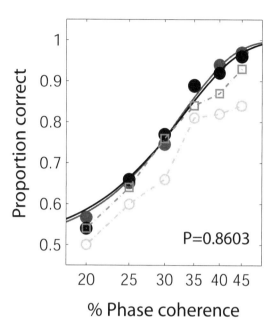

Figure 25.3   Comparison of behavioral and neuronal performance. Psychometric (solid grey) and neurometric (solid black) functions for one subject. The abscissas represent the percentage of phase coherence of our stimuli, and the ordinate indicates the subject's performance as proportion correct. We fit both data with separate Weibull functions (Quick (1974)). The psychophysical and neuronal data are statistically indistinguishable as assessed by a likelihood-ratio test after we fit the best single Weibull function jointly to the two datasets. The *p*-value in the bottom right corner represents the output of this test. A *p*-value greater than 0.05 indicates that a single function fits the two datasets as well as the two separate functions. The dotted grey lines connect the A_z values computed for each of the two training windows separately (earlier window, lighter grey circles; later window, darker grey squares).

components were found by fitting a parametric function to the extracted component $y(t)$. For simplicity, we use a Gaussian profile that is parameterized by its height β, width σ, delay μ, and baseline offset α:

$$\hat{y}(t) = \alpha + \frac{\beta}{\sigma\sqrt{2\pi}}e^{-\frac{(t-\mu)^2}{2\sigma^2}}. \tag{25.1}$$

Response-locking of discriminating components is determined by computing the linear regression coefficients that predict the latency of the component activity as measured by μ from the response times given by r as described by (25.2). The proportionality factor from the response time peak latency regression (θ) is defined to be the degree of response-locking (percentage) for each component. This metric quantifies the extent to which the component is correlated with the response across trials. It ranges from 0 percent for pure stimulus lock to 100 percent for pure response lock. A factor $\theta = 100\%$ indicates that slow

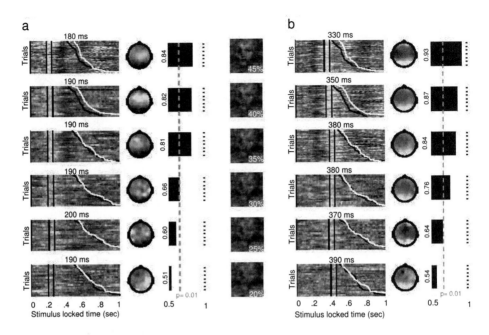

Figure 25.4 Discriminant component activity that shows the difference between face vs. car trials at each coherence level for one subject for (a) the early (N170) and (b) the late ($\approx 300 - 400$ ms) window. White represents positive and black negative activity. Each row of these maps represents the output of the linear discriminator for a single trial, using a 60-ms training window (vertical black lines) with onset times specified at the top of each panel. All trials are aligned to the onset of visual stimulation, as indicated by the vertical black line at time 0 ms, and sorted by response time. The black sigmoidal curves represent the subject's response times for face trials. The representation of the topology of the discriminating activity is shown by the scalp plots to the right (dorsal view). White represents positive correlation of the sensor readings to the extracted activity and black negative correlation. The A_z values for each time window at each coherence level are represented by the bar graphs. The significance of the difference activity is represented by the dotted line ($p = 0.01$).

responses show a corresponding late activity, and fast responses show a corresponding early activity. A factor of $\theta = 0\%$ indicates that the timing of the activity does not change with response time and is therefore stimulus locked.

$$\hat{\mu}_j = \theta r_j + b \tag{25.2}$$

where $\hat{\mu}_j$ and r_j are the predicted peak latencies and response times for the jth trial and b is an offset term for the regression. This is shown for one subject in figure 25.6.

The group results for the discriminating component activity across nine participants is shown in figure 25.7. Scalp projections of discriminating components were normalized prior to averaging. Group averaged results show a shift of activity from frontal to parietal regions over the course of 200 ms, which is consistent with previous studies of visual oddball BCIs (Makeig et al. (1999, 2004)). Additional analysis and discussion is provided in Gerson et al. (2005).

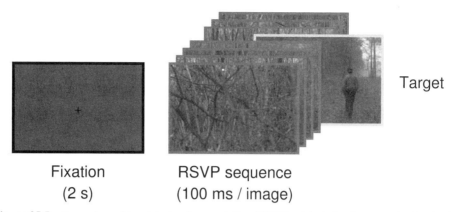

Fixation
(2 s)

RSVP sequence
(100 ms / image)

Target

Figure 25.5   Example rapid serial visual presentation (RSVP) trial. A fixation cross lasting 2 s is followed by a sequence of fifty images. Each sequence has a 50% probability of containing one target image. This target can appear only within the middle thirty images to ensure that a one-second image buffer precedes and follows the target.

To estimate the progression of response-locking across all subjects, it is necessary to account for response time variability among subjects. It is not appropriate to average results since components are not temporally aligned across subjects. Rather, histograms of response times were equalized to one subject (subject 2), and component peak times were scaled accordingly. Scaled response times and component peak times were concatenated across subjects. These registered group response times were then projected onto the scaled component peak times to estimate the degree of response-locking across subjects. The group response lock increased from 28 percent at -200 ms to 78 percent at 50 ms after the response.

The features of discriminating components are believed to reflect visual processing, attention, and decision stages. Modeling the peak latency, amplitude, and duration of each trial allows us to study the extent to which each stage varies with response time. Consistent with Kammer et al. (1999), figure 25.7 indicates that significant processing delays may be introduced by early processing stages. Within 200 ms prior to response ($\approx$ 250 ms following stimulus), activity is already, on average, between 25 and 35% response-locked. Due to our method, it is not possible to determine whether this response-locking is a result of components at this onset time or earlier onset times, since discriminating components were not significant for earlier onset (peak) times. Thus, we conclude it is possible that some of this early response-locking may be due to early visual processes (0–250 ms poststimulus). For our nine subjects, correlation analysis reveals that discriminating component activity progressively becomes more response-locked with subsequent processing stages. Along with scalp projections derived from discriminant analysis, the covariability of peak latency with response time describes which cortical regions introduce processing delays, providing insight into the nature of information flow through the brain during visual discrimination.

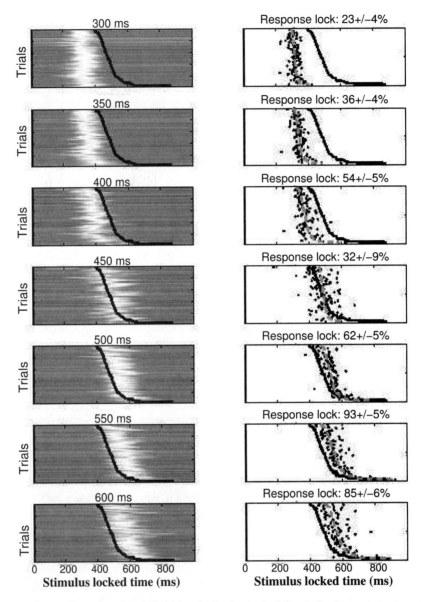

Figure 25.6 Detailed temporal analysis of stimulus-locked discriminating activity for subject 2. Each row in the left column shows the fit of discriminating activity to a Gaussian profile described by (25.1). On the top of each of these panels is the onset time of the window used for discrimination. Right columns of each panel display the peak latency (μ) (black dots) of each trial. The projection of response times onto these peak latencies is shown with a thin black curve, with thick black curves representing response times. The parameters for this projection indicate the degree of response locking for each component. Purely stimulus- and response-locked conditions are indicated by 0% and 100% response lock, respectively. On top of these panels are reported the percent response lock and corresponding error in the fit of the peak latencies across trials as well as the mean onset time of the component. The standard deviation of peak latencies is 62 ms.

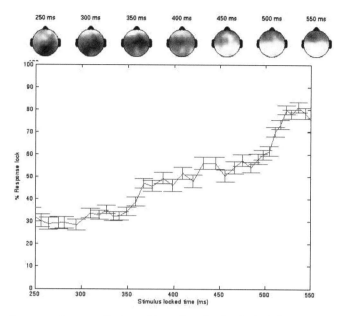

Figure 25.7   Group results over all nine subjects for stimulus-locked discriminating components. Top row shows scalp distribution of discriminating activity averaged over all subjects. Bottom row shows the degree of response-locking over time. Error bars reflect standard error of the regression parameter associated with response-locking percent. For all subjects the first discriminating activity is frontal and correlated more with the stimulus than response. By the time it arrives in parietal areas, a delay has been introduced.

25.6   EEG-Based Image Triage

Finally, we describe an EEG system capable of using neural signatures detected during RSVP to triage sequences of images, reordering them so target images are placed near the beginning of the sequence. We term our system "cortically coupled computer vision" since we leverage the robust recognition capabilities of the human visual system (e.g., invariance to pose, lighting, scale), and use a noninvasive cortical interface (e.g., EEG) to intercept signatures of recognition events—the visual processor performs perception and recognition and the EEG interface detects the result (e.g., decision) of that processing.

The RSVP triage task is similar to the task described in figure 25.5; however, following the image sequence, a series of self-paced feedback slides were presented indicating the position of target images within the sequence before and after EEG-based triage. Participants completed two blocks of fifty sequences with a brief rest period lasting no more than five minutes between blocks. During the second block, participants were instructed to quickly press the left button of a generic three-button mouse with their right index finger as soon as they recognized target images. They were instructed to press the button twice, as quickly as possible, if one target image immediately followed the other. Participants did not respond with a button press during the first block.

To classify EEG online, we use a Fisher linear discriminator to estimate a spatial weighting vector that maximally discriminates between sensor array signals evoked by target and non-target images. During each experimental condition (with and without motor response), 5,000 images were presented to the subject in sequences of 100 images. EEG evoked by the first 2,500 images (50 targets, 2,450 non-targets) was used to train the classifier. During the experimental sessions, a training window between 400 and 500 ms following stimulus onset was used to extract training data. Weights were updated adaptively with each trial during the training period. Classification threshold is adjusted to give optimum performance for the observed prevalence (class-prior). These weights and threshold were fixed at the end of the training period and applied to the subsequent testing dataset (images 2,501–5,000).

To boost offline triage performance, after the experiment multiple classifiers with different training window onsets were used. The training window onsets ranged from 0 to 900 ms in steps of 50 ms. The duration of the training windows was 50 ms. Once these classifiers were trained, the optimal weighting of these classifier outputs was found using logistic regression to discriminate between target and non-target images.

Again, only EEG data evoked by the first 2,500 images was used to train the classifiers and then find the interclassifier weights. These weights were then applied to the testing dataset evoked by the second set of 2,500 images (images 2,501–5,000).

Following the experiment, all image sequences were concatenated to create training and testing sequences that each contain 2,500 images (50 targets and 2,450 non-targets). These image sequences are resorted according to the output of our classifier with multiple training windows for EEG evoked by every image.

For comparison, sequences were triaged based on the button response. Images were resorted according to

$$p(\text{target}|RT) = \frac{p(RT|\text{target})p(\text{target})}{p(RT|\text{target})p(\text{target}) + p(RT|\text{non-target})p(\text{non-target})} \tag{25.3}$$

where RT is the onset of a button response that occurs within one second of image onset. $p(\text{target}|RT) = 0$ when no response occurred within one second of image onset. The priors $p(\text{target}) = 0.02$ and $p(\text{non-target}) = 0.98$. $p(RT|\text{target})$ are Gaussian distributions with a mean and variance determined from the response times from the training sequences. Since more than one response is likely to follow a target image if the two target images are presented within one second of each other, for training sequences response times were assigned to target images based on the position of the target image within the sequence. In other words, if the target appeared first in the sequence and two button responses occurred within one second of this target's onset, the first response was assigned to that target image and the second response was assigned to the second target image. For testing sequences, if two or more responses occur within one second of the onset of any image, the response with the greatest $p(\text{target}|RT)$ is assigned to the image. $p(RT|\text{non-target})$ is a mixture of 13 Gaussians, each with the same variance as that used for $p(RT|\text{target})$ and with means assigned by shifting the mean from $p(RT|\text{target})$ 600 ms in the past to 700 ms in the future in increments of 100 ms, excluding the actual mean of $p(RT|\text{target})$. This mixture model contains a sufficient number of Gaussians so that the mixture is consistent within

Table 25.1   Triage performance and behavioral results.

Subject	EEG (no motor)	EEG (motor)	Button	EEG (motor) and button	RT (training) (ms)	RT (testing) (ms)	% Correct (training)	% Correct (testing)
1	0.92	0.91	0.87	0.94	418 ± 133	413 ± 101	88	86
2	0.94	0.96	0.86	0.97	412 ± 64	450 ± 64	94	74
3	0.90	0.87	0.96	0.96	445 ± 79	423 ± 59	86	94
4	0.91	0.92	0.98	0.98	433 ± 74	445 ± 59	98	98
5	0.91	0.93	0.98	0.98	398 ± 86	402 ± 58	96	96
Group	0.91 ± 0.02	0.92 ± 0.03	0.93 ± 0.06	0.97 ± 0.02	421 ± 91	426 ± 71	92 ± 5	90 ± 10

the one-second interval following image onset. $p(RT|\text{non-target})$ was designed to model responses occurring within one second of the onset of a non-target image presented within one second prior to or following a target image.

Triage results for one subject (subject 2) are shown in figure 25.8. Figure 25.8a shows the number of targets as a function of the number of distractor images both before and after triage based on button press and EEG. The area under the curve generated by plotting the fraction of targets as a function of the fraction of distractor images presented is used to quantify triage performance. Triage performance for five subjects is listed in table 25.1. This area is 0.50 for all unsorted image sequences since target images are randomly distributed throughout the sequences. Ideal triage performance results in an area of 1.00. There is no significant difference in performance between button-based and EEG-based triage ($0.93 \pm 0.06, 0.92 \pm 0.03, p = 0.69, N = 5$). Interestingly, there is no significant difference in performance between EEG-based triage for the motor and no-motor response conditions ($0.92 \pm 0.03, 0.91 \pm 0.02, p = 0.81, N = 5$).

Figure 25.8b–f are rasters showing the position of the target images (black squares) and non-target images (white squares) in the concatenated image sequence. Based on these rasters and the EEG- and button-based triage performance for the five subjects listed in table 25.1, it is clear that both EEG- and button-based triage systems are capable of a high level of performance. The button-based triage performance begins to fail, however, when subjects do not consistently respond to target stimuli, and response times exceed one second. Subject 2, for instance, correctly responded to only 74 percent of targets during the testing session. In fact, this subject did not respond to twelve of fifty target images and the response time for one target image exceeded one second. Excessively late responses cannot effectively be classified using our Bayesian methods since it is not clear whether these button presses were in response to the target image or a subsequent non-target images. The EEG response evoked by images with either no response or a late response is, however, still consistent with EEG evoked by the target images with predictable response times. The EEG-based triage system is therefore capable of detecting the recognition of these target images and subsequently resorting these target images appropriately. For this reason, we exploit the information provided by both EEG and button press using another perception to boost triage performance. This approach is effective for increasing triage performance for subjects that either did not respond or had a delayed motor response to a significant number of target images (e.g., subjects 1 and 2).

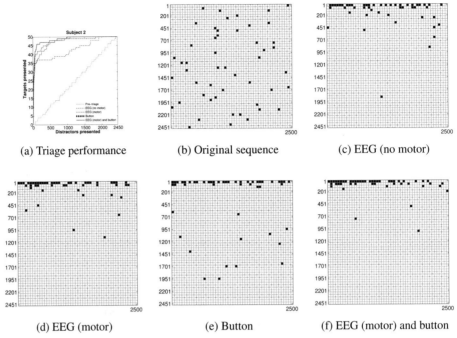

(a) Triage performance   (b) Original sequence   (c) EEG (no motor)

(d) EEG (motor)   (e) Button   (f) EEG (motor) and button

Figure 25.8   Triage performance for subject 2. (a) Number of target images presented as a function of the number of distractor images presented. An ideal triage system will place 50 (100%) of target images before all 2,450 distractor images. The light grey curve shows the original sequence. Button-based triage is shown by the dashed curve. The dash-dot curve shows EEG-based triage during the experiment without motor response. The dotted curve shows EEG-based triage during the experiment with motor response and the thick black curve shows triage based on EEG (motor) and the button response. (b–f) Rasters showing the position of non-target (white squares) and target (black squares) within the (b) original image sequence, (c) EEG (no motor)-based triage sequence, (d) EEG (motor)-based triage sequence, (e) button-based triage sequence, and (f) combined EEG (motor) and button-based triage sequence. The first and last images in each sequence are shown by the squares in the upper left and lower right of each raster respectively.

25.7   Conclusion

Invasive and noninvasive electrophysiological recordings obtained during RSVP of natural image stimuli have shed light on the speed, variability, and spatiotemporal dynamics of visual processing. Recent advances in high-spatial density EEG, real-time signal processing, machine learning, and human-computer interface design have enabled these basic neuroscience findings to be used in the development of systems that could support high-throughput image triage. Further basic and applied neuroscience research by our group will consider issues related to learning/priming/habituation, the effect of subject expertise, image type and category, and correlated spatiotemporal structure, which is prevalent in video sequences. We continue to develop "application-level" demonstrations that focus on intercepting neural correlates of visual discrimination and recognition events that effectively bypass the "slow and noisy" motor response loop.

Acknowledgments

This work was supported in part by grants from the Defense Advanced Research Projects Agency, the Office of Naval Research Multidisciplinary University Research Initiative, the National Geospatial-Intelligence Agency, and the National Institutes of Health.

Notes

E-mail for correspondence: ps629@columbia.edu

References

Altschuller, E. L., A. Vankov, E. M. Hubbard, E. Roberts, V. S. Ramachandran, and J. A. Pineda. 2000. Mu wave blocking by observation of movement and its possible use as a tool to study theory of other minds. *Society of Neuroscience Abstracts* 26(68).

Andersen, R. A., J. W. Burdick, S. Musallam, B. Pesaran, and J. G. Cham. 2004a. Cognitive neural prosthetics. *Trends in Cognitive Sciences* 8(11):486–493.

Andersen, R. A., J. W. Burdick, S. Musallam, H. Scherberger, B. Pesaran, D. Meeker, B. D. Corneil, I. Fineman, Z. Nenadic, E. Branchaud, J. G. Cham, B. Greger, Y. C. Tai, and M. M. Mojarradi. 2004b. Recording advances for neural prosthetics. In *Proceedings of the 26th International Conference of the Engineering in Medicine and Biology Society* vol. 7: 5352–5355. IEEE.

Andersen, R. A., L. H. Snyder, D. C. Bradley, and J. Xing. 1997. Multimodal representation of space in the posterior parietal cortex and its use in planning movements. *Annual Review of Neuroscience* 20(303–330):591–596.

Anderson, C. W., J. N. Knight, T. O'Connor, M. J. Kirby, and A. Sokolov. 2006. Geometric subspace methods and time-delay embedding for EEG artifact removal and classification. *IEEE Transactions on Neural Systems and Rehabilitation Engineering* 14(2): 142–146.

Anderson, C. 2005. Taxonomy of feature extraction and translation methods for bci (Web page). http://www.cs.colostate.edu/eeg/taxonomy.html.

Anderson, C. W. and M. J. Kirby. 2003. EEG subspace representations and feature selection for brain-computer interfaces. In *Proceedings of the 1st IEEE Workshop on Computer Vision and Pattern Recognition for Human Computer Interaction (CVPRHCI)*, Madison, Wis.

Anderson, C. W. 1997. Effects of variations in neural network topology and output averaging on the discrimination of mental tasks from spontaneous EEG. *Journal of Intelligent Systems* 7:165–190.

Annett, J. 1995. Motor imagery: perception or action? *Neuropsychologia* 33(11):1395–1417.

Arkin, R. C. 1998. Behavior-based robotics. MIT Press.

Ashe, J. 1997. Force and the motor cortex. *Behavioural Brain Research* 87(2):255–269.

Babiloni, C., A. Brancucci, L. Arendt-Nielsen, F. Babiloni, P. Capotosto, F. Carducci, F. Cincotti, L. Romano, A. C. Chen, and P. M. Rossini. 2004. Alpha event-related desynchronization preceding a go/no-go task: a high-resolution eeg study. *Neuropsychology* 18(4):719–728.

Babiloni, F., F. Cincotti, L. Bianchi, G. Pirri, J. d. R. Millán, J. Mouriño, S. Salinari, and M. G. Marciani. 2001. Recognition of imagined hand movements with low resolution surface Laplacian and linear classifiers. *Medical Engineering & Physics* 23(5):323–328.

Babiloni, F., F. Cincotti, L. Lazzarini, J. d. R. Millán, J. Mouriño, M. Varsta, J. Heikkonen, L. Bianchi, and M. G. Marciani. 2000. Linear classification of low-resolution EEG patterns produced by imagined hand movements. *IEEE Transactions on Rehabilitation Engineering* 8:186–188.

Babiloni, C., F. Carducci, F. Cincotti, P. M. Rossini, C. Neuper, G. Pfurtscheller, and F. Babiloni. 1999. Human movement-related potentials vs. desynchronization of EEG alpha rhythm: a high-resolution EEG study. *NeuroImage* 10(6):658–665.

Baillet, S., J. C. Mosher, and R. M. Leahy. 2001. Electromagnetic brain mapping. *IEEE Signal Processing Magazine* 18(6):14–30.

Balbale, U. H., J. E. Huggins, S. L. BeMent, and S. P. Levine. 1999. Multi-channel analysis of human event-related cortical potentials for the development of a direct brain interface. In *Proceedings of the First Joint BMES/EMBS Conference. IEEE Engineering in Medicine and Biology* vol. 1.

Barnett, V. and T. Lewis. 1994. Outliers in statistical data. New York: Wiley, 3rd edition.

Bashashati, A., R. K. Ward, and G. E. Birch. 2005. A new design of the asynchronous brain computer interface using the knowledge of the path of features. In *2nd International IEEE-EMBS Conference on Neural Engineering*. IEEE-EMBS.

Batista, A. P., C. A. Buneo, L. H. Snyder, and R. A. Andersen. 1999. Reach plans in eye-centered coordinates. *Science* 285(5425):257–260.

Bauer, G., F. Gerstenbrand, and E. Rumpl. 1979. Varieties of the locked-in syndrome. *Journal of Neurology* 221(2):77–91.

Bayliss, J. D., S. A. Inverso, and A. Tentler. 2004. Changing the P300 brain computer interface. *Cyberpsychology & Behavior: The Impact of the Internet, Multimedia and Virtual Reality on Behavior and Society* 7(6):694–704.

Bayliss, J. D. 2003. Use of the evoked potential P3 component for control in a virtual apartment. *IEEE Transactions on Neural Systems and Rehabilitation Engineering* 11 (2):113–116.

Bayliss, J. D. and D. H. Ballard. 2000. A virtual reality testbed for brain-computer interface research. *IEEE Transactions on Rehabilitation Engineering* 8(2):188–190.

BCI Competition III. 2005. Available from http://ida.first.fhg.de/projects/bci/competition_iii/results/.

BCI Competition III. 2005a. Data set IIIa of the BCI competition. Available from http://ida.first.fhg.de/projects/bci/competition_iii/results/#graz1.

BCI Competition III. 2005b. Data set IIIb of the BCI competition. Available from http://ida.first.fhg.de/projects/bci/competition_iii/results/#graz2.

Beck, D. M. and N. Lavie. 2005. Look here but ignore what you see: Effects of distractors at fixation. *Journal of Experimental Psychology: Human Perception and Performance* 31(3):592–607.

Bell, A. J. and T. J. Sejnowski. 1995. An information-maximization approach to blind separation and blind deconvolution. *Neural Computation* 7(6):1129–1159.

Belouchrani, A., K. A. Meraim, J.-F. Cardoso, and E. Moulines. 1997. A blind source separation technique based on second order statistics. *IEEE Transactions on Signal Processing* 45(2):434–444.

Benabid, A. L., P. Pollak, C. Gervason, D. Hoffmann, D. M. Gao, M. Hommel, J. E. Perret, and J. de Rougemont. 1991. Long-term suppression of tremor by chronic stimulation of the ventral intermediate thalamic nucleus. *Lancet* 337(8738):403–406.

Bennett, K. P. and O. L. Mangasarian. 1992. Robust linear programming discrimination of two linearly inseparable sets. *Optimization Methods and Software* 1:23–34.

Berger, T. W. and D. L. Glanzman, editors. 2005. Toward replacement parts for the brain: Implantable biomimetic electronics as neural prostheses. Cambridge, Mass.: MIT Press.

Birbaumer, N. 2006a. Breaking the silence: brain-computer interfaces (BCI) for communication and motor control. *Psychophysiology* 43(6):517–532.

Birbaumer, N. 2006b. Brain-computer-interface research: coming of age. *Clinical Neurophysiology* 117(3):479–483.

Birbaumer, N. and R. F. Schmid. 2006. Biologische Psychologie, chapter Methoden der Biologischen Psychologie, 483–511. Berlin: Springer, 6 edition.

Birbaumer, N. 2005. Nur das Denken bleibt. Neuroethik des Eingeschlossen-Seins. In *Neurowissenschaften und Menschenbild*, edited by E. Engels and E. Hildt. Paderborn: Mentis-Verlag.

Birbaumer, N. and L. Cohen. 2005. A brain-computer-interface (BCI) for chronic stroke. In *35th Annual Meeting of the Society for Neuroscience*, Washington, DC.

Birbaumer, N., R. Veit, M. Lotze, M. Erb, C. Hermann, W. Grodd, and H. Flor. 2005. Deficient fear conditioning in psychopathy: a functional magnetic resonance imaging study. *Archives of General Psychiatry* 62(7):799–805.

Birbaumer, N., T. Hinterberger, A. Kübler, and N. Neumann. 2003. The thought translation device (TTD): neurobehavioral mechanisms and clinical outcome. *IEEE Transactions on Neural Systems and Rehabilitation Engineering* 11(2):120–123.

Birbaumer, N., A. Kübler, N. Ghanayim, T. Hinterberger, J. Perelmouter, J. Kaiser, I. Iversen, B. Kotchoubey, N. Neumann, and H. Flor. 2000. The thought translation device (TTD) for completely paralyzed patients. *IEEE Transactions on Rehabilitation Engineering* 8(2):190–193.

Birbaumer, N., N. Ghanayim, T. Hinterberger, I. Iversen, B. Kotchoubey, A. Kübler, J. Perelmouter, E. Taub, and H. Flor. 1999. A spelling device for the paralysed. *Nature* 398:297–298.

Birbaumer, N., T. Elbert, A. G. Canavan, and B. Rockstroh. 1990. Slow potentials of the cerebral cortex and behavior. *Physiological Review* 70(1):1–41.

Birch, G. E., S. G. Mason, and J. F. Borisoff. 2003. Current trends in brain-computer interface research at the Neil Squire Foundation. *IEEE Transactions on Neural Systems and Rehabilitation Engineering* 11(2):123–126.

Birch, G. E., Z. Bozorgzadeh, and S. G. Mason. 2002. Initial on-line evaluations of the LF-ASD brain-computer interface with able-bodied and spinal-cord subjects using imagined voluntary motor potentials. *IEEE Transactions on Neural Systems and Rehabilitation Engineering* 10(4):219–224.

Birch, G. E., J. R. Watzke, and C. Bolduc. 1995. Research and development of adaptive equipment for persons with significant disabilities and the elderly; activities conducted by the Neil Squire Foundation. *Technology and Disability* 4:169–173.

Birch, G. E., P. D. Lawrence, and R. D. Hare. 1993. Single-trial processing of event-related potentials using outlier information. *IEEE Transactions on Biomedical Engineering* 40 (1):59–73.

Bishop, C. M. 1995. Neural networks for pattern recognition. Oxford, UK: Clarendon Press.

Blanchard, G., M. Sugiyama, M. Kawanabe, V. Spokoiny, and K.-R. Müller. 2006. In search of non-Gaussian components of a high-dimensional distribution. *Journal of Machine Learning Research* 7:247–282.

Blanchard, G. and B. Blankertz. 2004. BCI competition 2003 – data set IIa: Spatial patterns of self-controlled brain rhythm modulations. *IEEE Transactions on Biomedical Engineering* 51(6):1062–1066.

Blankertz, Benjamin, Guido Dornhege, Matthias Krauledat, Gabriel Curio, and Klaus-Robert Müller. 2007. The non-invasive Berlin Brain-Computer Interface: Fast acquisition of effective performance in untrained subjects. *Neuroimage*. In press.

Blankertz, B., G. Dornhege, M. Krauledat, K.-R. Müller, V. Kunzmann, F. Losch, and G. Curio. 2006a. The Berlin Brain-Computer Interface: EEG-based communication without subject training. *IEEE Transactions on Neural Systems and Rehabilitation Engineering* 14(2):147–152.

Blankertz, B., G. Dornhege, S. Lemm, M. Krauledat, G. Curio, and K.-R. Müller. 2006b. The Berlin Brain-Computer Interface: Machine learning based detection of user specific brain states. *Journal of Universal Computer Science* 12(6):581–607.

Blankertz, B., K. R. Müller, D. Krusienski, J. R. Wolpaw, A. Schlögl, G. Pfurtscheller, J. d. R. Millán, M. Schröder, and N. Birbaumer. 2006c. The BCI competition III: Validating alternative approaches to actual BCI problems. *IEEE Transactions on Neural Systems and Rehabilitation Engineering* 14(2):153–159.

Blankertz, B. 2005a. BCI Competition III results (Web page). http://ida.first.fhg.de/projects/bci/competition_iii/results/.

Blankertz, B., G. Dornhege, M. Krauledat, K.-R. Müller, and G. Curio. 2005. The Berlin Brain-Computer Interface: report from the feedback sessions. Technical Report 1, Fraunhofer FIRST.

Blankertz, B. 2005b. BCI Competitions. Web page. http://ida.first.fhg.de/projects/bci/competitions/.

Blankertz, B., K. R. Müller, G. Curio, T. M. Vaughan, G. Schalk, J. R. Wolpaw, A. Schlögl, C. Neuper, G. Pfurtscheller, T. Hinterberger, M. Schröder, and N. Birbaumer. 2004. The BCI Competition 2003: progress and perspectives in detection and discrimination of EEG single trials. *IEEE Transactions on Biomedical Engineering* 51(6):1044–1051.

Blankertz, B. 2003. BCI Competition 2003 results (Web page). http://ida.first.fhg.de/projects/bci/competition_ii/results/.

Blankertz, B., G. Dornhege, C. Schäfer, R. Krepki, J. Kohlmorgen, K.-R. Müller, V. Kunzmann, F. Losch, and G. Curio. 2003. Boosting bit rates and error detection for the classification of fast-paced motor commands based on single-trial EEG analysis. *IEEE Transactions on Neural Systems and Rehabilitation Engineering* 11(2):127–131.

Blankertz, B., G. Curio, and K.-R. Müller. 2002. Classifying single trial EEG: towards brain computer interfacing. In *Advances in Neural Information Processing Systems (NIPS 01)*, edited by T. G. Diettrich, S. Becker, and Z. Ghahramani vol. 14: 157–164, Cambridge, Mass. The MIT Press.

Blatt, G. J., R. A. Andersen, and G. R. Stoner. 1990. Visual receptive-field organization and cortico-cortical connections of the lateral intraparietal area (area LIP) in the macaque. *The Journal of Comparative Neurology* 299(4):421–445.

Bock, O., S. Schneider, and J. Bloomberg. 2001. Conditions for interference versus facilitation during sequential sensorimotor adaptation. *Experimental Brain Research* 138(3):359–365.

Borisoff, J. F., S. G. Mason, A. Bashashati, and G. E. Birch. 2004. Brain-computer interface design for asynchronous control applications: improvements to the LF-ASD asynchronous brain switch. *IEEE Transactions on Biomedical Engineering* 51(6):985–992.

Bortz, H. and G. A. Lienert. 1998. Kurzgefasste statistik für die klassische forschung, chapter 6: Übereinstimmungsmaße für subjektive Merkmalsurteile, 265–270. Berlin Heidelberg: Springer.

Boser, B. E., I. M. Guyon, and V. N. Vapnik. 1992. A training algorithm for optimal margin classifiers. In *Proceedings of the 5th Annual ACM Workshop on Computational Learning Theory*, edited by D. Haussler: 144–152.

Brain-Computer Interface Technology: Theory and Practice—First International Meeting Program and Papers. 1999. Wadsworth Center Brain-Computer Interface Project.

Brain-Computer Interface Technology: Third International Meeting. 2005. Rensselaerville, New York. June 14-19.

Branchaud, E., J. G. Cham, Z. Nenadic, R. A. Andersen, and J. W. Burdick. 2005. A miniature robot for autonomous single neuron recordings. In *Proceedings of the 2005 IEEE International Conference on Robotics and Automation* vol. 2: 5352–5355 Vol. 7. IEEE.

Braun, C., M. Staudt, C. Schmitt, H. Preissl, N. Birbaumer, and C. Gerloff. submitted. Crossed cortico-spinal motor control after capsular stroke. *Journal of Neurophysiology*.

Braun, C., R. Schweizer, T. Elbert, N. Birbaumer, and E. Taub. 2000. Differential activation in somatosensory cortex for different discrimination tasks. *Journal of Neuroscience* 20 (1):446–450.

Breiman, L., J. Friedman, J. Olshen, and C. Stone. 1984. Classification and regression trees. Wadsworth.

Britten, K. H., W. T. Newsome, M. N. Shadlen, S. Celebrini, and J. A. Movshon. 1996. A relationship between behavioral choice and visual responses of neurons in macaque MT. *Visual Neuroscience* 13(1):87–100.

Britten, K. H., M. N. Shadlen, W. T. Newsome, and J. A. Movshon. 1992. The analysis of visual motion: a comparison of neuronal and psychophysical performance. *Journal of Neuroscience* 12(12):4745–4765.

Brockwell, A. E., A. L. Rojas, and R. E. Kass. 2004. Recursive Bayesian decoding of motor cortical signals by particle filtering. *Journal of Neurophysiology* 91(4):1899–1907.

Bronstein, M. M., A. M. Bronstein, M. Zibulevsky, and Y. Y. Zeevi. 2005. Blind deconvolution of images using optimal sparse representations. *IEEE Trans Image Process* 14(6):726–736.

Brookings, J. B., G. F. Wilson, and C. R. Swain. 1996. Psychophysiological responses to changes in workload during simulated air traffic control. *Biological Psychology* 42(3): 361–377.

Brunner, C., R. Scherer, B. Graimann, G. Supp, and G. Pfurtscheller. In revision. Online control of a brain-computer interface using phase synchronization. *IEEE Transactions on Biomedical Engineering*.

Brunner, C., B. Graimann, J. E. Huggins, S. P. Levine, and G. Pfurtscheller. 2005. Phase relationships between different subdural electrode recordings in man. *Neuroscience Letters* 375(2):69–74.

Bunce, S. C., M. Izzetoglu, K. Izzetoglu, B. Onaral, and K. Pourrezaei. 2006. Functional near-infrared spectroscopy. *IEEE Engineering in Medicine and Biology Magazine* 25 (4):54–62.

Burges, C. J. C. 1998. A tutorial on support vector machines for pattern recognition. *Data Mining and Knowledge Discovery* 2(2):121–167.

Buttfield, A., P. W. Ferrez, and J. d. R. Millán. 2006. Towards a robust BCI: error recognition and online learning. *IEEE Transactions on Neural Systems and Rehabilitation Engineering* 14(2):164–168.

Cacace, A. T. and D. J. McFarland. 2003. Spectral dynamics of electroencephalographic activity during auditory information processing. *Hearing Research* 176(1–2):25–41.

Caminiti, R., P. B. Johnson, and A. Urbano. 1990. Making arm movements within different parts of space: dynamic aspects in the primary motor cortex. *Journal of Neuroscience* 10(7):2039–2058.

Campbell, C. and K.P. Bennett. 2001. A linear programming approach to novelty detection. In *Advances in Neural Information Processing Systems (NIPS 00)*, edited by T.K. Leen, T.G. Dietterich, and V. Tresp vol. 13: 395–401, Cambridge, Mass. The MIT Press.

Cardoso, J.-F. and A. Souloumiac. 1993. Blind beamforming for non gaussian signals. *IEE Proceedings-F.* 140(46):362–370.

Carmena, J. M., M. A. Lebedev, R. E. Crist, J. E. O'Doherty, D. M. Santucci, D. F. Dimitrov, P. G. Patil, C. S. Henriquez, and M. A. Nicolelis. 2003. Learning to control a brain-machine interface for reaching and grasping by primates. *PLoS Biology* 1(2):E42.

Carter, C. S., T. S. Braver, D. M. Barch, M. M. Botvinick, D. Noll, and J. D. Cohen. 1998. Anterior cingulate cortex, error detection, and the online monitoring of performance. *Science* 280(5364):747–749.

Cham, J. G., E. A. Branchaud, Z. Nenadic, B. Greger, R. A. Andersen, and J. W. Burdick. 2005. Semi-chronic motorized microdrive and control algorithm for autonomously isolating and maintaining optimal extracellular action potentials. *Journal of Neurophysiology* 93(1):570–579.

Chapelle, O., P. Haffner, and V. Vapnik. 1999. Support vector machines for histogram based image classification. *IEEE Transactions on Neural Networks* 10(5):1055–1064.

Chapin, J. K. 2006. Talk presented at IEEE 2006 International Conference of the Engineering in Medicine and Biology Society, New York City, USA.

Chapin, J. K., K. A. Moxon, R. S. Markowitz, and M. A. Nicolelis. 1999. Real-time control of a robot arm using simultaneously recorded neurons in the motor cortex. *Nature Neuroscience* 2(7):664–670.

Chen, W. and S. Ogawa. 2000. Principles of BOLD functional MRI. In *Functional MRI*, edited by C. Moonen and P. Bandettini. Berlin Heidelberg: Springer.

Cheng, M., X. Gao, S. Gao, and D. Xu. 2002. Design and implementation of a brain-computer interface with high transfer rates. *IEEE Transactions on Biomedical Engineering* 49(10):1181–1186.

Cohen, J. and J. Polich. 1997. On the number of trials needed for P300. *International Journal of Psychophysiology* 25(3):249–255.

Cohen, J. 1960. A coefficient of agreement for nominal scales. *Educational and Psychological Measurement* 20:37–46.

Coin3D. High-level 3d graphics toolkit for developing cross-platform real-time 3d visualization and visual simulation software. Available from http://www.coin3d.org.

Collobert, R. and S. Bengio. 2001. SVMTorch: support vector machines for large-scale regression problems. *Journal of Machine Learning Research* 1(2):143–160.

Connolly, J. D., R. A. Andersen, and M. A. Goodale. 2003. FMRI evidence for a "parietal reach region" in the human brain. *Experimental Brain Research* 153(2):140–145.

Cover, T. M. and J. M. Van Campenhout. 1977. On the possible ordering in the measurement selection problem. *IEEE transactions on systems, man, and cybernetics* SMC-7: 657–661.

Cover, T. M. 1969. Learning in pattern recognition. In *Methodologies of Pattern Recognition*, edited by Satoshi Watanabe. New York: Academic Press.

Coyle, S., T. Ward, C. Markham, and G. McDarby. 2004. On the suitability of near-infrared (NIR) systems for next-generation brain-computer interfaces. *Physiological Measurement* 25(4):815–822.

Crammer, K. and Y. Singer. 2001. On the algorithmic implementation of multiclass kernel-based vector machines. *Journal of Machine Learning Research* 2(2):265–292.

Creasey, G. H., C. H. Ho, R. J. Triolo, D. R. Gater, A. F. DiMarco, K. M. Bogie, and M. W. Keith. 2004. Clinical applications of electrical stimulation after spinal cord injury. *The Journal of Spinal Cord Medicine* 27(4):365–375.

Crochiere, R. E. 1980. A weighted overlap-add method of short-time fourier analysis/synthesis. *IEEE Transactions on Acoustics, Speech, & Signal Processing* ASSP-28 (1):99–102.

Cruz-Neira, C., D. J. Sandin, and T. A. DeFanti. 1993. Surround-screen projection-based virtual reality: the design and implementation of the CAVE. In *Proceedings of the 20th annual conference on Computer graphics and interactive techniques*: 135–142.

Cui, R. Q., D. Huter, W. Lang, and L. Deecke. 1999. Neuroimage of voluntary movement: topography of the Bereitschaftspotential, a 64-channel DC current source density study. *Neuroimage* 9(1):124–134.

Cunnigham, H. A. and R. B. Welch. 1994. Multiple concurrent visual-motor mappings: implication for models of adaptation. *Journal of Experimental Psychology. Human Perception and Performance* 20(5):987–999.

Curran, E. A. and M. J. Stokes. 2003. Learning to control brain activity: A review of the production and control of EEG components for driving brain-computer interface (BCI) systems. *Brain and cognition* 51(3):326–336.

Dakin, S. C., R. F. Hess, T. Ledgeway, and R. L. Achtman. 2002. What causes non-monotonic tuning of fMRI response to noisy images? *Current Biology* 12(14):R476–477.

Davidson, R. J., D. Pizzagalli, J. B. Nitschke, and K. Putnam. 2002. Depression: perspectives from affective neuroscience. *Annual Review of Psychology* 53:545–574.

Decety, J., D. Perani, M. Jeannerod, V. Bettinardi, B. Tadary, R. Woods, J. C. Mazziotta, and F. Fazio. 1994. Mapping motor representations with positron emission tomography. *Nature* 371(6498):600–602.

DeCharms, R. C., F. Maeda, G. H. Glover, D. Ludlow, J. M. Pauly, D. Soneji, J. D. Gabrieli, and S. C. Mackey. 2005. Control over brain activation and pain learned by using real-time functional MRI. *Proceedings of the National Academy of Sciences of the United States of America* 102(51):18626–18631.

DeCharms, R. C., K. Christoff, G. H. Glover, J. M. Pauly, S. Whitfield, and J. D. Gabrieli. 2004. Learned regulation of spatially localized brain activation using real-time fMRI. *Neuroimage* 21(1):436–443.

Delorme, A. and S. Makeig. 2004. EEGLAB: an open source toolbox for analysis of single-trial EEG dynamics including independent component analysis. *Journal of Neuroscience Methods* 134(1):9–21.

Delorme, A. and S. Makeig. 2003. EEG changes accompanying learned regulation of 12-Hz EEG activity. *IEEE Transactions on Neural Systems and Rehabilitation Engineering* 11(2):133–137.

Donchin, E., K. M. Spencer, and R. Wijesinghe. 2000. The mental prosthesis: assessing the speed of a P300-based brain-computer interface. *IEEE Transactions on Rehabilitation Engineering* 8(2):174–179.

Donoghue, J. 2002. Connecting cortex to machines: Recent advances in brain interfaces. *Nature Neuroscience* 5:1085–1088.

Dornhege, G. 2006. Increasing information transfer rates for brain-computer interfacing. PhD thesis, University of Potsdam.

Dornhege, G., B. Blankertz, M. Krauledat, F. Losch, G. Curio, and K.-R. Müller. 2006a. Optimizing spatio-temporal filters for improving brain-computer interfacing. In *Advances in Neural Information Processing Systems (NIPS 05)* vol. 18: 315–322, Cambridge, Mass. The MIT Press.

Dornhege, G., B. Blankertz, M. Krauledat, F. Losch, and G. and K. R. Müller. 2006b. Combined optimization of spatial and temporal filters for improving brain-computer interfacing. *IEEE Transactions on Biomedical Engineering* 53(11):2274–2281.

Dornhege, G., B. Blankertz, G. Curio, and K. R. Müller. 2004a. Boosting bit rates in noninvasive EEG single-trial classifications by feature combination and multi-class paradigms. *IEEE Transactions on Biomedical Engineering* 51(6):993–1002.

Dornhege, G., B. Blankertz, G. Curio, and K. R. Müller. 2004b. Increase information transfer rates in BCI by CSP extension to multi-class. In *Advances in Neural Information Processing Systems (NIPS 03)*, edited by S. Thrun, L. Saul, and B. Schölkopf, vol. 16. Cambridge, Mass.: The MIT Press.

Dornhege, G., B. Blankertz, and G. Curio. 2003a. Speeding up classification of multi-channel brain-computer interfaces: common spatial patterns for slow cortical potentials. In *Proceedings of the 1st International IEEE EMBS Conference on Neural Engineering. Capri 2003*: 595–598.

Dornhege, G., B. Blankertz, G. Curio, and K. R. Müller. 2003b. Combining features for BCI. In *Advances in Neural Information Processing Systems (NIPS 02)*, edited by S. Becker, S. Thrun, and K. Obermayer vol. 15: 1115–1122, Cambridge, Mass. The MIT Press.

Drake, K. L., K. D. Wise, J. Farraye, D. J. Anderson, and S. L. BeMent. 1988. Performance of planar multisite microprobes in recording extracellular single-unit intracortical activity. *IEEE Transactions on Biomedical Engineering* 35(9):719–732.

Duda, R. O., P. E. Hart, and D. G. Stork. 2001. Pattern classification. New York: John Wiley and Sons Publishing Company, 2nd edition.

Duncan-Johnson, C. C. and E. Donchin. 1977. On quantifying surprise: the variation of event-related potentials with subjective probability. *Psychophysiology* 14(5):456–467.

Duque, J., F. Hummel, P. Celnik, N. Murase, R. Mazzocchio, and L. G. Cohen. 2005. Transcallosal inhibition in chronic subcortical stroke. *Neuroimage* 28(4):940–946.

Dworkin, B. R. and N. E. Miller. 1986. Failure to replicate visceral learning in the acute curarized rat preparation. *Behavioral Neuroscience* 100(3):299–314.

Eaton, J. W. Octave. Available at http://www.octave.org/.

Eckmiller, R. 1997. Learning retina implants with epiretinal contacts. *Ophthalmic research* 29(5):281–289.

Edell, D. J., V. V. Toi, V. M. McNeil, and L. D. Clark. 1992. Factors influencing the biocompatibility of insertable silicon microshafts in cerebral cortex. *IEEE Transactions on Biomedical Engineering* 39(6):635–643.

Eichhorn, J., A. Tolias, A. Zien, M. Kuss, C. E. Rasmussen, J. Weston, N. Logothetis, and B. Schölkopf. 2004. Prediction on spike data using kernel algorithms. In *Advances in Neural Information Processing Systems (NIPS 03)*, edited by S. Thrun, L. Saul, and B. Schölkopf vol. 16, Cambridge, MA. The MIT Press.

Elbert, T., B. Rockstroh, W. Lutzenberger, and N. Birbaumer. 1980. Biofeedback of slow cortical potentials. I. *Electroencephalography and Clinical Neurophysiology* 48(3):293–301.

EMEGS. Electromagnetic encaphalography software. Available at http://134.34.43.26/emegs/modules/news/.

Evarts, E. V. 1968. Relation of pyramidal tract activity to force exerted during voluntary movement. *Journal of Neurophysiology* 31(1):14–27.

Fabiani, G. E., D. J. McFarland, J. R. Wolpaw, and G. Pfurtscheller. 2004. Conversion of EEG activity into cursor movement by a brain computer interface (BCI). *IEEE Transactions on Neural Systems and Rehabilitation Engineering* 12(3):331–338.

Fabiani, M., G. Gratton, D. Karis, and E. Donchin. 1987. Definition, identification, and reliability of measurement of the P300 component of the event-related brain potential. *Advances in Psychophysiology* 2:1–78.

Falkenstein, M., J. Hoormann, S. Christ, and J. Hohnsbein. 2000. ERP components on reaction errors and their functional significance: a tutorial. *Biological Psychology* 51 (2–3):87–107.

Farwell, L. A. and E. Donchin. 1988. Talking off the top of your head: toward a mental prosthesis utilizing event-related brain potentials. *Electroencephalography and Clinical Neurophysiology* 70(6):510–523.

Felton, E. A., J. A. Wilson, R. G. Radwin, J. C. Williams, and P. C. Garell. 2005. Electrocorticogram-controlled brain-computer interfaces with patients with temporary subdural electrode implants. *Neurosurgery* 57(2).

Ferrez, P. W. and J. d. R. Millán. 2005. You are wrong!—Automatic detection of interaction errors from brain waves. In *19th International Joint Conference on Artificial Intelligence*.

FES. The cleveland functional electrical stimulation center. Available at http://fescenter.case.edu.

Fessler, J. A., S. Y. Chun, J. E. Huggins, and S. P. Levine. 2005. Detection of event-related spectral changes in electrocorticograms. In *Proceedings IEEE EMBS Conference on Neural Engineering*: 269–272.

FieldTrip. Available at http://www2.ru.nl/fcdonders/fieldtrip/1020.html.

Fisher, R. A. 1936. The use of multiple measurements in taxonomic problems. *Annals of Eugenics* 7:179–188.

Flach, P. A. 2004. The many faces of ROC analysis in machine learning. Tutorial presented at the 21st International Conference on Machine Learning. Available from http://www.cs.bris.ac.uk/~flach/ICML04tutorial/.

Flament, D. and J. Hore. 1988. Relations of motor cortex neural discharge to kinematics of passive and active elbow movements in the monkey. *Journal of Neurophysiology* 60 (4):1268–1284.

Fleiss, J. L. 1981. Statistical methods for rates and proportions. New York: John Wiley and Sons Publishing Company, 2nd edition.

Flotzinger, D., G. Pfurtscheller, C. Neuper, J. Berger, and W. Mohl. 1994. Classification of non-averaged EEG data by learning vector quantisation and the influence of signal preprocessing. *Medical & Biological Engineering & Computing* 32(5):571–576.

Foffani, G., A. M. Bianchi, A. Priori, and G. Baselli. 2004. Adaptive autoregressive identification with spectral power decomposition for studying movement-related activity in scalp EEG signals and basal ganglia local field potentials. *Journal of Neural Engineering* 1(3):165–173.

Franceschini, M. A., S. Fantini, J. H. Thompson, J. P. Culver, and D. A. Boas. 2003. Hemodynamic evoked response of the sensorimotor cortex measured noninvasively with near-infrared optical imaging. *Psychophysiology* 40(4):548–560.

Frecon, E., G. Smith, A. Steed, M. Stenius, and O. Stahl. 2001. An overview of the COVEN platform. *Presence-Teleoperators and Virtual Environments* 10(1):109–127.

Friedman, J. H. 1991. Multivariate adaptive regression splines. *Annals of Statistics* 19(1): 1–141.

Friedman, J. H. 1989. Regularized discriminant analysis. *Journal of the American Statistical Association* 84(405):165–175.

Friedman, J. H. 1988. Fitting functions to noisy data in high dimensions. In *Computing Science and Statistics: Proceedings of the 20th Symposium on the Interface*, edited by E. Wegman, D. Gantz, and J. Miller: 13–43, Alexandria, Va. American Statistical Association.

Fu, Q. G., D. Flament, J. D. Coltz, and T. J. Ebner. 1995. Temporal coding of movement kinematics in the discharge of primate primary motor and premotor neurons. *Journal of Neurophysiology* 73(2):836–854.

Fukunaga, K. 1990. Inroduction to statistical pattern recognition. San Diego: Academic Press, 2nd edition.

Gandolfo, F., C. S. R. Li, B. J. Benda, C. P. Schioppa, and E. Bizzi. 2000. Cortical correlates of learning in monkeys adapting to a new dynamical environment. *Proceedings of the National Academy of Sciences of the United States of America* 97(5):2259–2263.

Gao, Y., M. J. Black, E. Bienenstock, W. Wu, and J. P. Donoghue. 2003a. A quantitative comparison of linear and non-linear models of motor cortical activity for the encoding and decoding of arm motions. In *First International IEEE EMBS Conference on Neural Engineering*: 189–192.

Gao, X., D. Xu, M. Cheng, and S. Gao. 2003b. A BCI-based environmental controller for the motion-disabled. *IEEE Transactions on Neural Systems and Rehabilitation Engineering* 11(2):137–140.

Gao, Y., M. J. Black, E. Bienenstock, S. Shoham, and J. P. Donoghue. 2002. Probabilistic inference of hand motion from neural activity in motor cortex. In *Advances in Neural Information Processing Systems (NIPS 01)*, edited by T. G. Dietterich, S. Becker, and Z. Ghahramani vol. 14: 213–220, Cambridge, Mass. The MIT Press.

Garrett, D., D. A. Peterson, C. W. Anderson, and M. H. Thaut. 2003. Comparison of linear, nonlinear, and feature selection methods for EEG signal classification. *IEEE Transactions on Neural Systems and Rehabilitation Engineering* 11(2):141–144.

Gehring, W., M. Coles, D. Meyer, and E. Donchin. 1990. The error-related negativity: An event-related brain potential accompanying errors. *Psychophysiology* 27:34.

Georgopoulos, A. P., R. E. Kettner, and A. B. Schwartz. 1988. Primate motor cortex and free arm movements to visual targets in three-dimensional space. II. Coding of the direction of movement by a neuronal population. *Journal of Neuroscience* 8(8):2928–2937.

Georgopoulos, A. P., A. B. Schwartz, and R. E. Kettner. 1986. Neural population coding of movement direction. *Science* 233(4771):1416–1419.

Georgopoulos, A. P., J. F. Kalaska, and J. T. Massey. 1983. Spatial coding of movements: A hypothesis concerning the coding of movement direction by motor cortical populations. *Experimental Brain Research* 7:327–336.

Georgopoulos, A. P., J. F. Kalaska, R. Caminiti, and J. T. Massey. 1982. On the relations between the direction of two-dimensional arm movements and cell discharge in primate motor cortex. *Journal of Neuroscience* 2(11):1527–1537.

Gerson, A. D., L. C. Parra, and P. Sajda. 2005. Cortical origins of response time variability during rapid discrimination of visual objects. *Neuroimage* 28(2):342–353.

Gevins, A., M. E. Smith, H. Leong, L. McEvoy, S. Whitfield, R. Du, and G. Rush. 1998. Monitoring working memory load during computer-based tasks with EEG pattern recognition methods. *Human Factors* 40(1):79–91.

Gevins, A., M. E. Smith, L. McEvoy, and D. Yu. 1997. High-resolution EEG mapping of cortical activation related to working memory: effects of task difficulty, type of processing, and practice. *Cerebral Cortex* 7(4):374–385.

Girone, M., G. Burdea, M. Bouzit, V. Popescu, and J. E. Deutsch. 2000. Orthopedic rehabilitation using the "Rutgers ankle" interface. *Studies in Health Technology and Informatics* 70:89–95.

glib. GTK+ team: *General-purpose utility library*. Available at http://www.gtk.org.

Goncharova, I. I., D. J. McFarland, T. M. Vaughan, and J. R. Wolpaw. 2003. EMG contamination of EEG: spectral and topographical characteristics. *Clinical Neurophysiology* 114(9):1580–1593.

Gonsalvez, C. L. and J. Polich. 2002. P300 amplitude is determined by target-to-target interval. *Psychophysiology* 39(3):388–396.

GPL. Free Software Foundation: *The GNU General Public License*. Available at http://www.gnu.org/licenses/licenses.html.

Graimann, B., G. Townsend, J. E. Huggins, A. Schlögl, S. P. Levine, and G. Pfurtscheller. 2005. A comparison between using ECoG and EEG for direct brain communication. In *Proceedings of the EMBEC05*.

Graimann, B., J. E. Huggins, S. P. Levine, and G. Pfurtscheller. 2004. Towards a direct brain interface based on human subdural recordings and wavelet-packet analysis. *IEEE Transactions on Biomedical Engineering* 51(6):954–962.

Graimann, B., J. E. Huggins, A. Schlögl, S. P. Levine, and G. Pfurtscheller. 2003. Detection of movement-related desynchronization patterns in ongoing single-channel electrocorticogram. *IEEE Transactions on Neural Systems and Rehabilitation Engineering* 11(3): 276–281.

Graimann, B., J. E. Huggins, S. P. Levine, and G. Pfurtscheller. 2002. Visualization of significant ERD/ERS patterns in multichannel EEG and ECoG data. *Clinical Neurophysiology* 113(1):43–47.

Grave de Peralta Menendez, R., S. Gonzalez Andino, A. Khateb, A. Pegna, G. Thut, and T. Landis. 2005a. About the information content of local field potentials noninvasively estimated from the EEG. In *16th Meeting of the International Society for Brain Electromagnetic Topography*.

Grave de Peralta Menendez, R., S. Gonzalez Andino, L. Perez, P. W. Ferrez, and J. d. R. Millán. 2005b. Non-invasive estimation of local field potentials for neuroprosthesis control. *Cognitive Processing* 6:59–64.

Grave de Peralta Menendez, R., M. M. Murray, C. M. Michel, R. Martuzzi, and S. L. Gonzalez Andino. 2004. Electrical neuroimaging based on biophysical constraints. *Neuroimage* 21(2):527–539.

Grave de Peralta Menendez, R., S. L. Gonzalez Andino, S. Morand, C. M. Michel, and T. Landis. 2000. Imaging the electrical activity of the brain: ELECTRA. *Human Brain Mapping* 9(1):1–12.

Grave de Peralta Menendez, R. and S. L. Gonzalez Andino. 1998. A critical analysis of linear inverse solutions to the neuroelectromagnetic inverse problem. *IEEE Transactions on Biomedical Engineering* 45(4):440–448.

Green, D. M. and J. A. Swets. 1966. Signal detection theory and psychophysics. New York: Wiley.

Gruzelier, J. and T. Egner. 2005. Critical validation studies of neurofeedback. *Child and Adolescent Psychiatric Clinics of North America* 14(1):83–104.

g.tec. g.tec Guger Technologies. Available at http.//www.gtec.at.

GTK. GTK+ team: *The GIMP Toolkit*. Available at http://www.gtk.org.

Guger, C., G. Edlinger, W. Harkam, I. Niedermayer, and G. Pfurtscheller. 2003. How many people are able to operate an EEG-based brain-computer interface (BCI)? *IEEE Transactions on Neural Systems and Rehabilitation Engineering* 11(2):145–147.

Guger, C., A. Schlögl, C. Neuper, D. Walterspacher, T. Strein, and G. Pfurtscheller. 2001. Rapid prototyping of an EEG-based brain-computer interface (BCI). *IEEE Transactions on Neural Systems and Rehabilitation Engineering* 9(1):49–58.

Guger, C., H. Ramoser, and G. Pfurtscheller. 2000. Real-time EEG analysis with subject-specific spatial patterns for a brain computer interface (BCI). *IEEE Transactions on Rehabilitation Engineering* 8(4):447–456.

Guger, C., W. Harkam, C. Hertnaes, and G. Pfurtscheller. 1999. Prosthetic control by an EEG-based brain-computer interface (BCI). In *Proceedings if the 5th European Conference for the Advancement of Assistive Technology (AAATE)*, Düsseldorf, Germany.

Guyon, I., S. Gunn, M. Nikravesh, and L. Zadeh, editors. 2006a. Feature extraction, foundations and applications, chapter Filter Methods. Springer.

Guyon, I., S. Gunn, M. Nikravesh, and L. A. Zadeh, editors. 2006b. Feature extraction: Foundations and applications. Springer.

Guyon, I., J. Weston, S. Barnhill, and V. Vapnik. 2002. Gene selection for cancer classification using support vector machines. *Machine Learning* 46(1–3):389–422.

Gysels, E. and P. Celka. 2004. Phase synchronization for the recognition of mental tasks in a brain computer interface. *IEEE Transactions on Neural Systems and Rehabilitation Engineering* 12(4):406–415.

Halgren, E., T. Raij, K. Marinkovic, V. Jousmaki, and R. Hari. 2000. Cognitive response profile of the human fusiform face area as determined by MEG. *Cerebral Cortex* 10(1): 69–81.

Hamalainen, M. S. and R. J. Ilmoniemi. 1994. Interpreting magnetic fields of the brain: minimum norm estimates. *Medical & Biological Engineering & Computing* 32(1):35–42.

Hampel, F. R., E. M. Rochetti, P. J. Rousseeuw, and W. A. Stahel. 1986. Robust statistics. New York: Wiley.

Hanagasi, H. A., I. H. Gurvit, N. Ermutlu, G. Kaptanoglu, S. Karamursel, H. A. Idrisoglu, M. Emre, and T. Demiralp. 2002. Cognitive impairment in amyotrophic lateral sclerosis: evidence from neuropsychological investigation and event-related potentials. *Brain Research. Cognitive Brain Research* 14(2):234–244.

Hancock, K. M., A. R. Craig, H. G. Dickson, E. Chang, and J. Martin. 1993. Anxiety and depression over the first year of spinal cord injury: a longitudinal study. *Paraplegia* 31 (6):349–357.

Hankins, T. C. and G. F. Wilson. 1998. A comparison of heart rate, eye activity, EEG and subjective measures of pilot mental workload during flight. *Aviation, Space, and Environmental Medicine* 69(4):360–367.

Harland, C. J., T. D. Clark, and R. J. Prance. 2002. Remote detection of human eleectroencephalograms using ultrahigh input impedance electric potential sensors. *Applied Physics Letters* 81(17):3284–3286.

Harmeling, S., G. Dornhege, D. Tax, F. Meinecke, and K. R. Müller. 2006. From outliers to prototypes: ordering data. *Neurocomputing* 69(13–15).

Harmeling, S. 2005. Independent component analysis and beyond. PhD thesis, University of Potsdam, Potsdam.

Harmeling, S., A. Ziehe, M. Kawanabe, and K.-R. Müller. 2003. Kernel-based nonlinear blind source separation. *Neural Computation* 15:1089–1124.

Harmeling, S., A. Ziehe, M. Kawanabe, and K.-R. Müller. 2002. Kernel feature spaces and nonlinear blind source separation. In *Advances in Neural Information Processing Systems (NIPS 01)*, edited by T.G. Dietterich, S. Becker, and Z. Ghahramani vol. 14, Cambridge, Mass. The MIT Press.

Harris, F. J. 1978. On the Use of Windows for Harmonic Analysis with Discrete Fourier Transform. *Proceedings of the IEEE* 66:51–83.

Hasson, U., I. Levy, M. Behrmann, T. Hendler, and R. Malach. 2002. Eccentricity bias as an organization principle for human high-order object areas. *Neuron* 34(3):479–490.

Hastie, T., R. Tibshirani, and J. Friedman. 2001. The elements of statistical learning: data mining, inference, and prediction. New York: Springer-Verlag.

Hauser, A., P. E. Sottas, and J. d. R. Millán. 2002. Temporal processing of brain activity for the recognition of EEG patterns. In *Proceedings 12th International Conference on Artificial Neural Networks*.

Haynes, J. D. and G. Rees. 2006. Decoding mental states from brain activity in humans. *Nature Reviews Neuroscience* 7(7):523–534.

He, B., J. Lian, K. M. Spencer, J. Dien, and E. Donchin. 2001. A cortical potential imaging analysis of the P300 and novelty P3 components. *Human Brain Mapping* 12(2):120–130.

Heekeren, H. R., S. Marrett, P. A. Bandettini, and L. G. Ungerleider. 2004. A general mechanism for perceptual decision-making in human brain. *Nature* 431(7010):859–862.

Hellman, M. E. and J. Raviv. 1970. Probability of error, equivocation, and the Chernoff bound. *IEEE Transactions on Information Theory* IT-16(4):368–372.

Hernandez, A., A. Zainos, and R. Romo. 2000. Neuronal correlates of sensory discrimination in the somatosensory cortex. *Proceedings of the National Academy of Sciences of the United States of America* 97(11):6191–6196.

Hettich, S., C. L. Blake, and C. J. Merz. 1998. UCI repository of machine learning databases. http://www.ics.uci.edu/~mlearn/MLRepository.html. University of California, Irvine, Department of Information and Computer Sciences.

Hill, N. J., T. N. Lal, M. Schröder M, T. Hinterberger, B. Wilhelm, F. Nijboer, U. Mochty, G. Widman, C. Elger, B.Schölkopf, A. Kübler, and N. Birbaumer. 2006. Classifying EEG and ECoG signals without subject training for fast BCI implementation: comparison of nonparalyzed and completely paralyzed subjects. *IEEE Transactions on Neural Systems and Rehabilitation Engineering* 14(2):183–186.

Hill, N. J., T. N. Lal, K. Bierig, N. Birbaumer, and B. Schölkopf. 2005. An auditory paradigm for brain–computer interfaces. In *Advances in Neural Information Processing Systems 17*, edited by L. K. Saul, Y. Weiss, and L. Bottou: 569–576, Cambridge, Mass., USA. The MIT Press.

Hinterberger, T., N. Birbaumer, and H. Flor. 2005a. Assessment of cognitive function and communication ability in a completely locked-in patient. *Neurology* 64(7):1307–1308.

Hinterberger, T., R. Veit, B. Wilhelm, N. Weiskopf, J. J. Vatine, and N. Birbaumer. 2005b. Neural mechanisms underlying control of a brain-computer-interface. *The European Journal of Neuroscience* 21(11):3169–3181.

Hinterberger, T., B. Wilhelm, J. Mellinger, B. Kotchoubey, and N. Birbaumer. 2005c. A device for the detection of cognitive brain functions in completely paralyzed or unresponsive patients. *IEEE Transactions on Biomedical Engineering* 52(2):211–220.

Hinterberger, T., N. Neumann, M. Pham, A. Kübler, A. Grether, N. Hofmayer, B. Wilhelm, H. Flor, and N. Birbaumer. 2004a. A multimodal brain-based feedback and communication system. *Experimental Brain Research* 154(4):521–526.

Hinterberger, T., S. Schmidt, N. Neumann, J. Mellinger, B. Blankertz, G. Curio, and N. Birbaumer. 2004b. Brain-computer communication and slow cortical potentials. *IEEE Transactions on Biomedical Engineering* 51(6):1011–1018.

Hinterberger, T., N. Weiskopf, R. Veit, B. Wilhelm, E. Betta, and N. Birbaumer. 2004c. An EEG-driven brain-computer interface combined with functional magnetic resonance imaging MRI. *IEEE Transactions on Biomedical Engineering* 51(6):971–974.

Hinterberger, T., A. Kübler, J. Kaiser, N. Neumann, and N. Birbaumer. 2003a. A brain-computer interface (BCI) for the locked-in: comparison of different EEG classifications for the thought translation device. *Clinical Neurophysiology* 114(3):416–425.

Hinterberger, T., J. Mellinger, and N. Birbaumer. 2003b. The Thought Translation Device: Structure of a multimodal brain-computer communication system. In *Proceedings of the 1st International IEEE EMBS Conference on Neural Engineering*: 603–606, Capri Island, Italy.

Hinterberger, T., R. Veit, U. Strehl, T. Trevorrow, M. Erb, B. Kotchoubey, H. Flor, and N. Birbaumer. 2003c. Brain areas activated in fMRI during self-regulation of slow cortical potentials (SCPs). *Experimental Brain Research* 152(1):113–122.

Hinterberger, T., J. Kaiser, A. Kübler, N. Neumann, and N. Birbaumer. 2001. The Thought Translation Device and its applications to the completely paralyzed. In *Sciences of the Interfaces*, edited by H. Diebner, T. Druckrey, and P. Weibel. Genista-Verlag Tübingen.

Hjorth, B. 1970. EEG analysis based on time domain properties. *Electroencephalography and Clinical Neurophysiology* 29(3):306–310.

Hochberg, L. R., M. D. Serruya, G. M. Friehs, J. A. Mukand, M. Saleh, A. H. Caplan, A. Branner, D. Chen, R. D. Penn, and J. P. Donoghue. 2006. Neuronal ensemble control of prosthetic devices by a human with tetraplegia. *Nature* 442(7099):164–171.

Hoel, P., S. Port, and C. Stone. 1971. Introduction to statistical theory. Boston: Houghton Mifflin.

Holden, M. K. 2005. Virtual environments for motor rehabilitation: review. *Cyberpsychology & Behavior: the Impact of the Internet, Multimedia and Virtual Reality on Behavior and Society* 8(3):187–211. discussion 212–219.

Holroyd, C. B. and M. G. Coles. 2002. The neural basis of human error processing: reinforcement learning, dopamine, and the error-related negativity. *Psychological Review* 109(4):679–709.

Howard, M. W., D. S. Rizzuto, J. B. Caplan, J. R. Madsen, J. Lisman, R. Aschenbrenner-Scheibe, A. Schulze-Bonhage, and M. J. Kahana. 2003. Gamma oscillations correlate with working memory load in humans. *Cerebral Cortex* 13(12):1369–1374.

Huan, N.-J. and R. Palaniappan. 2004. Neural network classification of autoregressive features from electroencephalogram signals for brain computer interface design. *Journal of Neural Engineering* 1(3):142–150.

Huber, H. 2005. Der Einsatz virtueller Realitäten in der psychologischen Behandlung [the use of virtual realties in psychological threatment]. *Psychologie in Österreich* 25(1): 13–200.

Huber, P. J. 1981. Robust statistics. New York: John Wiley and Sons.

Huggins, J. E., S. P. Levine, S. L. BeMent, R. K. Kushwaha, L. A. Schuh, E. A. Passaro, M. M. Rohde, D. A. Ross, K. V. Elisevich, and B. J. Smith. 1999. Detection of event-related potentials for development of a direct brain interface. *Journal of Clinical Neurophysiology* 16(5):448–455.

Hundley, D. R., M. J. Kirby, and M. Anderle. 2002. Blind source separation using the maximum signal fraction approach. *Signal Processing* 82(10):1505–1508.

Hwang, E. J., O. Donchin, M. A. Smith, and R. Shadmehr. 2003. A gain-field encoding of limb position and velocity in the internal model of arm dynamics. *Public Library of Science: Biology* 1(2):E25.

Hyvarinen, A., J. Karhunen, and E. Oja. 2001. Independent component analysis. New York: Wiley.

Hyvärinen, A. 1999. Survey on independent component analysis. *Neural Computing Surveys* 2:94–128.

IEEE754. Ieee standard for binary floating-point arithmetic (ansi/ieee std 754-1985). It is also known as IEC 60559:1989, Binary floating-point arithmetic for microprocessor systems (originally the reference number was IEC 559:1989).

Ilmoniemi, R. J. 1993. Models of source currents in the brain. *Brain Topography* 5(4): 331–336.

Isaacs, R. E., D. J. Weber, and A. B. Schwartz. 2000. Work toward real-time control of a cortical neural prothesis. *IEEE Transactions on Rehabilitation Engineering* 8(2): 196–198.

Jack, D., R. Boian, A. S. Merians, M. Tremaine, G. C. Burdea, S. V. Adamovich, M. Recce, and H. Poizner. 2001. Virtual reality-enhanced stroke rehabilitation. *IEEE Transactions on Neural Systems and Rehabilitation Engineering* 9(3):308–318.

Jacob, R. J. K. 1990. What you look at is what you get: eye movement-based interaction techniques. In *Proceedings CHI'90*: 11–18.

James, W. 1983. The principles of psychology. New York: Holt. reprint: Cambridge, Mass.: Harvard University Press.

Jasper, H. H. 1958. Report of the committee on methods of clinical investigation of EEG. Appendix: The ten twenty electrode system of the international federation. *Electroencephalography and Clinical Neurophysiology* 10:371–375.

Jeannerod, M. and V. Frak. 1999. Mental imaging of motor activity in humans. *Current Opinion in Neurobiolology* 9(6):735–739.

Jeffreys, D. A. 1996. Evoked studies of face and object processing. *Visual Cognition* 3(1): 1–38.

Joachims, T. 1998. Text categorization with support vector machines: Learning with many relevant features. In *Proceedings of the European Conference on Machine Learning*, edited by Claire Nédellec and Céline Rouveirol: 137–142, Berlin. Springer.

Johnson, J. S. and B. A. Olshausen. 2003. Timecourse of neural signatures of object recognition. *Journal of Vision* 3(7):499–512.

Johnson, P. B., S. Ferraina, L. Bianchi, and R. Caminiti. 1996. Cortical networks for visual reaching: physiological and anatomical organization of frontal and parietal lobe arm regions. *Cerebral Cortex* 6(2):102–119.

Johnson, R. Jr. and E. Donchin. 1978. On how P300 amplitude varies with the utility of the eliciting stimuli. *Electroencephalography and Clinical Neurophysiology* 44(4): 424–437.

Jolliffe, I. T. 1986. Principal component analysis. New York: Springer Verlag.

Jurkiewicz, M. T., A. P. Crawley, M. C. Verrier, M. G. Fehlings, and D. J. Mikulis. 2006. Somatosensory cortical atrophy after spinal cord injury: a voxel-based morphometry study. *Neurology* 66(5):762–764.

Jutten, C. and J. Herault. 1991. Blind separation of sources, part I: An adaptive algorithm based on neuromimetic architecture. *Signal Processing* 24(1):1–10.

Kagerer, F. A., J. L. Contreras-Vidal, and G. E. Stelmach. 1997. Adaptation to gradual as compared with sudden visuo-motor distortions. *Experimental Brain Research* 115(3): 557–561.

Kaiser, J., J. Perelmouter, I. H. Iversen, N. Neumann, N. Ghanayim, T. Hinterberger, A. Kübler, B. Kotchoubey, and N. Birbaumer. 2001. Self-initiation of EEG-based communication in paralyzed patients. *Clinical Neurophysiology* 112(3):551–554.

Kalcher, J., D. Flotzinger, C. Neuper, S. Gölly, and G. Pfurtscheller. 1996. Graz brain-computer interface II: towards communication between man and computer based on on-line classification of three different EEG patterns. *Medical & Biological Engineering & Computing* 34(5):382–388.

Kalman, R. E. 1960. A new approach to linear filtering and prediction problems. *Trans. ASME, Journal of Basic Engineering* 82:35–45.

Kamitani, Y. and F. Tong. 2005. Decoding the visual and subjective contents of the human brain. *Nature Neuroscience* 8(5):679–685.

Kammer, T., L. Lehr, and K. Kirschfeld. 1999. Cortical visual processing is temporally dispersed by luminance in human subjects. *Neuroscience Letters* 263(2–3):133–136.

Kaper, M., A. Saalbach, A. Finke, H. M. Mueller, S. Weiss, and H. Ritter. 2005. Exploratory data analysis of EEG coherence using self-organizing maps. In *Proceedings of the International Conference on Neural Information Processing (ICONIP)*.

Kaper, M., P. Meinicke, U. Grossekathoefer, T. Lingner, and H. Ritter. 2004. BCI Competition 2003–Data set IIb: support vector machines for the P300 speller paradigm. *IEEE Transactions on Biomedical Engineering* 51(6):1073–1076.

Karim, A. A., T. Hinterberger, J. Richter, J. Mellinger, N. Neumann, A. Kübler, M. Bensch, M. Schröder, H. Flor, and N. Birbaumer. 2006. Neural internet: Web surfing with brain potentials for the completely paralysed. *Neurorehabilitation and Neural Repair* 20(4): 508–515.

Kassubek, J., A. Unrath, H. J. Huppertz, D. Lule, T. Ethofer, A. D. Sperfeld, and A. C. Ludolph. 2005. Global brain atrophy and corticospinal tract alterations in ALS, as investigated by voxel-based morphometry of 3-D MRI. *Amyotrophic Lateral Sclerosis and other Motor Neuron Disorders* 6(4):213–220.

Katz, R. T., A. J. Haig, B. B. Clark, and R. J. DiPaola. 1992. Long-term survival, prognosis, and life-care planning for 29 patients with chronic locked-in syndrome. *Archives of Physical Medicine and Rehabilitation* 73(5):403–408.

Kauhanen, K., T. Nykopp, J. Lehtonen, P. Jylanki, J. Heikkonen, P. Rantanen, H. Alaranta, and M. Sams. 2006. EEG and MEG brain-computer interface for tetraplegic patients. *IEEE Transactions on Neural Systems and Rehabilitation Engineering* 14(2):190–193.

Kauhanen, L., P. Rantanen, J. A. Lehtonen, I. Tarnanen, H. Alaranta, and M. Sams. 2004. Sensorimotor cortical activity of tetraplegics during attempted finger movements. *Biomedizinische Technik* 49(1):59–60.

Kay, S. M. 1988. Modern spectral estimation. New York: Prentice-Hall.

Keirn, Z. A. and J. I. Aunon. 1990. A new mode of communication between man and his surroundings. *IEEE Transactions on Biomedical Engineering* 37(12):1209–1214.

Keith, M. W., P. H. Peckham, G. B. Thrope, K. C. Stroh, B. Smith, J. R. Buckett, K. L. Kilgore, and J. W. Jatich. 1989. Implantable functional neuromuscular stimulation in the tetraplegic hand. *The Journal of Hand Surgery* 14(3):524–530.

Kelly, S. P., E. C. Lalor, R. B. Reilly, and J. J. Foxe. 2005. Visual spatial attention tracking using high-density SSVEP data for independent brain-computer communication. *IEEE Transactions on Neural Systems and Rehabilitation Engineering* 13(2):172–178.

Kennedy, P. R., M. T. Kirby, M. M. Moore, B. King, and A. Mallory. 2004. Computer control using human intracortical local field potentials. *IEEE Transactions on Neural Systems and Rehabilitation Engineering* 12(3):339–344.

Kennedy, P. R., R. A. Bakay, M. M. Moore, K. Adams, and J. Goldwaithe. 2000. Direct control of a computer from the human central nervous system. *IEEE Transactions on Rehabilitation Engineering* 8(2):198–202.

Kennedy, P. R. and R. A. Bakay. 1998. Restoration of neural output from a paralyzed patient by a direct brain connection. *Neuroreport* 9(8):1707–1711.

Kettner, R. E., A. B. Schwartz, and A. P. Georgopoulos. 1988. Primate motor cortex and free arm movements to visual targets in three-dimensional space. III. Positional gradients and population coding of movement direction from various movement origins. *Journal of Neuroscience* 8(8):2938–2947.

Kew, J. J., P. N. Leigh, E. D. Playford, R. E. Passingham, L. H. Goldstein, R. S. Frackowiak, and D. J. Brooks. 1993. Cortical function in amyotrophic lateral sclerosis. A positron emission tomography study. *Brain* 116(3):655–680.

Keysers, C., D.-K. Xiao, P. Foldiak, and D. I. Perrett. 2001. The speed of sight. *Journal of Cognitive Neuroscience* 13(1):90–101.

Kilgore, K. L. and R. F. Kirsch. 2004. Upper and lower extremity motor prosthesis. In *Neuroprosthetics Theory and Practice*, edited by K. W. Horch and G. S. Dhillon. New York: World Scientific Publishing Co.

Kim, S-.P., J. C. Sanchez, Y. N. Rao, D. Erdogmus, J. M. Carmena, M. A. Lebedev, M. A. L. Nicolelis, and J. C. Principe. 2006. A comparison of optimal MIMO linear and nonlinear models for brain-machine interfaces. *Journal of Neural Engineering* 3(2): 145–161.

Kim, J. N. and M. N. Shadlen. 1999. Neural correlates of decision making in the dorsolateral prefrontal cortex of the macaque. *Nature Neuroscience* 2(2):176–185.

Kipke, D. R., R. J. Vetter, J. C. Williams, and J. F. Hetke. 2003. Silicon-substrate intracortical microelectrode arrays for long-term recording of neuronal spike activity in cerebral cortex. *IEEE Transactions on Neural Systems and Rehabilitation Engineering* 11(2):151–155.

Kira, K. and L. A. Rendell. 1992. The feature selection problem: traditional methods and a new algorithm. In *10th National Conference on Artificial Intelligence*: 129–134.

Kirby, M. and C. Anderson. 2003. Geometric analysis for the characterization of nonstationary time-series. In *Springer Applied Mathematical Sciences Series Celebratory Volume for the Occasion of the 70th Birthday of Larry Sirovich*, edited by E. Kaplan, J. Marsden, and K. R. Katepalli Sreenivasan. Springer-Verlag.

Kirby, M., F. Weisser, and G. Dangelmayr. 1993. A model problem in the representation of digital image sequences. *Pattern Recognition* 26(1):63–73.

Kittler, J. 1978. Feature set search algorithms. In *Pattern Recognition and Signal Processing*, edited by C. H. Chen. Alphen aan den Rijn, The Netherlands: Sijthoff and Noordhoff, 2nd edition.

Kivinen, J. and M. K. Warmuth. 1995. Additive versus exponentiated gradient updates for linear prediction. In *Proceedings 27th Annual ACM Symposium Theory Computing*: 209–218.

Klassen, J., C. Tong, and J. R. Flanagan. 2005. Learning and recall of incremental kinematic and dynamic sensorimotor transformations. *Experimental Brain Research* 164(2):250–259.

Knight, J. N. 2003. Signal fraction analysis and artifact removal in EEG. Master's thesis, Department of Computer Science, Colorado State University. Available at http://www.cs.colostate.edu/eeg/publications/natethesis.pdf.

Kohavi, R. 1995. A study of cross-validation and bootstrap for accuracy estimation and model selection. In *IJCAI 95. Proceedings of the Fourteenth International Joint Conference on Artificial Intelligence*, edited by C. S. Mellish vol. 2: 1137–1145.

Kohonen, T. 1997. Self-organizing maps. Berlin, Germany: Springer-Verlag, 2nd edition.

Koles, Z. J. and A. C. K. Soong. 1998. EEG source localization: implementing the spatio-temporal decomposition approach. *Electroencephalography and Clinical Neurophysiology* 107(5):343–352.

Koles, Z. J., M. S. Lazar, and S. Z. Zhou. 1990. Spatial patterns underlying population differences in the background EEG. *Brain Topography* 2(4):275–284.

Kornhuber, H. H. and L. Deecke. 1965. Hirnpotentialänderungen bei Willkürbewegungen und passiven Bewegungen des Menschen: Bereitschaftspotential und reafferente Potentiale. *Pflügers Archiv* 284:1–17.

Kotchoubey, B. 2005. Apallic syndrome is not apallic: is vegetative state vegetative? *Neuropsychological Rehabilitation* 15:333–356.

Kotchoubey, B., S. Lang, G. Mezger, D. Schmalohr, M. Schneck, A. Semmler, V. Bostanov, and N. Birbaumer. 2005. Information processing in severe disorders of consciousness: vegetative state and minimally conscious state. *Clinical Neurophysiology* 116(10):2441–2453.

Kotchoubey, B., S. Lang, V. Bostanov, and N. Birbaumer. 2002. Is there a mind? Electrophysiology of unconscious patients. *News in Physiological Sciences* 1–17:38–42.

Kotchoubey, B., H. Schleichert, W. Lutzenberger, and N. Birbaumer. 1997. A new method for self-regulation of slow cortical potentials in a timed paradigm. *Applied Psychophysiology and Biofeedback* 22(2):77–93.

Kotchoubey, B., D. Schneider, H. Schleichert, U. Strehl, C. Uhlmann, V. Blankenhorn, W. Fröscher, and N. Birbaumer. 1996. Self-regulation of slow cortical potentials in epilepsy: a retrial with analysis of influencing factors. *Epilepsy Research* 25(3):269–276.

Kraemer, H. C. 1982. Kappa coefficient. In *Encyclopedia of Statistical Sciences*, edited by S. Kotz and N. L. Johnson. New York: John Wiley & Sons.

Krauledat, M., G. Dornhege, B. Blankertz, and K. R. Müller. 2005. Robustifying EEG data analysis by removing outliers. *Chaos and Complexity* 2(2).

Krauledat, M., G. Dornhege, B. Blankertz, G. Curio, and K. R. Müller. 2004. The Berlin Brain-Computer Interface for rapid response. *Biomedizinische Technik* 49(1):61–62.

Krausz, G., R. Scherer, G. Korisek, and G. Pfurtscheller. 2003. Critical decision-speed and information transfer in the "Graz Brain-Computer Interface". *Applied Psychophysiology and Biofeedback* 28(3):233–240.

Krepki, R., G. Curio, B. Blankertz, and K. R. Müller. 2007. Berlin Brain-Computer Interface—the HCI communication channel for discovery. *International Journal of Human-Computer Studies* 65:460–477.

Krepki, R. 2004. Brain-Computer Interfaces: Design and implementation of an online BCI system of the control in gaming applications and virtual limbs. PhD thesis, Technische Universität Berlin, Fakultät IV—Elektrotechnik und Informatik.

Kronegg, J. and T. Pun. 2005. Measuring the performance of brain-computer interfaces using the information transfer rate. Brain-Computer Interface Technology: Third International Meeting, June 14–19, 2005, Rensselaerville, New York.

Kronegg, J., S. Voloshynovskiy, and T. Pun. 2005. Analysis of bit-rate definitions for brain-computer interfaces. In *Proceedings International Conference on Human-Computer Interaction (HCI'05)*, Las Vegas.

Krusienski, D. J., E. W. Sellers, F. Cabestaing, S. Bayoudh, D. J. McFarland, T. M. Vaughan, and J. R. Wolpaw. 2006. A comparison of classification techniques for the P300 speller. *The Journal of Neural Engineering* 3(4):299–305.

Krusienski, D. J., E. W. Sellers, T. M. Vaughan, D. J. McFarland, and J. R. Wolpaw. 2005. P300 speller matrix classification via stepwise linear discriminant analysis. Poster presented at the Brain-Computer Interface Technology Third International Meeting, Rensselaerville, New York.

Kübler, A., S. Häcker, E. M. Braun, M. Hautzinger, and T. Meyer. In preparation. Individually defined quality of life, depression, and variation of positive reinforcement in patients with ALS.

Kübler, A., C. Weber, and N. Birbaumer. 2006. Locked-in—freigegeben für den Tod. wenn nur Denken und Fühlen bleiben—Neuroethik des Eingeschlossenseins. *Zeitschrift für Medizinische Ethik* 52:57–70.

Kübler, A. and N. Neumann. 2005. Brain-computer interfaces - the key for the conscious brain locked into a paralysed body. *Progress in Brain Research* 150:513–525.

Kübler, A., F. Nijboer, J. Mellinger, T. M. Vaughan, H. Pawelzik, G. Schalk, D. J. McFarland, N. Birbaumer, and J. R. Wolpaw. 2005a. Patients with ALS can use sensorimotor rhythms to operate a brain computer interface. *Neurology* 64(10):1775–1777.

Kübler, A., S. Winter, A. Ludolph, M. Hautzinger, and N. Birbaumer. 2005b. Severity of depressive symptoms and quality of life in patients with amyotrophic lateral sclerosis. *Neurorehabilitation and Neural Repair* 19(3):182–193.

Kübler, A., N. Neumann, B. Wilhelm, T. Hinterberger, and N. Birbaumer. 2004. Predictability of brain-computer communication. *International Journal of Psychophysiology* 18:121–129.

Kübler, A., S. Winter, and N. Birbaumer. 2003. The Thought Translation Device: Slow cortical potential biofeedback for verbal communication in paralysed patients. In *Biofeedback - A Practitioner's Guide*, edited by M. S. Schwartz and F. Andrasik. New York: Guilford Press, 3rd edition.

Kübler, A., B. Kotchoubey, J. Kaiser, J. R. Wolpaw, and N. Birbaumer. 2001a. Brain-computer communication: unlocking the locked in. *Psychological Bulletin* 127(3):358–375.

Kübler, A., N. Neumann, J. Kaiser, B. Kotchoubey, T. Hinterberger, and N. P. Birbaumer. 2001b. Brain-computer communication: self-regulation of slow cortical potentials for verbal communication. *Archives of Physical Medicine and Rehabilitation* 82(11):1533–1539.

Kübler, A. 2000. Brain-computer communication—development of a brain-computer interface for locked-in patients on the basis of the psychophysiological self-regulation training of slow cortical potentials (SCP). Tübingen: Schwäbische Verlagsgesellschaft.

Kübler, A., B. Kotchoubey, T. Hinterberger, N. Ghanayim, J. Perelmouter, M. Schauer, C. Fritsch, E. Taub, and N. Birbaumer. 1999. The Thought Translation Device: a neurophysiological approach to communication in total motor paralysis. *Experimental Brain Research* 124(2):223–232.

Kübler, A., B. Kotchoubey, H. P. Salzmann, N. Ghanayim, J. Perelmouter, V. Homberg, and N. Birbaumer. 1998. Self-regulation of slow cortical potentials in completely paralyzed human patients. *Neuroscience Letters* 252(3):171–174.

Kumar, N. and A. G. Andreou. 1998. Heteroscedastic discriminant analysis and reduced rank HMMs for improved speech recognition. *Speech Communication* 26(4):283–297.

Lachaux, J. P., E. Rodriguez, J. Martinerie, and F. J. Varela. 1999. Measuring phase synchrony in brain signals. *Human Brain Mapping* 8(4):194–208.

Lahrmann, H., C. Neuper, G. R. Müller, R. Scherer, and G. Pfurtscheller. 2005. Usefulness of an EEG-based brain-computer interface to establish communication in ALS. *Journal of the Neurological Sciences* 238(1):485.

Lakerfeld, J., B. Kotchoubey, and A. Kübler. Submitted. Cognitive function in late stage ALS patients.

Lal, T. N., O. Chapelle, J. Weston, and A. Elisseeff. In press. Embedded methods. In *Feature extraction, foundations and applications*, edited by I. Guyon, S. Gunn, M. Nikravesh, and L. Zadeh. Springer.

Lal, T. N. 2005. Machine learning methods for brain-computer interfaces. MPI Series in Biological Cybernetics, Bd. 12. Berlin: Logos Verlag.

Lal, T. N., T. Hinterberger, G. Widman, M. Schröder, N. J. Hill, W. Rosenstiel, C. E. Elger, B. Schölkopf, and N. Birbaumer. 2005a. Methods towards invasive human brain computer interfaces. In *Advances in Neural Information Processing Systems (NIPS 04)*, edited by Lawrence K. Saul, Yair Weiss, and Léon Bottou, vol. 17. Cambridge, Mass.: The MIT Press.

Lal, T. N., M. Schröder, J. Hill, H. Preissl, T. Hinterberger, J. Mellinger, M. Bogdan, W. Rosenstiel, T. Hofmann, N. Birbaumer, and B. Schölkopf. 2005b. A brain computer interface with online feedback based on magnetoencephalography. In *Proceedings of the 22nd International Conference on Machine Learning*: 465–472.

Lal, T. N., M. Schröder, T. Hinterberger, J. Weston, M. Bogdan, N. Birbaumer, and B. Schölkopf. 2004. Support vector channel selection in BCI. *IEEE Transactions on Biomedical Engineering* 51(6):1003–1010.

Lalor, E. C., S. P. Kelly, C. Finucane, R. Burke, R. Smith, R. B. Reilly, and G. McDarby. 2005. Steady-state VEP-based brain-computer interface control in an immersive 3D gaming environment. *EURASIP Journal on Applied Signal Processing* 19:3156–3164.

Lang, W., M. Lang, F. Uhl, Ch. Koska, A. Kornhuber, and L. Deecke. 1988. Negative cortical DC shifts preceding and accompanying simultaneous and sequential movements. *Experimental Brain Research* 71(3):579–587.

Laskov, P., C. Schäfer, I. Kotenko, and K.-R. Müller. 2004. Intrusion detection in unlabeled data with quarter-sphere support vector machines (extended version). *Praxis der Informationsverarbeitung und Kommunikation* 27:228–236.

Lauer, R. T., P. H. Peckham, K. L. Kilgore, and W. J. Heetderks. 2000. Applications of cortical signals to neuroprosthetic control: a critical review. *IEEE Transactions on Rehabilitation Engineering* 8(2):205–208.

Laureys, S., F. Pellas, P. Van Eeckhout, S. Ghorbel, C. Schnakers, F. Perrin, J. Berre, M. E. Faymonville, K. H. Pantke, F. Damas, M. Lamy, G. Moonen, and S. Goldman. 2005. The locked-in syndrome: what is it like to be conscious but paralyzed and voiceless? *Progress in Brain Research* 150:495–511.

Lebedev, M. A. and M. A. L. Nicolelis. 2006. Brain machine interfaces: Past, present and future. *Trends in Neurosciences* 29(9):536–546.

Lee, P. L., J. C. Hsieh, C. H. Wu, K. K. Shyu, S. S. Chen, T. C. Yeh, and Y. T. Wu. 2006. The brain computer interface using flash visual evoked potential and independent component analysis. *Annals of Biomedical Engineering* 34(10):1641–1654.

Lee, Y. J., O. L. Mangasarian, and W. H. Wolberg. 2000. Breast cancer survival and chemotherapy: A support vector machine analysis. *DIMACS Series in Discrete Mathematics and Theoretical Computer Science* 55:1–10.

Leeb, R., F. Lee, C. Keinrath, R. Scherer, H. Bischof, and G. Pfurtscheller. In revision. Brain-Computer Communication: Motivation, aim and impact of exploring a virtual apartment. *IEEE Transactions on Neural Systems and Rehabilitation Engineering.*

Leeb, R., C. Keinrath, D. Friedman, C. Guger, R. Scherer, C: Neuper, M. Garau, A. Antley, A. Steed, M. Slater, and G. Pfurtscheller. 2006. Walking by thinking: The brainwaves are crucial, not the muscles. *Presence-Teleoperators and Virtual Environments* 15(5): 500–514.

Leeb, R., R. Scherer, C. Keinrath, C. Guger, and G. Pfurtscheller. 2005. Exploring virtual environments with an EEG-based BCI through motor imagery. *Biomedizinische Technik. Biomedical engineering (Berl)* 50(4):86–91.

Leeb, R. and G. Pfurtscheller. 2004. Walking through a virtual city by thought. In *Proceedings of the 26th Annual International Conference of the IEEE Engineering in Medicine and Biology Society - EMBC 2004* vol. 6: 4503–4506, San Francisco.

Leeb, R., C. Keinrath, C. Guger, and G. Pfurtscheller. 2003. Combining brain-computer interface and virtual reality technologies. In *Proceedings Annual Conference of the German, Austrian and Swiss Association of Biomedical Engineering (BMT 2003), Biomed Tech (Berl)* vol. 48 (Suppl.Vol.1): 34–35.

Lemm, S., B. Blankertz, G. Curio, and K. R. Müller. 2005. Spatio-spectral filters for improved classification of single trial EEG. *IEEE Transactions on Biomedical Engineering* 52(9):1541–1548.

Leon-Carrion, J., P. van Eeckhout, M. del R. Dominguez-Morales, and F. J. Perez-Santamaria. 2002. The locked-in syndrome: a syndrome looking for a therapy. *Brain Injury* 16(7):571–582.

Leuthardt, E. C., K. J. Miller, G. Schalk, R. P. Rao, and J. G. Ojemann. 2006a. Electrocorticography-based brain computer interface–the Seattle experience. *IEEE Transactions on Neural Systems and Rehabilitation Engineering* 14(2):194–198.

Leuthardt, E. C., G. Schalk, D. Moran, and J. G. Ojemann. 2006b. The emerging world of motor neuroprosthetics: a neurosurgical perspective. *Neurosurgery* 59(1):1–14.

Leuthardt, E. C., G. Schalk, J. R. Wolpaw, J. G. Ojemann, and D. W. Moran. 2004. A brain-computer interface using electrocorticographic signals in humans. *Journal of Neural Engineering* 1(2):63–71.

Levine, S. P., J. E. Huggins, S. L. BeMent, R. K. Kushwaha, L. A. Schuh, M. M. Rohde, E. A. Passaro, D. A. Ross, K. V. Elsievich, and B. J. Smith. 2000. A direct brain interface based on event-related potentials. *IEEE Transactions on Rehabilitation Engineering* 8 (2):180–185.

Levine, S. P., J. E. Huggins, S. L. BeMent, R. K. Kushwaha, L. A. Schuh, E. A. Passaro, M. M. Rohde, and D. A. Ross. 1999. Identification of electrocorticogram patterns as the basis for a direct brain interface. *Journal of Clinical Neurophysiology* 16(5):439–447.

Linde, Y., A. Buzo, and R. M. Gray. 1980. An algorithm for vector quantizer design. *IEEE Transactions on Communications* COM-28(1):84–95.

Liu, J., A. Harris, and N. Kanwisher. 2002. Stages of processing in face perception: an MEG study. *Nature Neuroscience* 5(9):910–916.

Liu, J., M. Higuchi, A. Marantz, and N. Kanwisher. 2000. The selectivity of the occipitotemporal M170 for faces. *Neuroreport* 11(2):337–341.

Liu, X., D. B. McCreery, R. R. Carter, L. A. Bullara, T. G. Yuen, and W. F. Agnew. 1999. Stability of the interface between neural tissue and chronically implanted intracortical microelectrodes. *IEEE Transactions on Rehabilitation Engineering* 7(3):315–326.

Liu, A. K., J. W. Belliveau, and A. M. Dale. 1998. Spatiotemporal imaging of human brain activity using functional MRI constrained magnetoencephalography data: Monte Carlo simulations. *Proceedings of the National Academy of Sciences of the United States of America* 95(15):8945–8950.

Llinas, R., U. Ribary, D. Jeanmonod, E. Kronberg, and P. P. Mitra. 1999. Thalamocortical dysrhythmia: A neurological and neuropsychiatric syndrome characterized by magnetoencephalography. *Proceedings of the National Academy of Sciences of the United States of America* 96(26):15222–15227.

Loog, M. and R.P.W. Duin. 2004. Linear dimensionality reduction via a heteroscedastic extension of LDA: the Chernoff criterion. *IEEE Transactions on Pattern Analysis and Machine Intelligence* 26(6):732–739.

Lotze, M., C. Braun, N. Birbaumer, S. Anders, and L. G. Cohen. 2003. Motor learning elicited by voluntary drive. *Brain* 126(4):866–872.

Lotze, M., H. Flor, W. Grodd, W. Larbig, and N. Birbaumer. 2001. Phantom movements and pain. An fMRI study in upper limb amputees. *Brain* 124(11):2268–2277.

Lotze, M., W. Grodd, N. Birbaumer, M. Erb, E. Huse, and H. Flor. 1999a. Does use of a myoelectric prosthesis prevent cortical reorganization and phantom limb pain? *Nature Neuroscience* 2(6):501–502.

Lotze, M., P. Montoya, M. Erb, E. Hülsmann, H. Flor, U. Klose, N. Birbaumer, and W. Grodd. 1999b. Activation of cortical and cerebellar motor areas during executed and imagined hand movements: an fMRI study. *Journal of Cognitive Neuroscience* 11 (5):491–501.

Low, A., B. Rockstroh, R. Cohen, O. Hauk, P. Berg, and W. Maier. 1999. Determining working memory from ERP topography. *Brain Topography* 12(1):39–47.

Lulé, D., V. Diekmann, J. Kassubek, A. Kurt, N. Birbaumer, A. C. Ludolph, and E. Kraft. In press. Cortical reorganization in amyotrophic lateral sclerosis: motor imagery and motor function. *Annals of Neurology*.

Lulé, D., A. Kurt, R. Jurgens, J. Kassubek, V. Diekmann, E. Kraft, N. Neumann, A. C. Ludolph, N. Birbaumer, and S. Anders. 2005. Emotional responding in amyotrophic lateral sclerosis. *Journal of Neurology* 252(12):1517–1524.

Lundqvist, C., A. Siosteen, C. Blomstrand, B. Lind, and M. Sullivan. 1991. Spinal cord injuries. clinical, functional, and emotional status. *Spine* 16(1):78–83.

Luo, A. and P. Sajda. 2006. Learning discrimination trajectories in EEG sensor space: application to inferring task difficulty. *Journal of Neural Engineering* 3(1):L1–6.

Lutzenberger, W., T. Elbert, B. Rockstroh, and N. Birbaumer. 1982. Biofeedback produced slow brain potentials and task performance. *Biological Psychology* 14(1–2):99–111.

Lutzenberger, W., N. Birbaumer, T. Elbert, B. Rockstroh, W. Bippus, and R. Breidt. 1980. Self-regulation of slow cortical potentials in normal subjects and patients with frontal lobe lesions. *Progress in Brain Research* 54:427–430.

Lutzenberger, W., T. Elbert, B. Rockstroh, and N. Birbaumer. 1979. The effects of self-regulation of slow cortical potentials on performance in a signal detection task. *The International Journal of Neuroscience* 9(3):175–183.

Makeig, S., A. Delorme, M. Westerfield, T. P. Jung, J. Townsend, E. Courchense, and T. J. Sejnowski. 2004. Electroencephalographic brain dynamics following manually responded visual targets. *PLoS Biology* 2(6):e176.

Makeig, S. and A. Delourme. EEGLAB. Available at http://sccn.ucsd.edu/eeglab/.

Makeig, S., M. Westerfield, T.-P. Jung, J. Covington, J. Townsend, T. Sejnowski, and E. Courchesne. 1999. Functionally independent components of the late positive event-related potential during visual spatial attention. *Journal of Neuroscience* 19(7):2665–2680.

Margalit, E., J. D. Weiland, R. E. Clatterbuck, G. Y. Fujii, M. Maia, M. Tameesh, G. Torres, S. A. D'Anna, D. V. Piyathaisere S. Desai, A. Olivi, E. Jr. de Juan, and M. S. Humayun. 2003. Visual and electrical evoked response recorded from subdural electrodes implanted above the visual cortex in normal dogs under two methods of anesthesia. *Journal of Neuroscience Methods* 123(2):129–137.

Mason, S. G., A. Bashashati, M. Fatourechi, K. F. Navarro, and G. E. Birch. Submitted. A comprehensive survey of brain interface technology designs. *Annals of Biomedical Engineering*.

Mason, S. G. and G. E. Birch. 2005. Temporal control paradigms for direct brain interfaces—rethinking the definition of asynchronous and synchronous. In *Proceedings of HCI International*, Las Vegas.

Mason, S. G., J. Kronegg, J. E. Huggins, A. Schlögl, M. Fatourechi, R. Kaidar, R. Scherer, and A. Buttfield. 2005a. Asynchronous BCI performance evaluation. BCIinfo.org research papers. Available at http://bciinfo.org/Research_Info/documents/articles/AsynchBCIDiscussionSummaryBCI2005.pdf.

Mason, S. G., M. M. Jackson, and G. E. Birch. 2005b. A general framework for characterizing studies of brain interface technology. *Annals of Biomedical Engineering* 33(11):1653–1670.

Mason, S. G., R. Bohringer, J. F. Borisoff, and G. E. Birch. 2004. Real-time control of a video game with a direct brain-computer interface. *Journal of Clinical Neurophysiology* 21(6):404–408.

Mason, S. G. and G. E. Birch. 2003. A general framework for brain-computer interface design. *IEEE Transactions on Neural Systems and Rehabilitation Engineering* 11(1):70–85.

Mason, S. G. and G. E. Birch. 2000. A brain-controlled switch for asynchronous control applications. *IEEE Transactions on Biomedical Engineering* 47(10):1297–1307.

Maynard, E., C. Nordhausen, and R. Normann. 1997. The Utah intracortical electrode array: A recording structure for potential brain-computer interfaces. *Electroencephalography and Clinical Neurophysiology* 102(3):228–239.

Mazurek, M. E., J. D. Roitman, J. Ditterich, and M. N. Shadlen. 2003. A role for neural integrators in perceptual decision making. *Cerebral Cortex* 13(11):1257–1269.

Mazzone, P., A. Lozano, P. Stanzione, S. Galati, E. Scarnati, A. Peppe, and A. Stefani. 2005. Implantation of human pedunculopontine nucleus: a safe and clinically relevant target in Parkinson's disease. *Neuroreport* 16(17):1877–1881.

McFarland, D. J., C. W. Anderson, K. R. Müller, A. Schlögl, and D. J. Krusienski. 2006. BCI Meeting 2005—workshop on BCI signal processing: feature extraction and translation. *IEEE Transactions on Neural Systems and Rehabilitation Engineering* 14 (2):135–138.

McFarland, D. J., W. A. Sarnacki, T. M. Vaughan, and J. R. Wolpaw. 2005. Brain-computer interface (BCI) operation: signal and noise during early training sessions. *Clinical Neurophysiology* 116(1):56–62.

McFarland, D. J. and J. R. Wolpaw. 2005. Sensorimotor rhythm-based brain-computer interface (BCI): Feature selection by regression improves performance. *IEEE Transactions on Neural Systems and Rehabilitation Engineering* 13(3):372–379.

McFarland, D. J., W. A. Sarnacki, and J. R. Wolpaw. 2003. Brain-computer interface (BCI) operation: optimizing information transfer rates. *Biological Psychology* 63(3):237–251.

McFarland, D. J., L. M. McCane, and J. R. Wolpaw. 1998. EEG-based communication and control: short-term role of feedback. *IEEE Transactions on Rehabilitation Engineering* 6(1):7–11.

McFarland, D. J., L. M. McCane, S. V. David, and J. R. Wolpaw. 1997a. Spatial filter selection for EEG-based communication. *Electroencephalography and Clinical Neurophysiology* 103(3):386–394.

McFarland, D. J., T. Lefkowicz, and J. R. Wolpaw. 1997b. Design and operation of an EEG-based brain-computer interface (BCI) with digital signal processing technology. *Behavioral Research Methods Instruments and Computers* 29(3):337–345.

McFarland, D. J., G. W. Neat, R. F. Read, and J. R. Wolpaw. 1993. An EEG-based method for graded cursor control. *Psychobiology* 21:77–81.

Mehring, C., J. Rickert, E. Vaadia, S. Cardoso de Oliveira, A. Aertsen, and S. Rotter. 2003. Inference of hand movements from local field potentials in monkey motor cortex. *Nature Neuroscience* 6(12):1253–1254.

Meinicke, P., M. Kaper, F. Hoppe, M. Huemann, and H. Ritter. 2002. Improving transfer rates in brain computer interface: A case study. In *Advances in Neural Information Processing Systems (NIPS 01)*: 1107–1114, Cambridge, Mass. The MIT Press.

Meir, R. and G. Rätsch. 2003. An introduction to boosting and leveraging. In *Advanced Lectures on Machine Learning*, edited by S. Mendelson and A. Smola, LNAI. Springer.

Mellinger, J., G. Schalk, C. Braun, H. Preissl, W. Rosenstiel, N. Birbaumer, and A. Kübler. Under revision. An MEG-based brain-computer interface. *Neuroimage.*

Mellinger, J., G. Schalk, C. Braun, H. Preissl, N. Birbaumer, and A. Kübler. 2005. A brain-computer interface (BCI) based on magnetoenecephalography (MEG). *Psychophysiology* 42(1):88.

Mellinger, J., T. Hinterberger, M. Bensch, M. Schröder, and N. Birbaumer. 2003. Surfing the web with electrical brain signals: the brain web surfer (BWS) for the completely paralysed. In *Proceedings of the 2nd World Congress of the International Society of Physical and Rehabilitation Medicine - ISPRM*, edited by Nachum Ring, Haim; Soroker: 731–738, Bologna (Monduzzi).

Merzenich, M. M., D. N. Schindler, and M. W. White. 1974. Feasibility of multichannel scala tympani stimulation. *Laryngoscope* 84(11):1887–1893.

Miall, R. C., N. Jenkinson, and K. Kulkarni. 2004. Adaptation to rotated visual feedback: a re-examination of motor interference. *Experimental Brain Research* 154(2):201–210.

Middendorf, M., G. McMillan, G. Calhoun, and K. S. Jones. 2000. Brain-computer interfaces based on the steady-state visual-evoked response. *IEEE Transactions on Rehabilitation Engineering* 8(2):211–214.

Mika, S., G. Rätsch, J Weston, B. Schölkopf, A. Smola, and K.-R. Müller. 2003. Constructing descriptive and discriminative non-linear features: Rayleigh coefficients in kernel feature spaces. *IEEE Transaction on Pattern Analysis and Machine Intelligence* 25(5): 623–628.

Mika, S. 2002. Kernel fisher discriminants. PhD thesis, University of Technology, Berlin.

Mika, S., G. Rätsch, and K.-R. Müller. 2001. A mathematical programming approach to the Kernel Fisher algorithm. In *Advances in Neural Information Processing Systems (NIPS 00)*, edited by T. K. Leen, T. G. Dietterich, and V. Tresp vol. 13: 591–597, Cambridge, Mass. The MIT Press.

Mika, S., B. Schölkopf, A.J. Smola, K.-R. Müller, M. Scholz, and G. Rätsch. 1999. Kernel PCA and de–noising in feature spaces. In *Advances in Neural Information Processing Systems (NIPS 98)*, edited by M.S. Kearns, S.A. Solla, and D.A. Cohn: 536–542, Cambridge, Mass. MIT Press.

Millán, J. d. R. 2004. On the need for on-line learning in brain-computer interfaces. In *Proceedings of the International Joint Conference on Neural Networks*, Budapest, Hungary.

Millán, J. d. R., F. Renkens, J. Mouriño, and W. Gerstner. 2004a. Noninvasive brain-actuated control of a mobile robot by human EEG. *IEEE Transactions on Biomedical Engineering* 51(6):1026–1033.

Millán, J. d. R., F. Renkens, J. Mouriño, and W. Gerstner. 2004b. Brain-actuated interaction. *Artificial Intelligence* 159(1–2):241–259.

Millán, J. d. R. 2003. Adaptive brain interfaces. *Communications of the ACM* 46:74–80.

Millán, J. d. R. and J. Mouriño. 2003. Asynchronous BCI and local neural classifiers: an overview of the Adaptive Brain Interface project. *IEEE Transactions on Neural Systems and Rehabilitation Engineering* 11(2):159–161.

Millán, J. d. R. 2002. Brain-computer interfaces. In *Handbook of Brain Theory and Neural Networks*, edited by Michael A. Arbib. Cambridge, Mass.: The MIT Press, 2nd ed.

Millán, J. d. R., M. Franzé, J. Mouriño, F. Cincotti, and F. Babiloni. 2002a. Relevant EEG features for the classification of spontaneous motor-related tasks. *Biological Cybernetics* 86(2):89–95.

Millán, J. d. R., M. Franzé, J. Mouriño, F. Cincotti, and F. Babiloni. 2002b. Relevant EEG features for the classification of spontaneous motor-related tasks. *Biological Cybernetics* 86(2):89–95.

Millán, J. d. R., J. Mouriño, M. Franzé, F. Cincotti, M. Varsta, J. Heikkonen J, and F. Babiloni. 2002c. A local neural classifier for the recognition of EEG patterns associated to mental tasks. *IEEE Transactions on Neural Networks* 13(3):678–686.

Miller, N. E. 1969. Learning of visceral and glandular responses. *Science* 163(866): 434–445.

Miner, L. A., D. J. McFarland, and J. R. Wolpaw. 1998. Answering questions with an electroencephalogram-based brain-computer interface. *Archives of Physical Medicine and Rehabilitation* 79(9):1029–1033.

Moran, D. W. and A. B. Schwartz. 1999. Motor cortical representation of speed and direction during reaching. *Journal of Neurophysiology* 82(5):2676–2692.

Morrow, M. M. and L. E. Miller. 2003. Prediction of muscle activity by populations of sequentially recorded primary motor cortex neurons. *Journal of Neurophysiology* 89(4): 2279–2288.

Mosher, J. C., S. Baillet, and R. M. Leahy. 1999. EEG source localization and imaging using multiple signal classification approaches. *Journal of Clinical Neurophysiology* 16 (3):225–238.

Mouriño, J. 2003. EEG-based analysis for the design of adaptive brain interfaces. PhD thesis, Centre de Recerca en Enginyeria Biomdica, Universitat Politcnica de Catalunya, Barcelona, Spain.

Mouriño, J., J. d. R. Millán, F. Cincotti, S. Chiappa, R. Jané, and F. Babiloni. 2001. Spatial filtering in the training process of a brain computer interface. In *Proceedings 23rd Annual Int. Conf. of the IEEE Engineering in Medicine and Biology Society*.

Müller, K.-R. and B. Blankertz. 2006. Toward non-invasive brain-computer interfaces. *IEEE Signal Processing Magazine*.

Müller, K.-R., M. Krauledat, G. Dornhege, G. Curio, and B. Blankertz. 2004a. Machine learning techniques for brain-computer interfaces. *Biomedizinische Technik* 49(1):11–22.

Müller, G. R., R. Scherer, C. Neuper, H. Lahrmann, P. Staiger-Sälzer, and G. Pfurtscheller. 2004b. EEG-basierende Kommunikation: Erfahrungen mit einem Telemonitoringsystem zum Patiententraining. In *Proceedings of 38th Ann. Conv. of the German Society for Medical and Biological Engineering in VDE* vol. 49: 230–231. Suppl. vol. Biomed Techn (Berl.).

Müller, K.-R., C. W. Anderson, and G. E. Birch. 2003a. Linear and nonlinear methods for brain-computer interfaces. *IEEE Transactions on Neural Systems and Rehabilitation Engineering* 11(2):165–169.

Müller, G. R., C. Neuper, and G. Pfurtscheller. 2003b. Implementation of a telemonitoring system for the control of an EEG-based brain-computer interface. *IEEE Transactions on Neural Systems and Rehabilitation Engineering* 11(1):54–59.

Müller, K.-R., S. Mika, G. Rätsch, K. Tsuda, and B. Schölkopf. 2001. An introduction to kernel-based learning algorithms. *IEEE Transactions on Neural Networks* 12(2):181–201.

Müller, G. R., C. Neuper, and G. Pfurtscheller. 2001. "Resonance-like" frequencies of sensorimotor areas evoked by repetitive tactile stimulation. *Biomedizinische Technik* 46 (7–8):186–190.

Müller-Gerking, J., G. Pfurtscheller, and H. Flyvbjerg. 1999. Designing optimal spatial filters for single-trial EEG classification in a movement task. *Clinical Neurophysiology* 110(5):787–798.

Müller-Putz, G. R., R. Scherer, C. Neuper, and G. Pfurtscheller. 2006. Steady-state somatosensory evoked potentials: suitable brain signals for brain-computer interfaces? *IEEE Transactions on Neural Systems and Rehabilitation Engineering* 14(1):30–37.

Müller-Putz, G. R., R. Scherer, C. Brauneis, and G. Pfurtscheller. 2005a. Steady-state visual evoked potential (SSVEP)-based communication: impact of harmonic frequency components. *Journal of neural engineering* 2(4):123–130.

Müller-Putz, G. R., R. Scherer, G. Pfurtscheller, and R. Rupp. 2005b. EEG-based neuroprosthesis control: a step towards clinical practice. *Neuroscience Letters* 382(1–2): 169–174.

Murase, N., J. Duque, R. Mazzocchio, and L. G. Cohen. 2004. Influence of interhemispheric interactions on motor function in chronic stroke. *Annals of Neurology* 55(3): 400–409.

Musallam, S., B. D. Corneil, B. Greger, H. Scherberger, and R. A. Andersen. 2004. Cognitive control signals for neural prosthetics. *Science* 305(5681):258–262.

Mussa-Ivaldi, F. A. and L. E. Miller. 2003. Brain-machine interfaces: computational demands and clinical needs meet basic neuroscience. *Trends in Neurosciences* 26(6): 329–334.

Nagai, Y., H. D. Crittchley, E. Feathersone, P. B. Fenwick, M. R. Trimble, and R. J. Dolan. 2004. Brain activity relating to the contingent negative variation: an fMRI investigation. modulation by volitional control of peripheral autonomic arousal. *NeuroImage* 21(4): 1232–1241.

National Instruments. Available atr http://www.ni.com/.

Nelson, W. T., L. J. Hettinger, J. A. Cunningham, M. M. Roe, M. W. Haas, and L. B. Dennis. 1997. Navigating through virtual flight environments using brain-body-actuated control. In *Proceedings Virtual Reality Annual International Symposium*: 30–37.

Nenadic, Z. In press. Information discriminant analysis: Feature extraction with an information-theoretic objective. *IEEE Transactions on Pattern Analysis and Machine Intelligence*.

Nenadic, Z. and J. W. Burdick. 2006. A control algorithm for autonomous optimization of extracellular recordings. *IEEE Transactions on Biomedical Engineering* 53(5):941–955.

Nenadic, Z. and J. W. Burdick. 2005. Spike detection using the continuous wavelet transform. *IEEE Transactions on Biomedical Engineering* 52(1):74–87.

Neumann, N., A. Kübler, J. Kaiser, T. Hinterberger, and N. Birbaumer. 2003. Conscious perception of brain states: mental strategies for brain-computer communication. *Neuropsychologia* 41(8):1026–1036.

Neuper, C., R. Scherer, M. Reiner, and G. Pfurtscheller. 2005. Imagery of motor actions: differential effect of kinesthetic and visual-motor mode of imagery in single-trial EEG. *Brain Research. Cognitive Brain Research* 25(3):668–677.

Neuper, C., G. R. Müller, A. Kübler, N. Birbaumer, and G. Pfurtscheller. 2003. Clinical application of an EEG-based brain-computer interface: a case study in a patient with severe motor impairment. *Clinical Neurophysiology* 114(3):399–409.

Neuper, C. and G. Pfurtscheller. 2001. Event-related dynamics of cortical rhythms: frequency-specific features and functional correlates. *International Journal of Psychophysiology* 43(1):41–58.

Neuper, C. and G. Pfurtscheller. 1999. Motor imagery and ERD. In *Event-Related Desynchronization. Handbook of Electroencephalography and Clinical Neurophysiology*, edited by G. Pfurtscheller and F. H. Lopes da Silva. Amsterdam: Elsevier.

Neuper, C., A. Schlögl, and G. Pfurtscheller. 1999. Enhancement of left-right sensorimotor EEG differences during feedback-regulated motor imagery. *Journal of Clinical Neurophysiology* 16(4):373–382.

Neurotech Network of the Society to Increase Mobility. Available at http://www.neurotechnetwork.org/home.html.

Newsome, W. T., K. H. Britten, and J. A. Movshon. 1989. Neuronal correlates of a perceptual decision. *Nature* 341(6237):52–54.

Nicolelis, M. A. 2003. Brain-machine interfaces to restore motor function and probe neural circuits. *Nature Reviews Neuroscience* 4(5):417–422.

Nicolelis, M. A., D. Dimitrov, J. M. Carmena, R. Crist, G. Lehew, J. D. Kralik, and S. P. Wise. 2003. Chronic, multisite, multielectrode recordings in macaque monkeys. *Proceedings of the National Academy of Sciences of the United States of America* 100 (19):11041–11046.

Nicolelis, M. A. L. 2001. Actions from thoughts. *Nature* 409(6818):403–407.

Niedermeyer, E. 2005a. Maturation of the EEG: Development of waking and sleep patterns. In *Electroencephalography—Basic Principles, Clinical Applications, and Related Fields*, edited by E. Niedermeyer and F. H. Lopes da Silva. Philadelphia: Lippincott Williams & Wilkins, 5th edition.

Niedermeyer, E. 2005b. The normal EEG of the waking adult. In *Electroencephalography—Basic Principles, Clinical Applications, and Related Fields*, edited by E. Niedermeyer and F. H. Lopes da Silva. Philadelphia: Lippincott Williams & Wilkins, 5th edition.

Nielsen, K. D., A. F. Cabrera, and O. F. do Nascimento. 2006. EEG based BCI-towards a better control. Brain-computer interface research at Aalborg University. *IEEE Transactions on Neural Systems and Rehabilitation Engineering* 14(2):202–204.

Nijboer, F., E. Sellers, J. Mellinger an T. Matuz, U. Mochty, M. Jordan, D. Krusienski, J. R. Wolpaw, and A. Kübler. Submitted. A brain-computer interface (BCI) for people with amyotrophich lateral sclerosis (ALS).

Nijboer, F., A. Furdea, I. Gunst, J. Mellinger, D: McFarland, N. Birbaumer, and A. Kübler. In press. An auditory brain-computer interface. *Journal of Neuroscience Methods*.

Nijboer, F., U. Mochty, J. Mellinger, T. Matuz, M. Jordan, E. Sellers, T. M. Vaughan, D. J. McFarland, G. Schalk, J. R. Wolpaw, N. Birbaumer, and A. Kübler. 2005. Comparing sensorimotor rhythms, slow cortical potentials, and P300 for brain-computer interface (BCI) use by ALS patients—a within subjects design. Poster presented at Brain-Computer Interface Technology: Third International Meeting, Rensselaerville, New York, June 14-19.

Nunez, P. L., R. Srinivasan, A. F. Westdorp, R. S. Wijesinghe, D. M. Tucker, R. B. Silberstein, and P. J. Cadusch. 1997. EEG coherency I: statistics, reference electrode, volume conduction, Laplacians, cortical imaging, and interpretation at multiple scales. *Electroencephalography and Clinical Neurophysiology* 103(5):499–515.

Nykopp, T. 2001. Statistical modelling issues for the adaptive brain interface. Master's thesis, Helsinki University of Technology, Department of Electrical and Communications Engineering.

Obermaier, B., G. R. Müller, and G. Pfurtscheller. 2003. "Virtual keyboard" controlled by spontaneous EEG activity. *IEEE Transactions on Neural Systems and Rehabilitation Engineering* 11(4):422–426.

Obermaier, B., G. Müller, and G. Pfurtscheller. 2001. 'Virtual keyboard' controlled by spontaneous EEG activity. In *Artificial-Neural-Networks-ICANN-2001*, edited by G. Dorffner, H. Bischof, and K. Hornik: 636–641, Berlin. Springer. LNCS 2130.

OctaveForge. The GNU Octave Repository. Available at http://octave.sourceforge.net/.

OpenEEG. ModEEG – Open Source EEG amplifier. Available at http://openeeg.sourceforge.net/doc/modeeg/modeeg.html.

Oppenheim, A. V. and R. W. Schafer. 1989. Discrete-time signal processing. Prentice Hall Signal Processing Series. Prentice Hall.

Orr, G. B. and K.-R. Müller, editors. 1998. Neural networks: tricks of the trade, vol. LNCS 1524. Heidelberg: Springer.

Owen, A. M., M. R. Coleman, M. Boly, M. H. Davis, S. Laureys, and J. D. Pickard. 2006. Detecting awareness in the vegetative state. *Science* 313(5792):1402.

Pal. 2002. Computing discriminability and bias with the R software. Available from http://www.pallier.org/ressources/aprime/aprime.pdf.

Pang, C., J. G. Cham, Z. Nenadic, S. Musallam, Y. C. Tai, J. W. Burdick, and R. A. Andersen. 2005a. A new multi-site probe array with monolithically integrated parylene flexible cable for neural prostheses. In *Proceedings of the 27th Annual International Conference of the IEEE Engineering in Medicine and Biology Society* vol. 2: 5352 – 5355 Vol. 7. IEEE.

Pang, C., J. G. Cham, Z. Nenadic, Y. C. Tai, J. W. Burdick, and R. A. Andersen. 2005b. A new neural recording electrode array with parylene insulating layer. In *Proceedings of the 9th International Conference on Miniaturized Systems for Chemistry and Life Sciences (μTAS)* vol. 2: 675–677. IEEE.

Paninski, L., M. R. Fellows, N. G. Hatsopoulos, and J. P. Donoghue. 2004. Spatiotemporal tuning of motor cortical neurons for hand position and velocity. *Journal of Neurophysiology* 91(1):515–532.

Parra, L. C., C. D. Spence, A. D. Gerson, and P. Sajda. 2005. Recipes for the linear analysis of EEG. *Neuroimage* 28(2):326–341.

Parra, L. C., C. D. Spence, A. D. Gerson, and P. Sajda. 2003. Response error correction— a demonstration of improved human-machine performance using real-time EEG monitoring. *IEEE Transactions on Neural Systems and Rehabilitation Engineering* 11(2): 173–177.

Parra, L., C. Alvino, A. Tang, B. Pearlmutter, N. Yeung, A. Osman, and P. Sajda. 2002. Linear spatial integration for single-trial detection in encephalography. *Neuroimage* 17 (1):223–230.

Pascual-Marqui, R. D. LORETA – low resolution brain electromagnetic tomography. Available at http://www.unizh.ch/keyinst/NewLORETA/LORETA01.htm.

Patterson, J. R. and M. Grabois. 1986. Locked-in syndrome: a review of 139 cases. *Stroke* 17(4):758–764.

Paz, R., T. Boraud, C. Natan, H. Bergman, and E. Vaadia. 2003. Preparatory activity in motor cortex reflects learning of local visuomotor skills. *Nature Neuroscience* 6(8): 882–890.

Peckham, P. H., M. W. Keith, K. L. Kilgore, J. H. Grill, K. S. Wuolle, G. B. Thrope, P. Gorman, J. Hobby, M. J. Mulcahey, S. Carroll, V. R. Hentz, and A. Wiegner. 2001. Efficacy of an implanted neuroprosthesis for restoring hand grasp in tetraplegia: a multicenter study. *archphysmed* 82(10):1380–1388.

Perelmouter, J. and N. Birbaumer. 2000. A binary spelling interface with random errors. *IEEE Transactions on Neural Systems and Rehabilitation Engineering* 8(2):227–232.

Perelmouter, J., B. Kotchoubey, A. Kübler, E. Taub, and N. Birbaumer. 1999. Language support program for thought-translation devices. *Automedica* 18:67–84.

Perrin, F., J. Pernier, O. Bertrand, and J. Echallier. 1990. Corrigendum eeg 02274. *Electroencephalography and Clinical Neurophysiology* 76:565.

Perrin, F., J. Pernier, O. Bertrand, and J. Echallier. 1989. Spherical splines for potential and current density mapping. *Electroencephalography and Clinical Neurophysiology* 72 (2):184–187.

Pesaran, B., J. S. Pezaris, M. Sahani, P. P. Mitra, and R. A. Andersen. 2002. Temporal structure in neuronal activity during working memory in macaque parietal cortex. *Nature Neuroscience* 5(8):805–811.

Pfingst, B. E. 2000. Auditory prostheses. In *Neural Prostheses for Restoration of Sensory and Motor Function*, edited by J. K. Chapin and K. A. Moxon. Boca Raton, Florida: CRC Press, Inc.

Pfurtscheller, G., R. Scherer, R. Leeb, C. Keinrath, C. Neuper, F. Lee, B. Graimann, A. Schlögl, and H. Bischof. 2007. Viewing moving objects in virtual reality can change the dynamics of sensorimotor EEG rhythms. *Presence-Teleoperators and Virtual Environments* 16(1):111–118.

Pfurtscheller, G., C. Brunner, A. Schlögl, and F. H. Lopes da Silva. 2006a. Mu-rhythm (de)synchronization and EEG single-trial classification of different motor imagery tasks. *Neuroimage* 31(1):153–159.

Pfurtscheller, G., R. Leeb, C. Keinrath, D. Friedman, C. Neuper, C. Guger, and M. Slater. 2006b. Walking from thought. *Brain Research* 1071(1):145–152.

Pfurtscheller, G., G. R. Müller-Putz, A. Schlögl, B. Graimann, R. Scherer, R. Leeb, C. Brunner, C. Keinrath, F. Lee, G. Townsend, C. Vidaurre, and C. Neuper. 2006c. 15 years of BCI research at Graz University of technology: current projects. *IEEE Transactions on Neural Systems and Rehabilitation Engineering* 14(2):205–210.

Pfurtscheller, G. 2005. EEG event-related desynchronization (ERD) and event related synchronization (ERS). In *Electroencephalography—Basic Principles, Clinical Applications, and Related Fields*, edited by E. Niedermeyer and F. H. Lopes da Silva. Philadelphia: Lippincott Williams & Wilkins, 5th edition.

Pfurtscheller, G., C. Neuper, and N. Birbaumer. 2005a. Human brain-computer interface. In *Motor Cortex in Voluntary Movements: a distributed system for distributed functions. Series: Methods and New Frontiers in Neuroscience*, edited by A. Riehle and E. Vaadia. New York: CRC Press.

Pfurtscheller, G., C. Neuper, C. Brunner, and F. Lopes da Silva. 2005b. Beta rebound after different types of motor imagery in man. *Neuroscience Letters* 378(3):156–159.

Pfurtscheller, G., B. Graimann, J. E. Huggins, S. P. Levine, and L. A. Schuh. 2003a. Spatiotemporal patterns of beta desynchronization and gamma synchronization in corticographic data during self-paced movement. *Clinical Neurophysiology* 114(7):1226–1236.

Pfurtscheller, G., G. R. Müller, J. Pfurtscheller, H. J. Gerner, and R. Rupp. 2003b. "Thought"—control of functional electrical stimulation to restore hand grasp in a patient with tetraplegia. *Neuroscience Letters* 351(1):33–36.

Pfurtscheller, G., C. Neuper, G. R. Müller, B. Obermaier, G. Krausz, A. Schlögl, R. Scherer, B. Graimann, C. Keinrath, D. Skliris, M. Wörtz, G. Supp, and C. Schrank. 2003c. Graz-BCI: State of the art and clinical applications. *IEEE Transactions on Neural Systems and Rehabilitation Engineering* 11(2):177–180.

Pfurtscheller, G. and C. Neuper. 2001. Motor imagery and direct brain-computer communication. *Proceedings of the IEEE* 89(7):1123–1134.

Pfurtscheller, G., C. Guger, G. Müller, G. Krausz, and C. Neuper. 2000a. Brain oscillations control hand orthosis in a tetraplegic. *Neuroscience Letters* 292(3):211–214.

Pfurtscheller, G., C. Neuper, C. Guger, W. Harkam, H. Ramoser, A. Schlögl, B. Obermaier, and M. Pregenzer. 2000b. Current trends in Graz brain-computer interface (BCI) research. *IEEE Transactions on Neural Systems and Rehabilitation Engineering* 8(2): 216–219.

Pfurtscheller, G., C. Neuper, H. Ramoser, and J. Müller-Gerking. 1999. Visually guided motor imagery activates sensorimotor areas in humans. *Neuroscience Letters* 269(3): 153–156.

Pfurtscheller, G. and F. H. Lopes da Silva. 1999. Event-related EEG/MEG synchronization and desynchronization: basic principles. *Clinical Neurophysiology* 110(11):1842–1857.

Pfurtscheller, G., C. Neuper, A. Schlögl, and K. Lugger. 1998. Separability of EEG signals recorded during right and left motor imagery using adaptive autoregressive parameters. *IEEE Transactions on Rehabilitation Engineering* 6(3):316–325.

Pfurtscheller, G. and C. Neuper. 1997. Motor imagery activates primary sensorimotor area in humans. *Neuroscience Letters* 239(2–3):65–68.

Pfurtscheller, G., C. Neuper, D. Flotzinger, and M. Pregenzer. 1997. EEG-based discrimination between imagination of right and left hand movement. *Electroencephalography and Clinical Neurophysiology* 103(6):642–651.

Pfurtscheller, G., J. Kalcher, C. Neuper, D. Flotzinger, and M. Pregenzer. 1996. On-line EEG classification during externally-paced hand movements using a neural network-based classifier. *Electroencephalography and Clinical Neurophysiology* 99(5):416–425.

Pfurtscheller, G., D. Flotzinger, M. Pregenzer, J. R. Wolpaw, and D. J. McFarland. 1995. EEG-based brain computer interface (BCI). Search for optimal electrode positions and frequency components. *Medical Progress through Technology* 21(3):111–121.

Pfurtscheller, G., D. Flotzinger, and J. Kalcher. 1993. Brain-computer interface—a new communication device for handicapped persons. *Journal of Microcomputer Applications* 16(3):293–299.

Pfurtscheller, G. 1989. Functional topography during sensorimotor activation studied with event-related desynchronization mapping. *Journal of Clinical Neurophysiology* 6(1): 75–84.

Pfurtscheller, G. and A. Aranibar. 1979. Evaluation of event-related desynchronization (ERD) preceding and following self-paced movements. *Electroencephalography and Clinical Neurophysiology* 46(2):138–146.

Pfurtscheller, G. and A. Aranibar. 1977. Event-related cortical desynchronization detected by power measurements of scalp EEG. *Electroencephalography and Clinical Neurophysiology* 42(6):817–826.

Pham, M., T. Hinterberger, N. Neumann, A. Kübler, N. Hofmayer, A. Grether, B. Wilhelm, J. J. Vatine, and N. Birbaumer. 2005. An auditory brain-computer interface based on the self-regulation of slow cortical potentials. *Journal for Neurorehabilitation and Neural Repair* 19(3):206–218.

Pham, D.-T. 1996. Blind separation of instantaneous mixture of sources via the Gaussian mutual information criterion. *IEEE Transactions on Signal Processing* 44(11):2668–2779.

Philiastides, M. G., R. Ratcliff, and P. Sajda. 2006. Neural representation of task difficulty and decision making during perceptual categorization: a timing diagram. *Journal of Neuroscience* 26(35):8965–8975.

Philiastides, M. G. and P. Sajda. 2006. Temporal characterization of the neural correlates of perceptual decision making in the human brain. *Cerebral Cortex* 16(4):509–518.

Piccione, F., F. Giorgi, P. Tonin, K. Priftis, S. Giove, S. Silvoni, G. Palmas, and F. Beverina. 2006. P300-based brain computer interface: Reliability and performance in healthy and paralysed participants. *Clinical Neurophysiology* 117(3):531–537.

Pierce, J. R. 1980. An introduction to information theory: symbols, signals and noise. New York: Dover Publications, 2nd edition.

Pineda, J. A., D. S. Silverman, A. Vankov, and J. Hestenes. 2003. Learning to control brain rhythms: making a brain-computer interface possible. *IEEE Transactions on Neural Systems and Rehabilitation Engineering* 11(2):181–184.

Platt, M. L. and P. W. Glimcher. 1999. Neural correlates of decision variables in parietal cortex. *Nature* 400(6741):233–238.

Poggio, T. and F. Girosi. 1990. Networks for approximation and learning. *Proceedings of the IEEE* 78(9):1481–1497.

Polich, J., editor. 2003. Detection of change: Event-related potential and fMRI findings. Boston: Kluwer Academic Publishers.

Polich, J. 1989. Habituation of P300 from auditory stimuli. *Psychobiology* 17:19–28.

Pope, A. T., E. H. Bogart, and D. S. Bartolome. 1995. Biocybernetic system evaluates indices of operator engagement on automated task. *Biological Psychology* 40(1–2):187–195.

Posner, M. I. 1980. Orienting of attention. *Quarterly Journal of Experimental Psychology* 32(1):3–25.

Pregenzer, M. and G. Pfurtscheller. 1999. Frequency component selection of an EEG-based brain to computer interface. *IEEE Transactions on Rehabilitation Engineering* 7(4):413–419.

Pregenzer, M., G. Pfurtscheller, and D. Flotzinger. 1996. Automated feature selection with a distinction sensitive learning vector quantizer. *Neurocomputing* 11(1):19–29.

Pregenzer, M., G. Pfurtscheller, and D. Flotzinger. 1994. Selection of electrode positions for an EEG-based brain computer interface (BCI). *Biomedizinische Technik* 39(10): 164–169.

Principe, J. C., J. W. Fisher III, and D. Xu. 2000. Information theoretic learning. In *Unsupervised Adaptive Filtering*, edited by Simon Haykin. New York: Wiley.

Prinzel, L. J., F. G. Freeman, M. W. Scerbo, P. J. Mikulka, and A. T. Pope. 2000. A closed-loop system for examining psychophysiological measures for adaptive task allocation. *International Journal of Aviation Psychology* 10(4):393–410.

Puce, A., T. Allison, M. Asgari, J. C. Gore, and G. McCarthy. 1996. Differential sensitivity of human visual cortex to faces, letterstrings, and textures: A functional magnetic resonance imaging study. *Journal of Neuroscience* 16(16):5205–5215.

Pudil, P., J. Novovicová, and J. Kittler. 1994. Floating search methods in feature selection. *Pattern Recognition Letters* 15(11):1119–1125.

Pulvermüller, F., B. Mohr, H. Schleichert, and R. Veit. 2000. Operant conditioning of left-hemispheric slow cortical potentials and its effect on word processing. *Biological Psychology* 53(2–3):177–125.

QT4. QT library version 4. Available at http://www.trolltech.com/.

Quick, R. F. 1974. A vector magnitude model of contrast detection. *Kybernetik* 16(2): 65–67.

Ramoser, H., J. Müller-Gerking, and G. Pfurtscheller. 2000. Optimal spatial filtering of single trial EEG during imagined hand movement. *IEEE Transactions on Rehabilitation Engineering* 8(4):441–446.

Raymond, J., I. Sajid, L. A. Parkinson, and J. H. Gruzelier. 2005. Biofeedback and dance performance: a preliminary investigation. *Applied Psychophysiology and Biofeedback* 30(1):64–73.

Renyi, A. 1961. On measures of entropy and information. In *Proceedings of the Fourth Berkeley Symposium Mathematical Statistics and Probability*: 547–561, Berkeley Calif. University of California Press.

Rieke, F., D. Warland, R. de Ruyter van Steveninck, and W. Bialek. 1999. Spikes— exploring the neural code. Cambridge Mass: The MIT Press.

Rijsbergen, C. J. 1979. Information retrieval. Available at http://www.dcs.gla.ac.uk/˜iain/keith/.

Ringholz, G. M., S. H. Appel, M. Bradshaw, N. A. Cooke, D. M. Mosnik, and P. E. Schulz. 2005. Prevalence and patterns of cognitive impairment in sporadic ALS. *Neurology* 65 (4):586–590.

Rizzolatti, G., L. Fogassi, and V. Gallese. 2001. Neurophysiological mechanisms underlying the understanding and imitation of action. *Nature reviews. Neuroscience* 2(9): 661–670.

Rizzuto, D. S., A. N. Mamelak, W. W. Sutherling, I. Fineman, and R. A. Andersen. 2005. Spatial selectivity in human ventrolateral prefrontal cortex. *Nature Neuroscience* 8(4): 415–417.

Roberts, S. J. and W. D. Penny. 2000. Real-time brain-computer interfacing: a preliminary study using Bayesian learning. *Medical & Biological Engineering & Computing* 38(1): 56–61.

Rockstroh, B., N. Birbaumer, T. Elbert, and W. Lutzenberger. 1984. Operant control of EEG and event-related and slow brain potentials. *Biofeedback and Self-Regulation* 9(2): 139–160.

Rockstroh, B., T. Elbert, W. Lutzenberger, and N. Birbaumer. 1982. The effects of slow cortical potentials on response speed. *Psychophysiology* 19(2):211–217.

Rohde, M. M., S. L. BeMent, J. E. Huggins, S. P. Levine, R. K. Kushwaha, and L. A. Schuh. 2002. Quality estimation of subdurally recorded, event-related potentials based on signal-to-noise ratio. *IEEE Transactions on Biomedical Engineering* 49(1):31–40.

Romo, R., A. Hernandez, A. Zainos, C. Brody, and E. Salinas. 2002. Exploring the cortical evidence of a sensory-discrimination process. *Philosophical Transactions of the Royal Society of London. Series B, Biological sciences* 357(1424):1039–1051.

Ron Angevin, R., A. Reyes-Lecuona, and A. Diaz-Estrella. 2004. The use of virtual reality to improve BCI training techniques. In *Proceedings of the 2nd International Brain-Computer Interface Workshop and Training Course* vol. 49 (Suppl.Vol.1): 79–80, Graz, Austria. Biomed Tech (Berl).

Rose, F. D., B. M. Brooks, and A. A. Rizzo. 2005. Virtual reality in brain damage rehabilitation: review. *Cyberpsychology & Behavior: the Impact of the Internet, Multimedia and Virtual Reality on Behavior and Society* 8(3):241–262. discussion 263–71.

Rossion, B., C. A. Joyce, G. W. Cottrell, and M. J. Tarr. 2003. Early laterization and orientation tuning for face, word, object processing in the visual cortex. *NeuroImage* 20 (3):1609–1624.

Rottig, D., B. Leplow, K. Eger, A. C. Ludolph, M. Graf, and S. Zierz. 2006. Only subtle cognitive deficits in non-bulbar amyotrophic lateral sclerosis patients. *Journal of Neurology* 253(3):333–339.

Roweis, S. T. and L. K. Saul. 2000. Nonlinear dimensionality reduction by locally linear embedding. *Science* 290(5500):2323–2326.

rtsBCI. Graz brain-computer interface real-time open source package. Available at http://sourceforge.net/projects/biosig/.

Saad, D., editor. 1998. On-line learning in neural networks. Cambridge University Press.

Sajda, P., A. Gerson, K. R. Müller, B. Blankertz, and L. Parra. 2003. A data analysis competition to evaluate machine learning algorithms for use in brain-computer interfaces. *IEEE Transactions on Neural Systems and Rehabilitation Engineering* 11(2):184–185.

Salanova, V., H. H. Morris, P. C. Van Ness, H. Luders, D. Dinner, and E. Wyllie. 1993. Comparison of scalp electroencephalogram with subdural electrocorticogram recordings and functional mapping in frontal lobe epilepsy. *Archives of Neurology* 50(3):294–299.

Sammon, Jr., J. W. 1969. A nonlinear mapping for data structure analysis. *IEEE Transactions on Computers* C-18(5):401–409.

Sanchez-Vives, M. V. and M. Slater. 2005. From presence to consciousness through virtual reality. *Nature reviews. Neuroscience* 6(4):332–339.

Santhanam, G., S. I. Ryu, B. M. Yu, A. Afshar, and K. V. Shenoy. 2006. A high-performance brain-computer interface. *Nature* 442(7099):195–198.

Saon, G. and M. Padmanabhan. 2000. Minimum Bayes error feature selection for continuous speech recognition. In *Advances in Neural Information Processing Systems (NIPS 99)*: 800–806, Cambridge, Mass. The MIT Press.

Scerbo, M. W., F. G. Freeman, and P. J. Mikulka. 2003. A brain-based system for adaptive automation. *Theoretical Issues in Ergonomics Science* 4(1–2):200–219.

Schack, B., N. Vath, H. Petsche, H. G. Geissler, and E. Moller. 2002. Phase-coupling of theta-gamma EEG rhythms during short-term memory processing. *International Journal of Psychophysiology* 44(2):143–163.

Schalk, G., D. J. McFarland, T. Hinterberger, N. Birbaumer, and J. R. Wolpaw. 2004. BCI2000: a general-purpose brain-computer interface (BCI) system. *IEEE Transactions on Biomedical Engineering* 51(6):1034–1043.

Schalk, G., J. R. Wolpaw, D. J. McFarland, and G. Pfurtscheller. 2000. EEG-based communication: presence of an error potential. *Clinical Neurophysiology* 111(12):2138–2144.

Scheffers, M. K., R. Johnson, and D. S. Ruchkin. 1991. P300 in patients with unilateral temporal lobectomies: the effects of reduced stimulus quality. *Psychophysiology* 28(3): 274–284.

Scherberger, H., M. R. Jarvis, and R. A. Andersen. 2005. Cortical local field potential encodes movement intentions in the posterior parietal cortex. *Neuron* 46(2):347–354.

Scherer, R., F. Lee, R. Leeb, A. Schlögl, H. Bischof, and G. Pfurtscheller. In revision. Towards asynchronous (uncued) brain-computer communication: Navigation through virtual worlds. *IEEE Transactions on Biomedical Engineering*.

Scherer, R., G. R. Müller, C. Neuper, B. Graimann, and G. Pfurtscheller. 2004a. An asynchronously controlled EEG-based virtual keyboard: improvement of the spelling rate. *IEEE Transactions on Biomedical Engineering* 51(6):979–984.

Scherer, R., A. Schlögl, G. R. Müller-Putz, and G. Pfurtscheller. 2004b. Inside the Graz-BCI: rtsBCI. In *Biomedizinische Technik: Proceedings of the 2nd International Brain-Computer Interface Workshop and Training Course (Graz)*: 81–82. Boenick, U. and Bolz, A. (Berlin Schiele & Schön).

Scherer, R., B. Graimann, J. E. Huggins, S. P. Levine, and G. Pfurtscheller. 2003. Frequency component selection for an ECoG-based brain-computer interface. *Biomedizinische Technik* 48(1–2):31–36.

Scherg, M. 1994. From EEG source localization to source imaging. *Acta neurologica Scandinavica. Supplementum* 152:29–30.

Scherg, M. 1992. Functional imaging and localization of electromagnetic brain activity. *Brain Topography* 5(2):103–111.

Schlögl, A. 2006. A general data format (GDF) for biomedical signals. Available at http://arxiv.org/abs/cs.DB/0608052.

Schlögl, A., F. Lee, H. Bischof, and G. Pfurtscheller. 2005. Characterization of four-class motor imagery EEG data for the BCI-competition 2005. *Journal of Neural Engineering* 2(4):L14–L22.

Schlögl, A., C. Keinrath, R. Scherer, and G. Pfurtscheller. 2003. Information transfer of an EEG-based brain-computer interface. In *Proceedings of the 1st International IEEE EMBS Conference on Neural Engineering*: 641–644.

Schlögl, A., C. Neuper, and G. Pfurtscheller. 2002. Estimating the mutal information of an EEG-based Brain-Computer Interface. *Biomedizinische Technik* 47(1–2):3–8.

Schlögl, A. 2000a. The electroencephalogram and the adaptive autoregressive model: theory and applications. Aachen, Germany: Shaker Verlag.

Schlögl, A. 2000b. The electroencephalogram and the adaptive autoregressive model: theory and applications. PhD thesis, Technical University Graz, Graz.

Schlögl, A. Missing values and NaN-toolbox for Matlab. Available at http://www.dpmi.tu-graz.ac.at/~schloegl/matlab/NaN/.

Schlögl, A. Time series analysis toolbox for Matlab. Available at http://www.dpmi.tu-graz.ac.at/~schloegl/matlab/tsa/.

Schlögl, A., P. Anderer, M. J. Barbanoj, G. Gruber G. Klösch, J. L. Lorenzo, O. Filz, M. Koivuluoma, I. Rezek, S. J. Roberts, A. Värri, P. Rappelsberger, G. Pfurtscheller, and G. Dorffner. 1999a. Artifact processing of the sleep EEG in the "SIESTA"-project. In *Proceedings EMBEC'99*: 1644–1645, Vienna, Austria.

Schlögl, A., P. Anderer, S. J. Roberts, M. Pregenzer, and G. Pfurtscheller. 1999b. Artefact detection in sleep EEG by the use of Kalman filtering. In *Proceedings EMBEC'99*: 1648–1649, Vienna, Austria.

Schlögl, A., B. Kemp, T. Penzel, D. Kunz, S.-L. Himanen, A. Värri, G. Dorffner, and G. Pfurtscheller. 1999c. Quality control of polysomnographic sleep data by histogram and entropy analysis. *Clinical Neurophysiology* 110(12):2165–2170.

Schlögl, A. and G. Pfurtscheller. 1998. Considerations on adaptive autoregressive modelling in EEG analysis. In *Proc. of 1st Int. Symposium on Communication Systems and Digital Signal Processing CSDSP'98*, edited by Z. Ghassemlooy and M. R. Saatchi vol. 1: 367–370.

Schlögl, A., D. Flotzinger, and G. Pfurtscheller. 1997a. Adaptive autoregressive modeling used for single-trial EEG classification. *Biomedizinische Technik* 42(6):162–167.

Schlögl, A., K. Lugger, and G. Pfurtscheller. 1997b. Using adaptive autoregressive parameters for a brain-computer-interface experiment. In *Proceedings of the 19th Annual International Conference of the IEEE Engineering in Medicine and Biology Society* vol. 4: 1533–1535.

Schölkopf, B. and A. Smola. 2002. Learning with kernels. Cambridge, Mass.: The MIT Press.

Schölkopf, B., J. C. Platt, J. Shawe-Taylor, A. J. Smola, and R. C. Williamson. 2001. Estimating the support of a high-dimensional distribution. *Neural Computation* 13(7): 1443–1471.

Schölkopf, B., B. Smola, and K. R. Müller. 1998. Nonlinear component analysis as a kernel eigenvalue problem. *Neural Computation* 10(5):1299–1319.

Schraudolph, N. N. 1999. Local gain adaptation in stochastic gradient descent. In *ICANN99. Ninth International Conference on Artificial Neural Networks* vol. 2: 569–574.

Schröder, M., T. N. Lal, T. Hinterberger, M. Bogdan, N. J. Hill, N. Birbaumer, W. Rosenstiel, and B. Schölkopf. 2005. Robust EEG channel selection across subjects for brain computer interfaces. *EURASIP Journal on Applied Signal Processing, Special Issue: Trends in Brain Computer Interfaces* 19:3103–3112.

Schultz, W. 2004. Neural coding of basic reward terms of animal learning theory, game theory, microeconomics and behavioural ecology. *Current Opinion in Neurobiolology* 14(2):139–147.

Schwartz, A. B. 2004a. Direct cortical control of 3D neuroprosthetic devices. In *4th Forum of European Neuroscience*, Lisbon, Portugal.

Schwartz, A. B. 2004b. Cortical neural prosthetics. *Annual Review of Neuroscience* 27: 487–507.

Schwartz, A., D. M. Taylor, and S. I. Tillery. 2001. Extraction algorithms for cortical control of arm prosthetics. *Current Opinion in Neurobiology* 11(6):701–707.

Schwartz, A. B., R. E. Kettner, and A. P. Georgopoulos. 1988. Primate motor cortex and free arm movements to visual targets in three-dimensional space. I. Relations between single cell discharge and direction of movement. *Journal of Neuroscience* 8(8):2913–2927.

Sellers, E. W. and E. Donchin. 2006. A P300-based brain-computer interface: initial tests by ALS patients. *Clinical Neurophysiology* 117(3):538–548.

Sellers, E. W., D. J. Krusienski, D. J. McFarland, T. M. Vaughan, and J. R. Wolpaw. 2006a. A P300 event-related potential brain-computer interface (BCI): The effects of matrix size and inter stimulus interval on performance. *Biological Psychology* 73(3):242–252.

Sellers, E. W., A. Kübler, and E. Donchin. 2006b. Brain computer interface research at the University of South Florida Cognitive Psychophysiology Laboratory: the P300 Speller. *IEEE Transactions on Neural Systems and Rehabilitation Engineering* 14(2):221–224.

Sellers, E. W., T. M. Vaughan, D. J. McFarland, D. J. Krusienski, S. A. Mackler, R. A. Cardillo, G. Schalk, S. A. Binder-Macleod, and J. R. Wolpaw. 2006c. Daily use of a brain-computer interface by a man with ALS. Poster presented at the Society for Neuroscience annual meeting, Atlanta, GA.

Sellers, E., G. Schalk, and E. Donchin. 2003. The P300 as a typing tool: tests of brain computer interface with an ALS patient. *Psychophysiology* 40:77.

Serby, H., E. Yom-Tov, and G. F. Inbar. 2005. An improved p300-based brain-computer interface. *IEEE Transactions on Neural Systems and Rehabilitation Engineering* 13(1): 89–98.

Serruya, M. D., N. G. Hatsopoulos, L. Paninski, M. R. Fellows, and J. P. Donoghue. 2002. Instant neural control of a movement signal. *Nature* 416(6877):141–142.

Shadlen, M. N. and W. T. Newsome. 2001. Neural basis of perceptual decision making in the parietal cortex (area LIP) of the rhesus monkey. *Journal of Neurophysiology* 86(4): 1916–1936.

Shannon, C. E. and W. Weaver. 1949. The mathematical theory of communication. Urbana: University of Illinois Press.

Shenoy, P., M. Krauledat, B. Blankertz, R. P. N. Rao, and K.-R. Müller. 2006. Towards adaptive classification for BCI. *Journal of Neural Engineering* 3(1):R13–R23.

Shenoy, K. V., D. Meeker, S. Cao, S. A. Kureshi, B. Pesaran, C. A. Buneo, A. P. Batista, P. P. Mitra, J. W. Burdick, and R. A. Andersen. 2003. Neural prosthetic control signals from plan activity. *Neuroreport* 14(4):591–596.

Sheridan, T. B. 1992. Telerobotics, automation, and human supervisory control. Cambridge, Mass.: The MIT Press.

Shpigelman, L., Y. Singer, R. Paz, and E. Vaadia. 2003. Spikernels: Embedding spiking neurons in inner product spaces. In *Advances in Neural Information Processing Systems (NIPS 02)*, edited by S. Becker, S. Thrun, and K. Obermayer vol. 15, Cambridge, MA. The MIT Press.

Singh, K. and S. H. Scott. 2003. A motor learning strategy reflects neural circuitry for limb control. *Nature Neuroscience* 6(4):399–403.

Sitaram, R., H. Zhang, C. Guan, M. Thulasidas, Y. Hoshi, A. Ishikawa, K. Shimizu, and N. Birbaumer. 2007. Temporal classification of multichannel near-infrared spectroscopy signals of motor imagery for developing a brain-computer interface. *NeuroImage* 34(4): 1416–1427.

Sitaram, R., A. Caria, R. Veit, K. Uludag, T. Gaber, A. Kübler, and N. Birbaumer. 2006. Functional magnetic resonance imaging based BCI for neurorehabilitation. Paper presented at the 3rd International Brain-Computer Interface Workshop and Training Course, Graz, Austria.

Sitaram, R., Y. Hoshi, and C. Guan, editors. 2005. Near infrared spectroscopy based brain-computer interfaces, vol. 5852. Bellingham, Wash.: Society of Photo-Optical Instrumentation Engineers.

Skrandies, W. 2005. Brain mapping of visual evoked activity—topographical and functional components. *Acta Neurologica Taiwanica* 14(4):164–178.

Slater, M., A. Steed, and Y. Chrysanthou. 2002. Computer graphics and virtual environments: from realism to real-time. Harlow, UK: Addison-Wesley.

Slater, M. and M. Usoh. 1993. Presence in immersive virtual environments. In *Proceedings IEEE Virtual Reality Annual International Symposium*: 90–96, Seattle, Wash.

Smith, E. and M. Delargy. 2005. Locked-in syndrome. *British Medical Journal* 330(7488): 406–409.

Smith, M. E., A. Gevins, H. Brown, A. Karnik, and R. Du. 2001. Monitoring task loading with multivariate EEG measures during complex forms of human-computer interaction. *Human Factors* 43(3):366–380.

Smola, A. J. and B. Schölkopf. 1998. A tutorial on support vector regression. NeuroCOLT Technical Report NC-TR-98-030, Royal Holloway College, University of London, UK.

Snyder, L. H., A. P. Batista, and R. A. Andersen. 1997. Coding of intention in the posterior parietal cortex. *Nature* 386(6621):167–170.

Solodkin, A., P. Hlustik, E. E. Chen, and S. L. Small. 2004. Fine modulation in network activation during motor execution and motor imagery. *Cerebral Cortex* 14(11):1246–1255.

Sonnenburg, S., G. Rätsch, and B. Schölkopf. 2005. Large scale genomic sequence SVM classifiers. In *Proceedings of the International Conference on Machine Learning, ICML.*

Spalding, M. C., M. Velliste, B. Jarosiewicz, and A. B. Schwartz. 2005. 3-D cortical control of an anthropomorphic robotic arm for reaching and retrieving. Program No. 401.3. 2005 Abstract Viewer/Itinerary Planner. Washington, DC. Online. Society for Neuroscience.

Spataro, L., J. Dilgen, S. Retterer, A. J. Spence, M. Isaacson, J. N. Turner, and W. Shain. 2005. Dexamethasone treatment reduces astroglia responses to inserted neuroprosthetic devices in rat neocortex. *Experimental Neurology* 194(2):289–300.

Speckmann, E. J., H. Caspers, and C. W. Elger. 1984. Neuronal mechanisms underlying the generation of field potentials. Berlin: Springer.

Squires, K. C., E. Donchin, R. I. Herning, and G. McCarthy. 1977. On the influence of task relevance and stimulus probability on event-related-potential components. *Electroencephalography and Clinical Neurophysiology* 42(1):1–14.

Squires, K. C., C. Wickens, N. K. Squires, and E. Donchin. 1976. The effect of stimulus sequence on the waveform of the cortical event-related potential. *Science* 193(4258): 1142–1146.

Stanislaw, H. and N. Todorow. 1999. Calculation of signal detection measures. *Behaviour Research Methods, Instruments & Computers* 31(1):137–149.

Sterman, M. B. and C. A. Mann. 1995. Concepts and applications of EEG analysis in aviation performance evaluation. *Biological Psychology* 40(1–2):115–130.

Sterman, M. B. 1977. Sensorimotor EEG operant conditioning: experimental and clinical effects. *Pavlovian Journal of Biological Sciences* 12(2):63–92.

Stipacek, A., R. H. Grabner, C. Neuper, A. Fink, and A. C. Neubauer. 2003. Sensitivity of human EEG alpha band desynchronization to different working memory components and increasing levels of memory load. *Neuroscience Letters* 353(3):193–196.

Strehl, U., T. Trevorrow, R. Veit, T. Hinterberger, B. Kotchoubey, M. Erb, and N. Birbaumer. 2006. Deactivation of brain areas during self-regulation of slow cortical potentials in seizure patients. *Applied Psychophysiology and Biofeedback* 31(1):85–94.

Studierstube. Augmented reality project. Available at http://www.studierstube.org.

Sugiyama, S. and K.-R. Müller. 2005. Input-dependent estimation of generalization error under covariate shift. *Statistics and Decisions* 23(4):249–279.

Super, H., H. Spekreijse, and V. A. Lamme. 2001. Two distinct modes of sensory processing observed in monkey primary visual cortex. *Nature Neuroscience* 4(3):304–310.

Sutter, E. E. 1992. The brain response interface: communication through visually-induced electrical brain responses. *Journal of Microcomputer Applications* 15(1):31–45.

Sutton, R. S. and A. G. Barto. 1998. Reinforcement learning: An introduction. Cambridge, Mass.: The MIT Press.

Sutton, R. S. 1992. Adapting bias by gradient descent: an incremental version of delta-bar-delta. In *AAAI 92. Proceedings Tenth National Conference on Artificial Intelligence*: 171–176.

Sykacek, P., S. Roberts, M. Stokes, E. Curran, M. Gibbs, and L. Pickup. 2003. Probabilistic methods in BCI research. *IEEE Transactions on Neural Systems and Rehabilitation Engineering* 11(2):192–195.

Talwar, S. K., S. Xu, E. S. Hawley, S. A. Weiss, K. A. Moxon, and J. K. Chapin. 2002. Rat navigation guided by remote control. *Nature* 417(6884):37–38.

Tarr, M. J. and W. H. Warren. 2002. Virtual reality in behavioral neuroscience and beyond. *Nature Neuroscience* 5(Suppl):1089–1092.

Tax, D. M. J. and R. P. W. Duin. 2001. Uniform object generation for optimizing one-class classifiers. *Journal for Machine Learning Research* 155–173.

Taylor, D. M., S. I. H. Tillery, and A. B. Schwartz. 2003. Information conveyed through brain-control: cursor versus robot. *IEEE Transactions on Neural Systems and Rehabilitation Engineering* 11(2):195–199.

Taylor, D. M., S. I. H. Tillery, and A. B. Schwartz. 2002. Direct cortical control of 3D neuroprosthetic devices. *Science* 296(5574):1829–1832.

Taylor, D. M. and A. B. Schwartz. 2001. Using virtual reality to test the feasibility of controlling an upper limb fes system directly from multiunit activity in the motor cortex. In *Proceedings of the 6th Annual IFESS Conference*, Cleveland, Ohio.

Tenenbaum, J. B., V. de Silva, and J. C. Langford. 2000. A global geometric framework for nonlinear dimensionality reduction. *Science* 290(5500):2319–2323.

Tesche, C. D. and J. Karhu. 1997. Somatosensory evoked magnetic fields arising from sources in the human cerebellum. *Brain Research* 744(1):23–31.

Thomson, D. J. 1982. Spectrum estimation and harmonic analysis. *Proceedings of the IEEE* 70(9):1055–1096.

Thorpe, S., D. Fize, and C. Marlot. 1996. Speed of processing in the human visual system. *Nature* 381(6582):520–522.

Thulasidas, M., C. Guan, and J. Wu. 2006. Robust classification of eeg signal for brain-computer interface. *IEEE Transactions on Neural Systems and Rehabilitation Engineering* 14(1):24–29.

Tillery, S. I. and D. M. Taylor. 2004. Signal acquisition and analysis for cortical control of neuroprosthetics. *Current Opinion in Neurobiolology* 14(6):758–762.

Tillery, S. I. H., D. M. Taylor, and A. B. Schwartz. 2003. Training in cortical control of neuroprosthetic devices improves signal extraction from small neuronal ensembles. *Reviews in the Neurosciences* 14(1–2):107–119.

Tillery, S. H., D. Taylor, R. Isaacs, and A. Schwartz. 2000. Online control of a prosthetic arm from motor cortical signals. In *Society for Neuroscience Abstracts* vol. 26.

Todorov, E., R. Shadmehr, and E. Bizzi. 1997. Augmented feedback presented in a virtual environment accelerates learning of a difficult motor task. *Journal of motor behavior* 29 (2):147–158.

Tomioka, R., G. Dornhege, K. Aihara, and K. R. Müller. 2006. An iterative algorithm for spatio-temporal filter optimization. In *Proceedings of the 3rd International Brain-Computer Interface Workshop and Training Course 2006*: 22–23. Verlag der Technischen Universität Graz.

Torkkola, K. 2003. Feature extraction by non-paramatric mutual information maximization. *Journal of Machine Learning Research* 3(7–8):1415–1438.

Townsend, G., B. Graimann, and G. Pfurtscheller. 2006. A comparison of common spatial patterns with complex band power features in a four-class BCI experiment. *IEEE Transactions on Biomedical Engineering* 53(4):642–651.

Townsend, G., B. Graimann, and G. Pfurtscheller. 2004. Continuous EEG classification during motor imagery - simulation of an asynchronous BCI. *IEEE Transactions on Neural Systems and Rehabilitation Engineering* 12(2):258–265.

Trejo, L. J., R. Rosipal, and B. Matthews. 2006. Brain-computer interfaces for 1-D and 2-D cursor control: designs using volitional control of the EEG spectrum or steady-state visual evoked potentials. *IEEE Transactions on Neural Systems and Rehabilitation Engineering* 14(2):225–229.

Truccolo, W., U. T. Eden, M. R. Fellows, J. P. Donoghue, and E. N. Brown. 2005. A point process framework for relating neural spiking activity to spiking history, neural ensemble and extrinsic covariate effects. *Journal of Neurophysiology* 93(2):1074–1089.

Turk, M. and A. Pentland. 1991. Face recognition using eigenfaces. *Journal of Cognitive Neuroscience* 3(1):71–86.

Turner, J. N., W. Shain, D. H. Szarowski, M. Andersen, S. Martins, M. Isaacson, and H. Craighead. 1999. Cerebral astrocyte response to micromachined silicon implants. *Experimental Neurology* 156(1):33–49.

Oosterom, A.van. 1991. History and evolution of methods for solving the inverse problem. *Journal of Clinical Neurophysiology* 8(4):371–380.

van Schie, H. T., R. B. Mars, M. G. H. Coles, and H. Bekkering. 2004. Modulation of activity in medial frontal and motor cortices during error observation. *Nature Neuroscience* 7(5):549–554.

VanRullen, R. and S. J. Thorpe. 2001. The time course of visual processing: from early perception to decision-making. *Journal of Cognitive Neuroscience* 13(4):454–461.

Vapnik, V. N. 1998. Statistical learning theory. New York: Wiley.

Vapnik, V. N. 1995. The Nature of Statistical Learning Theory. New York: Springer Verlag.

Vaughan, T. M., D. J. McFarland, G. Schalk, W. A. Sarnacki, D. J. Krusienski, E. W. Sellers, and J. R. Wolpaw. 2006. The Wadsworth BCI research and development program: At home with BCI. *IEEE Transactions on Neural Systems and Rehabilitation Engineering* 14(2):229–233.

Vaughan, T. M. and J. R. Wolpaw, editors. 2006. The third international meething on brain-computer interface technology: Making a difference, vol. 14.

Vaughan, T. M., D. J. McFarland, G. Schalk, E. Sellers, and J. R. Wolpaw. 2003a. Multichannel data from a brain-computer interface (BCI) speller using a P300 (i.e., oddball) protocol. *Society for Neuroscience Abstracts* 28.

Vaughan, T. M., W. J. Heetderks, L. J. Trejo, W. Z. Rymer, M. Weinrich, M. M. Moore, A. Kübler, B. H. Dobkin, N. Birbaumer, E. Donchin, E. W. Wolpaw, and J. R. Wolpaw. 2003b. Brain-computer interface technology: A review of the Second International Meeting. *IEEE Transactions on Neural Systems and Rehabilitation Engineering* 11(2): 94–109.

Vaughan, T. M., D. J. McFarland, G. Schalk, W. A. Sarnacki, L. Robinson, and J. R. Wolpaw. 2001. EEG-based brain-computer interface: development of a speller application. *Society for Neuroscience Abstracts* 26.

Vaughan, G. V., B. Elliston, T. Tromey, and I. L. Taylor. GNU autoconf, automake and libtool. Available at http://sourceware.org/autobook/.

Vaughan, T. M., L. A. Miner, D. J. McFarland, and J. R. Wolpaw. 1998. EEG-based communication: analysis of concurrent EMG activity. *Electroencephalography and Clinical Neurophysiology* 107(6):428–433.

Vaughan, T. M., J. R. Wolpaw, and E. Donchin. 1996. EEG-based communication: prospects and problems. *IEEE Transactions on Rehabilitation Engineering* 4(4):425–430.

Vidaurre, C. 2006. On-line adaptive classification for brain-computer interfaces. PhD thesis, Dept. Ingeniería Eléctrica y Electrónica, Universidad Pública de Navarra.

Vidaurre, C., A. Schlögl, R. Cabeza, R. Scherer, and G. Pfurtscheller. 2006. A fully on-line adaptive BCI. *IEEE Transactions on Biomedical Engineering* 53(6):1214–1219.

Vidaurre, C., A. Schlögl, R. Cabeza, R. Scherer, and G. Pfurtscheller. 2005. Adaptive on-line classification for EEG-based brain computer interfaces with AAR parameters and band power estimates. *Biomedizinische Technik* 50(11):350–354.

Vidaurre, C., A. Schlögl, R. Cabeza, and G. Pfurtscheller. 2004a. About adaptive classifiers for brain computer interfaces. *Biomedizinische Technik* 49(1):85–86.

Vidaurre, C., A. Schlögl, R. Cabeza, and G. Pfurtscheller. 2004b. A fully on-line adaptive brain computer interface. *Biomedizinische Technik* 49(2):760–761.

VRjuggler. Open source virtual reality tool. Available at http://www.vrjuggler.org.

Wackermann, J. 1999. Towards a quantitative characterisation of functional states of the brain: from the non-linear methodology to the global linear description. *International Journal of Psychophysiology* 34(1):65–80.

Walter, W. G., R. Cooper, V. J. Aldridge, W. C. McCallum, and A. L. Winter. 1964. Contingent negative variation: An electric sign of sensorimotor association and expectancy in the human brain. *Nature* 25:380–384.

Wang, Y., R. Wang, X. Gao, B. Hong, and S. Gao. 2006. A practical VEP-based brain-computer interface. *IEEE Transactions on Neural Systems and Rehabilitation Engineering* 14(2):234–239.

Wang, T., H. Deng, and B. He. 2004. Classifying EEG-based motor imagery tasks by means of time-frequency synthesized spatial patterns. *Clinical Neurophysiology* 115 (12):2744–2753.

Wang, Y., P. Berg, and M. Scherg. 1999. Common spatial subspace decomposition applied to analysis of brain responses under multiple task conditions: a simulation study. *Clinical Neurophysiology* 110(4):604–614.

Webster, J. S., P. T. McFarland, L. J. Rapport, B. Morrill, L. A. Roades, and P. S. Abadee. 2001. Computer-assisted training for improving wheelchair mobility in unilateral neglect patients. *Archives of Physical Medicine and Rehabilitation* 82(6):769–775.

Weiskopf, N., K. Mathiak, S. W. Bock, F. Scharnowski, R. Veit, W. Grodd, R. Goebel, and N. Birbaumer. 2004a. Principles of a brain-computer interface (BCI) based on real-time functional magnetic resonance imaging (fMRI). *IEEE Transactions on Biomedical Engineering* 51(6):966–970.

Weiskopf, N., F. Scharnowski, R. Veit, R. Goebel, N. Birbaumer, and K. Mathiak. 2004b. Self-regulation of local brain activity using real-time functional magnetic resonance imaging (fMRI). *Journal of Physiology, Paris* 98(4–6):357–373.

Weiskopf, N., R. Veit, M. Erb, K. Mathiak, W. Grodd, R. Goebel, and N. Birbaumer. 2003. Physiological self-regulation of regional brain activity using real-time functional magnetic resonance imaging (fMRI): methodology and exemplary data. *NeuroImage* 19 (3):577–586.

Welch, G. and G. Bishop. 2001. An introduction to the Kalman filter. Technical Report 95–041, University of North Carolina at Chapel Hill.

Welch, P. 1967. The use of fast fourier transform for the estimation of power spectra: A method based on time averaging over short, modified periodograms. *IEEE Trans. Audio Electroacoustics* AU-15:70–73.

Wessberg, J., C. R. Stambaugh, J. D. Kralik, P. D. Beck, M. Laubach, J. K. Chapin, J. Kim, S. J. Biggs, M. A. Srinivasan, and M. A. Nicolelis. 2000. Real-time prediction of hand trajectory by ensembles of cortical neurons in primates. *Nature* 408(6810):361–365.

Wigmore, V., C. Tong, and J. R. Flanagan. 2002. Visuomotor rotations of varying size and direction compete for a single internal model in motor working memory. *Journal of experimental psychology. Human perception and performance* 28(2):447–457.

Wilhelm, B., M. Jordan, and N. Birbaumer. 2006. Communication in locked-in syndrome effects of imagery on salivary pH. *Neurology* 67(3):534–535.

Wilson, J. A., E. A. Felton, P. C. Garell, G. Schalk, and J. C. Williams. 2006. ECoG factors underlying multimodal control of a brain-computer interface. *IEEE Transactions on Neural Systems and Rehabilitation Engineering* 14(2):246–250.

Wolpaw, J. R. and D. J. McFarland. 2004. Control of a two-dimensional movement signal by a noninvasive brain-computer interface in humans. *Proceedings of the National Academy of Sciences of the United States of America* 101(51):17849–17854.

Wolpaw, J. R., D. J. McFarland, T. M. Vaughan, and G. Schalk. 2003. The Wadsworth Center brain-computer interface (BCI) research and development program. *IEEE Transactions on Neural Systems and Rehabilitation Engineering* 11(2):204–207.

Wolpaw, J. R., N. Birbaumer, D. J. McFarland, G. Pfurtscheller, and T. M. Vaughan. 2002. Brain-computer interfaces for communication and control. *Clinical Neurophysiology* 113(6):767–791.

Wolpaw, J. R., N. Birbaumer, W. J. Heetderks, D. J. McFarland, P. H. Peckham, G. Schalk, E. Donchin, L. A. Quatrano, C. J. Robinson, and T. M. Vaughan. 2000a. Brain-computer interface technology: a review of the first inernational meeting. *IEEE Transactions on Rehabilitation Engineering* 8(2):164–173.

Wolpaw, J. R., D. J. McFarland, and T. M. Vaughan. 2000b. Brain-computer interface research at the Wadsworth Center. *IEEE Transactions on Rehabilitation Engineering* 8 (2):222–226.

Wolpaw, J. R., H. Ramoser, D. J. McFarland, and G. Pfurtscheller. 1998. EEG-based communication: improved accuracy by response verification. *IEEE Transactions on Rehabilitation Engineering* 6(3):326–333.

Wolpaw, J. R., D. Flotzinger, G. Purtscheller, and D. J. McFarland. 1997. Timing of EEG-based cursor control. *Journal of Clinical Neurophysiology* 14(6):529–538.

Wolpaw, J. R. and D. J. McFarland. 1994. Multichannel EEG-based brain-computer communication. *Electroencephalography and Clinical Neurophysiology* 90(6):444–449.

Wolpaw, J. R., D. J. McFarland, G. W. Neat, and C. A. Forneris. 1991. An EEG-based brain-computer interface for cursor control. *Electroencephalography and Clinical Neurophysiology* 78(3):252–259.

Wood, F., S. Roth, and M. J. Black. 2006. Modeling neural population spiking activity with Gibbs distributions. In *Advances in Neural Information Processing Systems (NIPS 05)* vol. 17, Cambridge, MA. The MIT Press.

Wood, F., Prabhat, J. P. Donoghue, and M. J. Black. 2005. Inferring attentional state and kinematics from motor cortical firing rates. In *27th International Conference of the IEEE Engineering in Medicine and Biology Society*: 149–152.

Wood, F., M. J. Black, C. Vargas-Irwin, M. Fellows, and J. P. Donoghue. 2004. On the variability of manual spike sorting. *IEEE Transactions on Biomedical Engineering* 51 (6):912–918.

Wu, W., Y. Gao, E. Bienenstock, J. P. Donoghue, and M. J. Black. 2005. Bayesian population decoding of motor cortical activity using a Kalman filter. *Neural Computation* 18 (1):80–118.

Wu, W., M. J. Black, M. J. D. Mumford, Y. Gao, E. Bienenstock, and J. P. Donoghue. 2004a. Modeling and decoding motor cortical activity using a switching Kalman filter. *IEEE Transactions on Biomedical Engineering* 51(6):933–942.

Wu, W., A. Shaikhouni, J. P. Donoghue, and M. J. Black. 2004b. Closed-loop neural control of cursor motion using a Kalman filter. In *Conference Proceedings, 26th Annual International Conference of the IEEE Engineering in Medicine and Biology Society*: 4126–4129.

Xu, N., X. Gao, B. Hong, X. Miao, S. Gao, and F. Yang. 2004. BCI Competition 2003– Data set IIb: enhancing P300 wave detection using ICA-based subspace projections for BCI applications. *IEEE Transactions on Biomedical Engineering* 51(6):1067–1072.

Yamato, M., A. Monden, K. Matsumoto, K. Inoue, and K. Torii. 2000. Quick button selection with eye gazing for general GUI environment. In *International Conference on Software: Theory and Practice (ICS2000)*.

Yom-Tov, E. and G. F. Inbar. 2003. Detection of movement-related potentials from the electro-encephalogram for possible use in a brain-computer interface. *Medical & Biological Engineering & Computing* 41(1):85–93.

Yoo, S. S., T. Fairneny, N. K. Chen, S. E. Choo, L. P. Panych, H. Park, S. Y. Lee, and F. A. Jolesz. 2004. Brain-computer interface using fMRI: spatial navigation by thoughts. *Neuroreport* 15(10):1591–1595.

Zaveri, H. P., W. J. Williams, L. D. Iasemidis, and J. C. Sackellares. 1992. Time-frequency representation of electrocorticograms in temporal lobe epilepsy. *IEEE Transactions on Biomedical Engineering* 39(5):502–509.

Zenner, H. P., H. Leysieffer, M. Maassen, R. Lehner, T. Lenarz, J. Baumann, S. Keiner, P. K. Plinkert, and Jr. J. T. McElveen. 2000. Human studies of a piezoelectric transducer and a microphone for a totally implantable electronic hearing device. *The American Journal of Otology* 21(2):196–204.

Zhang, Z., Y. Wang, Y. Li, and X. Gao. 2004. BCI competition 2003—data set IV: An algorithm based on CSSD and FDA for classifying single-trial EEG. *IEEE Transactions on Biomedical Engineering* 51(6):1081–1086.

Ziehe, A. and K. R. Müller. 1998. TDSEP—an efficient algorithm for blind separation using time structure. In *Proceedings of the 8th International Conference on Artificial Neural Networks, ICANN'98*, edited by L. Niklasson, M. Bodén, and T. Ziemke, Perspectives in Neural Computing: 675–680, Berlin. Springer Verlag.

Zien, A., G. Rätsch, S. Mika, B. Schölkopf, T. Lengauer, and K.-R. Müller. 2000. Engineering support vector machine kernels that recognize translation initiation sites. *BioInformatics* 16(9):799–807.

Zrenner, E. 2002. Will retinal implants restore vision? *Science* 295(5557):1022–1025.

Contributors

Andersen, Richard A.
Division of Biology
California Institute of Technology
Pasadena, CA 91125

Anderson, Charles W.
Department of Computer Science
Colorado State University
Fort Collins, CO 80523

Andino, Sara Gonzalez
Electrical Neuroimaging Group
Department of Neurology
University Hospital Geneva (HUG)
1211 Geneva, Switzerland

Bensch, Michael
Wilhelm-Schickard-Institute for Computer Science
Eberhard-Karls-University Tübingen, Germany

Birbaumer, Niels
Institute of Medical Psychology and
Behavioural Neurobiology
Eberhard-Karls-University Tübingen
Gartenstr. 29
72074 Tübingen, Germany

National Institute of Health (NIH)
NINDS
Human Cortical Physiology Unit
Bethesda, USA

Birch, Gary E.
Neil Squire Society
220 - 2250 Boundary Rd.
Burnaby, B.C., V5M 3Z3, Canada

International Collaboration on
Repair Discoveries
The University of British Columbia
6270 University Blvd., Vancouver
British Columbia, V6T 1Z4, Canada

Department of Electrical and
Computer Engineering
The University of British Columbia
2356 Main Mall, Vancouver
V6T 1Z4, Canada

Bischof, Horst
Institute for Computer Graphics and Vision
Graz University of Technology
Inffeldgasse 16, A-8010 Graz, Austria

Black, Michael J.
Departments of Computer Science and Neuroscience
Brown University
Providence RI 02912

Blankertz, Benjamin
Fraunhofer–Institute FIRST   Technical University Berlin
Intelligent Data Analysis Group (IDA)   Str. des 17. Juni 135
Kekuléstr. 7, 12489 Berlin, Germany   10 623 Berlin, Germany

Borisoff, Jaimie F.
Neil Squire Society   International Collaboration on
220 - 2250 Boundary Rd.   Repair Discoveries
Burnaby, B.C., V5M 3Z3, Canada   The University of British Columbia
        6270 University Blvd., Vancouver
        British Columbia, V6T 1Z4, Canada

Braun, Mikio L.
Fraunhofer–Institute FIRST
Intelligent Data Analysis Group (IDA)
Kekuléstr. 7, 12489 Berlin, Germany

Brunner, Clemens
Institute for Knowledge Discovery
Laboratory of Brain-Computer Interfaces
Graz University of Technology
Inffeldgasse 16a, 8010 Graz, Austria

Bruns, Andreas
DaimlerChrysler AG
Group Research, HPC 50-G024
71059 Sindelfingen, Germany

Burdick, Joel W.
Division of Engineering and Applied Science
California Institute of Technology
Pasadena, CA 91125

Buttfield, Anna
IDIAP Research Institute   Ecole Polytechnique Fédérale de
1920 Martigny, Switzerland   Lausanne (EPFL), Switzerland

Cabeza, Rafael
Department of Electrical and Electronic Engineering
Public University of Navarre
Pamplona, Spain

Chun, Se Young
Department of Electrical Engineering and Computer Science
University of Michigan
Ann Arbor, USA

Crammer, Koby
School of Computer Science and Engineering
The Hebrew University Jerusalem
91904, Israel

Curio, Gabriel
Department of Neurology, Neurophysics Group
Campus Benjamin Franklin, Charité University Medicine Berlin
Hindenburgdamm 30, 12200 Berlin, Germany

Donoghue, John P.
Departments of Computer Science and Neuroscience
Brown University
Providence RI 02912

Dornhege, Guido
Fraunhofer–Institute FIRST
Intelligent Data Analysis Group (IDA)
Kekuléstr. 7, 12489 Berlin, Germany

Elger, Christian E.
Epilepsy Center
University of Bonn, Germany

Ferrez, Pierre W.
IDIAP Research Institute
1920 Martigny, Switzerland

Ecole Polytechnique Fédérale de
Lausanne (EPFL), Switzerland

Fessler, Jeffery A.
Department of Electrical Engineering and Computer Science
University of Michigan
Ann Arbor, USA

Friedman, Doron
Department of Computer Science
University College London
Gower Street
WC1E 6BT London, United Kingdom

Furdea, Adrian
Institute of Medical Psychology and Behavioural Neurobiology
Eberhard-Karls-University Tübingen, Gartenstr. 29
72074 Tübingen, Germany

Gerson, Adam D.
Department of Biomedical Engineering
Columbia University
New York, NY 10027, USA

Glatz, Andreas
Institute for Human-Computer Interfaces
University of Technology Graz
Krenngasse 37, A-8010 Graz

Graimann, Bernhard
Institute for Knowledge Discovery
Laboratory of Brain-Computer Interfaces
Graz University of Technology
Inffeldgasse 16a, 8010 Graz, Austria

Hagemann, Konrad
DaimlerChrysler AG
Group Research, HPC 50-G024
71059 Sindelfingen, Germany

Hill, N. Jeremy
Max-Planck-Institute for Biological Cybernetics
Tübingen, Germany

Hinterberger, Thilo
Institute of Medical Psychology and
Behavioural Neurobiology
Eberhard-Karls-University Tübingen
Gartenstr. 29
72074 Tübingen, Germany

Division of Psychology
University of Northampton
Northampton, UK

Höfler, Eva
Institute for Knowledge Discovery
Laboratory of Brain-Computer Interfaces
Graz University of Technology
Inffeldgasse 16a, 8010 Graz, Austria

Huggins, Jane E.
Departments of Physical Medicine and Rehabilitation and Biomedical Engineering
University of Michigan, Ann Arbor
1500 East Medical Center Drive, Ann Arbor
MI 48109-0032, USA

Hundley, Douglas R.
Department of Mathematics
Whitman College
Walla Walla, WA 99362

Jordan, Miguel
Institute of Medical Psychology and Behavioural Neurobiology
Eberhard-Karls-University Tübingen, Gartenstr. 29
72074 Tübingen, Germany

Keinrath, Claudia
Institute for Knowledge Discovery
Laboratory of Brain-Computer Interfaces
Graz University of Technology
Inffeldgasse 16a, 8010 Graz, Austria

Kincses, Wilhelm E.
DaimlerChrysler AG
Group Research, HPC 50-G024
71059 Sindelfingen, Germany

Kirby, Michael J.
Department of Mathematics
Colorado State University
Fort Collins, CO 80523

Knight, James N.
Department of Computer Science
Colorado State University
Fort Collins, CO 80523

Kohlmorgen, Jens
Fraunhofer–Institute FIRST
Intelligent Data Analysis Group (IDA)
Kekuléstr. 7, 12489 Berlin, Germany

Krauledat, Matthias
Fraunhofer–Institute FIRST   Technical University Berlin
Intelligent Data Analysis Group (IDA)   Str. des 17. Juni 135
Kekuléstr. 7, 12489 Berlin, Germany   10 623 Berlin, Germany

Kronegg, Julien
Computer Vision and Multimedia Laboratory
Computer Science Department
University of Geneva, Switzerland

Krusienski, Dean J.
Laboratory of Nervous System Disorders
Wadsworth Center
New York State Department of Health
Albany, NY 12201-0509

Kübler, Andrea
Institute of Medical Psychology and Behavioural Neurobiology
Eberhard-Karls-University Tübingen, Gartenstr. 29
72074 Tübingen, Germany

Kunzmann, Volker
Department of Neurology, Neurophysics Group
Campus Benjamin Franklin, Charité University Medicine Berlin
Hindenburgdamm 30, 12200 Berlin, Germany

Lal, Thomas Navin
Max-Planck-Institute for Biological Cybernetics
Tübingen, Germany

Lee, Felix Y.
Institute for Computer Graphics and Vision
Graz University of Technology
Inffeldgasse 16, A-8010 Graz, Austria

Leeb, Robert
Institute for Knowledge Discovery
Laboratory of Brain-Computer Interfaces
Graz University of Technology
Inffeldgasse 16a, 8010 Graz, Austria

Levine, Simon P.
Departments of Physical Medicine and Rehabilitation and Biomedical Engineering
University of Michigan, Ann Arbor
1500 East Medical Center Drive, Ann Arbor
MI 48109-0032, USA

Losch, Florian
Department of Neurology, Neurophysics Group
Campus Benjamin Franklin, Charité University Medicine Berlin
Hindenburgdamm 30, 12200 Berlin, Germany

Mason, Steve G.
Neil Squire Society
220 2250 Boundary Rd.
Burnaby, BC Canada

Matuz, Tamara
Institute of Medical Psychology and Behavioural Neurobiology
Eberhard-Karls-University Tübingen, Gartenstr. 29
72074 Tübingen, Germany

McFarland, Dennis J.
Laboratory of Nervous System Disorders
Wadsworth Center
New York State Department of Health
Albany, NY 12201-0509

Mellinger, Jürgen
Institute of Medical Psychology and Behavioural Neurobiology
Eberhard-Karls-University Tübingen, Otfried-Müeller-Str. 47
72076 Tübingen, Germany

Menendez, Rolando Grave de Peralta
Electrical Neuroimaging Group
Department of Neurology
University Hospital Geneva (HUG)
1211 Geneva, Switzerland

Millán, José del R.
IDIAP Research Institute   Ecole Polytechnique Fédérale de
1920 Martigny, Switzerland   Lausanne (EPFL), Switzerland

Mochty, Ursula
Institute of Medical Psychology and Behavioural Neurobiology
Eberhard-Karls-University Tübingen, Gartenstr. 29
72074 Tübingen, Germany

Müller, Klaus-Robert
Fraunhofer–Institute FIRST   Technical University Berlin
Intelligent Data Analysis Group (IDA)   Str. des 17. Juni 135
Kekuléstr. 7, 12489 Berlin, Germany   10 623 Berlin, Germany

Müller-Putz, Gernot R.
Institute for Knowledge Discovery
Laboratory of Brain-Computer Interfaces
Graz University of Technology
Inffeldgasse 16a, 8010 Graz, Austria

Naeem, Muhammad
Institute for Knowledge Discovery
Laboratory of Brain-Computer Interfaces
Graz University of Technology
Inffeldgasse 16a, 8010 Graz, Austria

Nenadic, Zoran
Department of Biomedical Engineering
Department of Electical Engineering and Computer Science
University of California
Irvine, CA 92697

Neuper, Christa
Department of Psychology
Section Applied Neuropsychology
University of Graz
Universitätsplatz 2, 8010 Graz, Austria

Nijboer, Femke
Institute of Medical Psychology and Behavioural Neurobiology
Eberhard-Karls-University Tübingen, Gartenstr. 29
72074 Tübingen, Germany

Parra, Lucas C.
Department of Biomedical Engineering
City College of New York
New York, NY 10031, USA

Paz, Rony
Interdisciplinary Center for
Neural Computation
The Hebrew University Jerusalem
91904, Israel

Department of Physiology
Hadassah Medical School
The Hebrew University Jerusalem
91904, Israel

Pfurtscheller, Gert
Institute for Knowledge Discovery
Laboratory of Brain-Computer Interfaces
Graz University of Technology
Inffeldgasse 16a, 8010 Graz, Austria

Philiastides, Marios G.
Department of Biomedical Engineering
Columbia University
New York, NY 10027, USA

Rao, Rajesh P. N.
Computer Science Department
University of Washington
Seattle, USA

Rizzuto, Daniel S.
Division of Biology
California Institute of Technology
Pasadena, CA 91125

Rosenstiel, Wolfgang
Wilhelm-Schickard-Institute for Computer Science
Eberhard-Karls-University Tübingen, Germany

Sajda, Paul
Department of Biomedical Engineering
Columbia University
New York, NY 10027, USA

Schalk, Gerwin
Wadsworth Center
New York State Department of Health
E1001 Empire State Plaza
Albany, New York 12201

Scherer, Reinhold
Institute for Knowledge Discovery
Laboratory of Brain-Computer Interfaces
Graz University of Technology
Inffeldgasse 16a, 8010 Graz, Austria

Schlögl, Alois
Institute of Human Computer Interfaces and
Laboratory of Brain-Computer Interfaces
Graz University of Technology
Krenngasse 37, 8010 Graz, Austria

Schölkopf, Bernhard
Max-Planck-Institute for Biological Cybernetics
Tübingen, Germany

Schrauf, Michael
DaimlerChrysler AG
Group Research, HPC 50-G024
71059 Sindelfingen, Germany

Sejnowski, Terrence J.
The Salk Institute for Biological Studies
10010 North Torrey Pines Road
La Jolla, CA 92037

Sellers, Eric W.
Laboratory of Nervous System Disorders
Wadsworth Center
New York State Department of Health
Albany, NY 12201-0509

Shenoy, Pradeep
Computer Science Department
University of Washington
Seattle, USA

Shpigelman, Lavi
School of Computer Science
and Engineering
The Hebrew University Jerusalem
91904, Israel

Interdisciplinary Center for
Neural Computation
The Hebrew University Jerusalem
91904, Israel

Singer, Yoram
School of Computer Science and Engineering
The Hebrew University Jerusalem
91904, Israel

Slater, Mel
Department of Computer Science
University College London
Gower Street
WC1E 6BT London, United Kingdom

Department Llenguatges i Sistemes
Informàtics
Universitat Politècnica de Catalunya
E-08028 Barcelona, Spain

Tangermann, Michael
Fraunhofer–Institute FIRST
Intelligent Data Analysis Group (IDA)
Kekuléstr. 7, 12489 Berlin, Germany

Taylor, Dawn M.
Department of Biomedical Engineering
Case Western Reserve University
Cleveland, OH, USA

Cleveland FES Center of Excellence
Louis Stokes Department of Veterans
Affairs Medical Center
Cleveland, OH, USA

Townsend, George
Institute for Knowledge Discovery
Laboratory of Brain-Computer Interfaces
Graz University of Technology
Inffeldgasse 16a, 8010 Graz, Austria

Vaadia, Eilon
Interdisciplinary Center for
Neural Computation
The Hebrew University Jerusalem
91904, Israel

Department of Physiology
Hadassah Medical School
The Hebrew University Jerusalem
91904, Israel

Vidaurre, Carmen
Department of Electrical and Electronic Engineering
Public University of Navarre
Pamplona, Spain

Widman, Guido
Epilepsy Center
University of Bonn, Germany

Wolpaw, Jonathan R.
Laboratory of Nervous System Disorders
Wadsworth Center
New York State Department of Health
Albany, NY 12201-0509

Wriessnegger, Selina
Department of Psychology
Section Applied Neuropsychology
University of Graz
Universitätsplatz 2, 8010 Graz, Austria

Zimmermann, Doris
Institute for Knowledge Discovery
Laboratory of Brain-Computer Interfaces
Graz University of Technology
Inffeldgasse 16a, 8010 Graz, Austria

Index